Cardiovascular Regenerative Medicine: Nanotechnology and Clinical Applications

Cardiovascular Regenerative Medicine: Nanotechnology and Clinical Applications

Editor: Amanda Ferrara

FOSTER ACADEMICS
www.fosteracademics.com

www.fosteracademics.com

Cataloging-in-Publication Data

Cardiovascular regenerative medicine : nanotechnology and clinical applications / edited by Amanda Ferrara.
p. cm.
Includes bibliographical references and index.
ISBN 978-1-64646-584-2
1. Cardiovascular system--Diseases. 2. Regenerative medicine. 3. Nanotechnology.
4. Cardiovascular system--Diseases--Treatment. 5. Cardiology. I. Ferrara, Amanda.
RC667 .C374 2023
616.1--dc23

Foster Academics,
118-35 Queens Blvd., Suite 400,
Forest Hills, NY 11375, USA

ISBN 978-1-64646-584-2 (Hardback)

Contents

Preface

Regenerative medicine is a field of medicine that develops methods to create, repair or replace diseased or harmed cells, tissues or organs. This discipline encompasses the development and application of therapeutic stem cells, the creation of artificial organs, as well as tissue engineering. The heart holds a limited ability of self-renewal and this limitation can be overcome with the usage of nanotechnologies and nanomaterials in cardiovascular tissue engineering. Cardiac regeneration uses cutting-edge research, such as cell-free and stem cell therapy to heal damaged heart tissue. Tools for repair have been developed to use the body's inherent capacity for regeneration to restore damaged cardiac tissue and function. Cardiac stem cell therapy has the potential to stimulate myocardial regeneration in patients suffering from ischemic heart disease. This book explores all the important aspects of cardiovascular regenerative medicine. It includes some of the vital pieces of work being conducted across the world, on various topics related to the use of nanotechnology as well as the clinical applications of this field. This book will provide comprehensive knowledge to the readers.

The researches compiled throughout the book are authentic and of high quality, combining several disciplines and from very diverse regions from around the world. Drawing on the contributions of many researchers from diverse countries, the book's objective is to provide the readers with the latest achievements in the area of research. This book will surely be a source of knowledge to all interested and researching the field.

In the end, I would like to express my deep sense of gratitude to all the authors for meeting the set deadlines in completing and submitting their research chapters. I would also like to thank the publisher for the support offered to us throughout the course of the book. Finally, I extend my sincere thanks to my family for being a constant source of inspiration and encouragement.

Editor

1

Injectable Hydrogel-Based Nanocomposites for Cardiovascular Diseases

Xiaoshan Liao[1,2†], Xushan Yang[1†], Hong Deng[1], Yuting Hao[1], Lianzhi Mao[1], Rongjun Zhang[1], Wenzhen Liao[1] and Miaomiao Yuan[2*]*

[1] Department of Nutrition and Food Hygiene, Guangdong Provincial Key Laboratory of Tropical Disease Research, School of Public Health, Southern Medical University, Guangzhou, China, [2] The Eighth Affiliated Hospital, Sun Yat-sen University, Shenzhen, China

***Correspondence:**
Wenzhen Liao
wenzhenliao@163.com
Miaomiao Yuan
yuanmm2019@163.com

† These authors have contributed equally to this work

Cardiovascular diseases (CVDs), including a series of pathological disorders, severely affect millions of people all over the world. To address this issue, several potential therapies have been developed for treating CVDs, including injectable hydrogels as a minimally invasive method. However, the utilization of injectable hydrogel is a bit restricted recently owing to some limitations, such as transporting the therapeutic agent more accurately to the target site and prolonging their retention locally. This review focuses on the advances in injectable hydrogels for CVD, detailing the types of injectable hydrogels (natural or synthetic), especially that complexed with stem cells, cytokines, nano-chemical particles, exosomes, genetic material including DNA or RNA, etc. Moreover, we summarized the mainly prominent mechanism, based on which injectable hydrogel present excellent treating effect of cardiovascular repair. All in all, it is hopefully that injectable hydrogel-based nanocomposites would be a potential candidate through cardiac repair in CVDs treatment.

Keywords: injectable hydrogel, nanocomposite, angiogenesis, stem cell homing, cardiovascular diseases

INTRODUCTION

Cardiovascular diseases (CVDs), the group of pathological disorders, including atherosclerosis, myocardial infarction (AMI), stroke and heart failure (HF), remains the leading cause of death globally (Ujcic-Voortman et al., 2012; Nichols et al., 2014; Cainzos-Achirica et al., 2019). In the United States, there were 12.3 million deaths caused primarily by CVD from 2003 to 2017, among which, ischemic heart disease accounted for 48.2%, followed by cerebrovascular disease or stroke (16.7%), and heart failure or cardiomyopathy (10.6%) (Cross et al., 2019). CVDs affects the life of quality of patients, and causes enormous health and economic burdens (Gersh et al., 2010) all over the world, both in the developing countries (Lopez-Jaramillo, 2008; Gersh et al., 2010; Celermajer et al., 2012; McAloon et al., 2016) and in the rich ones (Gersh et al., 2010).

To date, current clinical regimens largely rely on the administration of drugs and other therapeutic agents such as the stem cell and the growth factors (Madonna and De Caterina, 2011; Bagno et al., 2018), basing on the hypothesis that a certain disease consists of dysfunctional cells and molecules within healthy organs and body. As well known, on the one hand, drugs or other therapeutic materials need to overcome physiological barriers to reach targets sites and during the process of transporting them, potential adverse effects may be produced; on the other hand, another hamper is the retention time of agents in the injury site is not adequate for new vessel growth. Therefore, the use of drug delivery systems (DDS) is necessary for enhancing the efficacy and safety of therapeutic agents (Matoba et al., 2017).

In the past decades, DDS has been investigated for improving the transportation efficiency of drugs or other agents of interest (Miyake et al., 1998). Currently, great advance about DDS has been made, for example, electrospun polymeric nanofibers (Torres-Martinez et al., 2018), Lipid-based DDSs (Semalty et al., 2009) and Metallic nanoparticles (Mody et al., 2010), Electrospun polymeric nanofibers (Torres-Martinez et al., 2018), as one of promising DDSs, has the capacity to improve drug's bioavailability and release them in a controlled way via making the low solubility drugs loaded into the fibers. Besides, the high surface-to-volume ratio of the fibers can promote cell adhesion and proliferation, drug loading, and mass transfer processes. However, because of its high cost, the matter of manufacturing drug loaded electrospun mats has to be considered before wide utilization. As one of the lipid-based DDS, pharmacosomes (Semalty et al., 2009) were able to improve dissolution and absorption efficiency through the lipophilic membrane tissue owing to its amphiphilic property (Wang et al., 2011), so that the bioavailability of drugs was greatly improved. However, the targeting of the lipid-based DDS is still a challenge. Metallic nanoparticles (Mody et al., 2010) such as iron oxide nanoparticles have been widely used in targeted drug delivery since they were able to conjugate with antibodies and drugs of interest via modification of different chemical functional groups. However, the toxicity of these magnetic nanoparticles to certain kinds of neuronal cells remain unclear (Pisanic et al., 2007).

Recently, the utilization of injectable hydrogel-based DDSs has attracted considerable attention in many medicine fields, including chemotherapeutics (Norouzi et al., 2016), tissue engineering and regenerative medicine such as cartilage (Li J. et al., 2019) and spinal cord (Macaya and Spector, 2012). Injectable hydrogel has mechanical properties to closely match the targeting organ, and can also be loaded with cellular and a cellular therapeutics to modulate the wound environment and enhance regeneration (Frith et al., 2013; Seo et al., 2017; Cipriani et al., 2018; Mao et al., 2019). In the past years, hydrogels have been paid considerable attention as potential candidates for restoration of ischemia myocardial, in particular, those stem from natural extracellular matrix (ECM) components (e.g., collagen, fibronectin, as well as glycosaminoglycans) could favor greatly endothelial cells adhesion and their transformation to microvessels *in vitro* (Moon et al., 2010) attributing to their high water content and structural similarity to the natural ECM (Peppas et al., 2006; Seliktar, 2012). Additionally, when in an extremly swollen state, hydrogel-based materials such as chitosan hydrogels show good ability to deliver cells and bioactive agents (Liu et al., 2006). Besides, owing to its pH- and temperature-responsive properties, injectable hydrogel exhibits good capacities as a minimally invasive biomaterial scaffolding (Van Vlierberghe et al., 2011) applied for CVDs. Here, we review the wide application of various kinds of injectable hydrogel and the major strategies for the cardiovascular disease therapy.

SINGLE USE OF INJECTABLE HYDROGELS

It is of significant potential for injectable hydrogels to be applied for cardiovascular diseases. The single use of injectable hydrogels characterized by minimally invasive has a suitable effect in cardiovascular disease treatment (Johnson and Christman, 2012). Injectable hydrogels are able to form a network structure at a certain temperature, to provide a morphological environment for supporting myocardial cells and retaining self-differentiated growth factors to promote myocardial repair (MacArthur et al., 2017). The current research and development focused on injectable hydrogels mainly divided into two categories: natural hydrogels and synthetic hydrogels.

Natural Hydrogel

Natural hydrogels are attracting attention because of their non-toxicity, immunogenicity, and excretion of metabolites (Li L. et al., 2019). Generally, natural hydrogels are composed of polysaccharides or proteins whose water-swelling properties making them easy to adsorb and contain nutrients and small molecules (Ahmed, 2015) and improving cell survival and exercise performance (Ahearne, 2014).

Among them, the application of ECM (Extracellular matrix) hydrogel is the representative of natural hydrogel (Francis et al., 2017). Once the nanofiber hydrogel is formed by thermal induction at physiological temperature, the decellularized myocardial matrix hydrogels are possible to quickly create a natural cellular microenvironment for heart tissue and promote myocardial cell repair (Stoppel et al., 2016). Currently, ECM hydrogels are transformed into clinically available injectable biomaterial therapy stages by clinical trials (Wang and Christman, 2016). However, ECM is currently encountered with the lack of effective extraction methods with the reason that the use of chemical reagents for decellularization to remove the nucleus and cytokines of tissue organs can cause damage and denaturation of ECM proteins. Some scholars have proposed the use of supercritical carbon dioxide to extract to reduce damage while with an inevitable challenge of higher cost (Seo et al., 2018).

Therefore, there are many scholars who have developed other natural hydrogels and studied their role in promoting cardiovascular disease repair to replace ECM. Currently developed hydrogels biomaterials include chitosan natural hydrogels (Li J. et al., 2013), hyaluronic acid hydrogels (Yoon et al., 2009), sodium alginate hydrogels (Rocca et al., 2016), and so on. As an immunological linear neutral polysaccharide, hyaluronic acid has multiple acid and hydroxyl groups in the molecule, which can be modified into different forms of hydrogels, including soft or hard hydrogels, as well as nanoparticles and electrospinning. HA-based biomaterial (Burdick and Prestwich, 2011; Larraneta et al., 2018). The presence of reduced left ventricular volume of the glue, increased ejection fraction and the increased wall thickness evaluated by nuclear magnetic resonance (MRI) combined with finite element (FE) models following the treatment of injectable hyaluronic acid hydrogels confirmed the cardiovascular properties of injectable hyaluronic acid hydrogels, including mechanical properties and degradation properties which have been strongly verified before (Rodell et al., 2016).

Perivascular macrophages maintain the balance between endothelial cells and vascular permeability, but when exposed to foreign substances, they activate the inflammatory response and break the balance leading to vascular embolism (Lapenna et al., 2018). Fortunately, chitosan not only has a group that can be modified to change its properties (Vukajlovic et al., 2019), but also has good compatibility with macrophages (Aussel et al., 2019), suggesting that chitosan can treat cardiovascular diseases through vascular repair. Chitosan injectable hydrogels can also be used to remove free radicals due to their antioxidant properties and degradability, resulting in anti-inflammatory effects to promote heart and blood vessel repair (Dorsey et al., 2015). Similarly, due to the easy modification of chitosan, a suitable biocompatible conductive polypyrrole (PPy)-chitosan hydrogel was designed to effectively maintain myocardial function by connecting isolated cardiomyocytes to increase the electrical conductivity of cardiac tissue (Mihic et al., 2015).

In addition, the easily degradable, non-toxic sodium alginate hydrogel can be modified without modification and induced specific properties for a wide range of applications (Hadley and Silva, 2019). Once the degradable alginate hydrogel was designed to own a microstructure to sustain the release of angiopoietin, it can promote cardiac repair (Rocca et al., 2016) and that is why it widely used in cardiac engineering (Ruvinov and Cohen, 2016). According to the rapid development of alginate hydrogel, a multicenter prospective randomized controlled trial called AUGMENT-HF followed up for 1 year was conducted and found that patients with advanced heart failure (HF) using calcium alginate-injected hydrogel presented better cardiac function and clinical outcome rather than who accepting clinical standard medicine therapy (SMT) (Mann et al., 2016).

Furthermore, the sericin-injected hydrogel also performed an excellent biodegradability whose advantage is promoting the recovery of acute myocardial infarction (MI) by promoting inflammation and promoting cardiomyocytes and vascular repair, with limited application due to the high cost and weaker mechanical properties (Song et al., 2016). In order to improve mechanical properties, silk fibroin (SF) is used as a raw material for hydrogel to increase hydrogel toughness and obtain an appropriate degradation rate for better therapeutic effects (Kambe and Yamaoka, 2019). The following is a classification description of several common natural hydrogel materials (**Figure 1**).

Obviously, natural injectable hydrogels own good cardiovascular repair and biocompatibility, while the defects in uncontrolled function, rapid degradation rate, long gel formation time (Ahearne, 2014; Pena et al., 2018) and high production cost play (Song et al., 2016) a tough role of obstacle in the way to cardiovascular application. Therefore, the development of synthetic hydrogels had become researchers' hot spot.

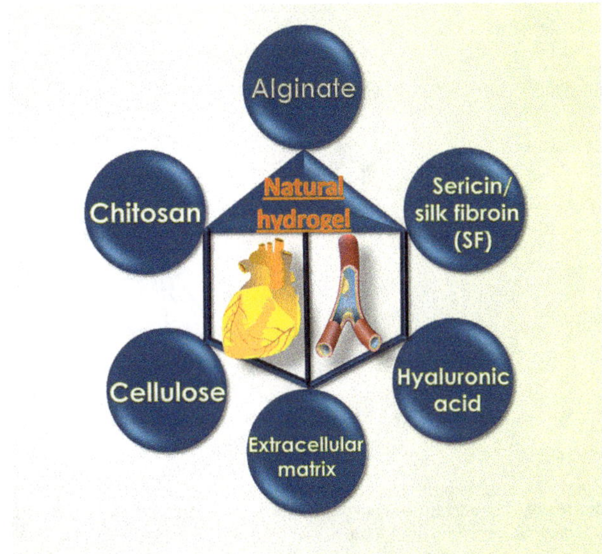

FIGURE 1 | Common types of natural injectable hydrogels materials.

Synthetic Hydrogels

Compared to natural hydrogels, synthetic hydrogels perform a strong mechanical properties and a possibility of being linked to new functional groups by physical and chemical means to achieve the desired function (Highley et al., 2016; Pena et al., 2018). Besides, extensively alternative synthetic materials range and the low risk of immune rejection implanted in the body (Wang R. M. et al., 2017) also facilitates the development of synthetic hydrogels. However, synthetic hydrogels are encountered with low adhesion, due to the lack of cell attachment sites, and poor biocompatibility (Do et al., 2015).

The biochemical properties of hydrogels would be altered to be suitable to play a role in cardiovascular regeneration engineering due to the addition of chemical groups, the following is the introduction of several common synthetic hydrogels (**Figure 2**). The addition of 2-methylene-1,3-dioxepane (MDO) provided biodegradability, and the introduction of tetraaniline endowed copolymers with desirable electrical properties and antioxidant activities, were added to an *in situ* hydrogel composing of poly (NIPAM-based) copolymer that presented superior biocompatibility and conductivity (Cui et al., 2014). Furthermore, the biomimetic hydrogel visible-crosslinking with the GelMA provided biodegradability perform a good biocompatibility, while the biosafety of which has been questioned to some extent (Noshadi et al., 2017). It is worth noting that a functional polyion complex added by static cross-linking create a controlled release system of NO to inflammatory tissues to remove the ROS by redox reaction to promote angiogenesis and prolong the retention period for more than 10 days, which solved the problem of short retention time of natural hydrogel (Vong et al., 2018). Equally, the cross-linking with oxygen-suppressing microspheres to release oxygen to infarcted tissue increase myocardial cell survival rate (Fan et al., 2018). Clearly, the plasticity of synthetic hydrogels provides an effective way to treatment based on cardiovascular disease pathways. Moreover, the commercialization of synthetic hydrogels has developed rapidly owing to its designability. An

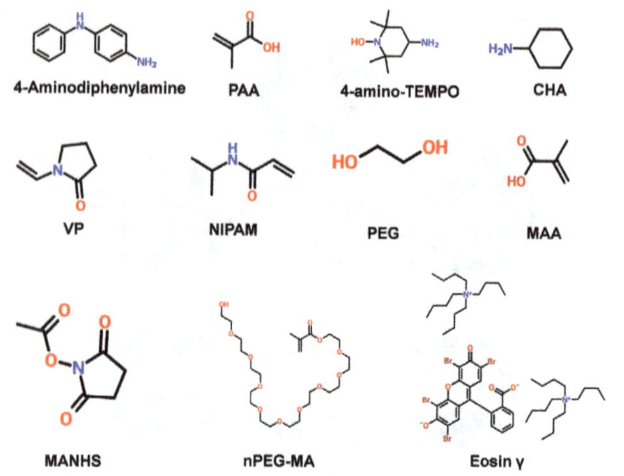

FIGURE 2 | Commonly used chemical structure of synthetic materials. 4-Aminodiphenylamine; PAA (Poly acrylic acid); 4-amino-TEMPO; CHA (cyclohexylamine); VP (*N*-vinylpyrrolidone); NIPAM (*N*-Isopropyl acrylamide); PEG (poly ethylene glycol); MAA (Meth acrylic acid); MANHS (methacrylic acid *N*-hydroxysuccinimide ester); nPEG-MA [Poly ethylene glycol (n) monomethacrylate]; Eosin γ [Eosin γ bis(tetrabutylammonium salt) + 2-(2,4,5,7-tetrabromo-3-oxido-6-oxoxanthen-9 yl)benzoate,tetrabutylazanium].

injectable bioabsorbable stent (IK-5001) was used in patients with clinical MI before a 6-month follow-up, the result evaluated by laboratory examinations showed that IK-5001 was well tolerated without damage to the myocardium (Süselbeck, 2014). Undoubtedly, the prominent superiority of synthetic hydrogels are low manufacturing cost, low immunogenicity and controllability, which provides a huge space for the design and development, while biocompatibility, degradability and biosafety of synthetic hydrogels are issues worthily to be discussed.

Since injectable hydrogels have proven to be a good treatment in clinical practice (Wang H. et al., 2018) while the method is also encountered with the lack of suitable injectable hydrogel materials owing to the respective characteristics of natural hydrogels or synthetic hydrogels. Therefore, the exploration of clinically appropriate injectable hydrogel materials is also one of the research priorities (**Table 1**).

INJECTABLE HYDROGEL-BASED NANOCOMPOSITES

It is urgent to develop an injectable hydrogel with a stronger intervention effect as the result of the suitable cardiovascular repair effect of a single natural or synthetic hydrogel usually dissatisfy the needs of clinical treatment. Generally, the hydrogels cross-linking with other substances present a better effect on the cardiovascular repair than which of hydrogel alone (Singelyn and Christman, 2011). It is significant that the nanofiber network structure of hydrogels provides a possibility of the combination with nanocomposites (Johnson et al., 2011). At the same time, in addition to the degradability of the injectable hydrogel (Tous et al., 2011), the particle size of the hydrogel (Yoon et al., 2014) is equally important to cardiovascular repair effects so that nanocomposite with hydrogel considered as a carrier plays a great potential role in the field of cardiovascular tissue engineering (Kurdi et al., 2010). We will review the common types of active nanomaterials complexed in injectable hydrogels for tissue repair as followed (**Figure 3**).

Nanoparticles and Nanotubes

Limitations of clinical application of natural hydrogels and the lack of cell sites of synthetic hydrogel was ameliorated by the introduction of nanoparticles and nanotubes. Biocompatibility of nanoparticle composite injectable hydrogel have been demonstrated that the addition of nanoformulations into the ECM maintained the functional behaviors and balance of electrical conductivity into cardiomyocytes (Zhang et al., 2019). The addition of nanotubes not only avoided the low conductivity of natural injectable hydrogels, but also retained the strong mechanical properties of synthetic injectable hydrogels. A pHEMA [poly(2-hydroxyethyl methacrylate)] hydrogel consisting of RNT (rosette nanotubes) and CNF (carbon nanofibers) was designed to increase the conductivity of the myocardium and the mechanical properties to promote the adhesion of cardiomyocytes to enhance cells survival rate (Meng et al., 2013). In addition, the Au-loaded Laponite nanoparticles/ECM injectable hydrogel with superior electrical conductivity to reduces the long-short structure of the hydrogel to create a good environment for the cells (Zhang et al., 2019). Nanotube-injectable hydrogel can increase cell adhesion sites and ameliorate the arrangement structure of hydrogels to ensure cell-to-cell integrity to increase the survival rate of cardiomyocytes. For instance, carbon nanotube-incorporated collagen hydrogels can improve arrangement to promote cell–cell integrity and accelerate the regeneration of functional tissues in 3-D hydrogels (Sun et al., 2017). Recently, in addition to superior biocompatibility and electrical conductivity as well as appropriate adhesion sites, the nanotube composite injectable hydrogels were designed to provide sites for bioactive substance adhesion. In terms of vascular tissue engineering applications, Pacelli et al. (2017) proposes a Nanodiamond-based injectable hydrogel for controlled release of angiogenic factors since the chemical functional group on the surface of the ND efficiently interact with the VEGF and facilitate sustained release from the Polymer staggered network structure. The design of the bioactive substance adhesion site not only provides convenience for retaining the active factors produced by the cardiomyocytes itself, but also provides the possibility for carrying foreign biologically active factors. Significantly, the combination of bio-nanomaterials and tissue engineering is a definite effective means for cardiac tissue engineering.

Drugs

Based on the insufficient therapeutic effect of oral medicine and cardiac stent treatment (Johnson and Christman, 2012), the drug-delivered injectable hydrogel treatment method, a minimally invasive surgical treatment, was proposed. Drugs or natural active substances can be introduced into the site of

TABLE 1 | Preclinical efficacy studies in the last 5 years using natural or synthetic injectable hydrogels for treating myocardial infarction.

Biomaterial	Type of hydrogel	Animal model	Type of MI model/ Processing time point after successful MI model	End-point after treatment	Injection site	Results compared to control	References
Gelatinized alginate hydrogel	Natural	Rats	Acute myocardial infarction model/48 h	48 h/after 4 weeks	Myocardium	Associated with improved left ventricular function after MI in rats, and may provide a long-term supply of Angiotensin-(1-7)	Rocca et al., 2016
pcECM	Natural	Rats	Chronic myocardial infarction/12 weeks	4 weeks or 8 weeks	Myocardium	Preserved heart functions and alleviated MI damage	Efraim et al., 2017
Sericin	Natural	Mice	Acute myocardial infarction model/Immediate	6 weeks	Myocardium	Reduces scar formation and infarct size, increases wall thickness and neovascularization, and inhibits the MI-induced inflammatory responses and apoptosis	Song et al., 2016
hpECM	Natural	Rats	Acute myocardial infarction model/30 min	1 h	Myocardium	A significant reduction in scar volume along with normal electrical activity of the surviving tissue, as determined by optical mapping	Francis et al., 2017
Chitosan CSCl-RoY hydrogel	Synthetic	Rats	Acute myocardial infarction model	/	Myocardium	Improve angiogenesis at MI region and improve the cardiac functions	Shu et al., 2015
	Synthetic	Mice	Acute myocardial infarction model	4 weeks	Myocardium	Remarkably decreased the infarction size and improved the heart function	Vong et al., 2018
Type I collagen hydrogel	Synthetic	Rats	Acute myocardial infarction model/10 min	2 h, 1 and 28 days	Myocardium	Enhance the grafted cell survival in the myocardium, which contributed to the increased neovascularization, decreased interstitial fibrosis	Xia et al., 2015
TEMPO Gel	Synthetic	Rats	Acute myocardial infarction model/30 min	24 h	Myocardium	Reduced infarction/reperfusion injury and preserved left ventricle geometry	Zhu et al., 2018
HA	Synthetic	Ovine	Acute myocardial infarction model/30 min	8 weeks	Myocardium	Contractility in the BZ was significantly higher and ES fiber stress was also greatly reduced	Wang H. et al., 2018.

MI, myocardial infarction; pcECM, porcine cardiac extracellular matrix cells; hpECM, human placenta-derived hydrogel; CSCL- Ro γ, chloride-Roγ hydrogel; TEMPO Gel, 2,2,6,6-tetramethylpiperidine-1-oxyl hydrogel; HA, hyaluronic acid; BZ, extension of the border zone; ES, end-systolic.

inflammation through using injectable hydrogels as carriers. Oxidative stress usually occurs with MI and lead to excessive generation of free radicals, which damages transplanted cell membrane lipid, proteins and DNA, seriously affecting the treatment of MI. Drug delivery with hydrogel can change the harsh environment of diseased tissue (Hasan et al., 2015). Hydrogels have a highly porous structure in which irregular pores are connected to each other throughout the structure (Trombino et al., 2019), and the drug or a biologically active substance like a liposome-encapsulated alpha-tocopherol (Qu et al., 2019) or Ferulic acid (FA) (Cheng et al., 2016) is uniformly distributed in the porous structure. The inlaid structure of the hydrogel creates a sustained release system to sustained-release to resists oxidative stress inflammatory response and improved cardiomyocyte survival rate. In addition to repairing blood vessels and promoting myocardial cell repair through the antioxidant action of biologically active substances, targeted therapy for drug delivery to damaged myocardium is also an effective means of treating adverse tissue remodeling. For instance, metalloproteinase inhibitor-containing injectable hydrogel was used to locally inhibit matrix metalloproteinases (MMPs), with the aim of reducing adverse tissue remodeling contributed by excess MMP activity (Purcell et al., 2014). At present, drug-encapsulated hydrogel treatment mainly focuses on finding suitable natural or chemical drugs that change the environment of tissue lesions, and designing suitable injectable hydrogel delivery systems. Moreover, the sustained-release effect of the DDS also affects the treatment of cardiovascular disease (Singh et al., 2019). It is worth noting that an injecting TIIA@PDA Nanoparticle-Cross-linked ROS-Sensitive Hydrogels as a nanoscale DDS roperly control of the drug release amount because TIIA@PDA NPs can be seized via the chemical bond between thiolate and quinone groups on PDA (Wang W. et al., 2019). There generally are a variety of sites of hydrogels that

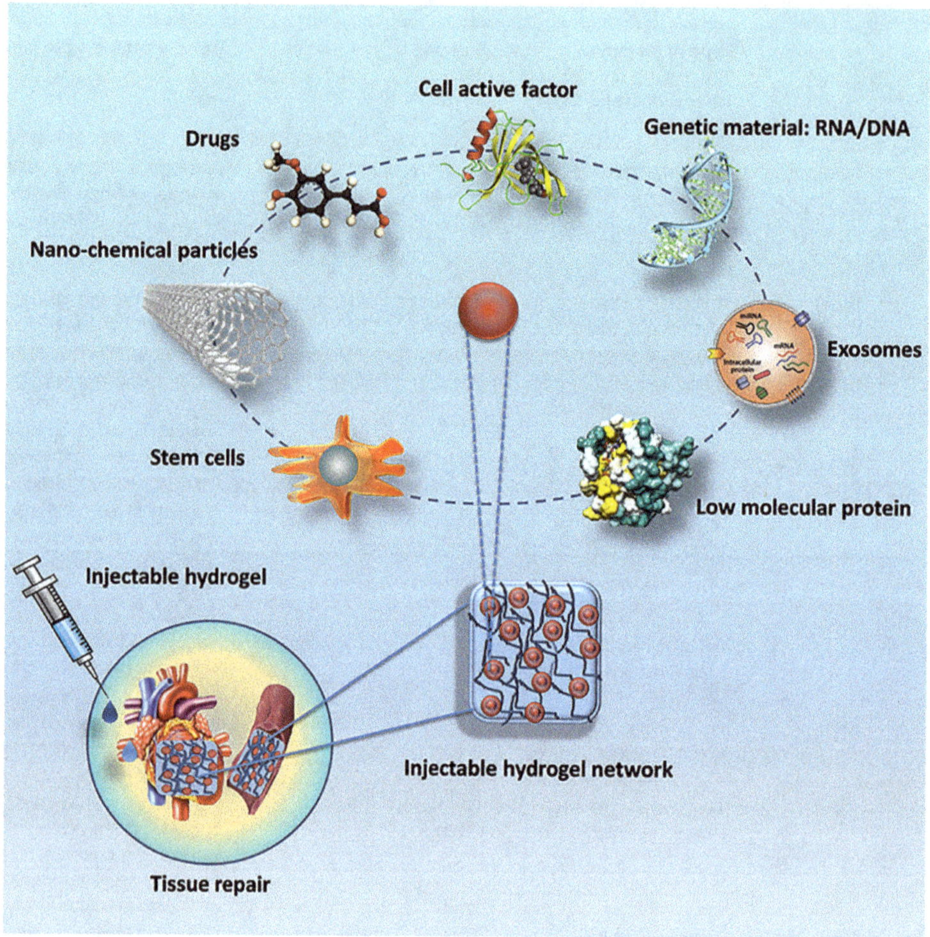

FIGURE 3 | Common types of active nanomaterials complexed in injectable hydrogels for tissue repair.

can be modified by reactive groups, such that the drug or active material to forms a composite gel by a cross-linking reaction such as a click chemistry or a supramolecular assembly of a guest-host pair (Highley et al., 2016). This design provides ideas for the development of sustained-release injectable hydrogels and it is an inevitable challenge of controlled release of the drug to be solved by the injectable hydrogel nanoscale DDS.

Stem Cells

Stem cell therapy, a treatment that has developed concurrently with drug-loaded injectable hydrogels therapy, is well known to play a very important role in cardiac engineering (Cheraghi et al., 2016). Hydrogels protect cells from host inflammation and enable functional integration with damaged myocardium by providing physical support for transplanted cells to maintain their location in the injured area (Sepantafar et al., 2016). Therefore, hydrogels for CVDs ought to be suitable for CMs owing to superior function in tissue repair (**Figure 4**). One of the aspects of current research on injectable hydrogels for transporting cells is to design a hydrogel that is more compatible with cells (Lovett et al., 2009). A polyethylene glycol (PEG) PEGylated fibrin proposed by Geuss et al. (2015) and an injectable hydrogel combained poly (propylene fumarate-co-sebacate-co-ethylene glycol) with PEGDA designed by Komeri and Muthu (2016) are also suitable for cardiomyocytes. In addition, hydrogel for CVDs should be electrically conductive to generate electrical signals to the myocardium (Sepantafar et al., 2016). An Injectable, flexible, antioxidant and electroconductive hydrogel with suitable biocompatibility, which is equivalent to CMs and provides a porous network structure suitable for embedding of CMs and sustained- generated electrical signal (Komeri and Muthu, 2017).

Myocardium contains approximately four basic cell types: 60–80% heart Fibroblast, 20–40% Cardiomyocyte (CM), smooth muscle cells (SMC) and endothelial cells (EC) (Dolnikov et al., 2006). It is necessary to recruit cardiac precursor cells to compensate for cell loss for high levels of cell slippage occurring during MI (Leri et al., 2005). Injectable hydrogel-based cell therapy techniques provide sufficient cell populations to support the ability to electromechanically couple to Cardiomyocytes (CMS) of host tissues, as well as provide appropriate vascular and connective tissue (Li and Weisel, 2014). The application and effects of various cell re-myocardia repair projects have been fully studied by researchers, among which embryonic stem cells (Lu et al., 2009) and CMs (Habib et al., 2011) are commonly used

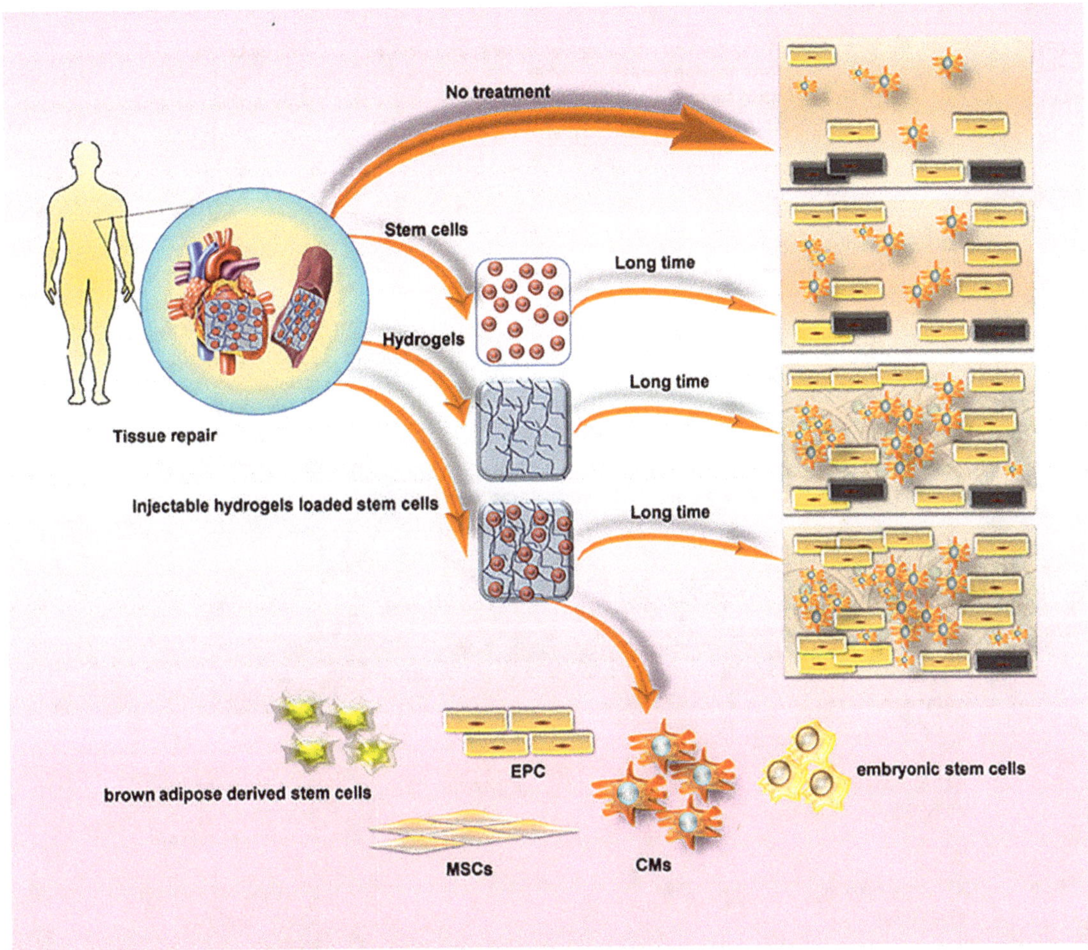

FIGURE 4 | Comparison about the method of cardiovascular regeneration of hydrogel. **(A)** Cells Delivery produces paracrine effects, while hydrogels reduce the reduction of myocardial wall thickness, preserve heart function, prevent the formation of fibrous tissue, and provide a suitable environment for cell survival. Injectable hydrogels loaded cells suppress the reduction of wall thickness by Inhibiting physical tension to provide a suitable environment, and significantly improve the efficacy of cell therapy. **(B)** Commonly used cell types: CMs, cardiomyocytes; EPC, endothelial progenitor cells; brown adipose derived stem cells; embryonic stem cells; MSCs, mesenchymal stem cells.

materials for cardiac engineering. In addition, mesenchymal stem cells (MSCs) are able to differentiate into cardiomyocytes for acute myocardial repair so that some researchers tried to combine the injectable hydrogel with MSCs to explore more effective therapeutic effects owing to the extremely low differentiation rate of MSCs in the heart and the function of hydrogel-injected network that provide a suitable environment and induce MSC differentiation (Li Z. et al., 2012). A tunable bioactive semi-interpenetrating polymer network (sIPN) hydrogels have been developed with matrix metalloproteinase (MMP) to create an assistive microenvironment for delivery of bone marrow-derived mesenchymal stem cells (BMSCs) into the Inflammatory myocardium. The cardiac function of the mice with the injection of hydrogel used as a carrier was improved which provided the basis for the long-term use of transplantation therapy for cardiac stem cells (Wall et al., 2010). Furthermore, an injectable hyaluronic acid (HA) shear-thinning hydrogel (STG) loaded endothelial progenitor cell (EPC) construct (STG-EPC) resulted in prolonged cell retention time and angiogenesis following injection into a myocardial infarction mouse model (Alarcin et al., 2018). In addition to the above-mentioned cells, researchers also used hydrogels to load human amniotic fluid stem cells (Yeh et al., 2010), cardiosphere-derived cells (Li Z. et al., 2011), brown adipose derived stem cells (Wang H. et al., 2014), autologous bone marrow cells (Chen et al., 2014) to promote cardiomyocyte differentiation and angiogenesis and so on (**Table 2**), and the achieved successful results among the cells above indicate that cell nanocomposites based on injectable hydrogels are a useful strategy for cardiac tissue engineering.

It is worth noting that the emerging 3D printing technology also provides a new idea for the design of injectable hydrogel cell nanocomposites (**Table 3**), since fine detail can be included on the micron level with high complexity which provide cells for a superior microenvironment with 3D printing (3DP) technology (Do et al., 2015; Kuo et al., 2015). There is no doubt that the cell composites based on the injectable hydrogel

TABLE 2 | Studies in the last 5 years using injectable hydrogels combined with cells for treating myocardial infarction.

Biomaterial	Type of cells	Animal model	Type of MI model/Processing time point after successful MI model	End-point after treatment	Injection site	Results compared to control	References
HA	Endothelial progenitor cell	Rats	Immediate acute myocardial infarction model	1/4 weeks	Myocardium	Minimize postischemic remodeling	Gaffey et al., 2015, 2019
FA	iPS	Mice	Immediate acute myocardial infarction model	1, 2, 4 weeks	Myocardium	Improved the retention and survival of iPS; less adverse heart remodeling and stimulation of neovascularization	Li H. et al., 2018
Chitosan	MSCs	Rats	1 weeks acute myocardial infarction model	24 h	Myocardium	Increased graft size and cell retention, promoted MSCs to differentiate into cardiomyocytes and increased the effects of MSCs on neovas-culature formation	Xu et al., 2017

HA, hyaluronic acid; FA, folic acid; iPS, induced pluripotent stem cells; MSCs, mesenchymal stem cells.

TABLE 3 | Studies of using injectable hydrogels to formulate 3D structure for treating cardiovascular diseases.

Biomaterial	Formed 3D material	Loaded cells	Loaded time	Survival rate	References
Alginate	3D hydrogel-based vascular	L929 mouse fibroblasts	7 days	>90%	Gao et al., 2017
3D printable MEGEL/ PEGDA3350/alginate hydrogel	3D hydrogel culture environment	HADMSC/ HAVIC/ HASSMC/	3 days	95%/93%/93%	Kang et al., 2017
Chitosan	3D hydrogel culture environment	NSCs/ECs	2 days	Survival rate in 3D hydrogel culture environment than that in 2D	Han H. W. et al., 2019
Plated PEGylated fibrin	3D hydrogel culture environment	HL-1 CMs	3 days	Increased cell retention and reduced scar tissue	Geuss et al., 2015

3D printable MEGEL/PEGDA3350/alginate hydrogel, extrusion 3D printable mixture of methacrylated gelatin/poly-ethylene glycol diacrylate/alginate (MEGEL/PEGDA3350/alginate); PEG, Polyethylene glycol; HADMSC, human adipose derived mesenchymal stem cells; HAVIC, human aortic valve interstitial cells; HASSMC, human aortic valve sinus smooth muscle cells; NSCs, neural stem cells; ECs: endothelial cells; CMs, cardiomyocytes.

of 3D printing technology will be one of the hotspots of cardiac tissue engineering in the future (Alonzo et al., 2019; Han H. W. et al., 2019).

Cell Active Factor

The common injectable hydrogels-based treatments for cardiovascular disease are drug-loaded therapy and stem cell therapy, but both have limitations. The drugs currently in use are usually angiotensin receptor blockers, beta-blockers, angiotensin-converting enzyme (ACE) inhibitors and aldosterone antagonists, which possibly cause severe adverse reactions in patients, including sleep disturbances, hypotension and difficulty breathing (Jin and Yu, 2018). In order to clinically reduce the incidence of adverse reactions of CVDs, cell active factor therapy, including small molecule protein and exosomes, is considered as a cell-free treatment alternative to drug therapy (Cohen et al., 2014).

Endogenous and exogenous low molecular proteins are usually used in clinically applied cell-free therapies with difficult control of delivery and local release. Obviously, the application of injectable hydrogel probably significantly improved the biological activity of small molecule protein. An injectable hydrogel with a light-sensitive bond and photoresolvability, including polyethylene glycol and heparin-based polymers, successfully wrapped fibroblast growth factor 2 (FGF-2), whose activity was comparable to that before embedding and significantly altered the release profile of FGF-2 (Kharkar et al., 2017). It is worth noting that some researchers attempted to embed horseradish peroxidase (HRP) with a bioactive peptide with a phenolic hydroxyl group into hydrogel to cause a coupling reaction to enhance the function of the active peptide (Wang L. S. et al., 2014). The combination of injectable hydrogel and small molecule protein, which can not only improve its biological activity but also significantly increase the retention time of active protein in the myocardium and achieve sustained release, promotes cardiovascular repair by promoting cell homing and regulating key proteins. MacArthur et al. (2013) successfully loaded the synthetic analog of stromal cell-derived factor 1-α (engineered stromal cell-derived factor analog [ESA]) into an injectable hyaluronic acid hydrogel and successfully induced the persistence of endothelial progenitor cells Homing. Moreover, a delivery system of MMP-2 specific inhibitor peptide CTTHWGFTLC (CTT), which enables CCT to be released continuously within 4 weeks, effectively preventing ECM degradation worsens the condition (Fan et al., 2017). The fusion protein (TAT-HSP27), consisting of the heat shock protein 27 (HSP27) and transcriptional activator (TAT), loaded into microsphere/hydrogel combination delivery devices for controlled release behavior for prolonged periods because the heat shock proteins is a favorable target for protecting cardiomyocytes under environmental stimulation (Lee et al., 2009). Similarly, researchers designed low molecular protein injectable hydrogel nanocomposites with sustained release function according to the mechanism of action of different low molecular proteins: an Poly(ethylene glycol) dimethacrylate(PEGDMA) hydrogel storing local increasing mechano growth factor (MGF), a member of the IGF-1 family with an anti-apoptotic E domain playing a role of a stem cell homing factor (Doroudian et al., 2014), a temperature-sensitive chitosan chloride-RoY (CSCl-RoY) hydrogel (Shu et al., 2015), a hydrogel loading Neuregulin-1β (NRG) which is a member of the epidermal growth factor family (Cohen et al., 2014), a hydrogel loading high-mobility group box 1 (HMGB1) (He et al., 2013), and so on. Song M's findings on association between stem cell homing factor (SDF-1) and angiogenic peptides (Ac-SDKP) also demonstrate a better therapeutic effect in combination with bioactive substances (Song et al., 2014).

In addition to the aforementioned small molecule regulatory proteins, certain growth factors, including Thymosin β4 (Tβ4), especially vascular endothelial growth factor (VEGF), should be delivered to heart tissue to reduced poor heart remodeling and improving ventricular function because of the poor cardiac remodeling that occurs later in the myocardial infarction (Anselmi et al., 2000). Thymosin β4 (Tβ4), a 43-amino acid peptide which performs angiogenic and cardioprotective properties, combined with injectable hydrogel resulted in stimulation of Vascular regeneration and cardiomyocyte migration (Shaghiera et al., 2018). Transportation of vascular endothelial growth factor (VEGF) and other angiogenic factors to promote angiogenesis are both potential treatment for cardiovascular disease and a vital aspect of tissue regeneration (Cao et al., 2009). The myocardial thickness and the density blood vessels of the rat myocardial infarction model were larger than that of the group without treating, following the injection of a novel temperature-susceptible aliphatic polyester hydrogel (HG) crosslinked with VEGF (Wu et al., 2011). Retention of highly vascularized cardiomyocytes is a limiting factor in growth factor therapy although it presents superior performance in cardiovascular repair (Rufaihah et al., 2017). The Dex-PCL-HEMA/PNIPAAm hydrogelcon containing VEGF developed by Zhu et al. (2016) and the injectable hydrogel amalgamated polyethylene glycol with fibrinogen (PEG-fibrinogen) loaded with VEGF-A designed by Rufaihah et al. (2013) both are able to release and store VEGF in a controlled manner and achieve better cardiac repair than VEGF alone. Moreover, in order to present a superior repair effect, an polyethylene glycol-fibrinogen (PF) hydrogels was manufactured for sustained dual transportation of VEGF and angiopoietin-1 (ANG-1) to promote myocardial therapy (Rufaihah et al., 2017). Recently, researchers' research hotspots have shifted from the development of nano-growth factor injectable hydrogels to exploring which nano-growth factor injectable hydrogel complexes present superior cardiac repair functions. Therefore, the growth factors, including hepatocyte growth factor (HGF) (Ruvinov et al., 2010), insulin-like growth factor 1 (IGF-1) (Koudstaal et al., 2014; Fang et al., 2015), etc. that have been explored in combination with injectable hydrogels and present good myocardial repair effects, are suitable in myocardial regeneration.

Though stem cell treatment is one of the effective strategies for the CVDs, the stem cell clinical transplantation is limited by the low cell implantation and survival rate (Li Z. et al., 2018). Exosomes have recently become recognized as new candidates for cell-free treatment (Emanueli et al., 2015; Davidson et al., 2017; Zhang et al., 2017). Exosomes, extracellular vesicles derived from endosomes and the vital mediators of intercellular communication (Ibrahim and Marbán, 2016), are released by major cardiac cells, including cardiomyocytes, fibroblasts and endothelial cells (Barile et al., 2017), to regulate cellular function (Poe and Knowlton, 2018). Direct use of paracrine factors is an attractive strategy that play a role in therapy via cytokine regulatory pathway, taking cell implantation or survival rate out of considered (Han C. S. et al., 2019). The development of injectable hydrogel nanocomposites for composite exosomes has raise researchers' attention since hydrogels are appropriate carrier materials. Significant improvement of exosome implantation on injured myocardium has been proven by that an injectable shear-thinning gel (STG) carrying EVs probably effectively improve myocardial function and increased the hemodynamics as well as the number of blood vessels (Chen et al., 2018). Furthermore, exosomes generated by human adipose-derived stem cells (hASCs), Gelatin and Laponite® were combined to formulate a shear-thinning, nanocomposite hydrogel (nSi Gel) which was considered as an injectable carrier of secretome (nSi Gel+), and the results indicate an increasing density of blood vessels around the myocardium, an improvement in myocardial function and a reduction in scar area (Waters et al., 2018). However, the residence time and stability of exosomes are the major challenges in the clinical application of exosomes in recent years. Therefore, good biocompatibility and retention time are the vital research directions of exosomes-delivered injectable hydrogels. The stability and cardiovascular application of chitosan-injectable hydrogel-encapsulated paracrine factors *in vivo* were demonstrated by the results which indicated that exosomes showed high retention rates and promote vascular repair and formation (Zhang K. et al., 2018). Since the principle of stem cell therapy is based on the release of paracrine factors around the myocardial injury tissue to interfere with the progression of myocardial infarction (Mirotsou et al., 2011), exosome nanocomplexes with injectable hydrogels plays a significant role as promising alternative therapies.

Genetic Material: RNA/DNA

Since stem cell and foreign active substance suppression is prone to collective immune rejection (Lu et al., 2010), embedding exogenous genetic material (DNA/RNA) into injectable hydrogels to produce autologous histocompatibility stem cells to promote myocardial regeneration, is an appreciated method in CVDs therapy. According to the pathway of MMP2 related to the cardiac harmful remodeling process, an injectable hydrogel complexed with siRNA up-regulate the hydrolytic activity of MMP2 protein to inhibit the harmful remodeling process of the heart and promote heart repair (Wang L. L. et al., 2018). In addition, an injectable Hyaluronan-Based hydrogel modulate remodeling of the myocardial extracellular matrix (ECM) by injecting a hyaluronic acid-based reservoir delivering exogenous microRNA-29B (miR-29B) (Monaghan et al., 2018). Noteworthily, protocols for injection-based delivery of Cre-CPP by ultrasound-guided injection to cardiac muscle in mice is mature owing to widely used technique of Cre-mediated DNA recombination at loxP sites (Chien et al., 2017), which provides a feasible mean for genetic material composite hydrogel. The study results above strongly demonstrated that genetic material (DNA/RNA) would be considered as the potential candidate for myocardial regeneration.

Composite Use of Nano-Bioactive Substances

Cell therapy is currently the most mature treatment in cardiac tissue engineering which encounters with the problems of immune rejection of foreign cells, low survival rate and short residence time (Lu et al., 2010) so that researchers have begun to combine biologically active substance with stem cells to increase stem cell functional activity. It is common to carry out the mixture of cell growth factor and stem cells: combined polyethylene glycol hydrogel (PEG), a hydrogel consisting of human induced pluripotent stem cell-derived cardiomyocyte (iPSC-CM) and erythropoietin (EPO) (Chow et al., 2017), a hydrogel consisting of insulin-like growth factor (IGF-1) and delivering mesenchymal stromal cell (MSC) (Wang et al., 2010), injectable linear engineering protein hydrogels encapsulating VEGF and human induced pluripotent stem cell-derived endothelial cells (hiPSC-EC) (Mulyasasmita et al., 2014) and the like. What raise researchers' attention is the combined use of multiple nano-bioactive substance. An injectable matrix metalloproteinase (MMP)-responsive, bioactive hydrogel used as an *in situ* forming scaffold to deliver thymosin β4 (Tβ4), along with vascular cells derived from human embryonic stem cells (hESC), which useful in engineering sustained tissue preservation (Kraehenbuehl et al., 2011). Noteworthily, Karam et al. (2014) proposed to integrate human adipose-derived stem cells (ADSCs) and pharmacologically active microcarriers (PAMs), a three-dimensional (3D) carrier of cells and growth factors, into an injectable hydrogel (HG), to obtain a system that stimulates the survival and/or differentiation of the grafted cells toward a cardiac phenotype. This study suggests that the use of 3D nanocomposites is one of the more effective means and a hot spot in cardiovascular repair development. From a gene therapy perspective, an injectable biocompatible hydrogel which can efficiently deliver a nanocomplex of graphene oxide (GO) and vascular endothelial growth factor-165 (VEGF) pro-angiogenic gene is significant for myocardial therapy (Paul et al., 2014), which suggested the feasibility of gene therapy combined with cardiac tissue engineering treatment is illustrate.

THE MAJOR MECHANISM USING BY INJECTABLE HYDROGEL IN CVDS

Although injectable hydrogel as a desirable candidate for CVDs with numerous outstanding properties has been widely used in clinical treatment, its mechanism of promotion restoration of CVDs remains unclear. Herein several possible paths are illustrated in the following parts.

The Promotion Effect of Recovery in CVDs via Angiogenesis

Recently, therapeutic angiogenesis, or the delivery of angiogenic agents such as growth factors (GFs) (Madonna and De Caterina, 2011), NO (Vong et al., 2018), and some drugs (Qi et al., 2018) to promote revascularization of ischemic tissue, holds great promise in the fields of treating CVDs. As shown in the **Figure 5**, a variety of GFs are indispensable for the different phrase of neovascularization. Nevertheless, this approach has been confronted with several obstacle when hydrogel used as

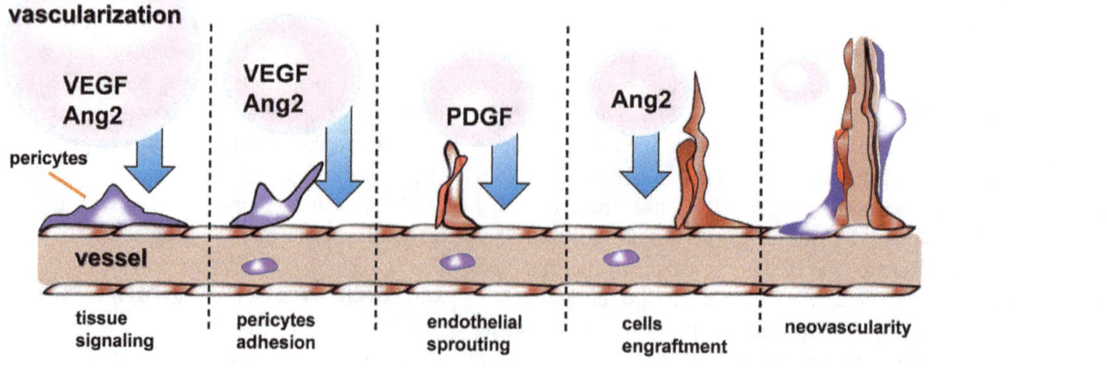

FIGURE 5 | Schematic illustrations of different growth factors signaling during angiogenesis.

a delivery device, among which, the difficulties of keeping angiogenic GFs retained locally at the injury site and released gradually to allow adequate time for growth of new blood vessels must be overcome before successful clinical implementation. Basing on the status, recently a growing body of evidences have shown evidence of injectable hydrogel's promising effects on cardiac recovery through addressing the problems mentioned above in the process of revascularization.

GFs therapy shows great promises in treating ischemia, but the retention of GFs in the highly vascularized myocardium is mainly obstacle of its widely application. Some researchers (Feng et al., 2017) designed an injectable hydrogel scaffold composed of Konjac glucomannan (KGM, a naturally derived polysaccharide with capability to activate macrophages/monocytes to secrete pro-angiogenic/-mitogenic GFs) and heparin (Hep, one of the glycosaminoglycan molecule that binds numerous pro-angiogenic GFs and sequester them). Therefore, the injectable hydrogel was capable of promote revascularization via first stimulating the secretion of endogenous pro-angiogenic growth factors (GFs) and next sequestering these GFs inside the scaffold. Furthermore, controlling the degradation kinetics of injectable hydrogel would be an effective strategy to prolong the retention of GFs. Gel-CDH/HA-mCHO (Hozumi et al., 2018) hydrogels, a new injectable hydrogel synthetized by carbohydrazide -modified Gel (Gel-CDH) and mono-aldehyde modified-HA (HA-mCHO), was degraded much more slowly because of stable Schiff's base formation between aldehyde and carbohydrazide groups. Additionally, the limited function of one single GF in the delivery system was one of the restrictions. Therefore, polyethylene glycol-fibrinogen (PF) hydrogels (Rufaihah et al., 2017) was employed and incorporating with vascular endothelial growth factor (VEGF) and angiopoietin-1 (ANG-1) to achieve the effect of dual delivery of GFs in a sustained release way. Besides, other materials also play the crucial roles on cardiovascular diseases. It is generally known the significance of nitric oxide (NO) but its therapeutic application is hampered because of its highly short half-life and rapidly consumed by excessive producing of ROS. Thereby, a new injectable hydrogel, namely NO-RIG (Vong et al., 2018), was prepared which consisted of PArg-PEG-PArg (NO releasing polymer) and PMNT-PEG-PMNT (ROS scavenging polymer), in a complex with polyanion PAAc, so that NO's effect on promoting angiogenesis were improved.

In addition to the adequate retention time of GFs at the targeted district, transporting the GFs to the injury site accurately is also important for inducing angiogenesis. Given the acidic microenvironment (Khabbaz et al., 2001; Kumbhani et al., 2004; Ding et al., 2011; Zhao et al., 2012; Wei et al., 2017) of ischemic myocardium, a pH- and temperature-responsive, injectable hydrogel has been synthesized (Garbern et al., 2011) with several pH- and temperature-responsive random copolymer, including *N*-isopropylacrylamide (NIPAAm), propylacrylic acid (PAA), and butyl acrylate (BA) by reversible addition fragmentation chain transfer polymerization. This polymer existed as a liquid at room temperature and pH 7.4 but becomes a gel at 37°C and pH 6.8. Thereby, the hydrogel successfully provided sustained release of basic fibroblast growth factor (bFGF) at the injury site locally and the angiogenesis effect of bFGF were improved. Similar, another new (Wu et al., 2011), temperature-sensitive, aliphatic polyester hydrogel (HG) conjugated with (VEGF) was designed and also shown good therapeutic effect on attenuating adverse cardiac remodeling and improved ventricular function when injected after an MI.

In a word, therapeutic angiogenesis showed remarkably therapeutic potential in cardiovascular disorders by changing the status of one single material delivering, prolonging the retention of pro-angiogenic factor and transmitting them accurately to the targeted site.

The Therapeutic Effect in CVDs Through Promoting Stem Cell Homing

Stem cell homing, the capability of stem cells to find their destination in a targeted organ through the bloodstream (Zhao and Zhang, 2016), was another promising therapeutic strategy in CVDs, especially in Myocardial infarction (MI). Here, an example of mesenchymal stromal cells (MSC) in **Figure 6** (Marquez-Curtis and Janowska-Wieczorek, 2013) was used to illustrate the mechanisms of stem cell transendothelial migration toward injured tissue. As we can see in the **Figure 6**, the effect of MSC homing was achieved by production of a series of some critical factors such as homing receptors including CXCR4. Although the mechanism of stem cell homing has been understood recently, the clinical utilization of stem cells was mainly hindered by their poor homing efficiency. In the recent years, a growing body of clinical evidence suggests that injectable hydrogel is a promising biomaterial that were capable of enhancing stem cell homing efficiency in treatment of numerous filed of regeneration medicine, such as in periodontal regeneration (He et al., 2019), cartilage regeneration (Lu et al., 2018), as well as corneal epithelium regeneration (Tang et al., 2017).

"Homing" directs stem cells migration through different signaling pathways, mediated by released chemokines or growth factor receptors on the surface of stem cells. Over the past decade, the most thoroughly studied stem cell homing factor is the chemokine SDF-1α/CXCL12 (Ghadge et al., 2011), based on which, a number of researchers committed themselves to develop some new delivery devices loaded with these promoting homing factors in order to improve the myocardium repair. Recently, a combined strategy (Naderi-Meshkin et al., 2016) was implemented via mixing human adipose tissue-derived MSCs (hASCs) into chitosan-glycerophosphate-hydroxyethyl cellulose (CH-GP-HEC) injectable hydrogel and as a result, site-directed homing efficacy and retention of ASCs increase by harnessing SDF1/CXCR4 axis. Similar, The E domain of mechano growth factor (MGF) (Doroudian et al., 2014) peptide is anti-apoptotic and a stem cell homing factor. As shown in a study, a microrod delivery device of poly (ethylene glycol) dimethacrylate (PEGDMA) hydrogel could absorb cells and decrease apoptosis of myocytes via incorporating MGF.

On the other hand, a comfortable microenvironment for stem cell survival is also of great significance. For example, as shown in a current report, ROS (Song et al., 2010) in MI microenvironment negatively regulated graft cell death and stem cell adhesion,

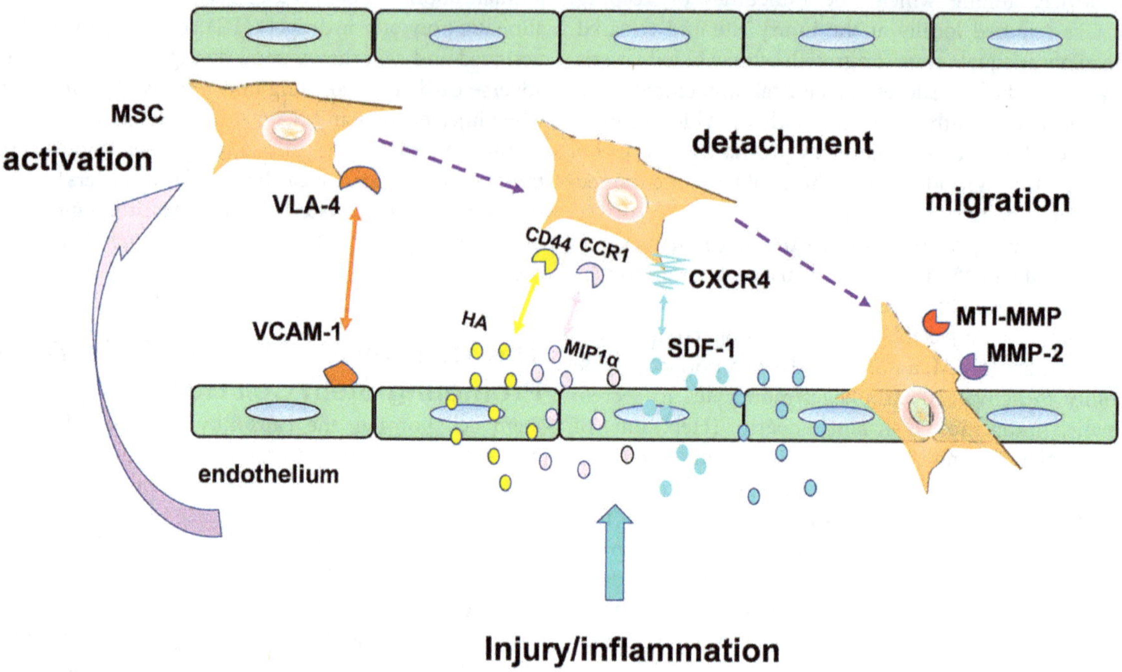

FIGURE 6 | Mechanisms of MSC transendothelial migration toward injured tissue.

finally caused anoikis of transplanted cells. Hence, changing the unfavorable MI microenvironment for stem cell homing and proliferation would have better therapeutic efficiency in cellular cardiomyoplasty. Chitosan hydrogel (Liu et al., 2012) were able to improve the MI microenvironment, enhance stem cell engraftment and survival through ROS scavenging. Furthermore, adequate blood vessel would be another crucial supportive condition for cell survival and proliferation. Thus, some scientists (Song et al., 2014) designed a biomimetic hydrogel incorporated with both stem cell homing factor (SDF-1) and angiogenic peptides (Ac-SDKP) in treating chronic myocardial infarction (CMI) and consequently, regeneration of cardiac function model were significantly promoted. By and large, the stem cell homing-based injectable hydrogel emerged as a promising therapy in treatment ischemic infarction.

All in all, as for treating CVDs, revascularization and stem cell homing are the two major effective strategies through injectable hydrogel as a delivery system in the recent years. Besides, there existing other approach that would hold great therapeutic potential in the field of CVDs treatment, for instance, taking advantage of an injectable hyaluronic acid (Zhang Y. et al., 2018) (HA) hydrogel to deliver miRNA in order to induce proliferation in cardiomyocytes through its inhibition of Hippo signaling via a direct binding site on the 3′ UTR, such as miR-302 (Wang L. L. et al., 2017) and miR-1825 (Pandey et al., 2017), developing a new hydrogel (Qi et al., 2018) from supramolecular assembling of a synthetic glycol peptide which endows the hydrogel with the capacity of endothelial cell adhesion and proliferation due to its high density of glucose moieties, as well as using Ferulic Acid (Kanki and Klionsky, 2009; Wu et al., 2012; Wiley et al., 2013) (a natural antioxidant that is most abundant in vegetables, especially in eggplants and maize bran) to form a new injectable hydrogel (Cheng et al., 2016) to effectively promote the recovery of Cisd2 deficiency induced damage.

SUMMARY AND PERSPECTIVE

Injectable hydrogels have shown promise in promoting cardiovascular disease repair for years from single hydrogels (natural or synthetic hydrogels) to hydrogel- based nanocomposite. To the begin, natural hydrogels were attracting attention because of their non-toxicity, immunogenicity, and excretion of metabolites (Li L. et al., 2019), such as. However, due to the lack of effective extraction methods (Francis et al., 2017), ECM were gradually replaced by other natural hydrogels, such as hyaluronic acid hydrogels (Yoon et al., 2009) (an immunological linear neutral polysaccharide with multiple acid and hydroxyl groups, which can be modified into different forms of hydrogels, including soft or hard hydrogels, as well as nanoparticles and electrospinning), chitosan natural hydrogels (which had good compatibility with macrophages and antioxidant properties and degradability) (Aussel et al., 2019), sodium alginate hydrogels (Hadley and Silva, 2019), and so on. On the other hand, synthetic hydrogels have been attached much importance since their strong mechanical properties and various and controllable function by physical and chemical means (Pena et al., 2018). Synthetic hydrogels are low manufacturing cost and could provide a huge space for the design and development, while their biocompatibility, degradability, biosafety and low adhesion for cell (Do et al., 2015) are issues worthily to be discussed.

Recently, since the porosity of hydrogel of hydrogels provides a possibility to combine with nanocomposites (Johnson et al., 2011), and the hydrogels cross-linking with other substances show better cardiovascular repair effect than which of hydrogel alone (Singelyn and Christman, 2011), several types of active nanomaterials complexed in injectable hydrogels for tissue repair have been explored. For instance, injectable hydrogel-based composite carrying drug and/or other bioactive materials have been explored and the effective have been achieved.

According to different treatment mechanisms and different aspects of concern, the invention of different nano-composite injectable hydrogels was designed. For example, drugs-delivered injectable hydrogels mainly improve the environment of myocardial tissue with excessive oxidative stress, and small molecule proteins-delivered and exosomes-delivered injectable hydrogels are mainly involved in the mechanism of hormone regulation in the process of self-repair of myocardium. Cell-delivered injectable hydrogels therapy is mainly to provide a large number of favorable healthy cells to promote the process of myocardial repair, while pure hydrogel therapy is mainly to provide the stent of myocardial cells. Recently, because of foreign material is prone to collective immune rejection, embedding foreign genetic material (DNA/RNA) into injectable hydrogels might be an appreciated method in CVDs therapy.

Although much progress has been made due to injectable hydrogel's wide application in the CVDs, some limitations remain challenges that need to be overcome before successful clinical implementation, for instance, the exploration of appropriate approach for injection (Chen et al., 2017), the method for controlling and tailoring release profiles of targeting agents confronting the complicated biological processes (Kharkar et al., 2013; Annabi et al., 2014; Yesilyurt et al., 2016), the substantial requirement for hydrogel's rheological and mechanical properties (Unterman et al., 2017), their capacities to be scaled up to a good manufacturing practice (cGMP) process (Ungerleider and Christman, 2014). It is of great hope that advances will be made along with our thorough study of the pathophysiology of CVDs and the accurate therapeutic mechanism by hydrogel in the treatment of CVDs in coming years. What is currently lacking is the comparison of the effects of different injectable hydrogels and that of their respective advantages in clinical applications. Although there are various designs of nanocomposite injectable hydrogels, their cost and clinical application are in controversy. Discussion and application of this composite product at this stage is Insufficient. In the future, we will focus on the rationality of the research design in this area and the possibility of clinical application.

AUTHOR CONTRIBUTIONS

All authors listed have made a substantial, direct and intellectual contribution to the work, and approved it for publication.

REFERENCES

Ahearne, M. (2014). Introduction to cell-hydrogel mechanosensing. *Interface Focus* 4:20130038. doi: 10.1098/rsfs.2013.0038

Ahmed, E. M. (2015). Hydrogel: preparation, characterization, and applications: a review. *J. Adv. Res.* 6, 105–121.

Alarcin, E., Lee, T. Y., Karuthedom, S., Mohammadi, M., Brennan, M. A., Lee, D. H., et al. (2018). Injectable shear-thinning hydrogels for delivering osteogenic and angiogenic cells and growth factors. *Biomater. Sci.* 6, 1604–1615. doi: 10.1039/c8bm00293b

Alonzo, M., AnilKumar, S., Roman, B., Tasnim, N., and Joddar, B. (2019). 3D Bioprinting of cardiac tissue and cardiac stem cell therapy. *Transl. Res.* 211, 64–83. doi: 10.1016/j.trsl.2019.04.004

Annabi, N., Tamayol, A., Uquillas, J. A., Akbari, M., Bertassoni, L. E., and Cha, C., et al. (2014). 25th anniversary article: Rational design and applications of hydrogels in regenerative medicine. *Adv. Mater.* 26, 85–123. doi: 10.1002/adma.201303233

Anselmi, M., Bolognese, L., Chierchia, S., Maggioni, A., and Marino, P. (2000). The role of myocardial viability in deriving benefit from reestablishing infarct-related artery flow after acute myocardial infarction. *Prog. Cardiovasc. Dis.* 42, 455–470.

Aussel, A., Boiziau, C., L'Azou, B., Siadous, R., Delmond, S., Montembault, A., et al. (2019). Cell and tissue responses at the interface with a chitosan hydrogel intended for vascular applications: in vitro and in vivo exploration. *Biomed. Mater.* 14:25009. doi: 10.1088/1748-605X/aafbf0

Bagno, L., Hatzistergos, K. E., Balkan, W., and Hare, J. M. (2018). Mesenchymal stem cell-based therapy for cardiovascular disease: progress and challenges. *Mol. Ther.* 26, 1610–1623. doi: 10.1016/j.ymthe.2018.05.009

Barile, L., Moccetti, T., Marbán, E., and Vassalli, G. (2017). Roles of exosomes in cardioprotection. *Eur. Heart J.* 38:w304. doi: 10.1093/eurheartj/ehw304

Burdick, J. A., and Prestwich, G. D. (2011). Hyaluronic acid hydrogels for biomedical applications. *Adv. Mater.* 23, H41–H56. doi: 10.1002/adma.201003963

Cainzos-Achirica, M., Fedeli, U., Sattar, N., Agyemang, C., Jenum, A. K., McEvoy, J. W., et al. (2019). Epidemiology, risk factors, and opportunities for prevention of cardiovascular disease in individuals of South Asian ethnicity living in Europe. *Atherosclerosis* 286, 105–113. doi: 10.1016/j.atherosclerosis.2019.05.014

Cao, L., Arany, P. R., Wang, Y. S., and Mooney, D. J. (2009). Promoting angiogenesis via manipulation of VEGF responsiveness with notch signaling. *Biomaterials* 30, 4085–4093. doi: 10.1016/j.biomaterials.2009.04.051

Celermajer, D. S., Chow, C. K., Marijon, E., Anstey, N. M., and Woo, K. S. (2012). Cardiovascular disease in the developing World. *J. Am. Coll. Cardiol.* 60, 1207–1216. doi: 10.1016/j.jacc.2012.03.074

Chen, C. H., Chang, M. Y., Wang, S. S., and Hsieh, P. C. (2014). Injection of autologous bone marrow cells in hyaluronan hydrogel improves cardiac performance after infarction in pigs. *Am. J. Physiol. Heart Circ. Physiol.* 306, H1078–H1086. doi: 10.1152/ajpheart.00801.2013

Chen, C. W., Wang, L. L., Zaman, S., Gordon, J., Arisi, M. F., Venkataraman, C. M., et al. (2018). Sustained release of endothelial progenitor cell-derived extracellular vesicles from shear-thinning hydrogels improves angiogenesis and promotes function after myocardial infarction. *Cardiovasc. Res.* 114, 1029–1040. doi: 10.1093/cvr/cvy067

Chen, M. H., Wang, L. L., Chung, J. J., Kim, Y.-H., Atluri, P., and Burdick, J. A. (2017). Methods to assess shear-thinning hydrogels for application as injectable biomaterials. *ACS Biomater Sci. Eng.* 3, 3146–3160. doi: 10.1021/acsbiomaterials.7b00734

Cheng, Y. H., Lin, F. H., Wang, C. Y., Hsiao, C. Y., Chen, H. C., Kuo, H. Y., et al. (2016). Recovery of oxidative stress-induced damage in Cisd2-deficient cardiomyocytes by sustained release of ferulic acid from injectable hydrogel. *Biomaterials* 103, 207–218. doi: 10.1016/j.biomaterials.2016.06.060

Cheraghi, M., Namdari, M., Eatemadi, A., and Negahdarib, B. (2016). Recent advances in cardiac regeneration: stem cell, biomaterial and growth factors. *Biomed. Pharmacother.* 87, 37–45.

Chien, W. M., Liu, Y., Dinca, A. A., and Chin, M. T. (2017). Injection-based delivery of cell-permeable peptide-tagged cre. *Methods Mol. Biol.* 1642, 99–107. doi: 10.1007/978-1-4939-7169-5_7

Chow, A., Stuckey, D. J., Kidher, E., Rocco, M., Jabbour, R. J., Mansfield, C. A., et al. (2017). Human induced pluripotent stem cell-derived cardiomyocyte encapsulating bioactive hydrogels improve rat heart function post myocardial infarction. *Stem Cell Rep.* 9, 1415–1422. doi: 10.1016/j.stemcr.2017.09.003

Cipriani, F., Kruger, M., de Torre, I. G., Sierra, L. Q., Rodrigo, M. A., Kock, L., et al. (2018). Cartilage regeneration in preannealed silk elastin-like co-recombinamers injectable hydrogel embedded with mature chondrocytes in an ex vivo culture platform. *Biomacromolecules* 19, 4333–4347. doi: 10.1021/acs.biomac.8b01211

Cohen, J. E., Purcell, B. P., MacArthur, J. J., Mu, A., Shudo, Y., Patel, J. B., et al. (2014). A bioengineered hydrogel system enables targeted and sustained intramyocardial delivery of neuregulin, activating the cardiomyocyte cell cycle and enhancing ventricular function in a murine model of ischemic cardiomyopathy. *Circ. Heart Fail.* 7, 619–626. doi: 10.1161/CIRCHEARTFAILURE.113.001273

Cross, S. H., Kaufman, B. G., Mentz, R. J., Kamal, A. H., Taylor, D. J., and Warraich, H. J. (2019). Trends in place of death for individuals with cardiovascular disease in the United States. *J. Am. Coll. Cardiol.* 74, 1943–1946. doi: 10.1016/j.jacc.2019.08.1015

Cui, H., Liu, Y., Cheng, Y., Zhang, Z., Zhang, P., Chen, X., et al. (2014). In vitro study of electroactive tetraaniline-containing thermosensitive hydrogels for cardiac tissue engineering. *Biomacromolecules* 15, 1115–1123. doi: 10.1021/bm4018963

Davidson, S. M., Takov, K., and Yellon, D. M. (2017). Exosomes and cardiovascular protection. *Cardiovasc. Drugs Ther.* 31, 77–86. doi: 10.1007/s10557-016-6698-6696

Ding, J., Zhuang, X., Xiao, C., Cheng, Y., Zhao, L., He, C., et al. (2011). Preparation of photo-cross-linked pH-responsive polypeptide nanogels as potential carriers for controlled drug delivery. *J. Mater. Chem.* 21, 11383–11391.

Do, A. V., Khorsand, B., Geary, S. M., and Salem, A. K. (2015). 3D printing of scaffolds for tissue regeneration applications. *Adv. Healthc. Mater.* 4, 1742–1762. doi: 10.1002/adhm.201500168

Dolnikov, K., Shilkrut, M., Zeevi Levin, N., Gerecht Nir, S., Amit, M., Danon, A., et al. (2006). Functional properties of human embryonic stem cell–derived cardiomyocytes: intracellular Ca2+ handling and the role of sarcoplasmic reticulum in the contraction. *Stem Cells* 24, 236–245.

Doroudian, G., Pinney, J., Ayala, P., Los, T., Desai, T. A., and Russell, B. (2014). Sustained delivery of MGF peptide from microrods attracts stem cells and reduces apoptosis of myocytes. *Biomed. Microdevices* 16, 705–715. doi: 10.1007/s10544-014-9875-z

Dorsey, S. M., McGarvey, J. R., Wang, H., Nikou, A., Arama, L., Koomalsingh, K. J., et al. (2015). MRI evaluation of injectable hyaluronic acid-based hydrogel therapy to limit ventricular remodeling after myocardial infarction. *Biomaterials* 69, 65–75. doi: 10.1016/j.biomaterials.2015.08.011

Efraim, Y., Sarig, H., Cohen Anavy, N., Sarig, U., de Berardinis, E., Chaw, S., et al. (2017). Biohybrid cardiac ECM-based hydrogels improve long term cardiac function post myocardial infarction. *Acta Biomater.* 50, 220–233. doi: 10.1016/j.actbio.2016.12.015

Emanueli, C., Shearn, A. I. U., Angelini, G. D., and Sahoo, S. (2015). Exosomes and exosomal miRNAs in cardiovascular protection and repair. *Vasc. Pharmacol.* 71, 24–30. doi: 10.1016/j.vph.2015.02.008

Fan, Z., Fu, M., Xu, Z., Zhang, B., Li, Z., Li, H., et al. (2017). Sustained release of a peptide-based matrix metalloproteinase-2 inhibitor to attenuate adverse cardiac remodeling and improve cardiac function following myocardial infarction. *Biomacromolecules* 18, 2820–2829. doi: 10.1021/acs.biomac.7b00760

Fan, Z., Xu, Z., Niu, H., Gao, N., Guan, Y., Li, C., et al. (2018). An injectable oxygen release system to augment cell survival and promote cardiac repair following myocardial infarction. *Sci. Rep.* 8:1371. doi: 10.1038/s41598-018-19906-w

Fang, R., Qiao, S., Liu, Y., Meng, Q., Chen, X., Song, B., et al. (2015). Sustained co-delivery of BIO and IGF-1 by a novel hybrid hydrogel system to stimulate endogenous cardiac repair in myocardial infarcted rat hearts. *Int. J. Nanomed.* 10, 4691–4703. doi: 10.2147/IJN.S81451

Feng, Y., Li, Q., Wu, D., Niu, Y., Yang, C., Dong, L., et al. (2017). A macrophage-activating, injectable hydrogel to sequester endogenous growth factors for in situ angiogenesis. *Biomaterials* 134, 128–142. doi: 10.1016/j.biomaterials.2017.04.042

Francis, M. P., Breathwaite, E., Bulysheva, A. A., Varghese, F., Rodriguez, R. U., Dutta, S., et al. (2017). Human placenta hydrogel reduces scarring in a rat model of cardiac ischemia and enhances cardiomyocyte and stem cell cultures. *Acta Biomater.* 52, 92–104. doi: 10.1016/j.actbio.2016.12.027

Frith, J. E., Cameron, A. R., Menzies, D. J., Ghosh, P., Whitehead, D. L., Gronthos, S., et al. (2013). An injectable hydrogel incorporating mesenchymal precursor cells and pentosan polysulphate for intervertebral disc regeneration. *Biomaterials* 34, 9430–9440. doi: 10.1016/j.biomaterials.2013.08.072

Gaffey, A. C., Chen, M. H., Trubelja, A., Venkataraman, C. M., Chen, C. W., Chung, J. J., et al. (2019). Delivery of progenitor cells with injectable shear-thinning hydrogel maintains geometry and normalizes strain to stabilize cardiac function after ischemia. *J. Thorac. Cardiovasc. Surg.* 157, 1479–1490. doi: 10.1016/j.jtcvs.2018.07.117

Gaffey, A. C., Chen, M. H., Venkataraman, C. M., Trubelja, A., Rodell, C. B., Dinh, P. V., et al. (2015). Injectable shear-thinning hydrogels used to deliver endothelial progenitor cells, enhance cell engraftment, and improve ischemic myocardium. *J. Thorac. Cardiovasc. Surg.* 150, 1268–1277. doi: 10.1016/j.jtcvs.2015.07.035

Gao, Q., Liu, Z., Lin, Z., Qiu, J., Liu, Y., Liu, A., et al. (2017). 3D bioprinting of vessel-like structures with multilevel fluidic channels. *ACS Biomater. Sci. Eng.* 3, 399–408. doi: 10.1021/acsbiomaterials.6b00643

Garbern, J. C., Minami, E., Stayton, P. S., and Murry, C. E. (2011). Delivery of basic fibroblast growth factor with a pH-responsive, injectable hydrogel to improve angiogenesis in infarcted myocardium. *Biomaterials* 32, 2407–2416. doi: 10.1016/j.biomaterials.2010.11.075

Gersh, B. J., Sliwa, K., Mayosi, B. M., and Yusuf, S. (2010). Novel therapeutic concepts * The epidemic of cardiovascular disease in the developing world: global implications. *Eur. Heart J.* 31, 642–648. doi: 10.1093/eurheartj/ehq030

Geuss, L. R., Allen, A. C., Ramamoorthy, D., and Suggs, L. J. (2015). Maintenance of HL-1 cardiomyocyte functional activity in PEGylated fibrin gels. *Biotechnol. Bioeng.* 112, 1446–1456. doi: 10.1002/bit.25553

Ghadge, S. K., Muhlstedt, S., Ozcelik, C., and Bader, M. (2011). SDF-1alpha as a therapeutic stem cell homing factor in myocardial infarction. *Pharmacol. Ther.* 129, 97–108. doi: 10.1016/j.pharmthera.2010.09.011

Habib, M., Shapira-Schweitzer, K., Caspi, O., Gepstein, A., Arbel, G., Aronson, D., et al. (2011). A combined cell therapy and in-situ tissue-engineering approach for myocardial repair. *Biomaterials* 32, 7514–7523. doi: 10.1016/j.biomaterials.2011.06.049

Hadley, D. J., and Silva, E. A. (2019). Thaw-induced gelation of alginate hydrogels for versatile delivery of therapeutics. *Ann. Biomed. Eng.* 47, 1701–1710. doi: 10.1007/s10439-019-02282-2285

Han, C. S., Zhou, J., Liang, C., Liu, B., Pan, X. B., Zhang, Y., et al. (2019). Human umbilical cord mesenchymal stem cell derived exosomes encapsulated in functional peptide hydrogels promote cardiac repair. *Biomater. Sci.* 7, 2920–2933. doi: 10.1039/c9bm00101h

Han, H. W., Hou, Y. T., and Hsu, S. H. (2019). Angiogenic potential of co-spheroids of neural stem cells and endothelial cells in injectable gelatin-based hydrogel. *Mater. Sci. Eng. C Mater. Biol. Appl.* 99, 140–149. doi: 10.1016/j.msec.2019.01.089

Hasan, A., Khattab, A., Islam, M. A., Hweij, K. A., Zeitouny, J., Waters, R., et al. (2015). Injectable hydrogels for cardiac tissue repair after myocardial infarction. *Adv. Sci.* 2:1500122. doi: 10.1002/advs.201500122

He, X. T., Li, X., Xia, Y., Yin, Y., Wu, R. X., Sun, H. H., et al. (2019). Building capacity for macrophage modulation and stem cell recruitment in high-stiffness hydrogels for complex periodontal regeneration: experimental studies in vitro and in rats. *Acta Biomater.* 88, 162–180. doi: 10.1016/j.actbio.2019.02.004

He, Y. Y., Wen, Y., Zheng, X. X., and Jiang, X. J. (2013). Intramyocardial delivery of HMGB1 by a novel thermosensitive hydrogel attenuates cardiac remodeling and improves cardiac function after myocardial infarction. *J. Cardiovasc. Pharmacol.* 61, 283–290. doi: 10.1097/FJC.0b013e31827ecd50

Highley, C. B., Prestwich, G. D., and Burdick, J. A. (2016). Recent advances in hyaluronic acid hydrogels for biomedical applications. *Curr. Opin. Biotechnol.* 40, 35–40. doi: 10.1016/j.copbio.2016.02.008

Hozumi, T., Kageyama, T., Ohta, S., Fukuda, J., and Ito, T. (2018). Injectable hydrogel with slow degradability composed of gelatin and hyaluronic acid cross-linked by schiff's base formation. *Biomacromolecules* 19, 288–297. doi: 10.1021/acs.biomac.7b01133

Ibrahim, A., and Marbán, E. (2016). Exosomes: fundamental biology and roles in cardiovascular physiology. *Annu. Rev. Physiol.* 78, 67–83. doi: 10.1146/annurev-physiol-021115-104929

Jin, L., and Yu, Y. (2018). Bioactive small molecules in the pathogenesis and pharmacology of cardiovascular diseases: from bench to bedside. *Curr. Top. Med. Chem.* 18, 1351–1353. doi: 10.2174/156802661816181107141558

Johnson, T. D., and Christman, K. L. (2012). Injectable hydrogel therapies and their delivery strategies for treating myocardial infarction. *Expert Opin. Drug Deliv.* 10, 59–72. doi: 10.1517/17425247.2013.739156

Johnson, T. D., Lin, S. Y., and Christman, K. L. (2011). Tailoring material properties of a nanofibrous extracellular matrix derived hydrogel. *Nanotechnology* 22:494015. doi: 10.1088/0957-4484/22/49/494015

Kambe, Y., and Yamaoka, T. (2019). Biodegradation of injectable silk fibroin hydrogel prevents negative left ventricular remodeling after myocardial infarction. *Biomater. Sci.* 7, 4153–4165. doi: 10.1039/c9bm00556k

Kang, L. H., Armstrong, P. A., Lee, L. J., Duan, B., Kang, K. H., and Butcher, J. T. (2017). Optimizing photo-encapsulation viability of heart valve cell types in 3D printable composite hydrogels. *Ann. Biomed. Eng.* 45, 360–377. doi: 10.1007/s10439-016-1619-1611

Kanki, T., and Klionsky, D. J. (2009). Mitochondrial abnormalities drive cell death in Wolfram syndrome 2. *Cell Res.* 19, 922–923. doi: 10.1038/cr.2009.94

Karam, J. P., Muscari, C., Sindji, L., Bastiat, G., Bonafe, F., Venier-Julienne, M. C., et al. (2014). Pharmacologically active microcarriers associated with thermosensitive hydrogel as a growth factor releasing biomimetic 3D scaffold for cardiac tissue-engineering. *J. Control. Release* 192, 82–94. doi: 10.1016/j.jconrel.2014.06.052

Khabbaz, K. R., Zankoul, F., and Warner, K. G. (2001). Intraoperative metabolic monitoring of the heart: II. Online measurement of myocardial tissue pH. *Ann. Thorac. Surg.* 72, S2227–S2234. doi: 10.1016/s0003-4975(01)03284-3282

Kharkar, P. M., Kiick, K. L., and Kloxin, A. M. (2013). Designing degradable hydrogels for orthogonal control of cell microenvironments. *Chem. Soc. Rev.* 42, 7335–7372. doi: 10.1039/c3cs60040h

Kharkar, P. M., Scott, R. A., Olney, L. P., LeValley, P. J., Maverakis, E., Kiick, K. L., et al. (2017). Controlling the release of small, bioactive proteins via dual mechanisms with therapeutic potential. *Adv. Healthc. Mater.* 6:1700713. doi: 10.1002/adhm.201700713

Komeri, R., and Muthu, J. (2016). In situ crosslinkable elastomeric hydrogel for long-term cell encapsulation for cardiac applications. *J. Biomed. Mater. Res. A* 104, 2936–2944. doi: 10.1002/jbm.a.35833

Komeri, R., and Muthu, J. (2017). Injectable, cytocompatible, elastic, free radical scavenging and electroconductive hydrogel for cardiac cell encapsulation. *Coll. Surf. B Biointerfaces* 157, 381–390. doi: 10.1016/j.colsurfb.2017.05.073

Koudstaal, S., Bastings, M. M., Feyen, D. A., Waring, C. D., van Slochteren, F. J., Dankers, P. Y., et al. (2014). Sustained delivery of insulin-like growth factor-1/hepatocyte growth factor stimulates endogenous cardiac repair in the chronic infarcted pig heart. *J. Cardiovasc. Transl. Res.* 7, 232–241. doi: 10.1007/s12265-013-9518-9514

Kraehenbuehl, T. P., Ferreira, L. S., Hayward, A. M., Nahrendorf, M., van der Vlies, A. J., Vasile, E., et al. (2011). Human embryonic stem cell-derived microvascular grafts for cardiac tissue preservation after myocardial infarction. *Biomaterials* 32, 1102–1109. doi: 10.1016/j.biomaterials.2010.10.005

Kumbhani, D. J., Healey, N. A., Birjiniuk, V., Crittenden, M. D., Josa, M., Treanor, P. R., et al. (2004). Determinants of regional myocardial acidosis during cardiac surgery. *Surgery* 136, 190–198. doi: 10.1016/j.surg.2004.04.015

Kuo, K. C., Lin, R. Z., Tien, H. W., Wu, P. Y., Li, Y. C., Melero-Martin, J. M., et al. (2015). Bioengineering vascularized tissue constructs using an injectable cell-laden enzymatically crosslinked collagen hydrogel derived from dermal extracellular matrix. *Acta Biomater.* 27, 151–166. doi: 10.1016/j.actbio.2015.09.002

Kurdi, M., Chidiac, R., Hoemann, C., Zouein, F., Zgheib, C., and Booz, G. W. (2010). Hydrogels as a platform for stem cell delivery to the heart. *Congest. Heart Fail.* 16, 132–135. doi: 10.1111/j.1751-7133.2010.00145.x

Lapenna, A., De Palma, M., and Lewis, C. E. (2018). Perivascular macrophages in health and disease. *Nat. Rev. Immunol.* 18, 689–702. doi: 10.1038/s41577-018-0056-59

Larraneta, E., Henry, M., Irwin, N. J., Trotter, J., Perminova, A. A., and Donnelly, R. F. (2018). Synthesis and characterization of hyaluronic acid hydrogels crosslinked using a solvent-free process for potential biomedical applications. *Carbohydr. Polym.* 181, 1194–1205. doi: 10.1016/j.carbpol.2017.12.015

Lee, J., Tan, C. Y., Lee, S. K., Kim, Y. H., and Lee, K. Y. (2009). Controlled delivery of heat shock protein using an injectable microsphere/hydrogel combination system for the treatment of myocardial infarction. *J. Control. Release* 137, 196–202. doi: 10.1016/j.jconrel.2009.04.008

Leri, A., Kajstura, J., and Anversa, P. (2005). Cardiac stem cells and mechanisms of myocardial regeneration. *Physiol. Rev.* 85, 1373–1416.

Li, H., Gao, J., Shang, Y., Hua, Y., Ye, M., Yang, Z., et al. (2018). Folic acid derived hydrogel enhances the survival and promotes therapeutic efficacy of iPS cells for acute myocardial infarction. *ACS Appl. Mater. Interfaces* 10, 24459–24468. doi: 10.1021/acsami.8b08659

Li, Z., Shen, D., Hu, S., Su, T., Huang, K., Liu, F., et al. (2018). Pretargeting and bioorthogonal click chemistry-mediated endogenous stem cell homing for heart repair. *ACS Nano* 12, 12193–12200. doi: 10.1021/acsnano.8b05892

Li, J., Chen, G., Xu, X., Abdou, P., Jiang, Q., Shi, D., et al. (2019). Advances of injectable hydrogel-based scaffolds for cartilage regeneration. *Regen. Biomater.* 6, 129–140. doi: 10.1093/rb/rbz022

Li, L., Yu, F., Zheng, L., Wang, R., Yan, W., Wang, Z., et al. (2019). Natural hydrogels for cartilage regeneration: modification, preparation and application. *J. Orthop. Transl.* 17, 26–41. doi: 10.1016/j.jot.2018.09.003

Li, J., Shu, Y., Hao, T., Wang, Y., Qian, Y., Duan, C., et al. (2013). A chitosan-glutathione based injectable hydrogel for suppression of oxidative stress damage in cardiomyocytes. *Biomaterials* 34, 9071–9081. doi: 10.1016/j.biomaterials.2013.08.031

Li, R., and Weisel, R. D. (2014). *Cardiac Regeneration and Repair: Biomaterials and Tissue Engineering*. Amsterdam: Elsevier.

Li, Z., Guo, X., Matsushita, S., and Guan, J. (2011). Differentiation of cardiosphere-derived cells into a mature cardiac lineage using biodegradable poly(N-isopropylacrylamide) hydrogels. *Biomaterials* 32, 3220–3232. doi: 10.1016/j.biomaterials.2011.01.050

Li, Z., Guo, X., Palmer, A. F., Das, H., and Guan, J. (2012). High-efficiency matrix modulus-induced cardiac differentiation of human mesenchymal stem cells inside a thermosensitive hydrogel. *Acta Biomater.* 8, 3586–3595. doi: 10.1016/j.actbio.2012.06.024

Liu, T. Y., Chen, S. Y., Lin, Y. L., and Liu, D. M. (2006). Synthesis and characterization of amphiphatic carboxymethyl-hexanoyl chitosan hydrogel: water-retention ability and drug encapsulation. *Langmuir* 22, 9740–9745. doi: 10.1021/la061471n

Liu, Z., Wang, H., Wang, Y., Lin, Q., Yao, A., Cao, F., et al. (2012). The influence of chitosan hydrogel on stem cell engraftment, survival and homing in the ischemic myocardial microenvironment. *Biomaterials* 33, 3093–3106. doi: 10.1016/j.biomaterials.2011.12.044

Lopez-Jaramillo, P. (2008). Defining the research priorities to fight the burden of cardiovascular diseases in Latin America. *J. Hypertens.* 26, 1886–1889. doi: 10.1097/HJH.0b013e328308ba8d

Lovett, M., Lee, K., Edwards, A., and Kaplan, D. L. (2009). Vascularization strategies for tissue engineering. *Tissue Eng. B Rev.* 15, 353–370. doi: 10.1089/ten.TEB.2009.0085

Lu, J., Shen, X., Sun, X., Yin, H., Yang, S., Lu, C., et al. (2018). Increased recruitment of endogenous stem cells and chondrogenic differentiation by a composite scaffold containing bone marrow homing peptide for cartilage regeneration. *Theranostics* 8, 5039–5058. doi: 10.7150/thno.26981

Lu, S., Wang, H., Lu, W., Liu, S., Lin, Q., Li, D., et al. (2010). Both the transplantation of somatic cell nuclear transfer- and fertilization-derived mouse embryonic stem cells with temperature-responsive chitosan hydrogel improve myocardial performance in infarcted rat hearts. *Tissue Eng. A* 16, 1303–1315. doi: 10.1089/ten.TEA.2009.0434

Lu, W. N., Lu, S. H., Wang, H. B., Li, D. X., Duan, C. M., Liu, Z. Q., et al. (2009). Functional improvement of infarcted heart by co-injection of embryonic stem cells with temperature-responsive chitosan hydrogel. *Tissue Eng. A* 15, 1437–1447. doi: 10.1089/ten.tea.2008.0143

MacArthur, J. J., Purcell, B. P., Shudo, Y., Cohen, J. E., Fairman, A., Trubelja, A., et al. (2013). Sustained release of engineered stromal cell-derived factor 1-alpha from injectable hydrogels effectively recruits endothelial progenitor cells and preserves ventricular function after myocardial infarction. *Circulation* 128(11 Suppl. 1), S79–S86. doi: 10.1161/CIRCULATIONAHA.112.000343

MacArthur, J. W., Steele, A. N., Goldstone, A. B., Cohen, J. E., Hiesinger, W., and Woo, Y. J. (2017). Injectable bioengineered hydrogel therapy in the treatment of ischemic cardiomyopathy. *Curr. Treat. Options Cardiovasc. Med.* 19:30. doi: 10.1007/s11936-017-0530-x

Macaya, D., and Spector, M. (2012). Injectable hydrogel materials for spinal cord regeneration: a review. *Biomed. Mater.* 7:12001. doi: 10.1088/1748-6041/7/1/012001

Madonna, R., and De Caterina, R. (2011). Stem cells and growth factor delivery systems for cardiovascular disease. *J. Biotechnol.* 154, 291–297. doi: 10.1016/j.jbiotec.2011.05.014

Mann, D. L., Lee, R. J., Coats, A. J., Neagoe, G., Dragomir, D., Pusineri, E., et al. (2016). One-year follow-up results from AUGMENT-HF: a multicentre randomized controlled clinical trial of the efficacy of left ventricular augmentation with Algisyl in the treatment of heart failure. *Eur. J. Heart Fail.* 18, 314–325. doi: 10.1002/ejhf.449

Mao, X., Cheng, R., Zhang, H., Bae, J., Cheng, L., Zhang, L., et al. (2019). Self-healing and injectable hydrogel for matching skin flap regeneration. *Adv. Sci.* 6:1801555. doi: 10.1002/advs.201801555

Marquez-Curtis, L. A., and Janowska-Wieczorek, A. (2013). Enhancing the Migration Ability of Mesenchymal Stromal Cells by Targeting the SDF-1/CXCR4 Axis. *Biomed. Res. Int.* 2013, 1–15. doi: 10.1155/2013/561098

Matoba, T., Koga, J. I., Nakano, K., Egashira, K., and Tsutsui, H. (2017). Nanoparticle-mediated drug delivery system for atherosclerotic cardiovascular disease. *J. Cardiol.* 70, 206–211. doi: 10.1016/j.jjcc.2017.03.005

McAloon, C. J., Boylan, L. M., Hamborg, T., Stallard, N., Osman, F., Lim, P. B., et al. (2016). The changing face of cardiovascular disease 2000-2012: an analysis of the world health organisation global health estimates data. *Int. J. Cardiol.* 224, 256–264. doi: 10.1016/j.ijcard.2016.09.026

Meng, X., Stout, D. A., Sun, L., Beingessner, R. L., Fenniri, H., and Webster, T. J. (2013). Novel injectable biomimetic hydrogels with carbon nanofibers and self assembled rosette nanotubes for myocardial applications. *J. Biomed. Mater. Res. A* 101, 1095–1102. doi: 10.1002/jbm.a.34400

Mihic, A., Cui, Z., Wu, J., Vlacic, G., Miyagi, Y., Li, S. H., et al. (2015). A conductive polymer hydrogel supports cell electrical signaling and improves cardiac function after implantation into myocardial infarct. *Circulation* 132, 772–784. doi: 10.1161/CIRCULATIONAHA.114.014937

Mirotsou, M., Jayawardena, T. M., Schmeckpeper, J., Gnecchi, M., and Dzau, V. J. (2011). Paracrine mechanisms of stem cell reparative and regenerative actions in the heart. *J. Mol. Cell Cardiol.* 50, 280–289. doi: 10.1016/j.yjmcc.2010.08.005

Miyake, F., Kamogawa, A., and Sakakibara, M. (1998). [Drug delivery system in cardiovascular drugs]. *Nihon Rinsho* 56, 737–741.

Mody, V. V., Siwale, R., Singh, A., and Mody, H. R. (2010). Introduction to metallic nanoparticles. *J. Pharm. Bioallied Sci.* 2, 282–289. doi: 10.4103/0975-7406.72127

Monaghan, M. G., Holeiter, M., Brauchle, E., Layland, S. L., Lu, Y., Deb, A., et al. (2018). Exogenous miR-29B delivery through a hyaluronan-based injectable system yields functional maintenance of the infarcted myocardium. *Tissue Eng. A* 24, 57–67. doi: 10.1089/ten.TEA.2016.0527

Moon, J. J., Saik, J. E., Poche, R. A., Leslie-Barbick, J. E., Lee, S. H., Smith, A. A., et al. (2010). Biomimetic hydrogels with pro-angiogenic properties. *Biomaterials* 31, 3840–3847. doi: 10.1016/j.biomaterials.2010.01.104

Mulyasasmita, W., Cai, L., Dewi, R. E., Jha, A., Ullmann, S. D., Luong, R. H., et al. (2014). Avidity-controlled hydrogels for injectable co-delivery of induced pluripotent stem cell-derived endothelial cells and growth factors. *J. Control. Release* 191, 71–81. doi: 10.1016/j.jconrel.2014.05.015

Naderi-Meshkin, H., Matin, M. M., Heirani-Tabasi, A., Mirahmadi, M., Irfan-Maqsood, M., Edalatmanesh, M. A., et al. (2016). Injectable hydrogel delivery plus preconditioning of mesenchymal stem cells: exploitation of SDF-1/CXCR4 axis toward enhancing the efficacy of stem cells' homing. *Cell Biol. Int.* 40, 730–741. doi: 10.1002/cbin.10474

Nichols, M., Townsend, N., Scarborough, P., and Rayner, M. (2014). Cardiovascular disease in Europe 2014: epidemiological update. *Eur. Heart J.* 35, 2950–2959. doi: 10.1093/eurheartj/ehu299

Norouzi, M., Nazari, B., and Miller, D. W. (2016). Injectable hydrogel-based drug delivery systems for local cancer therapy. *Drug Discov. Today* 21, 1835–1849. doi: 10.1016/j.drudis.2016.07.006

Noshadi, I., Hong, S., Sullivan, K. E., Shirzaei, S. E., Portillo-Lara, R., Tamayol, A., et al. (2017). In vitro and in vivo analysis of visible light crosslinkable gelatin methacryloyl (GelMA) hydrogels. *Biomater. Sci.* 5, 2093–2105. doi: 10.1039/c7bm00110j

Pacelli, S., Acosta, F., Chakravarti, A. R., Samanta, S. G., Whitlow, J., Modaresi, S., et al. (2017). Nanodiamond-based injectable hydrogel for sustained growth factor release: preparation, characterization and in vitro analysis. *Acta Biomater.* 58, 479–491. doi: 10.1016/j.actbio.2017.05.026

Pandey, R., Velasquez, S., Durrani, S., Jiang, M., Neiman, M., Crocker, J. S., et al. (2017). MicroRNA-1825 induces proliferation of adult cardiomyocytes and promotes cardiac regeneration post ischemic injury. *Am. J. Transl. Res.* 9, 3120–3137.

Paul, A., Hasan, A., Kindi, H. A., Gaharwar, A. K., Rao, V. T., Nikkhah, M., et al. (2014). Injectable graphene oxide/hydrogel-based angiogenic gene delivery system for vasculogenesis and cardiac repair. *ACS Nano* 8, 8050–8062. doi: 10.1021/nn5020787

Pena, B., Laughter, M., Jett, S., Rowland, T. J., Taylor, M., Mestroni, L., et al. (2018). Injectable hydrogels for cardiac tissue engineering. *Macromol. Biosci.* 18:e1800079. doi: 10.1002/mabi.201800079

Peppas, N. A., Hilt, J. Z., Khademhosseini, A., and Langer, R. (2006). Hydrogels in biology and medicine: from molecular principles to bionanotechnology. *Adv. Mater.* 18, 1345–1360. doi: 10.1002/adma.200501612

Pisanic, T. N., Blackwell, J. D., Shubayev, V. I., Finones, R. R., and Jin, S. (2007). Nanotoxicity of iron oxide nanoparticle internalization in growing neurons. *Biomaterials* 28, 2572–2581. doi: 10.1016/j.biomaterials.2007.01.043

Poe, A. J., and Knowlton, A. A. (2018). Exosomes and cardiovascular cell-cell communication. *Essays Biochem.* 62, 193–204. doi: 10.1042/EBC20170081

Purcell, B. P., Lobb, D., Charati, M. B., Dorsey, S. M., Wade, R. J., Zellars, K. N., et al. (2014). Injectable and bioresponsive hydrogels for on-demand matrix metalloproteinase inhibition. *Nat. Mater.* 13, 653–661. doi: 10.1038/nmat3922

Qi, J., Yan, Y., Cheng, B., Deng, L., Shao, Z., Sun, Z., et al. (2018). Enzymatic formation of an injectable hydrogel from a glycopeptide as a biomimetic scaffold for vascularization. *ACS Appl. Mater. Interfaces* 10, 6180–6189. doi: 10.1021/acsami.7b18535

Qu, Y., Tang, J., Liu, L., Song, L., Chen, S., and Gao, Y. (2019). alpha-Tocopherol liposome loaded chitosan hydrogel to suppress oxidative stress injury in cardiomyocytes. *Int. J. Biol. Macromol.* 125, 1192–1202. doi: 10.1016/j.ijbiomac.2018.09.092

Rocca, D. G. D., Willenberg, B. J., Qi, Y., Simmons, C. S., Rubiano, A., Ferreira, L. F., et al. (2016). An injectable capillary-like microstructured alginate hydrogel improves left ventricular function after myocardial infarction in rats. *Int. J. Cardiol.* 220, 149–154. doi: 10.1016/j.ijcard.2016.06.158

Rodell, C. B., Lee, M. E., Wang, H., Takebayashi, S., Takayama, T., Kawamura, T., et al. (2016). Injectable shear-thinning hydrogels for minimally invasive delivery to infarcted myocardium to limit left ventricular remodeling. *Circ. Cardiovasc. Interv.* 9:e004058. doi: 10.1161/CIRCINTERVENTIONS.116.004058

Rufaihah, A. J., Johari, N. A., Vaibavi, S. R., Plotkin, M., Di Thien, D. T., Kofidis, T., et al. (2017). Dual delivery of VEGF and ANG-1 in ischemic hearts using an injectable hydrogel. *Acta Biomater.* 48, 58–67. doi: 10.1016/j.actbio.2016.10.013

Rufaihah, A. J., Vaibavi, S. R., Plotkin, M., Shen, J., Nithya, V., Wang, J., et al. (2013). Enhanced infarct stabilization and neovascularization mediated by VEGF-loaded PEGylated fibrinogen hydrogel in a rodent myocardial infarction model. *Biomaterials* 34, 8195–8202. doi: 10.1016/j.biomaterials.2013.07.031

Ruvinov, E., and Cohen, S. (2016). Alginate biomaterial for the treatment of myocardial infarction: progress, translational strategies, and clinical outlook:

from ocean algae to patient bedside. *Adv. Drug Deliv. Rev.* 96, 54–76. doi: 10.1016/j.addr.2015.04.021

Ruvinov, E., Leor, J., and Cohen, S. (2010). The effects of controlled HGF delivery from an affinity-binding alginate biomaterial on angiogenesis and blood perfusion in a hindlimb ischemia model. *Biomaterials* 31, 4573–4582. doi: 10.1016/j.biomaterials.2010.02.026

Seliktar, D. (2012). Designing cell-compatible hydrogels for biomedical applications. *Science* 336, 1124–1128. doi: 10.1126/science.1214804

Semalty, A., Semalty, M., Rawat, B. S., Singh, D., and Rawat, M. S. (2009). Pharmacosomes: the lipid-based new drug delivery system. *Expert Opin. Drug Deliv.* 6, 599–612. doi: 10.1517/17425240902967607

Seo, B. B., Koh, J. T., and Song, S. C. (2017). Tuning physical properties and BMP-2 release rates of injectable hydrogel systems for an optimal bone regeneration effect. *Biomaterials* 122, 91–104. doi: 10.1016/j.biomaterials.2017.01.016

Seo, Y., Jung, Y., and Kim, S. H. (2018). Decellularized heart ECM hydrogel using supercritical carbon dioxide for improved angiogenesis. *Acta Biomater.* 67, 270–281. doi: 10.1016/j.actbio.2017.11.046

Sepantafar, M., Maheronnaghsh, R., Mohammadi, H., Rajabi-Zeleti, S., Annabi, N., Aghdami, N., et al. (2016). Stem cells and injectable hydrogels: synergistic therapeutics in myocardial repair. *Biotechnol. Adv.* 34, 362–379. doi: 10.1016/j.biotechadv.2016.03.003

Shaghiera, A. D., Widiyanti, P., and Yusuf, H. (2018). Synthesis and characterization of injectable hydrogels with varying Collagen(-)Chitosan(-)thymosin beta4 composition for myocardial infarction therapy. *J. Funct. Biomater.* 9:33. doi: 10.3390/jfb9020033

Shu, Y., Hao, T., Yao, F., Qian, Y., Wang, Y., Yang, B., et al. (2015). RoY peptide-modified chitosan-based hydrogel to improve angiogenesis and cardiac repair under hypoxia. *ACS Appl. Mater. Interfaces* 7, 6505–6517. doi: 10.1021/acsami.5b01234

Singelyn, J. M., and Christman, K. L. (2011). Modulation of material properties of a decellularized myocardial matrix scaffold. *Macromol. Biosci.* 11, 731–738. doi: 10.1002/mabi.201000423

Singh, A. P., Biswas, A., Shukla, A., and Maiti, P. (2019). Targeted therapy in chronic diseases using nanomaterial-based drug delivery vehicles. *Signal Transduct. Target. Ther.* 4, 1–21. doi: 10.1038/s41392-019-0068-63

Song, H., Cha, M. J., Song, B. W., Kim, I. K., Chang, W., Lim, S., et al. (2010). Reactive oxygen species inhibit adhesion of mesenchymal stem cells implanted into ischemic myocardium via interference of focal adhesion complex. *Stem Cells* 28, 555–563. doi: 10.1002/stem.302

Song, M., Jang, H., Lee, J., Kim, J. H., Kim, S. H., Sun, K., et al. (2014). Regeneration of chronic myocardial infarction by injectable hydrogels containing stem cell homing factor SDF-1 and angiogenic peptide Ac-SDKP. *Biomaterials* 35, 2436–2445. doi: 10.1016/j.biomaterials.2013.12.011

Song, Y., Zhang, C., Zhang, J., Sun, N., Huang, K., Li, H., et al. (2016). An injectable silk sericin hydrogel promotes cardiac functional recovery after ischemic myocardial infarction. *Acta Biomater.* 41, 210–223. doi: 10.1016/j.actbio.2016.05.039

Stoppel, W. L., Gao, A. E., Greaney, A. M., Partlow, B. P., Bretherton, R. C., Kaplan, D. L., et al. (2016). Elastic, silk-cardiac extracellular matrix hydrogels exhibit time-dependent stiffening that modulates cardiac fibroblast response. *J. Biomed. Mater. Res. A* 104, 3058–3072. doi: 10.1002/jbm.a.35850

Sun, H., Zhou, J., Huang, Z., Qu, L., Lin, N., Liang, C., et al. (2017). Carbon nanotube-incorporated collagen hydrogels improve cell alignment and the performance of cardiac constructs. *Int. J. Nanomed.* 12, 3109–3120. doi: 10.2147/IJN.S128030

Süselbeck, T. (2014). Intracoronary delivery of injectable bioabsorbable scaffold (IK-5001) to treat left ventricular remodeling after ST-elevation myocardial infarction: a first-in-man study. *Circ. Cardiovasc. Interv.* 7, 806–812.

Tang, Q., Luo, C., Lu, B., Fu, Q., Yin, H., Qin, Z., et al. (2017). Thermosensitive chitosan-based hydrogels releasing stromal cell derived factor-1 alpha recruit MSC for corneal epithelium regeneration. *Acta Biomater.* 61, 101–113. doi: 10.1016/j.actbio.2017.08.001

Torres-Martinez, E. J., Cornejo, B. J., Serrano, M. A., Perez, G. G., and Villarreal, G. L. (2018). A summary of electrospun nanofibers as drug delivery system: drugs loaded and biopolymers used as matrices. *Curr. Drug Deliv.* 15, 1360–1374. doi: 10.2174/1567201815666180723114326

Tous, E., Ifkovits, J. L., Koomalsingh, K. J., Shuto, T., Soeda, T., Kondo, N., et al. (2011). Influence of injectable hyaluronic acid hydrogel degradation behavior on infarction-induced ventricular remodeling. *Biomacromolecules* 12, 4127–4135. doi: 10.1021/bm201198x

Trombino, S., Servidio, C., Curcio, F., and Cassano, R. (2019). Strategies for hyaluronic acid-based hydrogel design in drug delivery. *Pharmaceutics* 11:407. doi: 10.3390/pharmaceutics11080407

Ujcic-Voortman, J. K., Baan, C. A., Seidell, J. C., and Verhoeff, A. P. (2012). Obesity and cardiovascular disease risk among Turkish and Moroccan migrant groups in Europe: a systematic review. *Obes. Rev.* 13, 2–16. doi: 10.1111/j.1467-789X.2011.00932.x

Ungerleider, J. L., and Christman, K. L. (2014). Concise review: injectable biomaterials for the treatment of myocardial infarction and peripheral artery disease: translational challenges and progress. *Stem Cells Transl. Med.* 3, 1090–1099. doi: 10.5966/sctm.2014-0049

Unterman, S., Charles, L. F., Strecker, S. E., Kramarenko, D., Pivovarchik, D., and Edelman, E. R., et al. (2017). Hydrogel nanocomposites with independently tunable rheology and mechanics. *ACS Nano.* 11, 2598–2610. doi: 10.1021/acsnano.6b06730

Van Vlierberghe, S., Dubruel, P., and Schacht, E. (2011). Biopolymer-based hydrogels as scaffolds for tissue engineering applications: a review. *Biomacromolecules* 12, 1387–1408. doi: 10.1021/bm200083n

Vong, L. B., Bui, T. Q., Tomita, T., Sakamoto, H., Hiramatsu, Y., and Nagasaki, Y. (2018). Novel angiogenesis therapeutics by redox injectable hydrogel - Regulation of local nitric oxide generation for effective cardiovascular therapy. *Biomaterials* 167, 143–152. doi: 10.1016/j.biomaterials.2018.03.023

Vukajlovic, D., Parker, J., Bretcanu, O., and Novakovic, K. (2019). Chitosan based polymer/bioglass composites for tissue engineering applications. *Mater. Sci. Eng. C Mater. Biol. Appl.* 96, 955–967. doi: 10.1016/j.msec.2018.12.026

Wall, S. T., Yeh, C. C., Tu, R. Y., Mann, M. J., and Healy, K. E. (2010). Biomimetic matrices for myocardial stabilization and stem cell transplantation. *J. Biomed. Mater. Res. A* 95, 1055–1066. doi: 10.1002/jbm.a.32904

Wang, F., Li, Z., Khan, M., Tamama, K., Kuppusamy, P., Wagner, W. R., et al. (2010). Injectable, rapid gelling and highly flexible hydrogel composites as growth factor and cell carriers. *Acta Biomater.* 6, 1978–1991. doi: 10.1016/j.actbio.2009.12.011

Wang, H., Rodell, C. B., Zhang, X., Dusaj, N. N., Gorman, J. R., Pilla, J. J., et al. (2018). Effects of hydrogel injection on borderzone contractility post-myocardial infarction. *Biomech. Model. Mechanobiol.* 17, 1533–1542. doi: 10.1007/s10237-018-1039-1032

Wang, L. L., Chung, J. J., Li, E. C., Uman, S., Atluri, P., and Burdick, J. A. (2018). Injectable and protease-degradable hydrogel for siRNA sequestration and triggered delivery to the heart. *J. Control. Release* 285, 152–161. doi: 10.1016/j.jconrel.2018.07.004

Wang, H., Shi, J., Wang, Y., Yin, Y., Wang, L., Liu, J., et al. (2014). Promotion of cardiac differentiation of brown adipose derived stem cells by chitosan hydrogel for repair after myocardial infarction. *Biomaterials* 35, 3986–3998. doi: 10.1016/j.biomaterials.2014.01.021

Wang, L. S., Lee, F., Lim, J., Du, C., Wan, A. C., Lee, S. S., et al. (2014). Enzymatic conjugation of a bioactive peptide into an injectable hyaluronic acid-tyramine hydrogel system to promote the formation of functional vasculature. *Acta Biomater.* 10, 2539–2550. doi: 10.1016/j.actbio.2014.02.022

Wang, L. L., Liu, Y., Chung, J. J., Wang, T., Gaffey, A. C., Lu, M., et al. (2017). Local and sustained miRNA delivery from an injectable hydrogel promotes cardiomyocyte proliferation and functional regeneration after ischemic injury. *Nat. Biomed. Eng.* 1, 983–992. doi: 10.1038/s41551-017-0157-y

Wang, R. M., Johnson, T. D., He, J., Rong, Z., Wong, M., Nigam, V., et al. (2017). Humanized mouse model for assessing the human immune response to xenogeneic and allogeneic decellularized biomaterials. *Biomaterials* 129, 98–110. doi: 10.1016/j.biomaterials.2017.03.016

Wang, R. M., and Christman, K. L. (2016). Decellularized myocardial matrix hydrogels: in basic research and preclinical studies. *Adv. Drug Deliv. Rev.* 96, 77–82. doi: 10.1016/j.addr.2015.06.002

Wang, W., Chen, J., Li, M., Jia, H., Han, X., Zhang, J., et al. (2019). Rebuilding postinfarcted cardiac functions by injecting TIIA@PDA nanoparticle-cross-linked ros-sensitive hydrogels. *ACS Appl. Mater. Interfaces* 11, 2880–2890. doi: 10.1021/acsami.8b20158

Wang, W., Ding, J., Xiao, C., Tang, Z., Li, D., Chen, J., et al. (2011). Synthesis of amphiphilic alternating polyesters with oligo (ethylene glycol) side chains and potential use for sustained release drug delivery. *Biomacromolecules* 12, 2466–2474. doi: 10.1021/bm200668n

Waters, R., Alam, P., Pacelli, S., Chakravarti, A. R., Ahmed, R., and Paul, A. (2018). Stem cell-inspired secretome-rich injectable hydrogel to repair injured cardiac tissue. *Acta Biomater.* 69, 95–106. doi: 10.1016/j.actbio.2017.12.025

Wei, L., Chen, J., Zhao, S., Ding, J., and Chen, X. (2017). Thermo-sensitive polypeptide hydrogel for locally sequential delivery of two-pronged antitumor drugs. *Acta Biomater.* 58, 44–53. doi: 10.1016/j.actbio.2017.05.053

Wiley, S. E., Andreyev, A. Y., Divakaruni, A. S., Karisch, R., Perkins, G., Wall, E. A., et al. (2013). Wolfram Syndrome protein, Miner1, regulates sulphydryl redox status, the unfolded protein response, and Ca2+ homeostasis. *EMBO Mol. Med.* 5, 904–918. doi: 10.1002/emmm.201201429

Wu, C. Y., Chen, Y. F., Wang, C. H., Kao, C. H., Zhuang, H. W., Chen, C. C., et al. (2012). A persistent level of Cisd2 extends healthy lifespan and delays aging in mice. *Hum. Mol. Genet.* 21, 3956–3968. doi: 10.1093/hmg/dds210

Wu, J., Zeng, F., Huang, X. P., Chung, J. C., Konecny, F., Weisel, R. D., et al. (2011). Infarct stabilization and cardiac repair with a VEGF-conjugated, injectable hydrogel. *Biomaterials* 32, 579–586. doi: 10.1016/j.biomaterials.2010.08.098

Xia, Y., Zhu, K., Lai, H., Lang, M., Xiao, Y., Lian, S., et al. (2015). Enhanced infarct myocardium repair mediated by thermosensitive copolymer hydrogel-based stem cell transplantation. *Exp. Biol. Med.* 240, 593–600. doi: 10.1177/1535370214560957

Xu, B., Li, Y., Deng, B., Liu, X., Wang, L., and Zhu, Q. (2017). Chitosan hydrogel improves mesenchymal stem cell transplant survival and cardiac function following myocardial infarction in rats. *Exp. Ther. Med.* 13, 588–594. doi: 10.3892/etm.2017.4026

Yeh, Y. C., Lee, W. Y., Yu, C. L., Hwang, S. M., Chung, M. F., Hsu, L. W., et al. (2010). Cardiac repair with injectable cell sheet fragments of human amniotic fluid stem cells in an immune-suppressed rat model. *Biomaterials* 31, 6444–6453. doi: 10.1016/j.biomaterials.2010.04.069

Yesilyurt, V., Webber, M. J., Appel, E. A., Godwin, C., Langer, R., and Anderson, D. G. (2016). Injectable self-healing glucose-responsive hydrogels with pH-regulated mechanical properties. *Adv. Mater.* 28, 86–91. doi: 10.1002/adma.201502902

Yoon, S. J., Fang, Y. H., Lim, C. H., Kim, B. S., Son, H. S., Park, Y., et al. (2009). Regeneration of ischemic heart using hyaluronic acid-based injectable hydrogel. *J. Biomed. Mater. Res. B Appl. Biomater.* 91, 163–171. doi: 10.1002/jbm.b.31386

Yoon, S. J., Hong, S., Fang, Y. H., Song, M., Son, K. H., Son, H. S., et al. (2014). Differential regeneration of myocardial infarction depending on the progression of disease and the composition of biomimetic hydrogel. *J. Biosci. Bioeng.* 118, 461–468. doi: 10.1016/j.jbiosc.2014.04.001

Zhang, K., Zhao, X., Chen, X., Wei, Y., Du, W., Wang, Y., et al. (2018). Enhanced therapeutic effects of mesenchymal stem cell-derived exosomes with an injectable hydrogel for hindlimb ischemia treatment. *ACS Appl. Mater. Interfaces* 10, 30081–30091. doi: 10.1021/acsami.8b08449

Zhang, Y., Cai, L., Li, D., Lao, Y., Liu, D., Li, M., et al. (2018). Tumor microenvironment-responsive hyaluronate-calcium carbonate hybrid nanoparticle enables effective chemotherapy for primary and advanced osteosarcomas. *Nano Res.* 11, 4806–4822.

Zhang, Y., Fan, W., Wang, K., Wei, H., Zhang, R., and Wu, Y. (2019). Novel preparation of Au nanoparticles loaded Laponite nanoparticles/ECM injectable hydrogel on cardiac differentiation of resident cardiac stem cells to cardiomyocytes. *J. Photochem. Photobiol. B* 192, 49–54. doi: 10.1016/j.jphotobiol.2018.12.022

Zhang, Y., Hu, Y., Zheng, L., and Wang, Q. (2017). Characteristics and roles of exosomes in cardiovascular disease. *DNA Cell Biol.* 36, 202–211. doi: 10.1089/dna.2016.3496

Zhao, L., Ding, J., Xiao, C., He, P., Tang, Z., Pang, X., et al. (2012). Glucose-sensitive polypeptide micelles for self-regulated insulin release at physiological pH. *J. Mater. Chem.* 22, 12319–12328.

Zhao, Y., and Zhang, H. (2016). Update on the mechanisms of homing of adipose tissue-derived stem cells. *Cytotherapy* 18, 816–827. doi: 10.1016/j.jcyt.2016.04.008

Zhu, H., Jiang, X., Li, X., Hu, M., Wan, W., Wen, Y., et al. (2016). Intramyocardial delivery of VEGF165 via a novel biodegradable hydrogel induces angiogenesis and improves cardiac function after rat myocardial infarction. *Heart Vessels* 31, 963–975. doi: 10.1007/s00380-015-0710-710

Zhu, Y., Matsumura, Y., Velayutham, M., Foley, L. M., Hitchens, T. K., and Wagner, W. R. (2018). Reactive oxygen species scavenging with a biodegradable, thermally responsive hydrogel compatible with soft tissue injection. *Biomaterials* 177, 98–112. doi: 10.1016/j.biomaterials.2018.05.044

2

Nanoparticle-Mediated Drug Delivery for Treatment of Ischemic Heart Disease

Chengming Fan[1†], Jyotsna Joshi[2†], Fan Li[2], Bing Xu[2], Mahmood Khan[3], Jinfu Yang[1] and Wuqiang Zhu[2,4*]*

[1] *Department of Cardiovascular Surgery, The Second Xiangya Hospital, Central South University, Changsha, China,* [2] *Department of Cardiovascular Diseases, Mayo Clinic, Scottsdale, AZ, United States,* [3] *Department of Emergency Medicine, The Ohio State University Wexner Medical Center, Columbus, OH, United States,* [4] *Department of Physiology and Biomedical Engineering, Mayo Clinic, Rochester, MN, United States*

***Correspondence:**
Chengming Fan
fchmfchm@163.com
Wuqiang Zhu
Zhu.Wuqiang@mayo.edu

† These authors have contributed equally to this work

The regenerative capacity of an adult cardiac tissue is insufficient to repair the massive loss of heart tissue, particularly cardiomyocytes (CMs), following ischemia or other catastrophic myocardial injuries. The delivery methods of therapeutics agents, such as small molecules, growth factors, exosomes, cells, and engineered tissues have significantly advanced in medical science. Furthermore, with the controlled release characteristics, nanoparticle (NP) systems carrying drugs are promising in enhancing the cardioprotective potential of drugs in patients with cardiac ischemic events. NPs can provide sustained exposure precisely to the infarcted heart via direct intramyocardial injection or intravenous injection with active targets. In this review, we present the recent advances and challenges of different types of NPs loaded with agents for the repair of myocardial infarcted heart tissue.

Keywords: nanoparticles, controlled release, myocardial infarction, cardiac repair, drug delivery systems

INTRODUCTION

Ischemic heart diseases, caused by coronary artery obstruction, account for almost 80% of deaths from cardiovascular diseases (Lloyd-Jones et al., 2010). Traditional clinical approaches for myocardial infarction rely on surgical revascularization procedures, such as coronary stenting or coronary artery bypass grafts (CABG). Although the novel therapeutics using cells (especially stem cells) (Gao et al., 2013; Madigan and Atoui, 2018; Terashvili and Bosnjak, 2019), genes (Oggu et al., 2017), exosomes (Davidson and Yellon, 2018), and growth factors (Crafts et al., 2015; Reboucas et al., 2016) are emerging and have shown significant research outcomes, numerous challenges still exist in translating those technologies into clinical practice (Egwim et al., 2017).

Nanoparticles have a long history. Faraday (1857) reported the synthesis of a colloidal Au NP solution for the first time. Similarly, Richard Feynman gave a talk in 1959 describing molecular machines built with atomic precision (Feynman, 1960). These were considered the very first reports on nanotechnology. Metal nanoparticles play a major role in the field of nanoparticle research (Jeevanandam et al., 2018). The 1950s and the 1960s saw the world turning its focus toward the use of nanoparticles in the field of drug delivery. Biological approaches for molecular nanotechnology were the first scientific conference held on the topic in the year 1996 (San Diego, CA, United States). Biological systems are organized at nanoscale dimensions and synthetic nanomaterials correlated in size with biological structures such as proteins, glycolipids, and DNA (Singh et al., 2011). Nanoparticles (NPs) are a type of nano-sized vesicles and can act as a sustained release delivery system of therapeutic agents and provide enhanced myocardial recovery in ischemic heart diseases (Binsalamah et al., 2011; Oduk et al., 2018). Nanoparticles can be classified either as organic (**Figures 1A,B**), inorganic (**Figures 1C–G**), or hybrid. Organic NPs usually show good biocompatibility, whereas inorganic NPs provide advantages in tailoring varied functions and properties (Vinhas et al., 2017). Organic nanoparticles are fabricated from proteins, carbohydrates, lipids, and other organic compounds to a characteristic dimension, such as a radius around 100 nm (Pan and Zhong, 2016), and are widely used NPs in cardiac therapy (**Table 1**). Inorganic NPs include carbon-based NPs, such as carbon nanotubes, buckyballs, and graphene, with remarkable features, strength and unique electrical properties (conducting, semiconducting, or insulating) (Vinhas et al., 2017). Besides, these inorganic NPs also include metal NPs, made of gold, silver, and iron oxide (Vinhas et al., 2017). **Table 2** lists recent studies that used inorganic NPs for cardiac therapy. In the organic-inorganic hybrid nanoparticles, the organic functional groups combine the unique properties of the inorganic counterparts to confer efficient utility for various *in vivo* biomedical and clinical applications (Haque and Chowdhury, 2018). The use of hybrid nanoparticles for the slow release of drugs has been gaining great interest, particularly, to improve the selectivity and efficacy of the drugs by combining features of both organic and inorganic components in one nanoparticle system (**Table 3**).

Here, we review the studies done over the last 10 years that investigated the applications of different NP types for repairing cardiac tissue after myocardial infarction and also summarize treatment efficacies of different NP types. Furthermore, some of the advances, challenges, and future strategies in this field are also provided.

ORGANIC NANOPARTICLES

Lipid-Based NPs

Typical lipid-based NP formulations (**Figure 1A**) include solid-lipid nanoparticles, nanostructured lipid carriers, lipid-drug conjugates, and nanoemulsions; all are primarily comprised of physiological lipid analogs with surfactants as stabilizers (Qi J. et al., 2017). According to the size of lipid-based nanoparticles, they are named as micelles (~15 nm), liposomes (~100 nm) or polymeric NPs (Paulis et al., 2012; Vinhas et al., 2017). Micelles consist of lipids and other amphiphilic artificial molecules that self-assemble in aqueous solution and form a monolayer with the hydrophobic phase inside that incorporates hydrophobic therapeutic agents (Katsuki et al., 2017). The enclosed space in the micelle is more confined than that in liposomes (Katsuki et al., 2017). Liposomes are heavily investigated in nanomedicine and are the first to get FDA approval for nanomedicine (Katsuki et al., 2017; Vinhas et al., 2017). Liposomes mainly consist of phospholipids that form bilayers with the aqueous phase inside, conferring superior biocompatibility to the liposomes (Katsuki et al., 2017). Polymeric nanoparticles, such as polylactic acid (PLA), polyglycolic acid (PGA), and poly lactic-co-glycolic acid (PLGA) are FDA-approved polymers. PLGA is a copolymer of PLA and PGA and is being tested for drug delivery systems for intractable diseases, including cardiovascular diseases (Pascual-Gil et al., 2017; Oduk et al., 2018).

Lipid NPs are broadly considered as promising candidates for the delivery of therapeutics in the infarcted heart. They possess morphology similar to that of cell membranes and can incorporate both lipophilic and hydrophilic substances (Saludas et al., 2018). They have successfully demonstrated the ability to deliver several biomaterials in the target tissue, such as low molecular weight drugs, imaging agents, peptides, proteins, and nucleic acids (Cheraghi et al., 2017). Paulis et al. (2012) reported that micelles are promising vehicles for the delivery of cardioprotective drugs, needed for the acute stage of MI, and also for the delivery of drugs that regulate infarct healing during the chronic stage of MI. On the other hand, liposomes are more suited for the delivery of pro-angiogenic drugs to the infarct microvasculature (Paulis et al., 2012).

Dendrimers

Dendrimers (**Figure 1B**) are the smallest of all the nanocarriers and they have their multiple end groups that are appropriate for a high degree of link targeting or the active agents (Morgan et al., 2005). Dendrimers are dendritically expanded macromolecules with monodisperse structure consisting of a central core, branching interior and exterior functional groups (Morgan et al., 2005). Dendrimers possess the advantage of enhancing the binding capacity upon modification of their exterior surface with some ligands or antibodies for active targeting (Thomas et al., 2013); also, they can carry drugs with poor solubility (Singh et al., 2016). Xue et al. (2018) reported that cardiomyocyte apoptosis and infraction size were significantly reduced following single intravenous administration of dendrimer (15 μg), loaded with microRNA-1 inhibitor, in the acute mice MI model.

Selective studies using organic nanoparticles for the delivery of therapeutics to repair infarcted myocardial tissue were listed as **Table 1**. Paulis et al. (2012) reported that micelles are promising vehicles for the delivery of cardioprotective drugs, needed for the acute stage of MI, and also for the delivery of drugs that regulate infarct healing during the chronic stage of MI. On the other hand, liposomes are more suited for the delivery of pro-angiogenic drugs to the infarct microvasculature. However, to achieve cardiac protection after myocardial infarction, some therapeutic cargoes were required. So far, a large number of agents were loaded into nanoparticles targeted for different purposes. Recent studies have demonstrated that encapsulating ROS, Puerarin or Baicalin into micelles or lipids to reduce infarct size of the animals' ischemic heart (Zhang et al., 2016; Dong et al., 2017; Vong et al., 2018). For cardiomyocyte apoptosis prevention, IGF1, liraglutide, Nitroxyl radical, Cyclosporine A, Pitavastatin or 2,2,6,6-tetramethyl piperidine-1-oxyl was embarked on lipid-based NPs and sent to the animals' ischemic heart (Chang et al., 2013; Yin et al., 2014; Asanuma et al., 2017; Mao et al., 2017; Qi Q. et al., 2017). Intravenous injection of collapsin response mediator protein-2 (CRMP2) lipid with the size of 50 nm was shown fibrosis reducing in the mice chronic MI heart (Zhou et al., 2015). For vasculogenesis enhancement, VEGF, FGF1, Ang-1, stromal cell-derived factor-1 (SDF-1) or CCR2 was loaded in

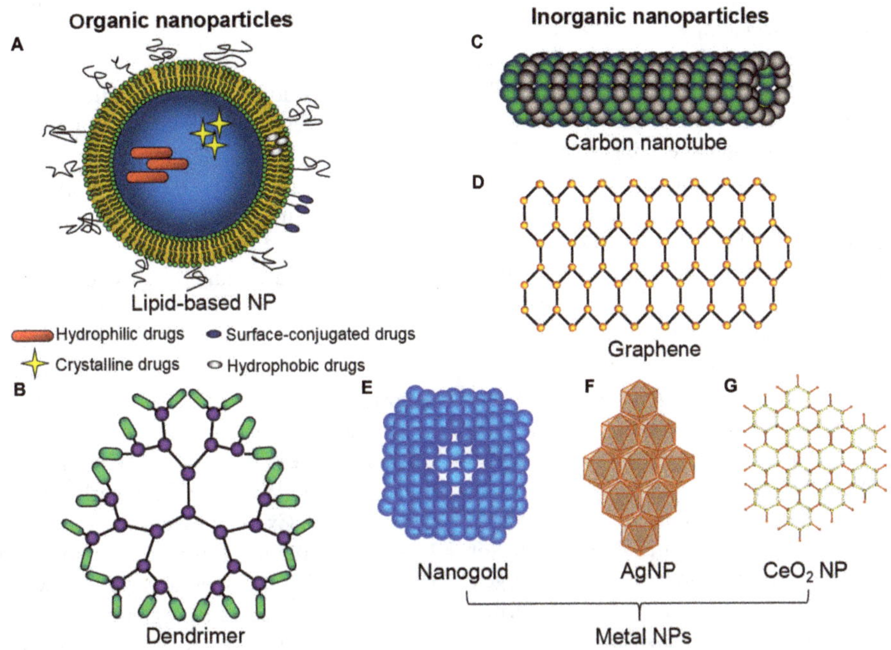

FIGURE 1 | Types of nanoparticles commonly used in cardiac therapeutic studies. A wide variety of NPs: organic **(A,B)**, inorganic **(C–G)** and hybrid NPs are commonly used. Organic nanoparticles (NPs) are fabricated from proteins, carbohydrates, lipids **(A)**, and other organic compounds **(B)**, to a characteristic dimension. Inorganic NPs include carbon-based NPs e.g., carbon nanotubes **(C)**, graphene **(D)** and metal NPs e.g., gold **(E)**, silver **(F)**, and iron oxide **(G)**.

NPs and delivered to the ischemic myocardial tissue to stimulate angiogenesis (Paul et al., 2011; Lu et al., 2015; Oduk et al., 2018; Ding et al., 2020; Fan et al., 2020). Interestingly, Wang et al. (2018) recently reported that no statistically significant improvements in cardiac function and infarct size were detected in mice acute MI heart with the intravenous administration of CCR2 targeting-nanoparticles (micelles) vs. non-targeted micelles. Recently, nanoparticle delivery through intravenous injection with targeting peptides has merged has a promising strategy. Xue et al. (2018) reported an early targeting therapy for myocardial infarcted mouse through the tail vein with anti-miR-1 antisense oligonucleotide (AMO-1) loaded and myocardium-targeting dendrimer: PEGylated dendrigraft poly-L-lysine with angiotensin II type 1 receptor (AT1-PEG-DGL AMO-1). They found that AT1-PEG-DGL quickly accumulated in the MI heart during the desired early period, significantly outperforming the group without AT1 targeting. Apoptotic cell death in the infarct border zone was significantly decreased and the myocardial infarct size was reduced by 64.1% with a single IV injection as compared with that in MI group (Xue et al., 2018).

INORGANIC NANOPARTICLES

Carbon-Based Nanoparticles

Carbon Nanotubes

Carbon nanotubes (CNT) (**Figure 1C**) are a subfamily of fullerenes and are composed of graphite sheets that are rolled up into tubular forms (Katsuki et al., 2017). As nano-carriers, they incorporate drugs in their inner space and present chemically modified external surfaces with biological molecules, such as nucleotides and proteins, to provide selective targeting (Katsuki et al., 2017). Based on their number of layers, carbon nanotubes are categorized as either single-walled or multi-walled (Sajid et al., 2016). The poor solubility of drugs, faster deactivation, and limited bioavailability can be addressed by using these carbon nanotubes which are preferentially used as drug carriers (Raphey et al., 2019). However, one of the major disadvantages of the CNT is the chance for their dissociation in biological fluids (Raphey et al., 2019). Nevertheless, carbon nanotube is a well-suited drug carrier for enhanced penetration in the cells and also for offering privileged drug actions (Zhang et al., 2011). Their unique optical, electrical, and mechanical properties make them a suitable candidate for potential therapeutic applications (Gorain et al., 2018). Moreover, a couple of studies have validated the promising potentials of CNT in cardiac tissue engineering, such as in the support of cardiomyocyte function and growth (Ahadian et al., 2017; Sun et al., 2017a) and acceleration of the gap junction formation (Martinelli et al., 2013; Shin et al., 2013). Aside these studies, other investigations have suggested that scaffold consisting of col-hydrogel and CNT could be promising injectable biomaterial to deliver drugs and cells for cardiac tissue regeneration in the infarcted myocardial tissues (Sun et al., 2017b; Gorain et al., 2018).

Graphene

The nanotechnology field is in constant research of novel materials that can be engineered for the precise, sensitive, and selective detection of biomarkers (Tang et al., 2020). Recently, the graphene-based family of materials has shown huge potential as their proposed biosensing applications have shown great diversity (Stankovich et al., 2006; Geim and Novoselov, 2007; Bitounis et al., 2013). The isolated two dimensional (2D) crystal structures composed of single atomic layers of graphite are called "graphene" (**Figure 1D**; Bitounis et al., 2013). In Novoselov et al. (2004) isolated and characterized a single sheet of graphene. Since then, research on graphene has been highly increasing and has attracted a deep interest in scientific fields (Bitounis et al., 2013; Paul et al., 2014). Feng et al. (2011) pioneered the successful use of graphene as a non-toxic nano-vehicle for efficient gene transfection. With all atoms exposed on its surface, graphene has an ultra-high surface area available for efficient loading of aromatic drug molecules via π-π stacking, providing a plethora of applications in drug delivery via stable complex formation and avoiding chemical conjugation (Sun et al., 2008; Zhang et al., 2010). Paul et al. (2014) reported that methacrylated gelatin hydrogel (GelMA) impregnated with functionalized graphene oxide (fGO) nanosheets, where the latter were complexed with pro-angiogenic human vascular endothelial growth factor plasmid DNA (pDNAVEGF), formed nanocomposite hydrogels (fGOVEGF/GelMA) that efficiently transfect the myocardial tissues and induce favorable therapeutic effects without invoking adverse cytotoxic effects. Nevertheless, adverse reactions induced by graphene-based materials on exposure will depend on multiple factors that need to be scrutinized (Bitounis et al., 2013). Therefore, clinical translation of graphene-based materials is still in its infancy, yet the field holds tremendous potential for the treatment of multiple diseases (Bitounis et al., 2013).

Metal Nanoparticles

Nanogold, also called gold nanoparticles (GNPs) or colloidal gold (**Figure 1E**), has been actively investigated in a wide variety of biomedical applications (Zhou Y. et al., 2018). The unique physical and chemical properties, such as ease of bio-conjugation, excellent stability, superior security, and strong biocompatibility of many GNPs make them promising candidates in nanomedicine (Sperling et al., 2008).

Silver nanoparticles (AgNPs) (**Figure 1F**) have been developed as potent anti-microbial agents and have a multitude of applications, such as in toothpastes, bedding, water purification, and nursing bottles (Priyadarsini et al., 2018). After oral exposure, it is shown that about 18% of silver could be absorbed in humans (Bostan et al., 2016). Animal studies showed that AgNPs exposure will cause enhanced superoxide anion production and cause deleterious effects in cardiac tissues (Ebabe Elle et al., 2013; Lin et al., 2017; Xu et al., 2018). Thus, toxicity concerns of AgNPs have limited their effective translation for the cardiac tissue repair.

Cerium oxide (CeO_2) nanoparticles (**Figure 1G**) have wide applications, such as in oxygen sensors and automotive catalytic converters (Niu et al., 2011). These nanoparticles are considered potent remedial options for the treatment of smoking-related diseases (El Shaer et al., 2017) since intravenous injection of these nanoparticles have shown a marked reduction in the myocardial oxidative stress and have also shown a significant reduction of the left ventricular dysfunction in the murine models of heart failure (Niu et al., 2011). The well-known mechanism underlying the action of these nanoparticles is attributed to their dual oxidation state, where the loss of oxygen and the reduction of Ce^{4+} to Ce^{3+} are accompanied by the creation of an oxygen vacancy (Niu et al., 2007).

Selective studies using inorganic nanoparticles for the delivery of therapeutics to repair infarcted myocardial tissue were listed as **Table 2**. Unlike the organic nanoparticles, the inorganic nanomaterials alone (without therapeutic agents loaded) could provide mechanical support even enhance cell electrical signaling in some conducting nanomaterials (Zhou J. et al., 2018). Zhou et al., created a conductive hydrogel by introducing graphene oxide (GO) nanoparticles into oligo(poly(ethylene glycol) fumarate) (OPF) hydrogels and delivered to the Sprague Dawley rats' acute MI heart by peri-infarct intramyocardial injection. They found that injected OPF/GO hydrogels can not only provide mechanical support but also electric connection between normal cardiomyocytes and the myocardium in the scar via activating the canonical Wnt signaling pathway, thus upregulating the generation of Cx43 and gap junction-associated proteins (Zhou J. et al., 2018). However, inorganic nanoparticles loaded with potential therapeutic agents have been widely studied. Similar to the studies of organic nanoparticles, scholars mainly aim at oxidative stress-reducing, inflammation attenuation, cardiomyocyte apoptosis prevention, fibrosis reducing and vasculogenesis enhancement (Han et al., 2018; Sharma et al., 2018). Copper has shown the anti-inflammatory, anti-oxidant potential and cardioprotective effect. Sharma et al. treated treat the I/R rat with low dose copper nanoparticles (CuNP) (1 mg/kg/day, p.o., 4 weeks) and myocardial protection was detected like the reduction of oxidative stress, inflammatory cytokines and apoptosis through phosphorylate GSK-3β kinase pathways (Sharma et al., 2018). Gold nanoparticles (AuNPs) delivered intravenously (400 μg/kg/day, 14 consecutive days) may also improve myocardial injury after myocardial infarction in rats with the decrease of eNOs immunoreaction, Bcl-2 and collagen fibers (Ahmed et al., 2017). However, in another mouse acute MI model, AuNPs intravenous administration (100 μl/day, 7 days) accumulated in infarcted hearts, decreased infarction size, inhibited cardiac fibrosis but has no effect on apoptosis and hypertrophy (Tian et al., 2018). Inflammation attenuation was shown in mouse MI models intramyocardial injection of 50 μl interleukin-4 plasmid DNA-functionalized macrophage-targeting graphene oxide complex (MGC/IL-4 pDNA) via a reduction in intracellular ROS and developing M2 macrophage phenotypes in macrophages (Han et al., 2018). Similar to the organic nanoparticles, intramyocardial injection of a nano-complex of graphene oxide loaded with vascular endothelial growth factor-165 (VEGF) gene in the rat acute MI model shows significant infarct size reduction and capillary density enhancement (Paul et al., 2014). Further studies are needed to elucidate the long-term biocompatibility and safety of these inorganic nanoparticles.

ORGANIC-INORGANIC HYBRID NANOPARTICLES

Recently, interests in the applications of various organic-inorganic hybrid nanoparticles (NPs) have risen tremendously.

TABLE 1 | List of selective studies using organic nanoparticles for the delivery of therapeutics to repair infarcted myocardial tissue.

Nanoparticles/ size (nm)	Therapeutic agents	MI Model	Dose/administration route	Results	References
Micelle/14.9 Liposome/101.5	None	Mouse, acute and chronic	50 μmol Gd/kg, intravenous	Micelles permeated the entire infarct area, Liposomes showed slower and restricted extravasation from the vasculature	Paulis et al., 2012
Micelles/ 90–100	ROS	Mouse, acute	3 mg, intramyocardial	Reduced infarct size and improved heart functions	Vong et al., 2018
PEG-PLGA/350	Liraglutide	Rat, chronic	380 μg, intramyocardial	Reduced infarct size, preserved wall thickness, stimulated angiogenesis, prevented cardiomyocyte apoptosis and improved heart functions	Qi Q. et al., 2017
PLGA/113	VEGF	Mouse, chronic	0.06, 2.6 or 0.6 pg, intramyocardial	Improved heart function, increased wall thickness, reduced infarct size and vasculogenesis	Oduk et al., 2018
PLGA/75	IGF1	Mouse, chronic	20 ng, intramyocardial	Prevented cardiomyocyte apoptosis, reduced infarct size, improved LV function and cardiac geometry	Chang et al., 2013
PK3/500	Nox2-siRNA	Mouse, chronic	5 ug/kg, intramyocardial	Improved fractional shortening	Somasuntharam et al., 2013
PK3/500	Nox2-miRNA	Mouse, chronic	5 ug/kg, intramyocardial	Improved fractional shortening and ejection fraction, reduced infarct size	Yang et al., 2017
Micelles/40	Nitroxyl radical	Dog, I/R	3 mg/kg, intravenous	Reduced infarct size and myocardial apoptosis	Asanuma et al., 2017
Micelles/ 34.7±14	CCR2	Mouse, acute	33 mg/kg, intravenous	No statistically significant improvements in cardiac function and infarct size	Wang et al., 2018
Silicon/ 100–200	siRNA, CCR2, MSCs	Mouse, chronic	25 mg/kg 1×10^5 cells, intravenous	Improved LV remodeling amelioration and vascular density	Lu et al., 2015
Lipid/ 50	siRNA CRMP2	Mouse, chronic	70 μg/kg, intravenous	Reduced post-MI heart failure, mortality and fibrosis	Zhou J. et al., 2018
Lipid/ <160	Cyclosporine A, ADSCs	Pig, chronic	2 mg/kg 4×10^7 cells, intravenous	Improved heart function, reduced infarct size and cardiomyocyte apoptosis	Yin et al., 2014
Silicon/ 180	ERK1/2 inhibitor	Rat, acute	33 μg, intravenous	Reduced hypertrophy	Ferreira et al., 2017
PLGA/ 100	Cyclosporine A	Mouse, I/R	1 mg/kg, intravenous	Improved LV remodeling	Ikeda et al., 2016
PLGA/ 200	Irbesartan	Mouse, I/R	3 mg/kg, intravenous	Reduced infarct size and LV remodeling	Nakano et al., 2016
PLGA/ 160	Pitavastatin	Rat, I/R	1 mg/kg, intravenous	Reduced cardiomyocyte apoptosis	Mao et al., 2017
PLGA/ 160	Pitavastatin	Mouse, I/R	1 mg/kg, intravenous	Improved LV remodeling	Nagaoka et al., 2015
PLGA/ 160	Pitavastatin	Pig, I/R	8–32 mg/kg, intravenous	Improved LV remodeling, reduced infarct size and cardiomyocyte apoptosis	Ichimura et al., 2016
PEI/ 45	siRNA Icam1, Icam1, Vcam1, Sele and Selp	Mouse, chronic	1 mg/kg, intravenous	Reduced matrix-degrading protease activity	Sager et al., 2016
Lipid/110	Puerarin	Rat, chronic	50 mg/kg, intravenous	Reduced infarct size and oxidative stress	Dong et al., 2017
Lipid/84	Baicalin	Rat, chronic	10 mg/kg, intravenous	Reduced infarct size and oxidative stress	Zhang et al., 2016
Lipid/130	Schisandrin B	Rat, chronic	10 mg/kg, intravenous	Reduced infarct size	Shao et al., 2017
Lipid/ <1000	Hemin	Mouse, chronic	2 mg/kg, intravenous	Improved infarct healing and repair	Ben-Mordechai et al., 2017
Lipid/105	Flavonoid	Rat, I/R	0.29 drug/lipid ratio, intravenous	Reduced infarct size	Tan et al., 2017
PEG-poly oxymethyl estyrene/40	2,2,6,6-tetramethyl piperidine-1-oxyl	Dog, I/R	3 mg/kg, intravenous	Reduced infarct size, apoptosis and ventricular fibrillation	Asanuma et al., 2017
Micellar/-	Rapamycin	Diabetic mouse, I/R	0.75 mg/kg/day, p.o. 10 weeks before I/R	Improved cardiac functions; reduced infarct size	Samidurai et al., 2017
Dendrimer/50	microRNA-1 inhibitor	Mouse, acute	15 μg, intravenous	Reduced cardiomyocyte apoptosis and infarct size	Xue et al., 2018

TABLE 2 | List of selective studies using inorganic nanoparticles for the delivery of therapeutics to repair infarcted myocardial tissue.

Nanoparticles/ size (nm)	Therapeutic agents	MI Model	Dose/administration route	Results	References
Graphene/30–40	VEGF	Rat, acute	300 μL, intramyocardial	Reduced infarct size, improved capillary density and cardiac performance	Paul et al., 2014
OPF/graphene oxide hydrogel	-	Rat, acute	100 μL, intramyocardial	Improved load-dependent ejection fraction/fractional shortening of heart function	Zhou J. et al., 2018
Graphene oxide complex/150	IL-4 pDNA	Mouse, acute	50 μL, intramyocardial	Attenuated inflammation, mitigated fibrosis and improved heart function	Han et al., 2018
Graphene oxide	Mesenchymal stem cell	Rat, I/R	One million MSCs	Improved the engraftment and therapeutic efficacy of MSCs, which promoted cardiac tissue repair and cardiac function	Park et al., 2015
Gold/10	PEG coated	Mouse, acute	100 μl/day, intravenous, 7 days	Decreased infarct size, improved systolic functions, inhibited cardiac fibrosis, no effect on apoptosis and hypertrophy	Tian et al., 2018
Copper/90–150	Cu	Rat, I/R	1 mg/kg/day, p.o.	Diminished oxidative stress, inflammatory cytokines and apoptosis, reduced infarct size	Sharma et al., 2018
Gold/50	Au	Rat, acute	(400 μg/kg/day) intravenous, 14 days	Improved myocardial injury	Ahmed et al., 2017
Cerium oxide/4–6	Ceria	Isoproterenol induced MI rat	(0.5 and 5 mg/kg/week), Intraperitonial, 5 weeks	Provided prophylactic effect against cardiac toxicity	El Shaer et al., 2017
Graphene oxide gold nanosheets (GO-Au)	chitosan-GO-Au scaffold	Rat, acute	5×2 mm scaffold	Improved the cardiac contractility and restored ventricular functions	Saravanan et al., 2018

TABLE 3 | List of selective studies using organic-inorganic nanoparticles for the delivery of therapeutics for the repair of myocardial infracted heart tissue.

Nanoparticles/ size (nm)	Therapeutic agents	MI Model	Dose/administration route	Results	References
DNAzyme-conjugated AuNPs/ 14± 3	Silence TNF-α	Rat, acute	100 μL, intramyocardial	Significant anti-inflammatory benefits and improved cardiac function	Somasuntharam et al., 2016
Organic-inorganic hybrid hollow mesoporous organosilica nanoparticles (HMONs)/20	Hepatocyte growth factor (HGF) gene-transfected BMMSCs	Rat, acute	2×10^6 HGF gene-transfected BMMSCs, intramyocardial	Decreased apoptotic cardiomyocytes, reduced infarct scar size, relieved interstitial fibrosis, increased angiogenesis, and improved cardiac functions	Zhu et al., 2016
Complex of recombinant baculovirus and Tat/DNA nanoparticles /500	Angiopoietin-1 gene	Rat, acute	300 μL, intramyocardial	Increased capillary density, reduced infarct size and improved cardiac functions	Paul et al., 2011

Hybrid NPs combine features of organic and inorganic building blocks and generate NPs with improved physicochemical properties, such as particle size and surface charge (Haque and Chowdhury, 2018). Hybrid organic-inorganic NPs hold great promise in overcoming the pitfalls being faced by existing inorganic materials in the delivery of therapeutics and contrast agents (Somasuntharam et al., 2016), such as unwanted interactions with serum proteins (particularly opsonins) and consequential removal from the circulation by macrophages of mononuclear phagocytic system, rapid renal clearance, prolonged body accumulation, and lack of targetability (Zhou and Zhang, 2019).

Magnetoliposomes (MLs) are composed of liposomes and magnetic NPs and are the first efficient hybrid liposome/NP systems produced for the drug delivery (Namdari et al., 2017). In this line, several experimental strategies have been investigated the potential scope of magnetic NPs to leverage the delivery of growth factors, cytokines, and biomolecules to the degenerating cardiac cells and tissues and enhance their regeneration (Allen and Cullis, 2013; Paul et al., 2014; Ottersbach et al., 2018).

Selective studies using organic-inorganic nanoparticles for the delivery of therapeutics to repair infarcted myocardial tissue were listed as **Table 3**. Somasuntharam et al. (2016) created deoxyribozyme (DNAzyme) functionalized AuNPs to catalytically silence tumor necrosis factor-α (TNF-α) as a potential therapeutic for acute myocardial infarction. After the intramyocardial injection, with the silencing of TNF-α, significant anti-inflammatory benefits, and cardiac function improvement were detected in the rat heart. With the same model, (Paul et al., 2011) design a new gene delivery method utilizing a self-assembled binary complex of negatively charged baculovirus (Bac) and positively charged endosomolytic histidine-rich Tat peptide/DNA nanoparticles (NP) together with Angiopoietin-1 (Ang-1) gene carried by. 3 weeks post intramyocardially delivery, cardiac function improvement, capillary density enhancement, and infarct sizes reduction were detected in Bac-NP(Ang1) compared to Bac(Ang1), NP(Ang1) and control groups due to enhanced myocardial Ang-1 expression at peri-infarct regions. Furthermore, (Zhu et al., 2016) designed and synthesized molecularly organic-inorganic hybrid hollow mesoporous organosilica nanoparticles (HMONs) for gene transfection (hepatocyte growth factor, HGF) in BMMSCs and subsequent *in vivo* cardiac repair. The fabricated organic-inorganic hybrid HMONs with large pore size represent a generalizable strategy to promote the ischemic myocardium therapeutic potential of HGF transfected BMMSCs including reduction of apoptotic cardiomyocytes, infarct scar size, and interstitial fibrosis while increasing angiogenesis (Zhu et al., 2016).

ARTIFICIAL DNA NANOSTRUCTURES

The success of DNA nanotechnology lies in the artificially constructed special nanostructure design systems for DNA computing (Lee et al., 2016). DNA nanostructures, owing to their precise control over chemistry, size, and shape, provide vast opportunity to unfold the convoluted mass of information relating to nanoparticle-biological interactions (Lee et al., 2016). Drug delivery and therapeutics is considered as one of the most promising applications of the structural DNA nanotechnology (Ke et al., 2018). In this line, artificial nucleic acid nano-devices could be utilized to provide targeted drug delivery in the tissues upon sensing their environment (Singh et al., 2016). Moreover, several studies have proposed various DNA nanostructures and strategies to load, deliver, and release biomolecular drugs for cardiac therapy (Paul et al., 2011).

COMPARISON OF THE NANOPARTICLES AS FOR ISCHEMIC MYOCARDIUM REPAIR

Nanoparticles of different types (for example, inorganic, organic and hybrid) designed to target ischemic cardiac cells are promising candidates for the treatment of myocardial infarction. Organic nanoparticles are offering numerous advantages which embrace the simplicity of their preparation from well-understood biodegradable, biocompatible polymers, and their high stability in biological fluids during storage (Virlan et al., 2016). Since the emergence of nanotechnology in the past decades, polymeric materials such as poly (d-lactic acid), polyethylene glycol (PEG) and poly lacticco-glycolic acid (PLGA) have emerged as a major class of biodegradable and controlled release systems for delivering biomolecules/proteins to the plaque site (Fredman et al., 2015; Kamaly et al., 2016).

The use of inorganic nanoparticles for applications in drug delivery presents a wide array of advantages, which include: (1) Ease of functionality with a range of surface and conjugation chemistries; (2) High payload loadings; (3) Tunable degradation rates; and (4) Enhanced penetration into tissue (Pandey and Dahiya, 2016). Magnetic nanoparticles were shown to accelerate the expression of critical gap junction proteins (for example, connexin 43) in cardiomyoblasts. These new cells demonstrated higher levels of both engraftment capacity and desirable paracrine factors compared with conventional therapeutic cells, thus significantly enhanced heart function and reduced scar size when delivered into the peri-infarcted area in rats (Han et al., 2015). Superparamagnetic iron oxide nanoparticles, with biocompatibility and capacity for simultaneous imaging and targeting, have emerged as the major particles for enhancing the engraftment of therapeutic cells in heart tissue. However, it was recently revealed that these nanoparticles increase tumor-associated macrophage activation (Zanganeh et al., 2016).

Intensive studies have thoroughly probed the toxicities of a wide range of nanoparticles (organic, inorganic, and polymeric) in different types of cells and organs. However, the cardiotoxicity of nanoparticles has been poorly investigated, and data are still limited to a few types of nanoparticle including metal oxides, silver, and carbon (Bostan et al., 2016). The main limiting issue for the design of safe and efficient nanoparticles for the treatment of ischemic heart disease is the lack of a deep understanding of the biological identity of nanoparticles. To accelerate the clinical translation of nanoparticles for use in cardiac nanotechnology,

TABLE 4 | Advantages and disadvantages of different nanoparticles for the delivery of therapeutics to repair infarcted myocardial tissue.

Type	Advantages	Disadvantages	References
Lipid-based NPs	Increased penetration and/or permeation, Biocompatible and biodegradable nature, Easy and scalable production process, Increased drug solubility, Possibility of specific follicular targeting, Good stability during storage period.	Loss of high amounts of drug, Lack of robust controlled drug release, Burst drug release may induce toxic effects, Macrophage drug clearance (rapid clearance).	Ghasemiyeh and Mohammadi-Samani, 2018
Dendrimers	Ease of fabrication, targeting ability, potential for repeat administration, low immune response and precise controllability of the functionality.	Great batch-to-batch variability and deterioration, the attachment of multiple molecules can often result in a population of conjugates with a wide distribution of the number of ligands.	Pearson et al., 2012
Carbon Nanotubes	Extremely small and lightweight, Resources required are plentiful, Resistant to temperature changes, Highly flexible and elastic, and Improve conductive mechanical properties.	Still don't understand how they work, Difficult to work with, Toxic qualities, Lack of solubility in most solvents, Susceptibility to oxidative environments, Difficulty in maintaining high quality and minimal impurities.	Pitroda et al., 2016
Metal Nanoparticles	Strong plasma absorption, Biological system imaging, Determine chemical information on metallic nanoscale substrate.	Instability, impurity, explosion and safety concerns (Toxicity),	Harish et al., 2018

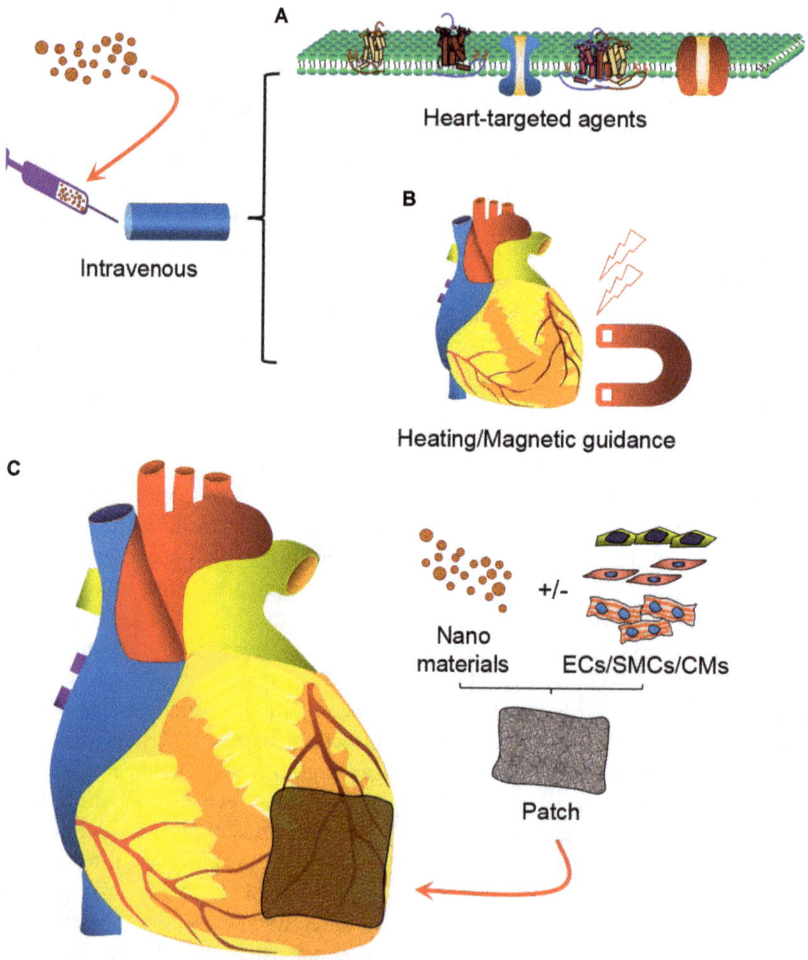

FIGURE 2 | Nanoparticle-based therapy for cardiovascular diseases. Therapeutic strategies may involve intravenous delivery of drug-loaded nanomaterials, modified with cardiac tissue-targeting moieties **(A)** or guided with non-invasive heating or magnetic field **(B)**. Furthermore, cardiac patch may be applied locally in the infarct region to provide simultaneous delivery of the nanoparticles and induced pluripotent stem cell-derived cardiovascular cells (cardiomyocytes, endothelial cells, and smooth muscle cells) **(C)** to provide robust myocardial tissue regeneration and functional improvements.

their biological identities must be precisely assessed and reported (Mahmoudi et al., 2017). The advantage and disadvantage of each NP category were summarized in **Table 4**.

CLINICAL APPLICATION

A large number of patents, pertinent to the invention of cardiovascular biomaterials, have been filed in the past decade. Importantly, an invention of the UV-crosslinkable gelatin methacrylate-based cardiac patch, impregnated with gold nano-rods, was recently patented (US20170143871 A1). The patent describes about patch that exhibits high surface area and electrical conductivity. Another recent invention describes a combination of gold nano-wires and engineered scaffolds for controlling the cellular function through electronic circuits (US20170072109 A1). Furthermore, a new strategy of nanoparticle-stem cell electrostatically conjugates for post-infarction treatment was patented in Japan (JP5495215 B2). A preparation method of nanomagnetic particles for the detection and treatment of coronary heart diseases was patented in China (CN102085380A). This method can be used for preparing magnetic nanoparticles for mid-late-stage treatment of coronary heart diseases; and good repairing and treatment effects on coronary heart diseases can be achieved. In another patent, a solid lipid nanoparticle of Gelan Xinning Ruanjiaonang (Chinese traditional medicine) for treating coronary heart disease was created and beneficial for clinical application (CN103027981B). The treatment effect of Gelan Xinning Ruanjiaonang for coronary heart disease is significantly improved with the solid lipid nanoparticle included. Despite several patented technologies for cardiovascular therapeutics, only a few have entered into the clinical trials, due to the stringent regulatory requirements (Lakshmanan and Maulik, 2018). Fortunately, some of the targeted drug nanocarriers for cardiac therapies successfully passed clinical trials (Galagudza et al., 2010) and are already commercially available (Chong et al., 2014). For instance, one of the clinical strategies that has been practiced since long for inducing angiogenesis in the ischemic tissues includes intramuscular transplantation of the micro-bubbles and causing ultrasound-mediated microbubble destruction for the delivery of entrapped bone marrow-derived mononuclear cells (BM-MNCs) to provide tissue regeneration (Tateishi-Yuyama et al., 2002).

CURRENT STATE-OF-THE-ART NANOTECHNOLOGY USED IN CARDIAC THERAPY AND FUTURE PERSPECTIVES

Despite initial encouraging results from nanotechnology-based cardiac protection, poor retention time, efficacy, side effects or off-target effects of the delivered NPs remain major obstacles for efficient myocardial regeneration (Chang et al., 2013; Somasuntharam et al., 2013; Yin et al., 2014; Zhou et al., 2015). Several delivery strategies like intracoronary, intramyocardial, or intravenous have been applied for cardiac repair. Traditionally, NPs were injected via intracoronary or intramyocardial route and they rely on open heart surgery (Chang et al., 2013; Somasuntharam et al., 2013). Most adverse effects were observed they were delivered either intravenously or orally (Yin et al., 2014; Zhou et al., 2015). So far, no strategy has been proven to replace the transmural scar tissue in the chronic infarcted heart tissues. However, the current state-of-the-art nanoparticle technologies have emerged as one of the most promising strategies for myocardial repair (Awada et al., 2016). With the application of heart targeted agents, efficacy could be highly improved, while lowering the adverse effects by delivering NPs by intravenous route (Nguyen J. et al., 2015; Ferreira et al., 2016). The active targeting agents include MMP-2 and MMP-9 targeting peptides (Nguyen M. M. et al., 2015), which may results in long-term retention at the site of infarction. The atrial natriuretic peptide (ANP) is a circulating cardiac hormone produced physiologically, which belongs to the natriuretic peptide family and has been shown to have cardioprotective properties through cGMP-dependent signaling involving guanylyl cyclase A (GC-A) receptors (Potter et al., 2009). Peptide CSTSMLKAC and CRSWNKADNRSC are cyclic structures and have shown alone selective targeting to the ischemic heart (Kanki et al., 2011; Ferreira et al., 2016). Furthermore, heart homing agents make oral administration or inhalation administration an alternative and promising approach (Miragoli et al., 2018; Sharma et al., 2018).

The majority of the *in vivo* studies have shown the great potential of the nanoparticle systems in improving the function and tissue regeneration of the infarcted myocardium. However, further improvement in the homing and delivery of these nanoparticles and their therapeutic effects, respectively, to the target tissues can be achieved via decoration of these nanoparticle systems using heart-targeting active molecules (**Figure 2A**) or using non-invasive physical cues (**Figure 2B**). Furthermore, future clinical strategy may involve the application of cardiac patch that not only delivers the therapeutic agents, but its scaffolding effect provides optimal mechanical support to the failing heart and also replaces lost cells and tissues with induced pluripotent stem cell-derived cardiovascular cells, such as cardiomyocytes, endothelial cells and smooth muscle cells (**Figure 2C**). Thus, it is expected that advances in drug therapy, nanomedicine, cell-therapy, and material science will provide robust functional improvement and tissue restoration in patients with myocardial infarction in the near future.

AUTHOR CONTRIBUTIONS

CF, JJ, and WZ wrote the manuscript. FL, BX, MK, JY, and WZ, revised the manuscript. All authors approved the submission and publication of the manuscript.

ACKNOWLEDGMENTS

The authors would like to thank Drs. Jianyi Zhang and Gangjian Qin in The University of Alabama at Birmingham for their continued support.

REFERENCES

Ahadian, S., Davenport Huyer, L., Estili, M., Yee, B., Smith, N., Xu, Z., et al. (2017). Moldable elastomeric polyester-carbon nanotube scaffolds for cardiac tissue engineering. *Acta Biomater.* 52, 81–91. doi: 10.1016/j.actbio.2016.12.009

Ahmed, S. M., Abdelrahman, S. A., and Salama, A. E. (2017). Efficacy of gold nanoparticles against isoproterenol induced acute myocardial infarction in adult male albino rats. *Ultrastruct. Pathol.* 41, 168–185. doi: 10.1080/01913123.2017.1281367

Allen, T. M., and Cullis, P. R. (2013). Liposomal drug delivery systems: from concept to clinical applications. *Adv. Drug Deliv. Rev.* 65, 36–48. doi: 10.1016/j.addr.2012.09.037

Asanuma, H., Sanada, S., Yoshitomi, T., Sasaki, H., Takahama, H., Ihara, M., et al. (2017). Novel synthesized radical-containing nanoparticles limit infarct size following ischemia and reperfusion in canine hearts. *Cardiovasc. Drugs Ther.* 31, 501–510. doi: 10.1007/s10557-017-6758-6

Awada, H. K., Hwang, M. P., and Wang, Y. (2016). Towards comprehensive cardiac repair and regeneration after myocardial infarction: aspects to consider and proteins to deliver. *Biomaterials* 82, 94–112. doi: 10.1016/j.biomaterials.2015.12.025

Ben-Mordechai, T., Kain, D., Holbova, R., Landa, N., Levin, L. P., Elron-Gross, I., et al. (2017). Targeting and modulating infarct macrophages with hemin formulated in designed lipid-based particles improves cardiac remodeling and function. *J. Control Release* 257, 21–31. doi: 10.1016/j.jconrel.2017.01.001

Binsalamah, Z. M., Paul, A., Khan, A. A., Prakash, S., and Shum-Tim, D. (2011). Intramyocardial sustained delivery of placental growth factor using nanoparticles as a vehicle for delivery in the rat infarct model. *Int. J. Nanomed.* 6, 2667–2678.

Bitounis, D., Ali-Boucetta, H., Hong, B. H., Min, D. H., and Kostarelos, K. (2013). Prospects and challenges of graphene in biomedical applications. *Adv. Mater.* 25, 2258–2268. doi: 10.1002/adma.201203700

Bostan, H. B., Rezaee, R., Valokala, M. G., Tsarouhas, K., Golokhvast, K., Tsatsakis, A. M., et al. (2016). Cardiotoxicity of nano-particles. *Life Sci.* 165, 91–99. doi: 10.1016/j.lfs.2016.09.017

Chang, M. Y., Yang, Y. J., Chang, C. H., Tang, A. C., Liao, W. Y., Cheng, F. Y., et al. (2013). Functionalized nanoparticles provide early cardioprotection after acute myocardial infarction. *J. Control Release* 170, 287–294. doi: 10.1016/j.jconrel.2013.04.022

Cheraghi, M., Negahdari, B., Daraee, H., and Eatemadi, A. (2017). Heart targeted nanoliposomal/nanoparticles drug delivery: an updated review. *Biomed. Pharmacother.* 86, 316–323. doi: 10.1016/j.biopha.2016.12.009

Chong, J. J., Yang, X., Don, C. W., Minami, E., Liu, Y. W., Weyers, J. J., et al. (2014). Human embryonic-stem-cell-derived cardiomyocytes regenerate non-human primate hearts. *Nature* 510, 273–277.

Crafts, T. D., Jensen, A. R., Blocher-Smith, E. C., and Markel, T. A. (2015). Vascular endothelial growth factor: therapeutic possibilities and challenges for the treatment of ischemia. *Cytokine* 71, 385–393. doi: 10.1016/j.cyto.2014.08.005

Davidson, S. M., and Yellon, D. M. (2018). Exosomes and cardioprotection – a critical analysis. *Mol. Aspects Med.* 60, 104–114. doi: 10.1016/j.mam.2017.11.004

Ding, Y., Zhao, A. S., Liu, T., Wang, Y. N., Gao, Y., Li, J. A., et al. (2020). An injectable nanocomposite hydrogel for potential application of vascularization and tissue repair. *Ann. Biomed. Eng.* 48, 1511–1523. doi: 10.1007/s10439-020-02471-7

Dong, Z., Guo, J., Xing, X., Zhang, X., Du, Y., and Lu, Q. (2017). RGD modified and PEGylated lipid nanoparticles loaded with puerarin: formulation, characterization and protective effects on acute myocardial ischemia model. *Biomed. Pharmacother.* 89, 297–304. doi: 10.1016/j.biopha.2017.02.029

Ebabe Elle, R., Gaillet, S., Vide, J., Romain, C., Lauret, C., Rugani, N., et al. (2013). Dietary exposure to silver nanoparticles in Sprague-Dawley rats: effects on oxidative stress and inflammation. *Food Chem. Toxicol.* 60, 297–301. doi: 10.1016/j.fct.2013.07.071

Egwim, C., Dixon, B., Ambrosy, A. P., and Mentz, R. J. (2017). Global variations in patient populations and outcomes in heart failure clinical trials. *Curr. Heart Fail Rep.* 14, 30–39. doi: 10.1007/s11897-017-0316-1

El Shaer, S. S., Salaheldin, T. A., Saied, N. M., and Abdelazim, S. M. (2017). In vivo ameliorative effect of cerium oxide nanoparticles in isoproterenol-induced cardiac toxicity. *Exp. Toxicol. Pathol.* 69, 435–441. doi: 10.1016/j.etp.2017.03.001

Fan, C., Tang, Y., Zhao, M., Lou, X., Pretorius, D., Menasche, P., et al. (2020). CHIR99021 and fibroblast growth factor 1 enhance the regenerative potency of human cardiac muscle patch after myocardial infarction in mice. *J. Mol. Cell Cardiol.* 141, 1–10. doi: 10.1016/j.yjmcc.2020.03.003

Faraday, M. (1857). The bakerian lecture: experimental relations of gold (and other metals) to light. *Philos. Trans. R. Soc. Lond.* 147, 145–181. doi: 10.1098/rstl.1857.0011

Feng, L., Zhang, S., and Liu, Z. (2011). Graphene based gene transfection. *Nanoscale* 3, 1252–1257.

Ferreira, M. P., Ranjan, S., Correia, A. M., Makila, E. M., Kinnunen, S. M., Zhang, H., et al. (2016). In vitro and in vivo assessment of heart-homing porous silicon nanoparticles. *Biomaterials* 94, 93–104. doi: 10.1016/j.biomaterials.2016.03.046

Ferreira, M. P. A., Ranjan, S., Kinnunen, S., Correia, A., Talman, V., Makila, E., et al. (2017). Drug-loaded multifunctional nanoparticles targeted to the endocardial layer of the injured heart modulate hypertrophic signaling. *Small* 13:1701276. doi: 10.1002/smll.201701276

Feynman, R. (1960). There's plenty of room at the bottom. *Caltech Eng. Sci.* 23, 22–36.

Fredman, G., Kamaly, N., Spolitu, S., Milton, J., Ghorpade, D., Chiasson, R., et al. (2015). Targeted nanoparticles containing the proresolving peptide Ac2-26 protect against advanced atherosclerosis in hypercholesterolemic mice. *Sci. Transl. Med.* 7:275ra220.

Galagudza, M. M., Korolev, D. V., Sonin, D. L., Postnov, V. N., Papayan, G. V., Uskov, I. S., et al. (2010). Targeted drug delivery into reversibly injured myocardium with silica nanoparticles: surface functionalization, natural biodistribution, and acute toxicity. *Int. J. Nanomed.* 5, 231–237.

Gao, L. R., Pei, X. T., Ding, Q. A., Chen, Y., Zhang, N. K., Chen, H. Y., et al. (2013). A critical challenge: dosage-related efficacy and acute complication intracoronary injection of autologous bone marrow mesenchymal stem cells in acute myocardial infarction. *Int. J. Cardiol.* 168, 3191–3199. doi: 10.1016/j.ijcard.2013.04.112

Geim, A. K., and Novoselov, K. S. (2007). The rise of graphene. *Nat. Mater.* 6, 183–191. doi: 10.1038/nmat1849

Ghasemiyeh, P., and Mohammadi-Samani, S. (2018). Solid lipid nanoparticles and nanostructured lipid carriers as novel drug delivery systems: applications, advantages and disadvantages. *Res. Pharm. Sci.* 13, 288–303.

Gorain, B., Choudhury, H., Pandey, M., Kesharwani, P., Abeer, M. M., Tekade, R. K., et al. (2018). Carbon nanotube scaffolds as emerging nanoplatform for myocardial tissue regeneration: a review of recent developments and therapeutic implications. *Biomed. Pharmacother.* 104, 496–508. doi: 10.1016/j.biopha.2018.05.066

Han, J., Kim, B., Shin, J. Y., Ryu, S., Noh, M., Woo, J., et al. (2015). Iron oxide nanoparticle-mediated development of cellular gap junction crosstalk to improve mesenchymal stem cells' therapeutic efficacy for myocardial infarction. *ACS Nano* 9, 2805–2819. doi: 10.1021/nn506732n

Han, J., Kim, Y. S., Lim, M. Y., Kim, H. Y., Kong, S., Kang, M., et al. (2018). Dual roles of graphene oxide to attenuate inflammation and elicit timely polarization of macrophage phenotypes for cardiac repair. *ACS Nano* 12, 1959–1977. doi: 10.1021/acsnano.7b09107

Haque, S. T., and Chowdhury, E. H. (2018). Recent progress in delivery of therapeutic and imaging agents utilizing organic-inorganic hybrid nanoparticles. *Curr. Drug Deliv.* 15, 485–496. doi: 10.2174/1567201814666171120114034

Harish, K. K., Nagasamy, V., Himangshu, B., and Anuttam, K. (2018). Metallic nanoparticle: a review. *Biomed. J. Sci. Tech. Res.* 4, 3765–3775.

Ichimura, K., Matoba, T., Nakano, K., Tokutome, M., Honda, K., Koga, J., et al. (2016). A translational study of a new therapeutic approach for acute myocardial infarction: nanoparticle-mediated delivery of pitavastatin into reperfused myocardium reduces ischemia-reperfusion injury in a preclinical porcine model. *PLoS One* 11:e0162425. doi: 10.1371/journal.pone.0162425

Ikeda, G., Matoba, T., Nakano, Y., Nagaoka, K., Ishikita, A., Nakano, K., et al. (2016). Nanoparticle-mediated targeting of cyclosporine a enhances cardioprotection against ischemia-reperfusion injury through inhibition of mitochondrial permeability transition pore opening. *Sci. Rep.* 6:20467.

Jeevanandam, J., Barhoum, A., Chan, Y. S., Dufresne, A., and Danquah, M. K. (2018). Review on nanoparticles and nanostructured materials: history, sources, toxicity and regulations. *Beilstein J. Nanotechnol.* 9, 1050–1074. doi: 10.3762/bjnano.9.98

Kamaly, N., Fredman, G., Fojas, J. J., Subramanian, M., Choi, W. I., Zepeda, K., et al. (2016). Targeted Interleukin-10 nanotherapeutics developed with a microfluidic chip enhance resolution of inflammation in advanced atherosclerosis. *ACS Nano* 10, 5280–5292. doi: 10.1021/acsnano.6b01114

Kanki, S., Jaalouk, D. E., Lee, S., Yu, A. Y., Gannon, J., and Lee, R. T. (2011). Identification of targeting peptides for ischemic myocardium by in vivo phage display. *J. Mol. Cell Cardiol.* 50, 841–848. doi: 10.1016/j.yjmcc.2011.02.003

Katsuki, S., Matoba, T., Koga, J. I., Nakano, K., and Egashira, K. (2017). Anti-inflammatory nanomedicine for cardiovascular disease. *Front. Cardiovasc. Med.* 4:87. doi: 10.3389/fcvm.2017.00087

Ke, Y., Castro, C., and Choi, J. H. (2018). Structural DNA nanotechnology: artificial nanostructures for biomedical research. *Annu. Rev. Biomed. Eng.* 20, 375–401. doi: 10.1146/annurev-bioeng-062117-120904

Lakshmanan, R., and Maulik, N. (2018). Development of next generation cardiovascular therapeutics through bio-assisted nanotechnology. *J. Biomed. Mater. Res. B Appl. Biomater.* 106, 2072–2083. doi: 10.1002/jbm.b.34000

Lee, D. S., Qian, H., Tay, C. Y., and Leong, D. T. (2016). Cellular processing and destinies of artificial DNA nanostructures. *Chem. Soc. Rev.* 45, 4199–4225. doi: 10.1039/c5cs00700c

Lin, C. X., Yang, S. Y., Gu, J. L., Meng, J., Xu, H. Y., and Cao, J. M. (2017). The acute toxic effects of silver nanoparticles on myocardial transmembrane potential, INa and IK1 channels and heart rhythm in mice. *Nanotoxicology* 11, 827–837.

Lloyd-Jones, D. M., Hong, Y., Labarthe, D., Mozaffarian, D., Appel, L. J., Van Horn, L., et al. (2010). Defining and setting national goals for cardiovascular health promotion and disease reduction: the American Heart Association's strategic Impact Goal through 2020 and beyond. *Circulation* 121, 586–613. doi: 10.1161/circulationaha.109.192703

Lu, W., Xie, Z., Tang, Y., Bai, L., Yao, Y., Fu, C., et al. (2015). Photoluminescent mesoporous silicon nanoparticles with siCCR2 improve the effects of mesenchymal stromal cell transplantation after acute myocardial infarction. *Theranostics* 5, 1068–1082. doi: 10.7150/thno.11517

Madigan, M., and Atoui, R. (2018). Therapeutic use of stem cells for myocardial infarction. *Bioengineering (Basel)* 5:28. doi: 10.3390/bioengineering5020028

Mahmoudi, M., Yu, M., Serpooshan, V., Wu, J. C., Langer, R., Lee, R. T., et al. (2017). Multiscale technologies for treatment of ischemic cardiomyopathy. *Nat. Nanotechnol.* 12, 845–855. doi: 10.1038/nnano.2017.167

Mao, Y., Koga, J. I., Tokutome, M., Matoba, T., Ikeda, G., Nakano, K., et al. (2017). Nanoparticle-mediated delivery of pitavastatin to monocytes/macrophages inhibits left ventricular remodeling after acute myocardial infarction by inhibiting monocyte-mediated inflammation. *Int. Heart J.* 58, 615–623. doi: 10.1536/ihj.16-457

Martinelli, V., Cellot, G., Toma, F. M., Long, C. S., Caldwell, J. H., Zentilin, L., et al. (2013). Carbon nanotubes instruct physiological growth and functionally mature syncytia: nongenetic engineering of cardiac myocytes. *ACS Nano* 7, 5746–5756. doi: 10.1021/nn4002193

Miragoli, M., Ceriotti, P., Iafisco, M., Vacchiano, M., Salvarani, N., Alogna, A., et al. (2018). Inhalation of peptide-loaded nanoparticles improves heart failure. *Sci. Transl. Med.* 10:eaan6205. doi: 10.1126/scitranslmed.aan6205

Morgan, M. T., Carnahan, M. A., Finkelstein, S., Prata, C. A., Degoricija, L., Lee, S. J., et al. (2005). Dendritic supramolecular assemblies for drug delivery. *Chem. Commun. (Camb)* 2005, 4309–4311.

Nagaoka, K., Matoba, T., Mao, Y., Nakano, Y., Ikeda, G., Egusa, S., et al. (2015). A new therapeutic modality for acute myocardial infarction: nanoparticle-mediated delivery of pitavastatin induces cardioprotection from ischemia-reperfusion injury via activation of PI3K/Akt pathway and anti-inflammation in a rat model. *PLoS One* 10:e0132451. doi: 10.1371/journal.pone.0132451

Nakano, Y., Matoba, T., Tokutome, M., Funamoto, D., Katsuki, S., Ikeda, G., et al. (2016). Nanoparticle-mediated delivery of irbesartan induces cardioprotection from myocardial ischemia-reperfusion injury by antagonizing monocyte-mediated inflammation. *Sci. Rep.* 6:29601.

Namdari, M., Cheraghi, M., Negahdari, B., Eatemadi, A., and Daraee, H. (2017). Recent advances in magnetoliposome for heart drug delivery. *Artif. Cells Nanomed. Biotechnol.* 45, 1–7.

Nguyen, J., Sievers, R., Motion, J. P., Kivimae, S., Fang, Q., and Lee, R. J. (2015). Delivery of lipid micelles into infarcted myocardium using a lipid-linked matrix metalloproteinase targeting peptide. *Mol. Pharm.* 12, 1150–1157. doi: 10.1021/mp500653y

Nguyen, M. M., Carlini, A. S., Chien, M. P., Sonnenberg, S., Luo, C., Braden, R. L., et al. (2015). Enzyme-responsive nanoparticles for targeted accumulation and prolonged retention in heart tissue after myocardial infarction. *Adv. Mater.* 27, 5547–5552. doi: 10.1002/adma.201502003

Niu, J., Azfer, A., Rogers, L. M., Wang, X., and Kolattukudy, P. E. (2007). Cardioprotective effects of cerium oxide nanoparticles in a transgenic murine model of cardiomyopathy. *Cardiovasc. Res.* 73, 549–559. doi: 10.1016/j.cardiores.2006.11.031

Niu, J., Wang, K., and Kolattukudy, P. E. (2011). Cerium oxide nanoparticles inhibit oxidative stress and nuclear factor-kappaB activation in H9c2 cardiomyocytes exposed to cigarette smoke extract. *J. Pharmacol. Exp. Ther.* 338, 53–61. doi: 10.1124/jpet.111.179978

Novoselov, K. S., Geim, A. K., Morozov, S. V., Jiang, D., Zhang, Y., Dubonos, S. V., et al. (2004). Electric field effect in atomically thin carbon films. *Science* 306, 666–669. doi: 10.1126/science.1102896

Oduk, Y., Zhu, W., Kannappan, R., Zhao, M., Borovjagin, A. V., Oparil, S., et al. (2018). VEGF nanoparticles repair the heart after myocardial infarction. *Am. J. Physiol. Heart Circ. Physiol.* 314, H278–H284.

Oggu, G. S., Sasikumar, S., Reddy, N., Ella, K. K. R., Rao, C. M., and Bokara, K. K. (2017). Gene delivery approaches for mesenchymal stem cell therapy: strategies to increase efficiency and specificity. *Stem Cell Rev.* 13, 725–740. doi: 10.1007/s12015-017-9760-2

Ottersbach, A., Mykhaylyk, O., Heidsieck, A., Eberbeck, D., Rieck, S., Zimmermann, K., et al. (2018). Improved heart repair upon myocardial infarction: combination of magnetic nanoparticles and tailored magnets strongly increases engraftment of myocytes. *Biomaterials* 155, 176–190. doi: 10.1016/j.biomaterials.2017.11.012

Pan, K., and Zhong, Q. (2016). Organic nanoparticles in foods: fabrication, characterization, and utilization. *Annu. Rev. Food Sci. Technol.* 7, 245–266. doi: 10.1146/annurev-food-041715-033215

Pandey, P., and Dahiya, M. (2016). A brief review on inorganic nanoparticles. *J. Crit. Rev.* 3, 18–26.

Park, J., Kim, B., Han, J., Oh, J., Park, S., Ryu, S., et al. (2015). Graphene oxide flakes as a cellular adhesive: prevention of reactive oxygen species mediated death of implanted cells for cardiac repair. *ACS Nano* 9, 4987–4999. doi: 10.1021/nn507149w

Pascual-Gil, S., Simon-Yarza, T., Garbayo, E., Prosper, F., and Blanco-Prieto, M. J. (2017). Cytokine-loaded PLGA and PEG-PLGA microparticles showed similar heart regeneration in a rat myocardial infarction model. *Int. J. Pharm.* 523, 531–533. doi: 10.1016/j.ijpharm.2016.11.022

Paul, A., Binsalamah, Z. M., Khan, A. A., Abbasia, S., Elias, C. B., Shum-Tim, D., et al. (2011). A nanobiohybrid complex of recombinant baculovirus and Tat/DNA nanoparticles for delivery of Ang-1 transgene in myocardial infarction therapy. *Biomaterials* 32, 8304–8318. doi: 10.1016/j.biomaterials.2011.07.042

Paul, A., Hasan, A., Kindi, H. A., Gaharwar, A. K., Rao, V. T., Nikkhah, M., et al. (2014). Injectable graphene oxide/hydrogel-based angiogenic gene delivery system for vasculogenesis and cardiac repair. *ACS Nano* 8, 8050–8062. doi: 10.1021/nn5020787

Paulis, L. E., Geelen, T., Kuhlmann, M. T., Coolen, B. F., Schafers, M., Nicolay, K., et al. (2012). Distribution of lipid-based nanoparticles to infarcted myocardium with potential application for MRI-monitored drug delivery. *J. Control Release* 162, 276–285. doi: 10.1016/j.jconrel.2012.06.035

Pearson, R. M., Sunoqrot, S., Hsu, H. J., Bae, J. W., and Hong, S. (2012). Dendritic nanoparticles: the next generation of nanocarriers? *Ther. Deliv.* 3, 941–959. doi: 10.4155/tde.12.76

Pitroda, J., Jethwa, B., and Dave, S. K. (2016). A critical review on carbon nanotubes. *Int. J. Construct. Res. Civil Eng.* 2, 36–42.

Potter, L. R., Yoder, A. R., Flora, D. R., Antos, L. K., and Dickey, D. M. (2009). Natriuretic peptides: their structures, receptors, physiologic functions and therapeutic applications. *Handb. Exp. Pharmacol.* 191, 341–366. doi: 10.1007/978-3-540-68964-5_15

Priyadarsini, S., Mukherjee, S., and Mishra, M. (2018). Nanoparticles used in dentistry: a review. *J. Oral Biol. Craniofac. Res.* 8, 58–67. doi: 10.1016/j.jobcr.2017.12.004

Qi, J., Zhuang, J., Lu, Y., Dong, X., Zhao, W., and Wu, W. (2017). In vivo fate of lipid-based nanoparticles. *Drug Discov. Today* 22, 166–172. doi: 10.1016/j.drudis.2016.09.024

Qi, Q., Lu, L., Li, H., Yuan, Z., Chen, G., Lin, M., et al. (2017). Spatiotemporal delivery of nanoformulated liraglutide for cardiac regeneration after myocardial infarction. *Int. J. Nanomed.* 12, 4835–4848. doi: 10.2147/ijn.s132064

Raphey, V. R., Henna, T. K., Nivitha, K. P., Mufeedha, P., Sabu, C., and Pramod, K. (2019). Advanced biomedical applications of carbon nanotube. *Mater. Sci. Eng. C Mater. Biol. Appl.* 100, 616–630.

Reboucas, J. S., Santos-Magalhaes, N. S., and Formiga, F. R. (2016). Cardiac regeneration using growth factors: advances and challenges. *Arq. Bras Cardiol.* 107, 271–275.

Sager, H. B., Dutta, P., Dahlman, J. E., Hulsmans, M., Courties, G., Sun, Y., et al. (2016). RNAi targeting multiple cell adhesion molecules reduces immune cell recruitment and vascular inflammation after myocardial infarction. *Sci. Transl. Med.* 8:342ra380.

Sajid, M. I., Jamshaid, U., Jamshaid, T., Zafar, N., Fessi, H., and Elaissari, A. (2016). Carbon nanotubes from synthesis to in vivo biomedical applications. *Int. J. Pharm.* 501, 278–299. doi: 10.1016/j.ijpharm.2016.01.064

Saludas, L., Pascual-Gil, S., Roli, F., Garbayo, E., and Blanco-Prieto, M. J. (2018). Heart tissue repair and cardioprotection using drug delivery systems. *Maturitas* 110, 1–9. doi: 10.1016/j.maturitas.2018.01.011

Samidurai, A., Salloum, F. N., Durrant, D., Chernova, O. B., Kukreja, R. C., and Das, A. (2017). Chronic treatment with novel nanoformulated micelles of rapamycin, Rapatar, protects diabetic heart against ischaemia/reperfusion injury. *Br. J. Pharmacol.* 174, 4771–4784. doi: 10.1111/bph.14059

Saravanan, S., Sareen, N., Abu-El-Rub, E., Ashour, H., Sequiera, G. L., Ammar, H. I., et al. (2018). Graphene oxide-gold nanosheets containing chitosan scaffold improves ventricular contractility and function after implantation into infarcted heart. *Sci. Rep.* 8:15069.

Shao, M., Yang, W., and Han, G. (2017). Protective effects on myocardial infarction model: delivery of schisandrin B using matrix metalloproteinase-sensitive peptide-modified, PEGylated lipid nanoparticles. *Int. J. Nanomed.* 12, 7121–7130. doi: 10.2147/ijn.s141549

Sharma, A. K., Kumar, A., Sahu, M., Sharma, G., Datusalia, A. K., and Rajput, S. K. (2018). Exercise preconditioning and low dose copper nanoparticles exhibits cardioprotection through targeting GSK-3beta phosphorylation in ischemia/reperfusion induced myocardial infarction. *Microvasc. Res.* 120, 59–66. doi: 10.1016/j.mvr.2018.06.003

Shin, S. R., Jung, S. M., Zalabany, M., Kim, K., Zorlutuna, P., Kim, S. B., et al. (2013). Carbon-nanotube-embedded hydrogel sheets for engineering cardiac constructs and bioactuators. *ACS Nano* 7, 2369–2380. doi: 10.1021/nn305559j

Singh, B., Garg, T., Goyal, A. K., and Rath, G. (2016). Recent advancements in the cardiovascular drug carriers. *Artif. Cells Nanomed. Biotechnol.* 44, 216–225. doi: 10.3109/21691401.2014.937868

Singh, M., Manikandan, S., and Kumaraguru, A. K. (2011). Nanoparticles: a new technology with wide applications. *Res. J. Nanosci. Nanotechnol.* 1, 1–11. doi: 10.3923/rjnn.2011.1.11

Somasuntharam, I., Boopathy, A. V., Khan, R. S., Martinez, M. D., Brown, M. E., Murthy, N., et al. (2013). Delivery of Nox2-NADPH oxidase siRNA with polyketal nanoparticles for improving cardiac function following myocardial infarction. *Biomaterials* 34, 7790–7798. doi: 10.1016/j.biomaterials.2013.06.051

Somasuntharam, I., Yehl, K., Carroll, S. L., Maxwell, J. T., Martinez, M. D., Che, P. L., et al. (2016). Knockdown of TNF-alpha by DNAzyme gold nanoparticles as an anti-inflammatory therapy for myocardial infarction. *Biomaterials* 83, 12–22. doi: 10.1016/j.biomaterials.2015.12.022

Sperling, R. A., Rivera Gil, P., Zhang, F., Zanella, M., and Parak, W. J. (2008). Biological applications of gold nanoparticles. *Chem. Soc. Rev.* 37, 1896–1908.

Stankovich, S., Dikin, D. A., Dommett, G. H., Kohlhaas, K. M., Zimney, E. J., Stach, E. A., et al. (2006). Graphene-based composite materials. *Nature* 442, 282–286.

Sun, H., Tang, J., Mou, Y., Zhou, J., Qu, L., Duval, K., et al. (2017a). Carbon nanotube-composite hydrogels promote intercalated disc assembly in engineered cardiac tissues through beta1-integrin mediated FAK and RhoA pathway. *Acta Biomater.* 48, 88–99. doi: 10.1016/j.actbio.2016.10.025

Sun, H., Zhou, J., Huang, Z., Qu, L., Lin, N., Liang, C., et al. (2017b). Carbon nanotube-incorporated collagen hydrogels improve cell alignment and the performance of cardiac constructs. *Int. J. Nanomedicine.* 12, 3109–3120. doi: 10.2147/ijn.s128030

Sun, X., Liu, Z., Welsher, K., Robinson, J. T., Goodwin, A., Zaric, S., et al. (2008). Nano-graphene oxide for cellular imaging and drug delivery. *Nano Res.* 1, 203–212. doi: 10.1007/s12274-008-8021-8

Tan, M. E., He, C. H., Jiang, W., Zeng, C., Yu, N., Huang, W., et al. (2017). Development of solid lipid nanoparticles containing total flavonoid extract from *Dracocephalum moldavica* L. and their therapeutic effect against myocardial ischemia-reperfusion injury in rats. *Int. J. Nanomed.* 12, 3253–3265. doi: 10.2147/ijn.s131893

Tang, C., Li, H., Hong, J., and Chai, X. (2020). Application of nanoparticles in the early diagnosis and treatment of tumors: current status and progress. *Trad. Med. Res.* 5, 34–43.

Tateishi-Yuyama, E., Matsubara, H., Murohara, T., Ikeda, U., Shintani, S., Masaki, H., et al. (2002). Therapeutic angiogenesis for patients with limb ischaemia by autologous transplantation of bone-marrow cells: a pilot study and a randomised controlled trial. *Lancet* 360, 427–435. doi: 10.1016/s0140-6736(02)09670-8

Terashvili, M., and Bosnjak, Z. J. (2019). Stem cell therapies in cardiovascular disease. *J. Cardiothorac. Vasc. Anesth.* 33, 209–222.

Thomas, T. P., Joice, M., Sumit, M., Silpe, J. E., Kotlyar, A., Bharathi, S., et al. (2013). Design and in vitro validation of multivalent dendrimer methotrexates as a folate-targeting anticancer therapeutic. *Curr. Pharm. Des.* 19, 6594–6605. doi: 10.2174/1381612811319370004

Tian, A., Yang, C., Zhu, B., Wang, W., Liu, K., Jiang, Y., et al. (2018). Polyethylene-glycol-coated gold nanoparticles improve cardiac function after myocardial infarction in mice. *Can. J. Physiol. Pharmacol.* 96, 1318–1327. doi: 10.1139/cjpp-2018-0227

Vinhas, R., Mendes, R., Fernandes, A. R., and Baptista, P. V. (2017). Nanoparticles-emerging potential for managing leukemia and lymphoma. *Front. Bioeng. Biotechnol.* 5:79. doi: 10.3389/fbioe.2017.00079

Virlan, M. J., Miricescu, D., Radulescu, R., Sabliov, C. M., Totan, A., Calenic, B., et al. (2016). Organic nanomaterials and their applications in the treatment of oral diseases. *Molecules* 21:207. doi: 10.3390/molecules21020207

Vong, L. B., Bui, T. Q., Tomita, T., Sakamoto, H., Hiramatsu, Y., and Nagasaki, Y. (2018). Novel angiogenesis therapeutics by redox injectable hydrogel – regulation of local nitric oxide generation for effective cardiovascular therapy. *Biomaterials* 167, 143–152. doi: 10.1016/j.biomaterials.2018.03.023

Wang, J., Seo, M. J., Deci, M. B., Weil, B. R., Canty, J. M., and Nguyen, J. (2018). Effect of CCR2 inhibitor-loaded lipid micelles on inflammatory cell migration and cardiac function after myocardial infarction. *Int. J. Nanomed.* 13, 6441–6451. doi: 10.2147/ijn.s178650

Xu, Q. H., Guan, P., Zhang, T., Lu, C., Li, G., and Liu, J. X. (2018). Silver nanoparticles impair zebrafish skeletal and cardiac myofibrillogenesis and sarcomere formation. *Aquat. Toxicol.* 200, 102–113. doi: 10.1016/j.aquatox.2018.04.018

Xue, X., Shi, X., Dong, H., You, S., Cao, H., Wang, K., et al. (2018). Delivery of microRNA-1 inhibitor by dendrimer-based nanovector: an early targeting therapy for myocardial infarction in mice. *Nanomedicine* 14, 619–631. doi: 10.1016/j.nano.2017.12.004

Yang, J., Brown, M. E., Zhang, H., Martinez, M., Zhao, Z., Bhutani, S., et al. (2017). High-throughput screening identifies microRNAs that target Nox2 and improve function after acute myocardial infarction. *Am. J. Physiol. Heart Circ. Physiol.* 312, H1002–H1012.

Yin, Q., Pei, Z., Wang, H., and Zhao, Y. (2014). Cyclosporine A-nanoparticles enhance the therapeutic benefit of adipose tissue-derived stem cell transplantation in a swine myocardial infarction model. *Int. J. Nanomed.* 9, 17–26.

Zanganeh, S., Hutter, G., Spitler, R., Lenkov, O., Mahmoudi, M., Shaw, A., et al. (2016). Iron oxide nanoparticles inhibit tumour growth by inducing pro-inflammatory macrophage polarization in tumour tissues. *Nat. Nanotechnol.* 11, 986–994. doi: 10.1038/nnano.2016.168

Zhang, L., Xia, J., Zhao, Q., Liu, L., and Zhang, Z. (2010). Functional graphene oxide as a nanocarrier for controlled loading and targeted delivery of mixed anticancer drugs. *Small* 6, 537–544. doi: 10.1002/smll.200901680

Zhang, S., Wang, J., and Pan, J. (2016). Baicalin-loaded PEGylated lipid nanoparticles: characterization, pharmacokinetics, and protective effects on acute myocardial ischemia in rats. *Drug Deliv.* 23, 3696–3703. doi: 10.1080/10717544.2016.1223218

Zhang, W., Zhang, Z., and Zhang, Y. (2011). The application of carbon nanotubes in target drug delivery systems for cancer therapies. *Nanoscale Res. Lett.* 6:555.

Zhou, J., Yang, X., Liu, W., Wang, C., Shen, Y., Zhang, F., et al. (2018). Injectable OPF/graphene oxide hydrogels provide mechanical support and enhance cell electrical signaling after implantation into myocardial infarct. *Theranostics* 8, 3317–3330. doi: 10.7150/thno.25504

Zhou, J., and Zhang, G. (2019). Antitumor applications of nano-traditional Chinese medicine. *Trad. Med. Res.* 4, 224–226.

Zhou, L. S., Zhao, G. L., Liu, Q., Jiang, S. C., Wang, Y., and Zhang, D. M. (2015). Silencing collapsin response mediator protein-2 reprograms macrophage phenotype and improves infarct healing in experimental myocardial infarction model. *J. Inflamm. (Lond.)* 12:11. doi: 10.1186/s12950-015-0053-8

Zhou, Y., Sun, H., Xu, H., Matysiak, S., Ren, J., and Qu, X. (2018). Mesoporous encapsulated chiral nanogold for use in enantioselective reactions. *Angew. Chem. Int. Ed. Engl.* 57, 16791–16795. doi: 10.1002/anie.201811118

Zhu, K., Wu, M., Lai, H., Guo, C., Li, J., Wang, Y., et al. (2016). Nanoparticle-enhanced generation of gene-transfected mesenchymal stem cells for in vivo cardiac repair. *Biomaterials* 74, 188–199. doi: 10.1016/j.biomaterials.2015.10.010

3

Delivery of Human Stromal Vascular Fraction Cells on Nanofibrillar Scaffolds for Treatment of Peripheral Arterial Disease

Caroline Hu[1†], Tatiana S. Zaitseva[2†], Cynthia Alcazar[1†], Peter Tabada[2], Steve Sawamura[2], Guang Yang[3,4], Mimi R. Borrelli[5], Derrick C. Wan[5], Dung H. Nguyen[5], Michael V. Paukshto[2] and Ngan F. Huang[1,3,4‡]*

[1] Veterans Affairs Palo Alto Health Care System, Palo Alto, CA, United States, [2] Fibralign Corporation, Inc., Union City, CA, United States, [3] The Stanford Cardiovascular Institute, Stanford University, Palo Alto, CA, United States, [4] Department of Cardiothoracic Surgery, Stanford University, Palo Alto, CA, United States, [5] Division of Plastic and Reconstructive Surgery, Stanford University, Palo Alto, CA, United States

***Correspondence:**
Ngan F. Huang
ngantina@stanford.edu

† These authors have contributed equally to this work

Cell therapy for treatment of peripheral arterial disease (PAD) is a promising approach but is limited by poor cell survival when cells are delivered using saline. The objective of this study was to examine the feasibility of aligned nanofibrillar scaffolds as a vehicle for the delivery of human stromal vascular fraction (SVF), and then to assess the efficacy of the cell-seeded scaffolds in a murine model of PAD. Flow cytometric analysis was performed to characterize the phenotype of SVF cells from freshly isolated lipoaspirate, as well as after attachment onto aligned nanofibrillar scaffolds. Flow cytometry results demonstrated that the SVF consisted of 33.1 ± 9.6% $CD45^+$ cells, a small fraction of $CD45^-/CD31^+$ (4.5 ± 3.1%) and 45.4 ± 20.0% of $CD45^-/CD31^-/CD34^+$ cells. Although the subpopulations of SVF did not change significantly after attachment to the aligned nanofibrillar scaffolds, protein secretion of vascular endothelial growth factor (VEGF) significantly increased by six-fold, compared to SVF cultured in suspension. Importantly, when SVF-seeded scaffolds were transplanted into immunodeficient mice with induced hindlimb ischemia, the cell-seeded scaffolds induced a significant higher mean perfusion ratio after 14 days, compared to cells delivered using saline. Together, these results show that aligned nanofibrillar scaffolds promoted cellular attachment, enhanced the secretion of VEGF from attached SVF cells, and their implantation with attached SVF cells stimulated blood perfusion recovery. These findings have important therapeutic implications for the treatment of PAD using SVF.

Keywords: angiogenesis, peripheral arterial disease, stem cell therapy, aligned scaffold, anisotropy, hindlimb ischemia

INTRODUCTION

Peripheral arterial disease (PAD) affects over 10 million people in the United States (Benjamin et al., 2018). It is associated with reduced blood flow to the arms and legs, leading to pain and even limb amputation. Major risk factors include smoking, diabetes mellitus, and aging. Severe cases of PAD lead to critical limb ischemia (CLI) that is characterized by rest pain, gangrene formation, and possible amputation of the limb (Davies, 2012). Current clinical treatments of PAD involve surgical interventions including bypass grafting and angioplasty to restore blood flow to the affected limb. However, a large portion of patients with severe disease lack suitable vessels for vascular intervention (Gerhard et al., 1995). Therefore, there is an urgent need for alternative approaches to stimulate angiogenesis.

Cell-based therapies hold promise for regenerating neovessels that support blood flow in the ischemic limb. Stem cells including bone marrow-derived mesenchymal stem cells (MSCs) are a potential therapy as they are easy to expand, resilient in hypoxic conditions, and secrete paracrine factors that have angiogenic effects (Kinnaird et al., 2004). Although some clinical studies report that the delivery of MSCs to the site of limb ischemia significantly improved rest pain and increased the ankle brachial index as a measurement of vascular function, limb amputation rates did not significantly change with treatment (Lu et al., 2011; Gupta et al., 2013). Similarly, clinical trials using mononuclear cells from bone marrow or peripheral blood have also showed mixed results (Rigato et al., 2017; Qadura et al., 2018). Consequently, alternative therapeutic cell types are desired for treatment of PAD.

The stromal vascular fraction (SVF) is a heterogeneous population of cells that is derived from subcutaneous fat (Levi et al., 2011; Blackshear et al., 2017). SVF contains various types of cells including adipose stromal and hematopoietic stem and progenitor cells, endothelial cells, erythrocytes, fibroblasts, lymphocytes, monocyte/macrophages, and pericytes (Zuk et al., 2001, 2002; Bourin et al., 2013). Cells from the SVF release a mix of cytokines and therapeutic growth factors such as vascular endothelial growth factor (VEGF) that promote angiogenesis (Thangarajah et al., 2009; Kapur and Katz, 2013; Comella et al., 2016). Compared to other cell types that require *in vitro* expansion, SVF can be derived autologously, extracted in a minimally invasive manner in a clinical setting (Levi et al., 2011), and transplanted back within hours. Consequently, SVF may have greater translational relevance than other stem cells types for treatment of limb ischemia. We have previously shown that collagen scaffolds seeded with human SVF and subcellular populations thereof significantly improved revascularization to dermal wounds (Brett et al., 2017b), which supports the safety of SVF-seeded collagen scaffolds.

Regardless of the kind of stem cell used, a major limitation to stem cell therapy is poor survival of the cells when transplanted in saline. As an alternative to saline as a cell delivery vehicle, biological scaffolds can localize cell delivery to the site of the scaffold, while also providing important extracellular matrix cues that modulate the survival and angiogenic capacity of the transplanted cells. In particular, cues derived from nano-scale anisotropic patterns of fibrillar collagen can modulate cellular organization, growth factor secretion, and upregulation of integrin gene expression (Huang et al., 2013a,b; Nakayama et al., 2015, 2019). We have previously demonstrated that parallel-aligned nanofibrillar scaffolds promote the survival and angiogenic capacity of transplanted primary human endothelial cells or human induced pluripotent stem cell-derived endothelial cells in a mouse model of PAD (Huang et al., 2013b; Nakayama et al., 2015). These studies suggest that nanoscale spatial patterning cues can directly modulate biological functions of therapeutic cells upon transplantation into the ischemic limb. Toward clinical translation, these nanofibrillar scaffolds have been demonstrated to improve angiogenesis (Huang et al., 2013b), arteriogenesis (Nakayama et al., 2015), and lymphangiogenesis (Hadamitzky et al., 2016) *in vivo*. Recently, these aligned collagen scaffolds have been demonstrated to be safe in a clinical study, without complication at a 1 year follow up (Rochlin et al., 2020). Accordingly, the delivery of SVF using aligned nanofibrillar scaffolds may synergistically enhance revascularization for treatment of PAD.

Therefore, the objective of this study was to characterize the adherent cells from human SVF on aligned nanofibrillar scaffolds, and to assess the therapeutic potential of aligned nanofibrillar scaffolds seeded with SVF in a murine model of PAD. We show that the subpopulation of SVF cells that adhered to the nanofibrillar scaffold had significantly higher release of VEGF, but without a significant change in the $CD45^-/CD31^-/CD34^+$ cell fraction, compared to bulk SVF cells in suspension. When implanted into mice with induced hindlimb ischemia as an experimental model of PAD, the SVF-seeded scaffolds significantly increased blood perfusion, compared to cell delivery in saline. These findings suggest that aligned nanofibrillar scaffolds promoted the adhesion of SVF cells that induce angiogenesis and blood perfusion recovery, which has important therapeutic implications for the treatment of PAD.

MATERIALS AND METHODS

Fabrication of Aligned Nanofibrillar Scaffolds

The aligned nanofibrillar collagen scaffolds were fabricated using shear-based fibrillogenesis technique as described previously (Huang et al., 2013b). In brief, purified monomeric type I collagen solution was concentrated to reach a liquid crystal state (Bobrov et al., 2002; Paukshto et al., 2008) and then sheared onto a rigid surface, creating thin film formed by parallel-aligned nanofibrils with 200–300 nm diameter (Muthusubramaniam et al., 2012). To make three-dimensional thread-like scaffolds, the membranes were dissociated from the rigid surface into a free-standing film that self-assembled by liquid–air surface tension into the thread-like scaffold (McMurtry et al., 2008). The scaffolds were then crosslinked by 1-ethyl-3-(3-dimethylaminopropyl)-1-carbodiimide (EDC) hydrochloride chemistry at 1 mg/ml and sterilized by e-beam per standard protocols (Fibralign Corporation). Surface topography of the scaffolds was assessed by routine scanning electron microscopy (SEM) (Huang et al., 2013b).

Isolation of SVF

Lipoaspirate was obtained from healthy female patients (n = 6) undergoing elective procedures in accordance with the Stanford University Institutional Review Board and kept at 4°C until processing. All samples were processed within 24 h from the time of collection. SVF cells were isolated based on established methods (Tevlin et al., 2016). Lipoaspirate was rinsed twice with equal volume of phosphate buffered saline (PBS) to separate fat from blood. Fresh collagenase digestion buffer was prepared using M199 medium containing 2.2 mg/ml type II collagenase (Sigma–Aldrich), 1000 U/ml DNAse, 0.5 μM calcium chloride, 0.1% bovine serum albumin, 1% polaxamer-188 (Sigma–Aldrich), and 2% hydroxyethyl piperazine ethanesulfonic acid (Life Technologies), and filtered using a 0.22-μm filter system. Aliquots of the rinsed fat (12.5 ml) were transferred into 50-ml Falcon tubes, and an equal volume of collagenase digestion buffer was added to the fat. The tube caps were sealed with Parafilm (Bemis NA). The fat/collagenase mixture was incubated at 37°C in a water bath for 10 min to activate the collagenase. The tubes with fat/collagenase mixture were placed into the orbital shaker set at 220 r/min for 45 min. Collagenase activity was then neutralized by addition of an equal volume of cold buffer consisted of PBS containing 2% fetal bovine serum, 1% poloxamer-188, and 1% penicillin/streptomycin (FACS buffer). The solution was then centrifuged at 1250 r/min at 4°C for 10 min. Supernatant was aspirated and the SVF pellets were resuspended again in FACS buffer again and filtered through a 100-μm cell strainer, before centrifuging again at 1250 r/min at room temperature for 10 min. The resulting cell pellet was resuspended in 15 ml FACS buffer and carefully layered over 15 ml of room-temperature equilibrated Histopaque (Sigma-Aldrich) in a new 50-ml Falcon tube. The cell suspension with Histopaque was centrifuged at 1500 r/min for 30 min at room temperature with acceleration set to low and deceleration settings inactivated. The cloudy interface was transferred to a new 50 ml Falcon tube, and 40 ml FACS buffer was added. The cell suspension was centrifuged at 1500 r/min at 4°C for 5 min. The pellet was resuspended for cell culture or for flow cytometry analysis.

Flow Cytometry

At indicated time points, cells were incubated for 30 min on ice in FACS buffer containing antibodies to CD34, CD31, and CD45 (BD Biosciences). Fluorescence-activated cell sorting was performed on a BD FACSAria II (BD Biosciences, San Jose, CA, United States), using a 100-μm nozzle. Propidium iodide was used as the live/dead discriminator. Compensation was performed using CD31-PB, CD45-PECy7, and CD43-FITC with antibody capture beads (Thermo Fisher). Acquisition was performed by BD FACSDiva (BD Biosciences). Analysis was performed using FlowJo (version 10). Gating for CD34-FITC positive utilized a full stain minus one control.

Cell Culture

Aligned nanofibrillar scaffolds (1-cm long) were placed in 24-well ultra-low attachment plate (Corning), and pre-incubated with 1 ml DMEM/10% FBS with 1% penicillin-streptomycin in CO_2 incubator for 45 min. At the end of the pre-incubation, media was removed, and 1 ml SVF suspension in DMEM/10% FBS with 1% penicillin-streptomycin was added to the wells containing scaffold samples. The scaffolds were incubated with SVF suspension 5% CO_2 and 37°C for 1 h, then the cell sample in each well was resuspended, and incubated again for 1 h. After the 2-h incubation, cell-seeded scaffold samples were transferred into new wells containing fresh media and incubated in CO_2 incubator at 37°C overnight. As a control, 1 ml SVF suspension in DMEM/10% FBS with 1% penicillin-streptomycin was incubated at 10^6 cells/ml/well in 24-well ultra-low attachment plate in CO_2 incubator at 37°C overnight. After overnight incubation, SVF cells cultured on scaffolds were dissociated using a 1:1 mixture of TrypLE (Fisher Scientific) and collagenase digestion buffer, pelleted, and resuspended in FACS buffer. SVF cells cultured in suspension were pelleted and resuspended in FACS buffer. Both scaffold- and suspension cultured SVF samples were analyzed by flow cytometry as described above.

VEGF Enzyme Linked Immunosorbent Assay (ELISA)

Following the overnight incubation of control cell suspension and cell-seeded scaffolds, media samples were collected and kept frozen at −80°C. Corresponding cell numbers were determined after counting by hemocytometer for cell suspension samples, and by DNA quantification for cell-seeded scaffold samples. VEGF concentration in media samples was measured by VEGF enzyme linked immunosorbent assay (ELISA) kit (R&D Systems) following manufacturer's instructions.

Preparation of Cell-Seeded Scaffolds and Control Cell Suspension for *in vivo* Implantation

Following the overnight incubation, cell-seeded scaffold samples were removed from the media, rinsed in PBS, placed in 1.5-ml Eppendorf tube filled with PBS, and transferred to the surgery room. Control samples were prepared from the SVF samples incubated in 24-well ultra-low attachment plate overnight. Cells were resuspended, centrifuged at 1250 r/min for 5 min at room temperature, and SVF suspension sample was prepared at 10^4 cells in 50 μl PBS per injection/animal. This cell number was based on pilot studies showed that 1-cm BioBridge scaffold could hold up to 10^4 cells. Quantification of scaffold-attached cells was performed by measuring DNA content in cell lysates using PicoGreen assay (Fisher Scientific), and calculation based on calibration curves obtained from series of cell samples with known cell numbers counted by hemocytometer.

Immunofluorescence Staining of SVF-Seeded Scaffolds

Cell-seeded scaffolds were fixed with 4% paraformaldehyde and permeabilized with 0.5% Triton-X-100, then blocked with 1% bovine serum albumin. Scaffolds were incubated with up to two of the following agents to determine the cellular makeup of the SVF. A 1:100 dilution of anti-human CD31 antibody (DAKO, M082301-2), 1:100 dilution anti-CD105 (endoglin) antibody (Santa Cruz Biotechnology, sc-18838), 1:200 dilution anti-human CD34 antibody (Novus Biologicals, NBP2-44568), and 1:100 dilution Alexa Fluor 488 Phalloidin (ThermoFisher, A12379) for F-actin visualization. Samples were washed in PBS and incubated with secondary antibodies conjugated to Alexa Fluor 488 or Alexa Fluor 594 (ThermoFisher). Scaffolds were washed in PBS and counterstained with Hoechst 33342 nuclear dye (Invitrogen, H3570). Scaffolds were then imaged with a confocal microscope (LSM710, Zeiss).

Hindlimb Ischemia and Blood Perfusion Assessment

Hindlimb ischemia was induced in 8–10 week old male NOD SCID mice (Jackson Laboratory) by unilaterally excising a portion of the femoral artery (Niiyama et al., 2009). The animals then received one of the following treatments: 10^4 SVF cells pre-seeded onto a 1-cm-long scaffold and delivered to the site of the ligated artery, or 1×10^4 SVF cell delivered to the adductor muscle of the ischemic leg by local intramuscular injection. Acellular scaffold and a PBS (50 μl) injection were included as reference control groups. Limb perfusion was measured up to 14 days post-surgery by using laser Doppler spectroscopy (PIM3, Perimed). Each animal was placed on a warming pad until they reached a core temperature of 37.5°C before imaging (Niiyama et al., 2009). Results were assessed by taking perfusion value of the ischemic foot, relative to that of the non-ischemic foot to obtain a mean perfusion ratio (Huang et al., 2010; Rufaihah et al., 2011; Nakayama et al., 2015; Hou et al., 2018). All animal studies were approved by the Stanford University Administrative Panel on Laboratory Animal Care.

Immunofluorescence Assessment of SVF Cell Retention

After 14 days, the gastrocnemius tissues were harvested, snap frozen in OCT, and cryosectioned in 10-μm thick sections. To visualize the persistence of human SVF cells, tissue sections were immunofluorescently stained with antibodies directed against human-specific nuclear matrix antigen (Millipore), human-specific CD34 (Novus Biologicals), and human-specific CD31 (Dako). After overnight incubation, the cells were washed in PBS and then incubated with secondary antibodies conjugated to Alexa Fluor 594 or Alexa Fluor 488. The immunofluorescently stained slides were imaged using an epifluorescence microscope (Observer Z1, Zeiss).

Statistics

Data are shown as mean ± standard deviation. Statistical analysis of SVF in suspension, in comparison to on aligned nanofibrillar scaffolds, was performed using the Wilcoxon non-parametric paired *t*-test. For *in vivo* studies, mean blood perfusion recovery among treatment groups was statistically analyzed using a one-way analysis of variance (ANOVA) with Bonferroni post-test. Statistical significance was accepted at $P < 0.05$.

RESULTS

Characterization of Freshly Isolated Bulk SVF by Flow Cytometry

Human SVF from six independent donors were analyzed by flow cytometry to characterize the phenotype of bulk SVF immediately after isolation (**Figure 1**). Using antibodies targeting phenotypic markers of vascular (CD31 and CD34) and hematopoietic (CD45) lineages, the SVF was found to be heterogeneous and having subpopulations of $CD45^+$, $CD45^-/CD31^+$, and $CD45^-/CD31^-/CD34^+$cells (**Figure 1A**). The mean distribution of these subpopulations among six donors was 33.1 ± 9.6% for $CD45^+$, 4.5 ± 3.1% for $CD45^-/CD31^+$, and 45.4 ± 20.0% for $CD45^-/CD31^-/CD34^+$ (**Figures 1B,C**), the latter subpopulation representing the largest segment of SVF. Among $CD45^-/CD31^+$ subset, 85.4 ± 33.7% of the cells co-expressed $CD34^+$.

Characterization of SVF Cellular Attachment on Aligned Nanofibrillar Scaffolds

Aligned nanofibrillar scaffolds were fabricated using shear-mediated extrusion technology that preferentially induced fibrillogenesis along one principle axis, creating 0.2-mm-wide thread-like scaffolds with longitudinally oriented bundles of nanofibrils. Each individual nanofibril was approximately 200 nm in diameter (**Figure 2A**), based on SEM imaging. After seeding of the freshly isolated bulk SVF onto the aligned nanofibrillar scaffolds for 1 day, the cell-seeded samples were fixed in 4% paraformaldehyde for immunofluorescence staining of phenotypic markers. As shown by the confocal microscopy images, overnight culture of freshly harvested SVF revealed diverse cellular morphologies, including elongated and adherent cells, loosely adherent cells with rounded morphology, as well as small cellular aggregates (**Figures 2B–D**). Some of the SVF expressed CD31 and CD34, in agreement with the flow cytometry data (**Figures 2B,C**). Additionally, CD105, which is expressed by both mesenchymal and endothelial lineages, was also found to be expressed by some cells attached to the aligned nanofibrillar scaffolds (**Figure 2D**). To quantitatively assess the phenotype of SVF 1 day after attachment to the nanofibrillar scaffold, in comparison to SVF in suspension culture, we performed flow cytometric analysis using the same phenotypic markers. Our results show that the percent population of vascular (CD31 and CD34) and hematopoietic (CD45) phenotypic markers did not significantly change over the course of 1 day of attachment to the scaffold (**Figure 3A**). Propidium iodide analysis confirmed > 80% viable cells in both treatment groups for all donor cells, which suggested high cell viability.

Although the cells remained phenotypically unchanged after attachment to aligned nanofibrillar scaffolds, the cells became functionally more angiogenic. Among individual SVF donor lines, the average VEGF level from the conditioned media derived from suspension cells was 4.3 ± 1.4 pg per 10^4 cells (**Figure 3B**). In stark contrast, the average VEGF secretion from cells seeded on the aligned collagen scaffold was 26.0 ± 23.5 pg per 10^4 cells, which represented a significant increase by more than a six-fold ($p < 0.05$). For all donor cell lines, there was a consistent increase in VEGF release on scaffold, compared to the bulk SVF suspension population, despite some degree of heterogeneity in the magnitude of VEGF increase among donor cells. These data suggested that aligned nanofibrillar scaffolds could promote angiogenic capacity of SVF.

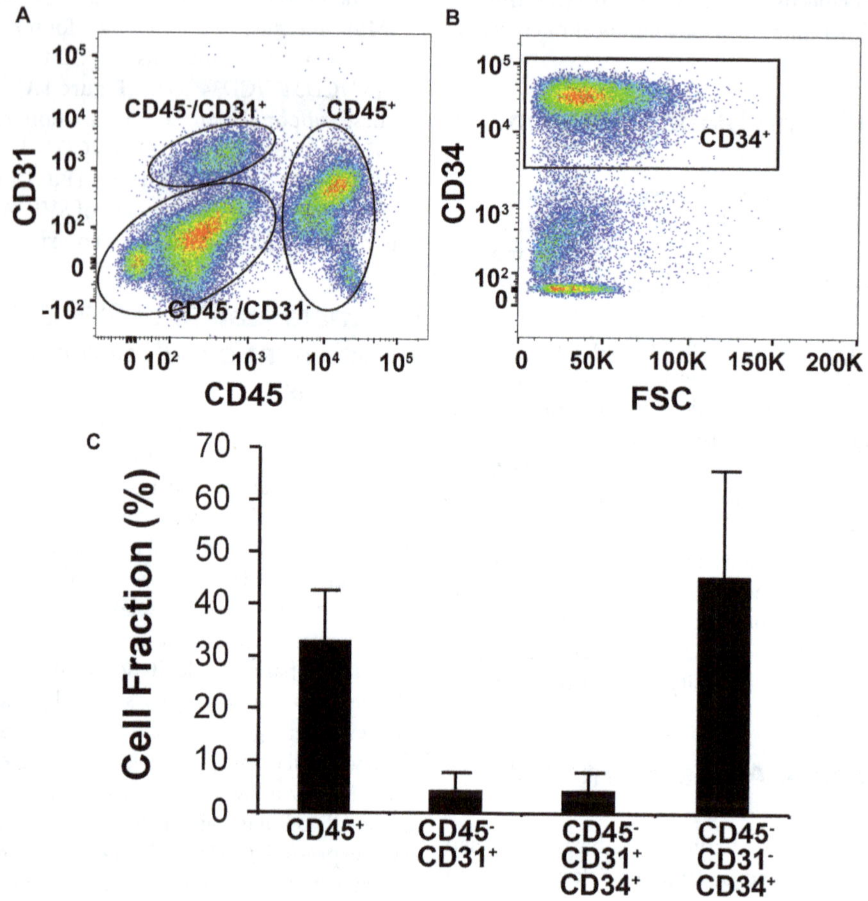

FIGURE 1 | Flow cytometric analysis of human stromal vascular fraction (SVF) cells. **(A)** Representative flow cytometric plot depicts subpopulations of cells based on the expression of CD31 and CD45. **(B)** Flow cytometric analysis of the $CD31^-/CD45^-$ subpopulation showing that the majority of the cells are $CD34^+$. **(C)** Mean cell fraction data among six independent donor SVF extractions.

Therapeutic Efficacy of Aligned Nanofibrillar Scaffolds Seeded With SVF in a Mouse Model of PAD

To determine if the enhanced production of VEGF by SVF on aligned scaffolds could impart a therapeutic benefit, we implanted SVF-seeded scaffolds into immune compromised NOD SCID mice with hindlimb ischemia as an experimental model of PAD. Therapeutic improvement was assessed by non-invasive measurement of blood perfusion recovery by laser Doppler spectroscopy over the course of 14 days after implantation. Quantitative analysis of mean perfusion recovery demonstrated a significant improvement in animals treated with the SVF-seeded scaffolds after 14 days (0.71 ± 0.21), in comparison to animals treated with PBS (0.34 ± 0.18) (**Figure 4**). In contrast, animals treated with injections of SVF or implantation of the acellular scaffold did not show statistically significant improvement in perfusion recovery, in comparison to animals treated with PBS (**Figure 4B**). Additionally, SVF could be visualized in some histological tissue sections using human specific nuclear matrix antigen near the site of implantation, suggesting the persistence of these cells (**Figure 5A**). The SVF cells appeared to retain the expression of CD34 and lacked the expression for CD31, based on staining with human-specific antibodies (**Figures 5B,C**). The persistence of CD34 and absence of CD31 is consistent with their cellular phenotype prior to transplantation, in which the majority of cells were CD34 with a low incidence of CD31 cells (**Figure 3**). Together, these results indicated that only SVF-seeded scaffolds promoted significant improvement in blood perfusion recovery, which concurs with the finding of SVF-seeded scaffolds releasing significantly more VEGF (**Figure 3B**).

DISCUSSION

The salient results of this study are that SVF-seeded aligned nanofibrillar scaffold significantly improved blood perfusion recovery, compared to a control PBS injection (**Figure 4**), and that SVF cells attached to aligned nanofibrillar scaffolds produced significantly more VEGF than SVF cells in suspension (**Figure 3**). This is the first preclinical study that demonstrates that SVF-seeded aligned nanofibrillar scaffold significantly improves blood perfusion, compared to the control PBS injection

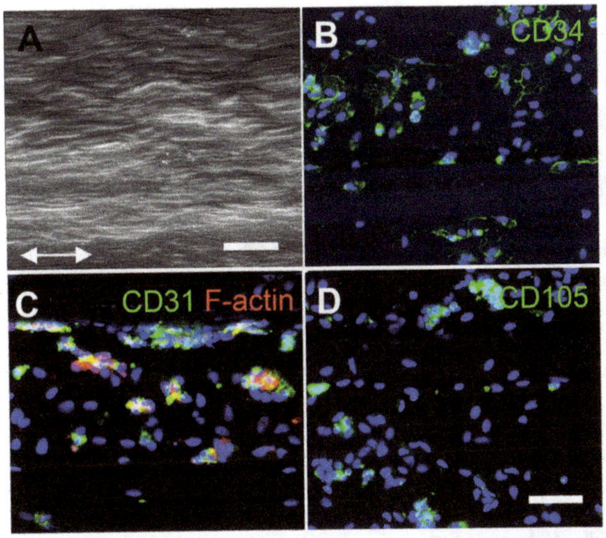

FIGURE 2 | Characterization of human SVF cells on aligned nanofibrillar collagen scaffolds. **(A)** Scanning electron microscopy image depicts nanofibrils arranged in parallel along the direction of the arrows. Confocal images show CD34 **(B)**, CD31 **(C)**, and CD105 **(D)** protein expression among adherent SVF cells on aligned nanofibrillar scaffolds after 1 day of attachment. Scale bars: 2 μm **(A)**; 50 μm **(B–D)**.

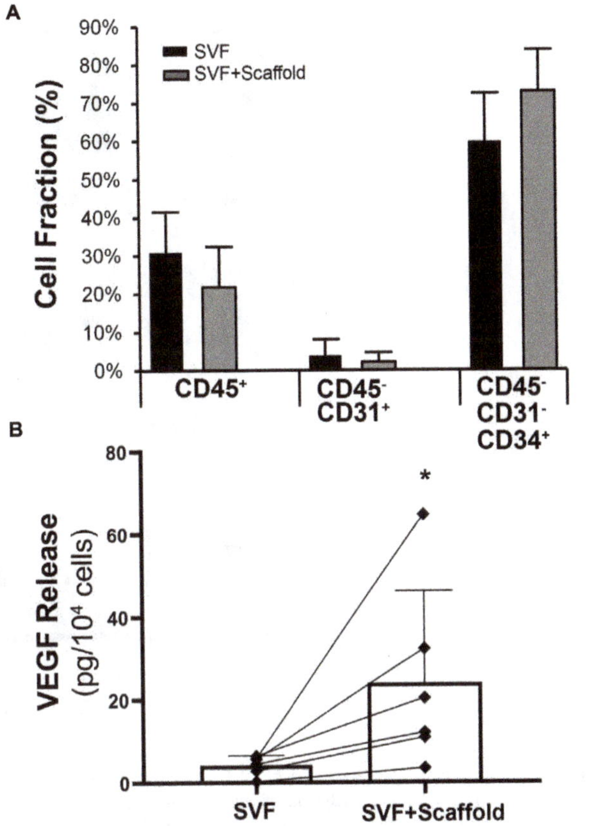

FIGURE 3 | Characterization of adherent SVF cells on aligned nanofibrillar scaffolds. **(A)** Phenotypic markers of adherent cells on aligned nanofibrillar scaffolds, compared to bulk SVF cells in suspension by flow cytometry ($n = 4$). **(B)** Quantification of VEGF protein release in the bulk SVF population, in comparison to the adherent cells seeded on aligned nanofibrillar scaffolds, for six independent donors. * denotes statistically significant relationship, compared to bulk SVF ($p < 0.05$).

group. In contrast, treatment with acellular scaffold alone had no therapeutic effect on the level of blood perfusion in the mouse ischemic limb. Likewise, treatment with SVF cellular injection alone did not have a significant benefit over PBS. Therefore, the combination of the SVF cells and aligned nanofibrillar scaffolds could be a promising therapeutic strategy to treat PAD.

Notably, cells attached to the scaffold *in vitro* produced significantly higher levels of VEGF, suggesting that cell attachment to the aligned collagen scaffold may be necessary for inducing VEGF production. This concurs with published literature showing that the gene expression of various pro-angiogenic factors such as VEGF could be regulated using hydrogels of various stiffnesses (Cai et al., 2016). Additionally, in our previous studies, we demonstrated that cellular attachment to aligned nanofibrillar scaffolds increased the gene expression of integrin α_1 subunit, which has been shown to be upregulated during angiogenesis (Nakayama et al., 2015). These studies highlight a potentially important role of nano-scale extracellular matrix interactions in mediating changes in cellular function. In a recent study, collagen biomaterial has been shown to enhance pro-angiogenic activity of CD34+ cells (McNeill et al., 2019). Together, the published literature supports our finding that mechanical and biophysical properties of biomaterials can modulate cellular secretion of angiogenic growth factors, which can contribute to pro-angiogenic capacity. However, further studies are warranted to elucidate the signaling mechanisms that govern how aligned nanofibrillar collagen scaffolds modulate cellular secretion of growth factors.

Another mechanism that may explain the increased blood perfusion with SVF-seeded scaffold treatment is cell survivability and persistence. In our previous studies, we observed that nanofibrillar scaffolds had increased the survival duration of endothelial cells, and this potentially also applies to other cell types such as SVF cells (Huang et al., 2013b; Nakayama et al., 2015). It is plausible that the nanofibrillar scaffold prolonged the survival of SVF cells, resulting in a longer duration of therapeutic effect (Hoareau et al., 2018).Besides VEGF, other interesting cellular signaling mechanisms may also be at play. Additionally, the small sample size and variability of blood perfusion recovery in this study may have precluded the possibility of observing significant improvements in the other treatment groups.

Previous studies have been conducted with the use of mononuclear cells as a therapy for CLI. Many of such preclinical and clinical studies used a heterogeneous population of mononuclear cells which showed mixed results in resolving limb pain, ulcers, and amputation rates in particular (Matoba

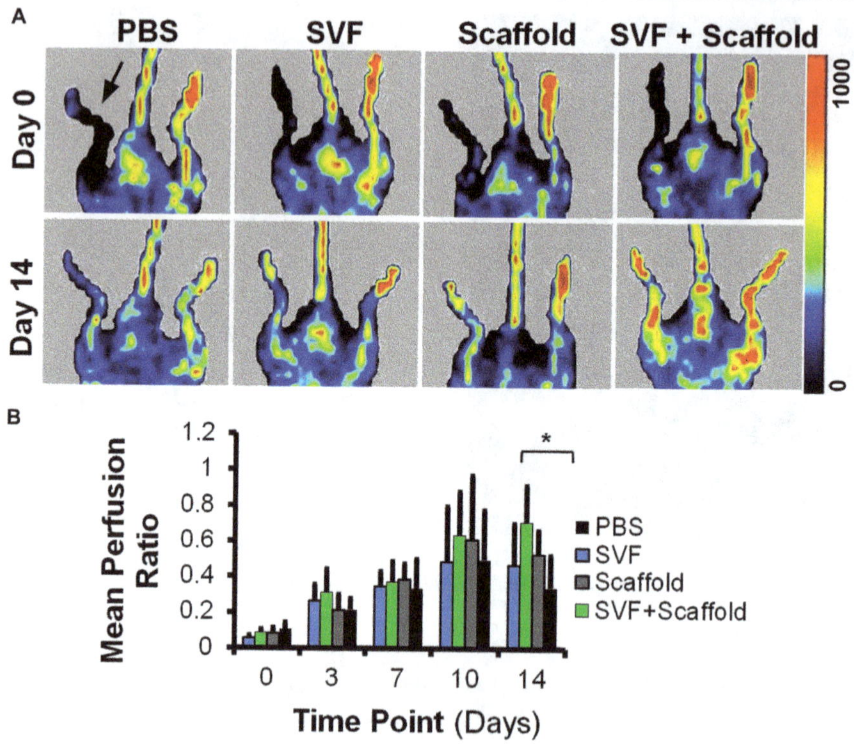

FIGURE 4 | Mean blood perfusion recovery after implantation of aligned nanofibrillar scaffolds seeded with SVF. **(A)** Representative laser Doppler spectroscopy images from day 0 and day 14. **(B)** Quantification of mean perfusion ratio (ischemic/control) over the course of 14 days (n = 5–9 per group). * denotes statistically significantly higher mean perfusion ratio in the SVF+Scaffold group, relative to the PBS group ($p < 0.05$). Arrow denotes ischemic limb.

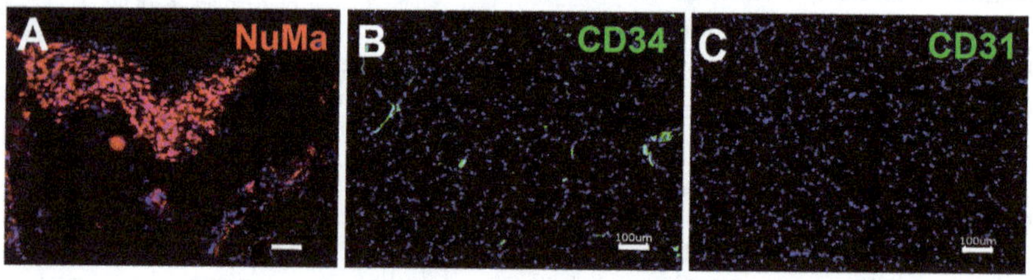

FIGURE 5 | Immunofluorescence staining of retained human SVF adjacent to the site of cell-seeded scaffold transplantation. **(A)** Human SVF are visualized using human specific nuclear matrix antigen (NuMA). Immunofluorescence imaging of human-specific antibodies targeting CD34 **(B)** and CD31 **(C)**. Scale bar: 50 μm **(A)**, 100 μm **(B,C)**.

et al., 2008; Teraa et al., 2015). Autologous stem cell therapy for PAD using mononuclear cells or MSC derived from bone marrow or peripheral blood improved the ulcer healing rate and reduced amputation rate, but no significant improvement in major limb salvage was reported (Gao et al., 2018). At least one clinical trial with the use of adipose-derived stem cells (ASC) to treat CLI is under way (Clinicaltrials.gov Identifier NCT03968198). ASC are multipotent cells that can differentiate in multiple cell types including endothelial cells (Cao et al., 2005). In addition to the multipotency of ASC, their benefits for vascular regeneration include paracrine secretion of cytokines and growth factors that may stimulate angiogenesis (Park et al., 2008). Pro-angiogenic potential of MSC is generally believed to be mediated by the secretion of multiple paracrine factors, and this property is largely similar between ASC (Park et al., 2008) and bone marrow derived MSC (Kwon et al., 2014).

The advantages of ASC over other stem cells include relative abundance of subcutaneous adipose tissue in many patients, ease of access without significant donor site morbidity (Tobita et al., 2011; Mizuno, 2013), and two orders of magnitude higher yield of cells per g tissue, compared to bone marrow (Mizuno, 2013; Ong and Sugii, 2013). However, MSC from both adipose tissue and bone marrow showed donor variability (Mohamed-Ahmed et al., 2018). Accordingly, the use of autologous ASCs showed a high variation in clinical outcome, due to differences in donor age, gender, and weight, and the anatomic harvest location and depth (Aksu et al., 2008; Baglioni et al., 2012).

Although this current study is not powered to evaluate donor-specific outcomes, it is plausible that inherent differences in the quality of donor SVF may lead to different *in vivo* angiogenic outcomes.

Freshly isolated SVF includes an abundant population of ASC, which can be identified as $CD34^{+}/CD31^{-}/CD45^{-}$ cells (Tevlin et al., 2016; Brett et al., 2017a), and are mostly of pericytic or mesenchymal phenotype (Traktuev et al., 2008). Non-hematopoietic SVF cells also have a small numbers of $CD31^{+}/CD34^{+}$ and $CD31^{+}/CD34^{-}$ cells, which are generally identified as endothelial progenitor and mature cells, respectively (Zimmerlin et al., 2013; Polancec et al., 2019), although the latter were also referred as co-expressing $CD34^{+}$ (Tallone et al., 2011).

Preclinical data showed that $CD34^{+}$ cells represent a main subset of stem/progenitor cells in peripheral blood mononuclear cell transplants that potentiate neovascularization in the ischemic area (Schatteman et al., 2000), and improve blood perfusion (Li et al., 2010) and wound healing (Tanaka et al., 2018). In the present study, $CD45^{-}/CD31^{-}/CD34^{+}$ comprised the majority of the SVF cells. To determine the contribution of $CD34^{+}$ SVF cells on revascularization in the setting of limb ischemia model, mechanistic studies in which $CD34^{+}$ cells are depleted can be performed in future studies. Nevertheless, clinical studies of mononuclear stem cell-based therapeutic angiogenesis employed to treat no-option CLI demonstrated that the number of transplanted $CD34^{+}$ cells was an independent predictor of positive outcome (Pan et al., 2019). In addition, in a study of donor variability of MSC proangiogenic efficacy, Kim et al. (2019) found that a subset of paracrine factors including VEGF serve as efficient biomarkers for predicting vascular regenerative efficacy of stromal/stem cells. Together, these studies together suggest a promising therapeutic benefit of $CD34^{+}$ cell therapy.

The SVF population in this study contained a relatively high fraction of $CD34^{+}$ cells, which are pro-angiogenic cells that are known to produce VEGF (Bautz et al., 2000). We also observed that the cells that attached to our nanofibrillar scaffold had a high amount of $CD34^{+}$ cells compared to cells containing other markers CD31 and CD45. Therefore, it is likely that the $CD34^{+}$ cells within the SVF contribute to the observed pro-angiogenic effects *in vitro* and *in vivo*.

CONCLUSION

This is the first study to evaluate an SVF-seeded aligned nanofibrillar scaffold as a potential therapy for PAD. *In vitro* the SVF seeded onto aligned scaffolds produced significantly higher levels of VEGF, compared to cells in suspension. Furthermore, *in vivo* the SVF-seeded scaffolds significantly increased blood perfusion after 14 days in a murine hindlimb ischemia model. SVF is a promising candidate for regenerative medicine due to its availability and as a source of pro-angiogenic cells. Our results suggest that aligned nanofibrillar scaffolds play an important role in enhancing the angiogenic potential of therapeutic cells and have important implications in the design of cell-based therapies for treatment of PAD in patients.

AUTHOR CONTRIBUTIONS

CH, TZ, CA, DN, DW, MP, and NH contributed to the conceptual design of the study. CH, TZ, CA, PT, SS, GY, and MB collected and analyzed the data. CH, TZ, CA, DN, DW, MP, and NH interpreted the data. CH, TZ, CA, MP, and NH wrote the manuscript, with input from all authors.

ACKNOWLEDGMENTS

We acknowledge the technical assistance Tanaka Tetsuo, Kiminami Hideaki, Nakagawa Yuuji, and Ishii Naoki from Terumo Corporation.

REFERENCES

Aksu, A. E., Rubin, J. P., Dudas, J. R., and Marra, K. G. (2008). Role of gender and anatomical region on induction of osteogenic differentiation of human adipose-derived stem cells. *Ann. Plast. Surg.* 60, 306–322. doi: 10.1097/sap.0b013e3180621ff0

Baglioni, S., Cantini, G., Poli, G., Francalanci, M., Squecco, R., Di Franco, A., et al. (2012). Functional differences in visceral and subcutaneous fat pads originate from differences in the adipose stem cell. *PLoS One* 7:e36569. doi: 10.1371/journal.pone.0036569

Bautz, F., Rafii, S., Kanz, L., and Mohle, R. (2000). Expression and secretion of vascular endothelial growth factor-a by cytokine-stimulated hematopoietic progenitor cells. Possible role in the hematopoietic microenvironment. *Exp. Hematol.* 28, 700–706. doi: 10.1016/s0301-472x(00)00168-5

Benjamin, E. J., Virani, S. S., Callaway, C. W., Chang, A. R., Cheng, S., Chiuve, S. E., et al. (2018). Heart disease and stroke statistics—2018 update: a report from the american heart association. *Circulation* 137, e67–e492.

Blackshear, C. P., Flacco, J. S., Vistnes, S. M., Chung, N. N., Irizarry, D., Brett, E. A., et al. (2017). Cell-based soft tissue reconstruction in a hydrogel scaffold. *Ann. Plast. Surg.* 79, 618–622. doi: 10.1097/sap.0000000000001194

Bobrov, Y., Fennell, L., Lazarev, P., Paukshto, M., and Remizov, S. (2002). Manufacturing of a thin-film LCD. *J. Soc. Inf. Display* 10, 317–321.

Bourin, P., Bunnell, B. A., Casteilla, L., Dominici, M., Katz, A. J., March, K. L., et al. (2013). Stromal cells from the adipose tissue-derived stromal vascular fraction and culture expanded adipose tissue-derived stromal/stem cells: a joint statement of the international federation for adipose therapeutics and science (ifats) and the international society for cellular therapy (isct). *Cytotherapy* 15, 641–648. doi: 10.1016/j.jcyt.2013.02.006

Brett, E., Tevlin, R., McArdle, A., Seo, E. Y., Chan, C. K. F., Wan, D. C., et al. (2017a). Human adipose-derived stromal cell isolation methods and use in osteogenic and adipogenic in vivo applications. *Curr. Protoc. Stem Cell Biol.* 43, 2H.1.1–2H.1.15.

Brett, E., Zielins, E. R., Chin, M., Januszyk, M., Blackshear, C. P., Findlay, M., et al. (2017b). Isolation of cd248-expressing stromal vascular fraction for targeted improvement of wound healing. *Wound Repair Regen.* 25, 414–422. doi: 10.1111/wrr.12542

Cai, L., Dewi, R. E., Goldstone, A. B., Cohen, J. E., Steele, A. N., Woo, Y. J., et al. (2016). Regulating stem cell secretome using injectable hydrogels with in situ network formation. *Adv. Healthc. Mater.* 5, 2758–2764. doi: 10.1002/adhm.201600497

Cao, Y., Sun, Z., Liao, L., Meng, Y., Han, Q., and Zhao, R. C. (2005). Human adipose tissue-derived stem cells differentiate into endothelial cells in vitro and improve postnatal neovascularization in vivo. *Biochem. Biophys. Res. Commun.* 332, 370–379. doi: 10.1016/j.bbrc.2005.04.135

Comella, K., Parcero, J., Bansal, H., Perez, J., Lopez, J., Agrawal, A., et al. (2016). Effects of the intramyocardial implantation of stromal vascular fraction in patients with chronic ischemic cardiomyopathy. *J. Transl. Med.* 14:158.

Davies, M. G. (2012). Criticial limb ischemia: epidemiology. *Methodist Debakey Cardiovasc. J.* 8, 10–14. doi: 10.14797/mdcj-8-4-10

Gao, L., Gregorich, Z. R., Zhu, W., Mattapally, S., Oduk, Y., Lou, X., et al. (2018). Large cardiac muscle patches engineered from human induced-pluripotent stem cell-derived cardiac cells improve recovery from myocardial infarction in swine. *Circulation* 137, 1712–1730. doi: 10.1161/circulationaha.117.030785

Gerhard, M., Baum, P., and Raby, K. E. (1995). Peripheral arterial-vascular disease in women: prevalence, prognosis, and treatment. *Cardiology* 86, 349–355. doi: 10.1159/000176899

Gupta, P. K., Chullikana, A., Parakh, R., Desai, S., Das, A., Gottipamula, S., et al. (2013). A double blind randomized placebo controlled phase i/ii study assessing the safety and efficacy of allogeneic bone marrow derived mesenchymal stem cell in critical limb ischemia. *J. Transl. Med.* 11:143.

Hadamitzky, C., Zaitseva, T. S., Bazalova-Carter, M., Paukshto, M. V., Hou, L., Strassberg, Z., et al. (2016). Aligned nanofibrillar collagen scaffolds – Guiding lymphangiogenesis for treatment of acquired lymphedema. *Biomaterials* 102, 259–267. doi: 10.1016/j.biomaterials.2016.05.040

Hoareau, L., Fouchet, F., Planesse, C., Mirbeau, S., Sindji, L., Delay, E., et al. (2018). Combined therapy for critical limb ischaemia: biomimetic plga microcarriers potentiates the pro-angiogenic effect of adipose tissue stromal vascular fraction cells. *J. Tissue Eng. Regen. Med.* 12, 1363–1373. doi: 10.1002/term.2667

Hou, L., Yang, G., Tang, S., Alcazar, C., Joshi, P., Strassberg, Z., et al. (2018). Small molecule derived from carboxyethylpyrrole protein adducts promotes angiogenesis in a mouse model of peripheral arterial disease. *J. Am. Heart Assoc.* 7:e009234.

Huang, N. F., Lai, E. S., Ribeiro, A. J., Pan, S., Pruitt, B. L., Fuller, G. G., et al. (2013a). Spatial patterning of endothelium modulates cell morphology, adhesiveness and transcriptional signature. *Biomaterials* 34, 2928–2937. doi: 10.1016/j.biomaterials.2013.01.017

Huang, N. F., Niiyama, H., Peter, C., De, A., Natkunam, Y., Fleissner, F., et al. (2010). Embryonic stem cell-derived endothelial cells engraft into the ischemic hindlimb and restore perfusion. *Arterioscler. Thromb. Vasc. Biol.* 30, 984–991. doi: 10.1161/atvbaha.110.202796

Huang, N. F., Okogbaa, J., Lee, J. C., Jha, A., Zaitseva, T., Paukshto, M., et al. (2013b). The modulation of endothelial cell morphology, function, and survival using anisotropic nanofibrillar collagen scaffolds. *Biomaterials* 34, 4038–4047. doi: 10.1016/j.biomaterials.2013.02.036

Kapur, S. K., and Katz, A. J. (2013). Review of the adipose derived stem cell secretome. *Biochimie* 95, 2222–2228. doi: 10.1016/j.biochi.2013.06.001

Kim, H. K., Lee, S. G., Lee, S. W., Oh, B. J., Kim, J. H., Kim, J. A., et al. (2019). A subset of paracrine factors as efficient biomarkers for predicting vascular regenerative efficacy of mesenchymal stromal/stem cells. *Stem Cells* 37, 77–88. doi: 10.1002/stem.2920

Kinnaird, T., Stabile, E., Burnett, M. S., Lee, C. W., Barr, S., Fuchs, S., et al. (2004). Marrow-derived stromal cells express genes encoding a broad spectrum of arteriogenic cytokines and promote in vitro and in vivo arteriogenesis through paracrine mechanisms. *Circ. Res.* 94, 678–685. doi: 10.1161/01.res.0000118601.37875.ac

Kwon, H. M., Hur, S. M., Park, K. Y., Kim, C. K., Kim, Y. M., Kim, H. S., et al. (2014). Multiple paracrine factors secreted by mesenchymal stem cells contribute to angiogenesis. *Vascul. Pharmacol.* 63, 19–28. doi: 10.1016/j.vph.2014.06.004

Levi, B., Wan, D. C., Glotzbach, J. P., Hyun, J., Januszyk, M., Montoro, D., et al. (2011). Cd105 protein depletion enhances human adipose-derived stromal cell osteogenesis through reduction of transforming growth factor beta1 (tgf-beta1) signaling. *J. Biol. Chem.* 286, 39497–39509. doi: 10.1074/jbc.m111.256529

Li, T. S., Kubo, M., Ueda, K., Murakami, M., Mikamo, A., and Hamano, K. (2010). Impaired angiogenic potency of bone marrow cells from patients with advanced age, anemia, and renal failure. *J. Thorac. Cardiovasc. Surg.* 139, 459–465. doi: 10.1016/j.jtcvs.2009.07.053

Lu, D., Chen, B., Liang, Z., Deng, W., Jiang, Y., Li, S., et al. (2011). Comparison of bone marrow mesenchymal stem cells with bone marrow-derived mononuclear cells for treatment of diabetic critical limb ischemia and foot ulcer: a double-blind, randomized, controlled trial. *Diab. Res. Clin. Pract.* 92, 26–36. doi: 10.1016/j.diabres.2010.12.010

Matoba, S., Tatsumi, T., Murohara, T., Imaizumi, T., Katsuda, Y., Ito, M., et al. (2008). Long-term clinical outcome after intramuscular implantation of bone marrow mononuclear cells (therapeutic angiogenesis by cell transplantation [tact] trial) in patients with chronic limb ischemia. *Am. Heart J.* 156, 1010–1018. doi: 10.1016/j.ahj.2008.06.025

McMurtry, D., Paukshto, M., and Bobrov, Y. (2008). *A Liquid Film Applicator Assembly and Rectilinear Shearing System Incorporating the Same: WO/2008/063631*. Geneva: World Intellectual Property Organization.

McNeill, B., Ostojic, A., Rayner, K. J., Ruel, M., and Suuronen, E. J. (2019). Collagen biomaterial stimulates the production of extracellular vesicles containing microrna-21 and enhances the proangiogenic function of cd34(+) cells. *FASEB J.* 33, 4166–4177. doi: 10.1096/fj.201801332r doi: 10.1096/fj.201801332r

Mizuno, H. (2013). Adipose-derived stem cells for regenerative medicine in the field of plastic and reconstructive surgery. *J. Oral Biosci.* 55, 132–136. doi: 10.1016/j.job.2013.04.005

Mohamed-Ahmed, S., Fristad, I., Lie, S. A., Suliman, S., Mustafa, K., Vindenes, H., et al. (2018). Adipose-derived and bone marrow mesenchymal stem cells: a donor-matched comparison. *Stem Cell Res. Ther.* 9:168.

Muthusubramaniam, L., Peng, L., Zaitseva, T., Paukshto, M., Martin, G. R., and Desai, T. A. (2012). Collagen fibril diameter and alignment promote the quiescent keratocyte phenotype. *J. Biomed. Mater. Res. A* 100, 613–621. doi: 10.1002/jbm.a.33284

Nakayama, K. H., Hong, G., Lee, J. C., Patel, J., Edwards, B., Zaitseva, T. S., et al. (2015). Aligned-braided nanofibrillar scaffold with endothelial cells enhances arteriogenesis. *ACS Nano* 9, 6900–6908. doi: 10.1021/acsnano.5b00545

Nakayama, K. H., Quarta, M., Paine, P., Alcazar, C., Karakikes, I., Garcia, V., et al. (2019). Treatment of volumetric muscle loss in mice using nanofibrillar scaffolds enhances vascular organization and integration. *Commun. Biol.* 2:170.

Niiyama, H., Huang, N. F., Rollins, M. D., and Cooke, J. P. (2009). Murine model of hindlimb ischemia. *J. Vis. Exp.* 23:1035.

Ong, W. K., and Sugii, S. (2013). Adipose-derived stem cells: fatty potentials for therapy. *Int. J. Biochem. Cell Biol.* 45, 1083–1086. doi: 10.1016/j.biocel.2013.02.013

Pan, T., Liu, H., Fang, Y., Wei, Z., Gu, S., Fang, G., et al. (2019). Predictors of responders to mononuclear stem cell-based therapeutic angiogenesis for no-option critical limb ischemia. *Stem Cell Res. Ther.* 10:15.

Park, B. S., Jang, K. A., Sung, J. H., Park, J. S., Kwon, Y. H., Kim, K. J., et al. (2008). Adipose-derived stem cells and their secretory factors as a promising therapy for skin aging. *Dermatol. Surg.* 34, 1323–1326. doi: 10.1111/j.1524-4725.2008.34283.x

Paukshto, M., McMurtry, D., Bobrov, Y., and Sabelman, E. (2008). *Oriented Collagen-Based Materials, Films and Methods of Making Same: WO/2008/131293*. Geneva: World Intellectual Property Organization.

Polancec, D., Zenic, L., Hudetz, D., Boric, I., Jelec, Z., Rod, E., et al. (2019). Immunophenotyping of a stromal vascular fraction from microfragmented lipoaspirate used in osteoarthritis cartilage treatment and its lipoaspirate counterpart. *Genes (Basel)* 10:474. doi: 10.3390/genes10060474

Qadura, M., Terenzi, D. C., Verma, S., Al-Omran, M., and Hess, D. A. (2018). Concise review: cell therapy for critical limb ischemia: an integrated review of preclinical and clinical studies. *Stem Cells* 36, 161–171. doi: 10.1002/stem.2751

Rigato, M., Monami, M., and Fadini, G. P. (2017). Autologous cell therapy for peripheral arterial disease: systematic review and meta-analysis of randomized, nonrandomized, and noncontrolled studies. *Circ. Res.* 120, 1326–1340. doi: 10.1161/circresaha.116.309045

Rochlin, D. H., Inchauste, S., Zelones, J., and Nguyen, D. H. (2020). The role of adjunct nanofibrillar collagen scaffold implantation in the surgical management of secondary lymphedema: review of the literature and summary of initial pilot studies. *J. Surg. Oncol.* 121, 121–128.

Rufaihah, A. J., Huang, N. F., Jame, S., Lee, J. C., Nguyen, H. N., Byers, B., et al. (2011). Endothelial cells derived from human ipscs increase capillary density and improve perfusion in a mouse model of peripheral arterial disease. *Arterioscler. Thromb. Vasc. Biol.* 31, e72–e79.

Schatteman, G. C., Hanlon, H. D., Jiao, C., Dodds, S. G., and Christy, B. A. (2000). Blood-derived angioblasts accelerate blood-flow restoration in diabetic mice. *J. Clin. Invest.* 106, 571–578. doi: 10.1172/jci9087

Tallone, T., Realini, C., Bohmler, A., Kornfeld, C., Vassalli, G., Moccetti, T., et al. (2011). Adult human adipose tissue contains several types of multipotent cells. *J. Cardiovasc. Transl. Res.* 4, 200–210. doi: 10.1007/s12265-011-9257-3

Tanaka, R., Masuda, H., Fujimura, S., Ito-Hirano, R., Arita, K., Kakinuma, Y., et al. (2018). Quality-quantity control culture enhances vasculogenesis and wound healing efficacy of human diabetic peripheral blood cd34+ cells. *Stem Cells Transl Med.* 7, 428–438. doi: 10.1002/sctm.17-0043

Teraa, M., Sprengers, R. W., Schutgens, R. E., Slaper-Cortenbach, I. C., van der Graaf, Y., Algra, A., et al. (2015). Effect of repetitive intra-arterial infusion of bone marrow mononuclear cells in patients with no-option limb ischemia: the randomized, double-blind, placebo-controlled rejuvenating endothelial progenitor cells via transcutaneous intra-arterial supplementation (juventas) trial. *Circulation* 131, 851–860. doi: 10.1161/circulationaha.114.012913

Tevlin, R., McArdle, A., Brett, E., Chung, M. T., Paik, K., Seo, E. Y., et al. (2016). A novel method of human adipose-derived stem cell isolation with resultant increased cell yield. *Plast. Reconstruct. Surg.* 138, 983e–996e.

Thangarajah, H., Vial, I. N., Chang, E., El-Ftesi, S., Januszyk, M., Chang, E. I., et al. (2009). Ifats collection: adipose stromal cells adopt a proangiogenic phenotype under the influence of hypoxia. *Stem Cells* 27, 266–274.

Tobita, M., Orbay, H., and Mizuno, H. (2011). Adipose-derived stem cells: current findings and future perspectives. *Discov. Med.* 11, 160–170.

Traktuev, D. O., Merfeld-Clauss, S., Li, J., Kolonin, M., Arap, W., Pasqualini, R., et al. (2008). A population of multipotent cd34-positive adipose stromal cells share pericyte and mesenchymal surface markers, reside in a periendothelial location, and stabilize endothelial networks. *Circ. Res.* 102, 77–85.

Zimmerlin, L., Donnenberg, V. S., Rubin, J. P., and Donnenberg, A. D. (2013). Mesenchymal markers on human adipose stem/progenitor cells. *Cytometry A* 83, 134–140.

Zuk, P. A., Zhu, M., Ashjian, P., De Ugarte, D. A., Huang, J. I., Mizuno, H., et al. (2002). Human adipose tissue is a source of multipotent stem cells. *Mol. Biol. Cell* 13, 4279–4295.

Zuk, P. A., Zhu, M., Mizuno, H., Huang, J., Futrell, J. W., Katz, A. J., et al. (2001). Multilineage cells from human adipose tissue: implications for cell-based therapies. *Tissue Eng.* 7, 211–228.

4

Application of the Nano-Drug Delivery System in Treatment of Cardiovascular Diseases

Yudi Deng [1,2†], Xudong Zhang [2†], Haibin Shen [2], Qiangnan He [2], Zijian Wu [2], Wenzhen Liao [2] and Miaomiao Yuan [1*]*

[1] The Eighth Affiliated Hospital, Sun Yat-sen University, Shenzhen, China, [2] Guangdong Provincial Key Laboratory of Tropical Disease Research, Department of Nutrition and Food Hygiene, School of Public Health, Southern Medical University, Guangzhou, China

***Correspondence:**
Wenzhen Liao
wenzhenliao@163.com
Miaomiao Yuan
yuanmm2019@163.com

† These authors have contributed equally to this work

Cardiovascular diseases (CVDs) have become a serious threat to human life and health. Though many drugs acting via different mechanism of action are available in the market as conventional formulations for the treatment of CVDs, they are still far from satisfactory due to poor water solubility, low biological efficacy, non-targeting, and drug resistance. Nano-drug delivery systems (NDDSs) provide a new drug delivery method for the treatment of CVDs with the development of nanotechnology, demonstrating great advantages in solving the above problems. Nevertheless, there are some problems about NDDSs need to be addressed, such as cytotoxicity. In this review, the types and targeting strategies of NDDSs were summarized, and the new research progress in the diagnosis and therapy of CVDs in recent years was reviewed. Future prospective for nano-carriers in drug delivery for CVDs includes gene therapy, in order to provide more ideas for the improvement of cardiovascular drugs. In addition, its safety was also discussed in the review.

Keywords: nano-drug delivery system, cardiovascular disease, targeting strategy, application progress, safety

INTRODUCTION

Cardiovascular diseases (CVDs) have become a serious worldwide public health problem, and the morbidity and mortality rank first above other diseases in the world (Gaurav et al., 2015). Faced with such a severe situation, developing drugs for the treatment of CVDs has become a top priority. Owing to the rapid development of nanoscience and outstanding performance of nanomaterials, nanotechnology has become a new solution to overcome the bottleneck of cardiovascular disease treatment. Nano-drug delivery systems (NDDSs) are a class of nanomaterials that have abilities to increase the stability and water solubility of drugs, prolong the cycle time, increase the uptake rate of target cells or tissues, and reduce enzyme degradation, thereby improve the safety and effectiveness of drugs (Quan et al., 2015; Gupta et al., 2019). NDDSs can be administered by various routes including inhalation, oral administration, or intravenous injection, remaining better bioavailability. In recent years, more scholars have started to develop nano-drug carrier system for the diagnosis and therapy of CVDs.

Additionally, as the application of nanomaterials increases, the exposure hazard of nanomaterials in clinical application also raises, resulting in the consequence that nanomaterials will have more opportunities to interact with blood vessels, blood, and their components, which will have an important impact on the human health. Therefore, this article mainly introduced the different types of NDDSs, their targeting strategies and application in CVDs, and the safety of nanomaterials was discussed as well.

TYPES OF THE NDDSs

NDDSs refer to material in which at least one dimension is in the range of nanometer scale (1–100 nm) or composed of them as basic units in three-dimensional space (Cooke and Atkins, 2016; Zhou et al., 2018). As an effective means to optimize the drug delivery, NDDSs have become a research hotspot in the field of pharmacy and modern biomedicine (Matoba et al., 2017). The investigation of NDDSs has been for more than 40 years, creating a mass of nano-drug carriers. According to the composition of the materials, the nanomaterials used in NDDSs can be divided into organic, inorganic and composite materials. The following is a description of several common NDDSs and their features (**Figure 1**, **Table 1**).

Liposomes

In general, liposomes are lipid vesicles formed by ordered phospholipid bilayer with cell-like structure (Landesman-Milo et al., 2013). As a type of drug carrier, liposomes show many advantages, such as non-toxic, non-immunogenicity, sustained-release drugs, prolonging drug action time, changing drug distribution *in vivo*, improving drug treatment index, reducing drug side effects, and so on (Yingchoncharoen et al., 2016). Liposomes can not only be easily developed for the entrapment of hydrophilic and ionic molecules, but compatible with hydrophobic drug (Chandrasekaran and King, 2014). Hydrophobic drugs can be surrounded by the bimolecular structure of phospholipids, and hydrophilic drugs, especially those containing genes, can be attached to the hydrophilic region of liposomes. The particle size, potential, and surface chemistry can be adjusted by modification of different lipid materials. Among various type of liposomes, cationic liposomes are positively charged, indicating that they may result in dose-dependent cytotoxicity and inflammatory responses, and as a kind of complexes, they may interact non-specifically with negatively charged serum proteins. Neutral lipids (Chapoy-Villanueva et al., 2015) and pH sensitive liposomes (Fan et al., 2017) are two ways to solve the above problems.

Polymer Micellar Co-delivery System

Polymer nanoparticles, another carriers for the delivery of drug, can be classified into non-biodegradable materials and biodegradable materials (Shi et al., 2019a,b). The synthetic polymer materials mainly include poly(lactic-co-glycolic acid) (PLGA), polyvinyl imine (PEI), polycaprolactone (PCL), polyvinyl alcohol (PVA), and so on (Danhier et al., 2012; Wei et al., 2018). These polymers exhibit biocompatibility, non-toxicity and no teratogenicity. Its degradation products, including oligomerization and final products, have no toxic effect on cells, and can coexist stably with most drugs. Natural polymers are mainly categorized into polysaccharides, peptides (Li et al., 2012), Chol and cyclodextrin inclusion complexes. Polymer nanoparticles usually formed by self-assembly of Amphiphilic block copolymers, are stable in the core and can be used to intercept insoluble drugs (Afsharzadeh et al., 2018). The stable structure of polymer nanoparticles is beneficial to the uniformity of particle size and the controlled release of drugs (Wang et al., 2011), and can effectively overcome the influence of gastrointestinal environment during oral administration. Their nanoscale and large surface area are conducive to uptake of drugs in cells and better bioavailability. Unfortunately, some polymer nanoparticles, have some drawbacks. For example, Chitosan, a natural polymer, is incompatible with biologic fluids, which can lead to particle degradation and reduce the working efficiency. Structural changes can be taken to solve its deficiency. Combining chitosan with polyethylene glycol, the conjugate has a unique endocytosis and macrophage phagocytosis mechanism (Yang et al., 2017). In addition, the modification of chitosan with a polypeptide can improve its working efficiency (Ping et al., 2017).

Dendritic Macromolecules

Macromolecules are synthetic, various-shaped and usually branched. Macromolecules shaped as sphere can be arranged in monodisperse space and mostly used as nano-carriers to be used for the administration and dissolution of insoluble targeted drugs. Dendritic macromolecules with unique branch structure, are also monodispersion and their molecular weight can be controlled. Besides, a large number of ready-made surface functional groups and hydrophobic environment are exist in the packaging, which make them an excellent drug delivery material (Kesharwani et al., 2012). Because of their excellent biological properties, dendritic macromolecules are widely used in biomedical and pharmaceutical fields, but the existence of surface cationic charge also limits their clinical application.

Metal Nanomaterials

The most commonly used metal nanomaterials are gold and silver nanomaterials, shaped in different structures that can be divided into/like nanoparticles, nanorods, nanocapsules, nanocuboid, and nanowire (Baeza et al., 2017). In addition to being used as nano-contrast agent for CT and surface-enhanced Raman spectroscopy, gold nanomaterials are also used in photothermal treatment of tumors and rheumatoid arthritis. As many studies shown, the application fields of silver nanomaterials mainly involved antibacterial, anti-infection and anti-tumor (Pietro et al., 2016). Moreover, some therapeutic drugs can be physically loaded into hollow gold or silver nanostructures (Liang et al., 2014), or chemically bonded to the surface of nanoparticles to achieve targeted delivery of the drugs. However, the removal of gold nanomaterials in human body is too slow, and the toxicity of silver ions *in vivo* limits the application of these metal nanomaterials in the treatment of chronic diseases.

Inorganic Non-metallic Nanomaterials

Inorganic non-metallic nanomaterials mainly include quantum dots, iron oxide, silicon, grapheme, and so on (Khafaji et al., 2019). Quantum dots (QDs), that is, semiconductor nanocrystals, are particularly focused on fluorescence imaging because of their unique luminous properties, while iron oxide nanoparticles are chiefly lay on the study of new MRI contrast agents (Jayagopal et al., 2009; Hauser et al., 2016; Su et al., 2017; Wei H. et al., 2017). Among them, mesoporous silicon nanomaterials have

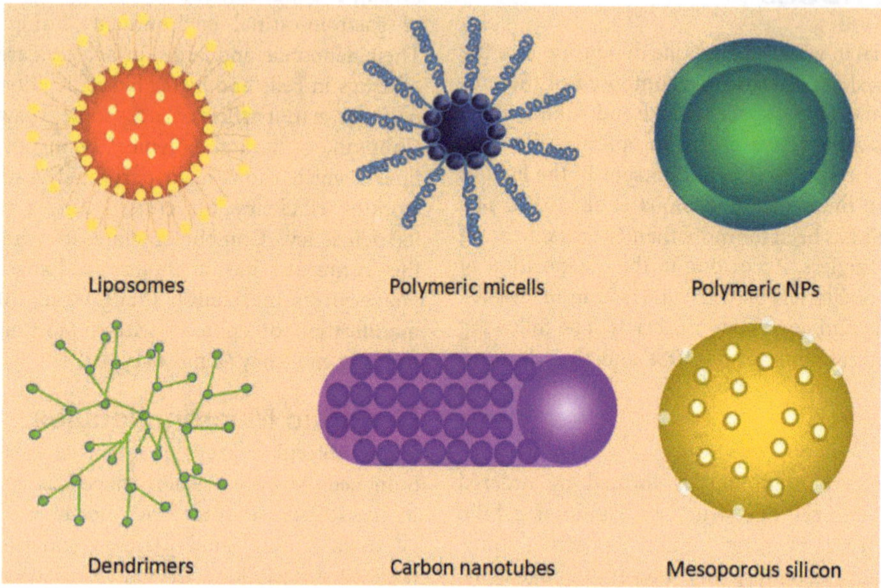

FIGURE 1 | Common types of nano-drug carriers.

TABLE 1 | Category and features of nano-drug carriers.

Category	Structure	Drug loading	Advantages	Limitations	References
Liposomes	Lipid bilayer	Physical encapsulation/Chemical connection	Great biocompatibility, none immunogenicity	Low stability, easy leakage of hydrophilic drug	Jain and Jain, 2018; Yue and Dai, 2018
Polymeric nanoparticles	Nanospheres/ Nanocapsules/Polymer-based nanoparticles with lipophilic core		Good stability, low leakage of drugs	Intravenous toxicity	Elsabahy and Wooley, 2012; Hu et al., 2018
Polymeric micelles	Core/shell architecture formed by self-assembly		Easily prepare, increase stability of hydrophobic drug	Low stability, depolymerization after dilution	Cagel et al., 2017
Metal nanomaterials	Nanoparticles, nanorods, nanocapsules, nanocuboid, and nanowire		Antibacterial properties, magneto-optical response characteristics	Toxicity, hard to degrade	Vimbela et al., 2017
Inorganic non-metallic nanomaterials	The same size with a adjustable pore size		Stable size, large surface area and pore volume, high drug loading	Extremely slow biodegradation rate	Yu F. et al., 2018

attracted more and more attention in the therapy of diseases in recent years due to its large surface area and porous structure (Wang W. et al., 2016). Those Inorganic nanomaterials can be used to improve the transport efficiency of drugs and genes in mammal cells through the integration of different functional groups. Meanwhile, they are suggested to be a kind of joint carrier with development potential. However, the bio-safety of inorganic non-metallic nanomaterials would be a considerable obstacle to their application in clinic (Perioli et al., 2019).

Composite Nanomaterials

In addition to the above nanomaterials, the preparation of composite nanomaterials with different properties is also under exploration in many studies. For example, metal or inorganic non-metallic nanomaterials are introduced into polymer or lipid nanomaterials to prepare multifunctional NDDSs containing both therapeutic drugs and contrast agents. Metal and inorganic nanomaterials are decorated or modified by organic materials to improve their physical and chemical properties, *in vivo* kinetic behavior and biocompatibility; and some NDDSs with special structure and diversified functions can be prepared by the combination of different metals and inorganic materials.

TARGETING STRATEGY OF THE NDDSs

The targeted design of NDDSs focuses on the diagnosis and therapy of cancer in the early stages of development, but recent researches argued that lesion cells or tissues of CVDs can also be targeted, even easier to targeted than tumor tissues with multiple physiological barriers. Compared with conventional preparations, the metabolic time of nano-transporter drugs in the blood circulation may be prolonged. By regulating pH value (Gao et al., 2018; Yi et al., 2018), temperature (Wei L. et al., 2017), light (Ding et al., 2011), ultrasound or biological enzyme (Zhang et al., 2019), the rate of those targeted nano-transporter drugs can be controlled to function longer.

Passive Target Transfer

Enhanced Vascular Permeability

Passive targeted transport mainly utilizes high permeability and high retention (EPR) effects (**Figure 2**) (Holback and Yeo, 2011). EPR refers to the fact that some molecules or particles tend to accumulate in tumor tissues (Dinarvand et al., 2011). The microvascular endothelial cell space in normal tissue is dense and intact, and NDDSs loaded with drug, generally in high molecular weight, are not easy to pass through the vascular wall. The tumor tissue is rich in blood vessels and poor in structural integrity (Torchilin, 2011). Those drug-loaded NDDSs in high molecular weight can selectively pass through the vascular wall and remain in the tumor tissue. A large number of studies have shown that nano-drug carriers with particle size <100 nm can be located and targeted to solid tumor tissues by EPR. Compared with the direct administration method, the nano-drug carrier can increase the accumulation of the drug in the tumor tissue by more than 10 times, greatly improving the bioavailability (Maeda et al., 2013). But it is discovered that EPR effect can also be used in various CVDs, not only for tumors. In some course of CVDs, for example, the occurrence and development of AS is a chronic inflammatory process, where vascular permeability is often increased, which is very similar to that of solid tumors. Vascular endothelial permeability provides an effective means for NDDSs to deliver from the lumen side to the interior of the plaque. The nano-drug carriers entering the circulation are also ingested by inflammatory cells (monocytes or macrophages), and these drug-carrying cells migrate to plaque inflammation, allowing drugs to be delivered in another way (Flogel et al., 2008).

Due to the size and surface characteristics of a portion of nanomaterials, they are rapidly cleared in the blood during intravenous injection, making nanomaterials unsuitable for drugs that require long cycle times. In this case, nano-coating technology can be applied to the nano-system for certain concealment, and the rate of administration of the coating agent can be also controlled and adjusted. This technology is particularly suitable for NDDSs in the treatment of CVDs. Developers on NDDSs have employed poly (ethylene glycol) (PEG) in particle design. In fact, PEG is a flexible hydrophilic polymer that can form a hydrated layer when grafted onto the surface, effectively reducing the adsorption of proteins on the surface (Jokerst et al., 2011). The tissue plasminogen activator is encapsulated in the nanoparticles, making the nanosystem concealed in some degree, thus protecting the tissue plasminogen activator from inactivation by plasma inhibitors and prolonging the half-life (Hemmati and Ghaemy, 2016).

Shear-Induced Targeting

Studies have shown that as the intima grew outward (toward the lumen) in CVDs, such as advanced AS or myocardial infarction, thrombosis or microthrombus occurs, stenosis of the blood vessels follows and blood flow rate through the plaque increases, and thus the fluid shear force increases. The mean blood fluid shear force in the normal vasculature is <70 dyne·cm^{-2}, while the blood fluid shear force in the AS plaque stenosis is up to 1,000 dyne·cm^{-2} (Korin et al., 2012). Therefore, the design of blood fluid shear-sensitive nanoparticles can achieve physicochemical targeting by utilizing the difference of blood fluid shear force between AS plaque and normal blood vessels. Holme et al. (2012) prepared a lenticular lipid nanoparticle vesicle with two sides convex. The drug-loaded nanometer can maintain structural stability in normal blood vessels, and the configuration change can be utilized to release the drug under the action of high blood fluid shear force through the blood circulation to the AS plaque. Inspired by the activation of platelets under the action of local high blood fluid shear forces in AS plaques and adhesion to plaque blood vessels, the researchers constructed a nanoparticle aggregate that can be assembled locally in plaques (Korin et al., 2012). First, the authors prepared PLGA nanoparticles with a particle size of about 180 nm and entrapped tissue plasminogen activator, and then obtained a PLGA nanoparticle aggregate with a particle size of 3.8 nm through spray drying. When the nanoparticles were exposed to the local high fluid shear stress of the AS plaque, they could be decomposed into 180 nm PLGA nanoparticles, and relied on the strong penetrability of the small particle size nanoparticles to enter the local thrombus of the plaque. The thrombolytic effect maximized the efficacy, significantly reduced the dose required for thrombolysis and the side effects of thrombolysis. In ischemic cardiomyopathy, the endothelial gap in ischemic myocardium widened, thus altering the shear of blood flow, and the concentration of polysaccharide from Ophiopogon japonicus in ischemic myocardium was twice as high as that in normal rats (Lin et al., 2010). Tan et al. found that both shear stress and blood flow shear rate of vascular wall could affect the aggregation of nanoparticles (Tan et al., 2011).

Magnetically Guided

Magnetically guided nanoparticle is an interesting "pseudo-passive" targeting method. Theoretically, the application of an external magnetic field can direct magnetic nanoparticles to the disease site (Prijic and Sersa, 2011). Recent evidence suggests that this strategy is beneficial for CVDs (Chandramouli et al., 2015). Alam et al. (2015) compared the effects of several nano drug carriers on atherosclerotic plaque imaging. Those Nanoparticles include iron oxide particles, superparamagnetic iron oxide nanoparticles, ultra-small superparamagnetic iron oxide nano-carrier, and very small superparamagnetic iron oxide nanoparticles. The results showed that the ultra-small superparamagnetic iron oxide nanoparticles have better vascular wall penetration ability and plaque retention than other groups. Some researchers have pointed out that the external magnetic field helps to transport particles from the cell-free layer which lacks red blood cells to the vessel wall (Freund and Shapiro, 2012).

Active Targeted Transhipment

On the basis of passive targeting, using the special pathological features of CVDs to develop an active targeting strategy for

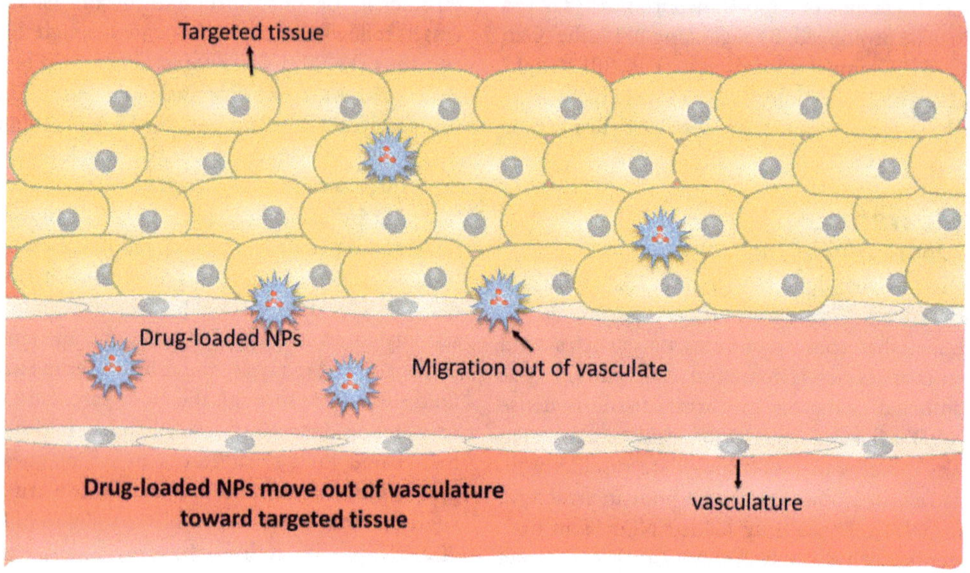

FIGURE 2 | Schematic representation of passive targeting. The occurrence and development of CVDs are chronic inflammatory processes in which vascular permeability is usually increased, and nanoparticles of appropriate size pass directly through the blood vessels and release the drug at the site of the disease.

CVDs can improve the targeted delivery efficiency of drugs to the lesions of CVDs, which aroused researchers strong interest. Active targeting is primarily directed to functional modification of NDDSs with one or more targets to allow the drug to reach a particular site (**Figure 3**) (Matoba and Egashira, 2014). That is to say, introducing a functional group or active substance that specifically interacts with diseased tissues or cells into the surface of the nano-drug carrier will enhance carriers targeting (Lee et al., 2006; Gullotti and Yeo, 2009). Some active targets are discussed in detail below (**Table 2**).

Active Targeting of Vascular Endothelial Cells

At different stages of CVDs, vascular endothelial cells are in an inflammatory activation state. Compared with normal vascular endothelial cells, some small molecules including intercellular adhesion molecule-1 (ICAM-1), vascular adhesion molecule-1 (VCAM-1), integrins, selectins, and so on, are often overexpressed, which provides the active target for NDDSs (Glass and Witztum, 2001). It is showed that the conjugation of lung-targeted single-stranded variable fragment/liposome together with platelet endothelial cell adhesion molecule-1 (PECAM-1) antibody increases liposome transport to the pulmonary vascular system and strengthen its anti-inflammatory effects (Hood et al., 2018). In 2013, Yang et al. decorated the surface of silica nanoparticles with anti-VCAM-1 monoclonal antibody. The nanoparticles were able to bind to sites of inflammation before they were taken up by endothelial cells (Yang et al., 2013).

Based on the pathological features of high expression of ICAM-1 in early vascular endothelial cells of AS, Paulis et al. (2012) modified the antibody anti-ICAM-1 which actively targets ICAM-1 on the surface of liposomes and used it to load contrast agents (gadolinium). Studies have shown that the liposome could achieve the activated targeting of vascular endothelial cells and AS plaques through the specific action of anti-ICAM-1 and ICAM-1. However, competitive binding of circulating white blood cells to the ICAM-1 site and blood flow shearing could reduce the targeting function of liposomes to AS plaques. The authors optimized the binding degree of liposome to ICAM-1 by screening liposome particle size, antibody and lipid ratio, and obtained higher active targeting efficiency.

E-selectin is a surface glycoprotein of endothelial cells, which can promote the attachment of monocytes/macrophages and lymphocytes to induce inflammatory response, and eventually cause the occurrence and development of CVDs, such as AS (Ma et al., 2016). E-selectin can also be used as a target for nano-transport drugs. Functional liposomes carrying mouse H18/7 mAb (specific antibody to E-selectin) were used to act on interleukin (IL)-1β-activated human umbilical vein endothelial cells and non-interleukin (IL)-1β-activated human umbilical cord Vein endothelial cells. It was found that the ability of functional liposomes to target activated human umbilical vein endothelial cells is 275 times that of the non-activated type (Flaht-Zabost et al., 2014).

AT1 rises in myocardial when myocardial infarction or heart failure happened. Dvir et al. (2011) designed a polyethylene glycol liposomes (142 ± 8 nm), that could carry therapeutic payloads (such as growth factors, cytokines, etc.) and released them in a controlled manner. The ligand attached on these liposomes is a string of amino chain sequenced Gly-Asp-Arg-Val-Tyr-Ile-His-Pro-Phe (binding sequence of AT1 receptor), which could direct the nanoparticles to the infarction heart.

Active Targeting of Macrophages or Foam Cells

Macrophages or foam cells play a key role in the development of AS. In the early stage of AS, mononuclear/macrophages were recruited to activate vascular endothelial cells, and

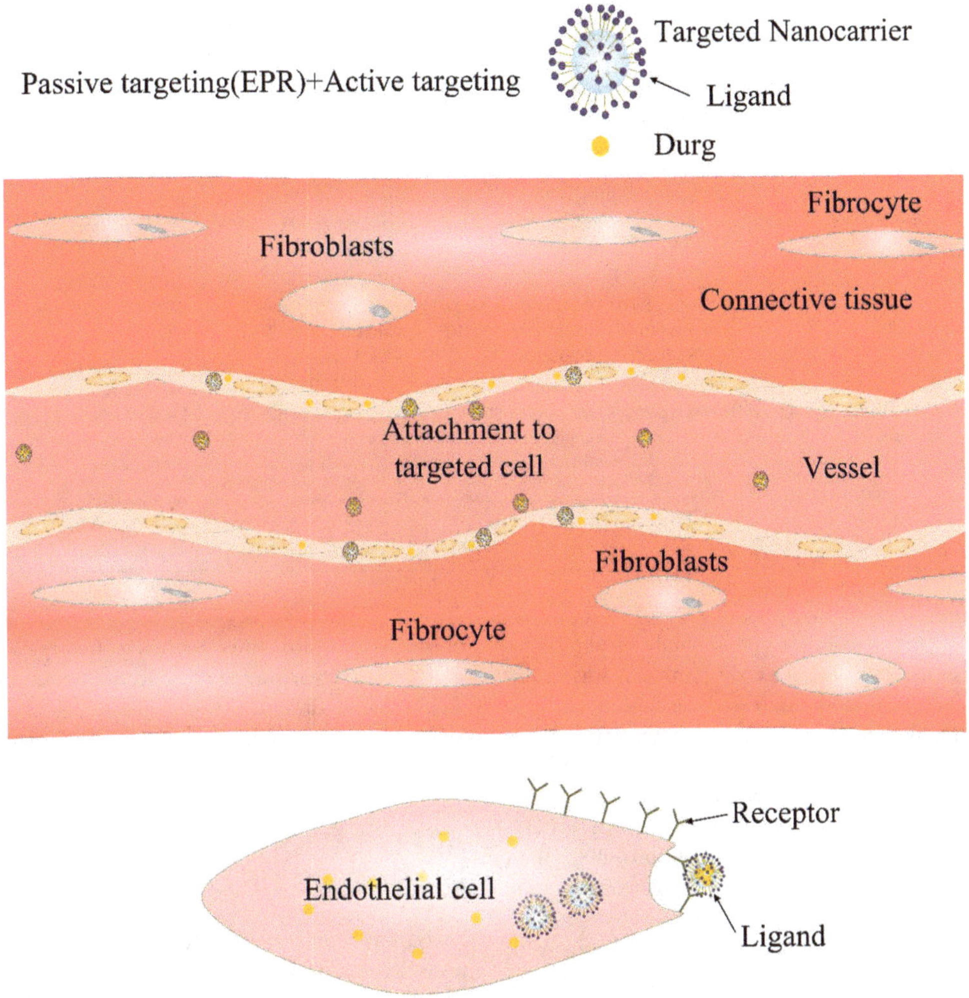

FIGURE 3 | Diagrammatic sketch of active targeting. The surface of the nano-carrier is grafted with a targeting ligand, which is strongly bound to the selective cell surface by ligand-receptor binding.

overexpressed some inflammation-related receptor molecules in an inflammatory environment, such as CD44 and interleukin-4 (IL-4) receptors, etc. Imaging and drug delivery for macrophages or foam cells using NDDSs will facilitate monitoring of disease progression and drug treatment in AS.

For example, Lee et al. (2015) linked 5β-cholic acid and fluorescent dye Cy5.5 to the carboxyl group of the HA skeleton by chemical bonding and formed nanoparticles (HA-NPs) by self-assembly. Compared with nanoparticles (HGC-NPs) constructed with chitosan backbones that did not target CD44 receptors, HA-NP could significantly increase the uptake of activated macrophages, and the plaque site of $ApoE^{-/-}$ mouse (AS model) was more targeted. Fluorescence co-localization studies indicated HA -NP was mainly distributed in macrophages in plaques.

Park et al. (2008) used phage library screening technology to optimize the amphiphilicity of the target IL-4 receptor peptide (CRKRLDRNC) which was modified on amphiphilic chitosan (with ethylene glycol chitosan as the backbone and 5β-cholate bonded) by chemical bond. Then nanoparticles with the function of targeted macrophages in AS plaque are obtained in a self-assembled method.

Targeting Vascular Basement Membrane Collagen

It has been reported that the vascular basement membrane of damaged blood vessels and inflammation sites is rich in collagen IV (Col IV) (Duner et al., 2015). In 2013, Kamaly et al. (2013) ligated the 7 amino acid oligopeptide molecule KLWVLPK (PLEA-β-PEG-Col IV) targeting collagen IV at the PEG end of the PLGA-β-PEG block copolymer and used it to package Act-26 (With anti-inflammatory and inhibition of leukocyte extravasation), thus nanoparticles (Ac2-26 Col IV NPs) targeting damaged blood vessels and collagen sites of inflammation sites were prepared. The results showed that Act-26 Col IV NPs reduced the migration and adhesion of neutrophils to the inflammation site and inhibited the development of inflammation. Further, in 2016, some researchers prepared nanoparticles (Col-IV IL-10 NPs) containing anti-inflammatory factor IL-10 by self-assembly using PLGA-p-PEG-Col IV and

TABLE 2 | Some molecules which can provide the active target for NDDSs.

Superfamily	Lectin adhesion molecules		Ig-superfamily cell adhesion molecules			Hyaluronic acid receptor
Cell adhesion molecule	**P-selectin**	**E-selectin**	**VCAM-1**	**ICAM-1**	**PECAM-1**	
CD classification	CD62P	CD62E	CD106	CD54	CD31	CD44
Surface expression	Inducible	Inducible	Inducible	Constitutive and up-regulated upon induction	Constitutive	Widely distributed, cell surface, transmembrane
Temporal expression	Expression is fast and transient; internalized within 20 min	Peak expression at 4 h (*in vitro*); declines to baseline within 24 h during inflammation	Very low copies/cell; increases to 10^4-10^5 copies/cell	10^4-10^5 copies/cell in normal tissue *d*; 3- to 5-fold increase in inflammation	10^6 copies/cell	–
Ligands	Leukocyte expressing sialyl-Lewis X	Leukocyte expressing sialyl-Lewis X	Leukocyte with β1 integrin VLA-4 (α4β1) and α4β7	Leukocyte with β2 integrins (e.g., LFA-1 and Mac-1)	Leukocyte with β1 and β3 integrins Heparin proteoglycans	Hyaluronic acid
Function	Leukocyte tethering and rolling		Leukocyte firm adhesion		Leukocytes transmigration; angiogenesis	Participation in heterogeneous adhesion

PDLA-PEG-OMe targeting collagen LV (Kamaly et al., 2016). After intravenous administration of $Ldlr^{-/-}$ mice, it was found that Col-IV IL-10 NP significantly increased the content of IL-10 in the plaque, and had better AS treatment effect than free IL-10.

In addition, multi-target nano-carriers with multiple inflammatory cell characteristics have been studied. PLNs incorporated these often ignored biophysical design criteria of platelet-mimetic discoid morphology and flexibility, then integrated these design parameters with the platelet-mimetic biochemical heteromultivalent interactive functions by dendritic presentation of multiple peptides that bind simultaneously to both activated natural platelets and injured endothelial sites (Anselmo et al., 2014).

Whether it is passive targeting or active targeting, the final targeting efficiency depends on the biological and physical properties of nanoparticles. The biological and physical properties includes particle size and distribution, targeting unit types, surface chemistry, morphology and density (Morachis et al., 2012). For the body, the development stage, type as well as location of CVDs and tumor, vascular wall shear rate, blood composition and its fluid type, together with other factors will greatly affect the targeting efficiency (Charoenphol et al., 2011). Although the application of active targeting NDDSs in clinical diagnosis and therapy is extremely attractive, its development is still facing great challenges. Those challenges are mainly reflected in two aspects: one is the limitation of the discovery of ideal target; the other is that there are still many bottleneck problems in the design and preparation of effective targeting nanosystem.

Multifunctional Responsiveness NDDSs

Multifunctional responsive NDDSs is a kind of drug carrier with better targeting ability, which is developed on the basis of the above two targeting modes of nano-drug carrier. In addition to having the previous targeting ability, this kind of carrier is generally composed of stimulating responsive materials, which can be released under the stimulation of the special environment of the focus site, thus reducing the release in the normal tissue and increasing the drug accumulation of the lesion tissue. At the same time, diagnostic molecules can be assembled or labeled on nano-carriers to compose an integrated diagnosis and therapy system.

APPLICATION OF THE NDDSs IN THE DIAGNOSIS OF CVDs

Early, rapid and accurate detection is important for effective prevention and treatment of CVDs. The application of molecular imaging in the diagnosis of CVDs has been paid more and more attention in recent years. In addition to the constant innovation of various imaging technologies, new contrast agents are the key to real-time, fast, high sensitivity and high resolution diagnostics. Compared with conventional contrast agents, nano-contrast agents have the following advantages: (1) *in vivo* stabilization, regulable distribution, and prolonging the half-life of contrast agents or drugs; (2) controllable physical and chemical properties (such as chemical composition, size) and imaging performance; (3) specific identification of certain biomolecules; (4) ability of multimodal imaging realization; (5) values in individualized diagnosis and therapy are expected to be realized (Attia et al., 2016). By designing specific nano-probes with the unique chemical signal molecules of diseased tissues determined by pathological studies, the contrast agent can be directed to the lesion area in the early stage of the disease for magnetic resonance imaging (MRI), X-ray imaging, fluorescence imaging, and contrast-enhanced ultrasound (US) imaging (**Figure 4**).

Magnetic Resonance Imaging

In many imaging methods, magnetic resonance imaging is non-invasive, safe, and high resolution, and it is good for soft tissue imaging. However, the sensitivity of MRI is not high (10^{-3}-10^{-9} M). The complexes of gadolinium commonly used in clinical

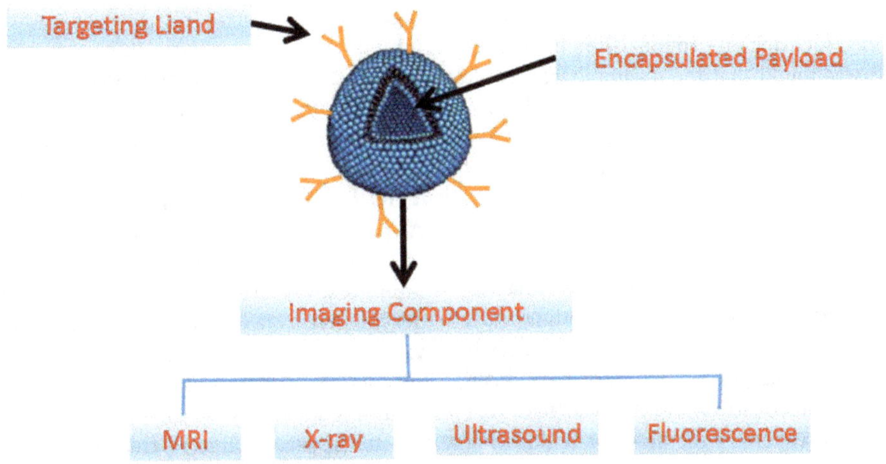

FIGURE 4 | Abridged general view map of targeted nanoparticles engineered for imaging and drug delivery. The components of a multifunctional nanocarrier include a ligand for cellular targeting, and an encapsulated payload for delivery of the therapeutic agents. The imaging components can be incorporated in the interior payload, on the targeting ligand or associated with the nanoparticle shell.

practice are used as T1-weighted imaging contrast agents, and gadolinium has certain nephrotoxicity. Fe_3O_4 nanoparticles are considered to be non-toxic T2-weighted imaging contrast agents (Corot et al., 2006). Compared with tinctures, they have high sensitivity, good tissue compatibility and superparamagnetism (Kim et al., 2007). Targeted contrast agents are used to accumulate MRI probes at a sufficiently high concentration (in micrograms to milligrams) in the target tissue to achieve a high signal to noise ratio.

It is discovered that vascular imaging can be performed in the early stage of cardiovascular disease formation, and drugs can be administered for treatment after the magnetic nanoparticles are injected into the body. Yoo et al. (2016) loaded the hydrophilic lipid (amphiphilic) gadolinium chelating agent diethylenetriamine pentaacetic acid (DTPA) into a dendritic polymer and then wrapped it in the kernel of amphiphilic micelles and connected with fibrin binding agent. Thus, its targeting to atherosclerotic plaque was enhance, and can be used for early detection of thrombus. Winter et al. chose paramagnetic nanoparticles targeting integrin $\alpha v\beta 3$ to inject intravenously into high fat fed New Zealand white rabbits to detect neovascularization in plaques in the early stage of AS (Winter et al., 2008).

X-Ray Imaging

Imaging with radionuclides plays a crucial role in the field of nuclear medicine (Mottu et al., 1999, 2002). Radionuclides are not only sensitive but also quantifiable. Positron emission tomography (PET) and single photon emission computed tomography (SPECT) are the most common types (Alie et al., 2015). At present, radionuclide-labeled nanomaterials can be used to monitor the embolization process and the distribution of nanomedicine to achieve targeted imaging (Mottu et al., 2002; Okamura et al., 2002; Torchilin, 2002; James et al., 2006). For example, the researchers used ^{186}Re-BMEDA (Bao et al., 2003) and ^{99m}Tc-PEGylate-labeled (Bao et al., 2004) doxorubicin liposomes to perform SPECT, which can trace the distribution of drugs in the body, and also promote drug release. The nanoparticles can be used to detect the formation of atherosclerotic plaques by CT and to judge the prognosis as well. Galperin et al. injected iodine nanoparticles contrast agent (N1177) into mice via vein. It was found that the contrast agent gathered in macrophage rich tissue, and the signal of atheromatous plaques could be significantly enhanced, and the enhancement time could last for more than 30 min (Galperin et al., 2007). In 2016, Chhour et al. (2016), used 11 mercaptoundecanoic acid (11-MUDA) to encapsulate gold nanoparticles, found that gold nanoparticles could accumulate in foam cells of atherosclerotic plaques and increase the contrast of imaging.

Fluorescence Imaging

Optical imaging is a powerful imaging method with the advantages of no radiation, no invasion, high resolution and good controllability, but its penetration is poor. Fluorescence imaging is usually performed by using fluorescein to generate fluorescence signals. Near-infrared fluorescence (NIRF) probes are widely used because of their strong penetrating power and safety. They have been used in small animal living imaging systems and clinical tumor transformation. At present, a large number of nano-drug carriers, such as liposomes, metal, or non-metallic nanoparticles can enclose NIRF to achieve optical imaging of blood vessels (Weissleder and Ntziachristos, 2003; Setua et al., 2010; Sevick-Muraca, 2012). Its application in cardiovascular disease imaging has been paid more and more attention. McCarthy et al. bound the group of near infrared light activated therapeutic (NILAT) with macrophage-targeted magnetic nanoparticles(MNP) and prepared a kind of diagnostic and therapeutic nanoparticles (McCarthy et al., 2006). The experiment results shown that within 24 h of administration, the nanoparticles were reached in area. Wang Y. et al. (2016) injected profilin-1 magnetic iron oxide nanoparticles (PF1-Cy5.5-DMSA-Fe_3O_4-NPs) focusing on profilin-1 into the vein of atherosclerotic mice. It was found that the magnetic iron oxide nanoparticles were aggregated in carotid atherosclerotic plaques. There was a good correlation between the MRI signal of the animals injected with PC-NPs and the fluorescence intensity of NIRF imaging *in vitro*.

Ultrasound Imaging

Compared with fluorescence imaging, ultrasound imaging has natural advantages in medical imaging including safe, convenient, and real-time. Nano-ultrasound imaging materials that can be targeted to vascular-related markers have been developed. For example, vascular ultrasound nanoparticles that can be targeted to high expression of the vascular endothelial growth factor receptor 2 (VEGFR2) not only provide a more clear ultrasound imaging of tumor blood vessels, but also promote drug localization in blood vessels (Rojas et al., 2018). Marsh et al. had developed perfluorocarbon nanoparticles targeting blood fibrin, carrying the thrombus drug streptokinase for the diagnosis and therapy in thrombus (Marsh et al., 2007). The drug-loaded particles are synthesized by evaporation/dispersion technique with a diameter of about 250 nm and can be used for ultrasonic imaging.

Multi-Modal Bioimaging

At present, multi-modal imaging technology using a combination of different types of imaging methods can integrate different imaging methods to produce synergistic effects, providing more comprehensive and accurate image information for accurate diagnosis and precise treatment of CVDs. For instance, it was found that ^{64}Cu-labeled SPIO-loaded doxorubicin nanoparticles could be used for MRI and PET (Yang et al., 2011). It has been reported that Cy5, sputum, and folic acid can be embedded in gold nanoparticles to achieve trimodal optical imaging, MRI and CT imaging in mice (Chen et al., 2016). This multimodal imaging and integration of diagnosis and treatment will be a new direction for the development of cardiovascular nanomedicine in the future.

APPLICATION OF THE NDDSs IN THE TREATMENT OF CVDs

The NDDSs in AS

AS is the most common type of CVDs, often leading to a stroke or heart attack. The formation of AS begins with endothelial dysfunction. Plaque-induced coronary artery stenosis can cause ischemic cardiomyopathy, while plaque rupture can cause acute myocardial infarction (Nabel and Braunwald, 2012; Wall, 2013). Mechanisms of plaque instability include enhanced vascular permeability, Platelet endothelial cell adhesion molecules (PECAM) expression, macrophage aggregation, and expression of proteases, which can be targets for intervention. The drug can be delivered to atherosclerotic plaques by nano-drug carrier, to effectively prolong the half-life of drug plasma, increase the concentration of lesions and reduce side effects. The treatment strategies of these nano-drug carriers including regulating lipoprotein level, reducing the degree of inflammation, inhibiting of neovascularization, preventing coagulation, and so on (**Table 3**). These treatment strategies are used as interventions to development of AS, reduce plaque area or stabilize vulnerable plaques (Chetprayoon et al., 2015; Bejarano et al., 2018).

The NDDSs in Hypertension

At present, many kinds of drugs are applied for the treatment of hypertension, including angiotensin converting enzyme inhibitors, vascular angiotensin antagonists, central sympathetic nerve drugs, adrenergic receptor blockers, diuretics and vasodilators (Sharma et al., 2016). However, all these antihypertensive therapeutic drugs have obvious defects, including short plasma half-life, low bioavailability, toxic and side effects (upper respiratory tract abstraction, angioedema, reflex tachycardia, extreme hypotensive effect, and so on) (Alam et al., 2017; Martin et al., 2017; Niaz et al., 2017). Conversely, nano-drug carriers can provide prominent advantages mentioned above (**Table 4**) (Kimura et al., 2009). Some researchers have made olmesartan into a nanoemulsion system. Compared with the conventional dose, the nanoemulsion group has better blood pressure lowering effect, longer maintenance time, and can produce nearly three times the dose reduction (Alam et al., 2017).

The NDDSs in Pulmonary Hypertension

Pulmonary hypertension, a progressive highly dangerous disease, is characterized by increased pulmonary vascular resistance and elevated pulmonary artery pressure. Prostaglandin I, Endothelin receptor antagonist, type 5 phosphodiesterase inhibitor, etc. are common vasodilators for pulmonary hypertension. These vasodilators have shown some effects, but the overall therapeutic ability is limited. For solving this problem, nano-mediated drug delivery system has gradually become an important alternative strategy (**Table 5**). Bosentan is a selective and competitive Endothelin receptor antagonist, which is loaded into nanoparticles and has a solubility of seven times as much as that of unprocessed bosentan (Ghasemian et al., 2016).

The NDDSs in Myocardial Infarction

Reperfusion is mainly used in the early stage of myocardial infarction, but it can cause apoptosis, calcium overload and reactive oxygen species. These factors cause the opening of the mitochondrial membrane permeability transition pore (MPTP) and the increase of mitochondrial outer membrane permeability, thereby promoting cardiomyocyte apoptosis and necrosis (Hausenloy and Yellon, 2013). Clinically, the drug therapy for myocardial ischemia mainly depends on growth factors, cytokines and some small molecular compounds. These drugs have the same disadvantages of the above traditional drugs. The high permeability of blood vessels and enrichment of monocytes in ischemic myocardium can be harnessed to deliver drugs by targeting ability of nano-drug carriers (**Table 6**).

The NDDSs in Other CVDs

As a new drug delivery platform, nano-drug delivery system also performs well in other CVDs. Coronary artery allogeneic

TABLE 3 | Application of the NDDSs in the AS.

Carrier	Ligand	Drug	Intervention mode	Model	References
Liposome	–	Glucocorticoids (PLP)	Intravenous injection (I.V.)	Rabbit	Lobatto et al., 2010
Dendrimeric nanoparticles	Mannose	Liver-x-receptor ligands(LXR-L)T091317	Intravenous injection (I.V.)	LDLR$^{-/-}$ mouse	He et al., 2018
Acetylated β-CD materials (Ac-bCDs)	–	Rapamycin (RAP)	Subcutaneous injection	ApoE$^{-/-}$ mouse	Dou et al., 2016
Polylactic acid-glycolic acid (PLGA)	Hyaluronan (HA), apolipoproteins A-1 (apoA-1)	Simvastatin	*In vitro*	Dynamic system of Endothelial macrophage Co-culture	Zhang et al., 2017
Peptide amphiphilic nanofiber	A1 apolipoprotein	Drug liver X receptor agonist GW 3965(LXR)	Intravenous injection (I.V.)	Mouse	Mansukhani et al., 2019
Acetal-CD (Ac-bCD) and ROS-sensitive CD-CD (Ox-bCD)	Acetaldehyde, sensitive to ROS	Rapamycin	Intraperitoneal injection (I.P.)	Mouse	Dou et al., 2017

TABLE 4 | Application of the NDDSs in the treatment of hypertension.

Carrier	Drug	Intervention mode	Model	References
Poly (D, L-lactide) (PLA)	Aliskiren	Gavage	Male spontaneously hypertensive rats (SHR)	Pechanova et al., 2019
Niosomes	Lacidipine (LAC)	Oral	Hypertensive rats	Qumbar et al., 2017
Lliposome	Valsartan	Cutaneous penetration	Experimental hypertensive rats	Ahad et al., 2016
Chitosan (CS) polymer	Captopril, amlodipine and valsartan	Oral	–	Niaz et al., 2016
Chitosan and polyethylene glycol composite sol.	Nitric oxide, NO precursor (nitrite)	Oral	–	Cabrales et al., 2010

angiopathy is an inflammatory proliferation process that undermines the long-term success of heart transplantation. Lipid nanoparticles coated with methotrexate or paclitaxel were injected intravenously into rabbits which fed cholesterol-rich diet and received an ectopic heart transplant, both of which reduced macrophage infiltration in the graft (Barbieri et al., 2017). Myocardial ischemia is mainly due to the decrease of aortic perfusion in the heart, resulting in insufficient oxygen supply and unstable myocardial energy metabolism, thus forming a pathological state that cannot support the normal work of the heart. Liposomes coated with phenytoin (PHT, a non-selective VGSC inhibitor) were prepared by thin film dispersion. The results showed that PHT-encapsulated liposomes partially inhibited I/R injury-induced CD43$^+$ inflammatory monocyte expansion and reduced infarct size and left ventricular fibrosis after intravenous injection of the rat myocardial I/R injury model (Zhou et al., 2013).

Vascular restenosis is the process of stenosis and obstruction after the interventional treatment of the blood vessels, such as angioplasty, arteriotomy, implantation of an endovascular stent, and so on (Wang et al., 2018). Some scientists (Banai et al., 2005; Kamath et al., 2006; Nakano et al., 2009; Schröder et al., 2018; Xi et al., 2018) have proposed that in the site of angioplasty, catheter-intervention techniques are used to infuse the drug-loaded nanoparticles into the injury site, enabling angioplasty, and topical administration in one step. The nanoparticles can enter the arterial wall through the damaged endothelium, localize, reside in and between cells, and then slowly release the drug (Wu et al., 2019). Therefore, the lesion vessel can be maintained at a relatively high concentration for a long period of time, which is beneficial to fully exerting the drug effect, and finally effectively prevents and treats vascular restenosis.

APPLICATION OF THE CO-LOADED NANO-SYSTEM IN THE CVDs

Drug combination therapy (including genes) is the treatment of two or more drugs to patients at the same time. In clinical practice, this therapy has been widely used for disease treatment. The purpose of this combination therapy is often due to the synergistic effect between drugs, or the therapeutic effect of multiple drugs is greater than that of a single drug. In recent years, many co-loaded nano-systems have been developed to carry common drugs and/or genes, especially siRNA to treat CVDs.

Application of RNAi in the Treatment of CVDs

RNA interference (RNAi) is a gene-specific silencing mechanism present in eukaryotic cells and an important measure for resisting foreign genes and infections during biological evolution. RNAi was first discovered in *Caenorhabditis elegans* (Braukmann et al., 2017), then in 2001, it was demonstrated to occur in mammalian cells (Lendeckel et al., 2001). RNA interference includes micro RNA (miRNA), small interfering RNA (siRNA),

TABLE 5 | Application of the NDDSs in pulmonary hypertension.

Carrier	Ligand	Drug	Intervention mode	Model	References
Nanostructured lipid carriers (NLCs)	–	Sildenafil (SC)	Endotracheal administration	A549 cells, rat	Nafee et al., 2018
Polymeric nanoparticles	Vitamin A	Nitric oxide(NO)	–	Hepatic stellate cells (HSCs)	Duong et al., 2015
Nanocomposite particle (nCmP)	–	Tacrolimus (TAC)	Direct intervention	A549 cells	Wang Z. et al., 2016
Liposome	Peptide CARSKNKDC (CAR)	Fasudil and superoxide dismutase (SOD)	Direct intervention, endotracheal administration	Pulmonary endothelial and smooth muscle cells, rat	Gupta et al., 2015
Poly(D,L-lactide-co-glycolide) nanoparticles	–	Silaenafil	Endotracheal administration	–	Beck-Broichsitter et al., 2012
Liposome	–	Cerivastatin	Endotracheal administration	Rat	Lee et al., 2018

TABLE 6 | Application of the NDDSs in myocardial infarction.

Carrier	Ligand	Drug	Intervention mode	Model	References
Poly(D,L-lactide-co-glycolide) (PLGA)	–	Insulin-like growth factor (IGF)-1	Injection in the heart	Mouse	Chang et al., 2013
Low molecular weight polyethyleneimine	Deoxycholic acid (PEI1.8-DA)	siRNA against Src homology region 2 domain-containing tyrosine phosphatase-1 (SHP-1)	Cardiac administration	Myocardial infarction (MI) rats	Dongkyu et al., 2013
Liposome	P-selectin	Vascular endothelial growth factor (VEGF)	–	Myocardial infarction (MI) rats	Scott et al., 2009
Distearyl phosphatidylethanolamine polyethylene glycol	Atrial natriuretic peptide (ANP)	Oleate adenosine prodrug (Ade-OA)	Intravenous injection (I.V.)	Acute myocardial infarction (AMI) rats	Yu J. et al., 2018
Polylactic co-glycolic acid nanoparticles	–	Vascular endothelial growth factor (VEGF)	Injection into the peri-infarct region	Infarcted mouse	Oduk et al., 2018
Lipid core nanoparticles (LDE)	–	Methotrexate (MTX)	Intraperitoneal injection(I.V.)	Myocardial infarction (MI) rats	Maranhao et al., 2017

Piwi-interacting RNA, and long non-coding (lncRNA). RNAi technology, also known as gene silencing, introduces double-stranded RNA (dsRNA) consisting of sense and antisense RNAs corresponding to a certain mRNA sequence into cells, degrading mRNA homologously complementary thereto, and inhibiting the expression of cell-specific genes. The rapid development of RNAi research has driven it from experimental technology to therapeutic development tools (Katyayani et al., 2017), and RNAi has potential value in the treatment of CVDs (Kwekkeboom et al., 2014; Tadin-Strapps et al., 2015; Hoelscher et al., 2017). At the same time, RNA interference therapy also has challenges in the treatment of CVDs, including the toxicity, targeting, time-effect, and effective delivery system of RNA, which limits its widespread use in the clinic and is urgently needed to be solved and improved (Cotten et al., 1992; Sioud, 2015; Kasner et al., 2016; Navickas et al., 2016; Zhou et al., 2016). **Table 7** indicated the future direction of cardiovascular RNA interference.

Co-loaded Gene and Drug Nano-System

For overcoming the problems in the delivery process and realizing the broad potential of RNAi-based therapeutics, safe and efficient nano delivery systems are needed. The apolipoprotein B (ApoB) siRNA was encapsulated into the liposome vector. After 48 h, the ApoB mRNA of the macaque liver decreased, and the maximum silencing rate exceeded 90%. ApoB protein, serum cholesterol, and low-density lipoprotein levels began to decrease 24 h after treatment and continued until day 11 (Zimmermann et al., 2006). Some researchers have used chitosan nanoparticles to construct and package small interfering RNA (siRNA) against PDGF-B mRNA expression vector, and then transfected into vascular smooth muscle cells (vSMC) of rabbit arterial wall damaged by balloon catheter, using therapeutic ultrasound for gene delivery. The results showed that the nanoparticles significantly inhibited the expressions of PCNA and PDGF-B mRNA in intimal vSMCs while the local intimal thickness and area were also reduced remarkably (Xia et al., 2013). Nox2-NADPH expression is significantly increased in the infarcted myocardium. Somasuntharam et al. (2013) demonstrated acid-degradable polyketal particles for Nox2-siRNA to the post-MI heart, which not only reduced siRNA degradation, but also inflammation.

Some pharmaceutical companies have developed new nano-dosages that deliver siRNA to the right cells at the right time (Hayden, 2014). Healthy volunteers (serum LDL levels of 3 mmol/L or higher) were injected intravenously with ALN-PCS or

TABLE 7 | Future directions in cardiovascular RNA interference.

Investigation	Novel strategies	Future perspectives	References
RNAi imaging *in vivo*	Prolyl hydroxylase domain protein 2 (PHD2)- short interfering RNA (shRNA) sequence followed by a hypoxia response element-containing promoter driving a firefly luciferase reporter gene	Imaging of RNAi distribution in space and time in experimental animal models	Huang and Wu, 2011
Cardiac-targeted RNAi	Cardiotropic adeno-associated virus 9 (AAV9)-based silencing of Ca^{2+} cycle regulator phospholamban for the treatment of severe heart failure via intravenous route	Cardiac-specific gene knockout for therapeutic purposes, and as an alternative for cardiac-specific inducible knockout models	Suckau et al., 2009
Induction of alloimmune tolerance by RNAI	In heart transplantation models, RNAi induced alloimmune tolerance through silencing of toll-like receptor (TLR) adaptors My D88 and TIR-domain-containing adapter-inducing interferon-β (TRIF)	*In vivo* treatment of recipients with siRNAs to My D88 and TRIF prolonged allograft survival	Zhang et al., 2012
Plaque stabilization by RNAI	Lentivirus-based RNAi to silence chymase increased plaque stability in *in vivo*	Chymase as a target for plaque stabilization in vasculature as an RNAi target	Guo et al., 2013
Monocyte-targeted RNAi	Nanoparticle-encapsulated synthetic siRNA for silencing of monocytic chemokine receptor C-C chemokine receptor type 2 (CCR2) in myocardial infarction	Non-viral RNAi delivery system targeting monocytes *in vivo*, with high translational potential	Majmudar et al., 2013

placebo developed by Alnylam Pharmaceuticals (Fitzgerald et al., 2014). ALN-PCS is a siRNA that inhibits the synthesis of PCSK9 and is assembled in lipid nanoparticles. PCSK9 protein in the human body cycle was reduced 70%, and LDL was reduced by 40% after intravenous injection of ALN-PCS.

The co-loaded gene and drug nano-system combined with nanotechnology and gene interference technology, the packaged substances have a synergistic effect, and the therapeutic effect is much better than the single treatment (**Figure 5**). Carvedilol, a kind of anti-hypertrophic drug that simultaneously blocks β-adrenergic receptors non-specifically in various organs, is widely used and effective. The non-specific genome-wide downregulation of p53 expression by specific siRNA efficiently abrogates cardiac hypertrophy. However, it can cause extensive tumorigenesis affecting bystander organs. Rana et al. (2015) encapsulated these bioactive molecules with stearic acid modified carboxymethyl chitosan (CMC) nanopolymers conjugated to a homing peptide for delivery *in vivo* to hypertrophied cardiomyocytes, resulted in effective regression of cardiac hypertrophy.

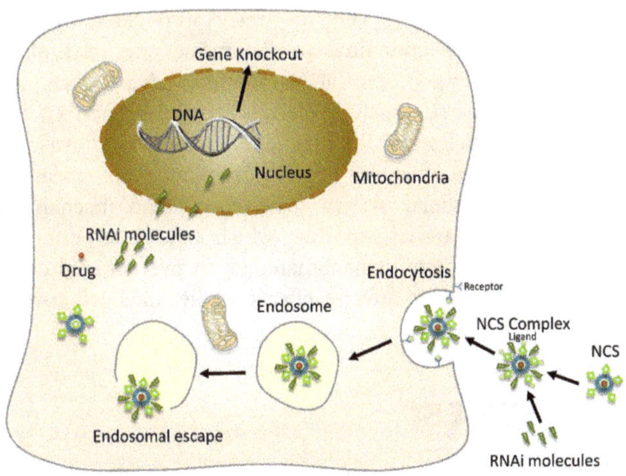

FIGURE 5 | Schematic diagram of nanoparticles-mediated gene and drug delivery. Nano-carrier system (NCS) encapsulates or adsorbs a drug, a therapeutic foreign gene molecule on its surface, and also couples a specific targeting molecule to the surface of the nano-carrier and then binds to a cell surface-specific receptor through a targeting molecule. This enables safe and effective targeted genes and drug treatment.

SAFETY OF THE NDDSs

As the researches of nanomaterials go further, an increasing number of nanomaterials are prepared as NDDSs, but the unclear toxicity and the lack of systematically study of materials themselves restrict their further application. When the particle size enters the nanometer scale, it will show strong surface effect, small scale effect, quantum scale effect and macroscopic quantum tunneling effect (Gatoo et al., 2014).

Relatively few studies discuss about toxicity of NDDSs, particular in cardiovascular toxicity. But the tissue of cardiovascular system is considered to be the key site of NDDSs induced toxicity, which can produce great impact on the disease prognosis. Studies have revealed that nanomaterials could enter the blood circulation through respiratory tract, digestive tract, skin and other mucous membranes, and inevitably interacted with the blood system, immune system and other organs or tissues including plasma proteins and immune proteins, blood cells and immune cells, and so on.

The safety evaluation of the NDDSs is mainly focused on the toxicological study of the health effect. At present, the cardiovascular toxicity of nanomaterials based on animal and cell level shown that the toxicity was closely related to a series of undesirable effects induced by nanomaterials, including oxidative stress, inflammation apoptosis, blood aggregation and cardiac signal transduction (Donnini et al., 2000; Savic et al., 2003; Chen and Von, 2005; Qinghua et al., 2005). Among them, inflammatory reaction and oxidative stress are recognized as the main mechanisms of cardiovascular toxicity of nanomaterials.

Inflammatory response can affect the occurrence and development of CVDs including hypertension, myocarditis, AS, acute myocardial infarction and heart failure. Some researchers have found that if nano-carriers have not been removed in time, they could reach all organs through blood, stimulate the body to produce a series of inflammatory cytokines, and eventually lead to cytotoxicity, which increases the risk of cardiovascular events (Suwa et al., 2002).

Nanomaterials have a large number of surface atoms and are highly reactive, which can generate free radicals and stimulate the formation of ROS, thereby interfering with antioxidant systems (Chen and Von, 2005). Oxidative stress can induce oxidative damage to macromolecular substances, such as DNA and proteins, which leads to cell growth inhibition, cell cycle abnormalities, and cell death.

The study on the toxic mechanism of cardiovascular system damage caused by nanomaterials in global is still in its infancy. There is very few relevant research evidence on the biological endpoints to determine the relationship between the physicochemical parameters (shape, size, size distribution, surface structure, electrochemical properties, etc.) of the nanoparticles and the toxic effects of the cardiovascular system. Therefore, scientists need to carry out more researches on the cardiovascular system toxic effects and mechanisms of typical nanomaterial exposure, which can make better use of the positive effects of nanomaterials to prevent, reduce or eliminate the possible adverse effects on health. Furthermore, it would provide theoretical and technical basis for the establishment of nanomaterial safety evaluation technology and standards.

SUMMARY AND PERSPECTIVE

In conclusion, the nano-carrier, as an efficient, specific and controllable intracellular drug delivery method, has shown unique advantages in the diagnosis and therapy of CVDs. It can effectively solve the problems of targeting, local drug delivery, controlled release, sustained release, and reducing toxicity while it is developing toward the multifunctional and integrated direction of diagnosis and therapy. With the innovation of nanotechnology and the deepening studies on molecular pathological mechanism of CVDs, the application of NDDSs will be promoted, and new techniques and methods will be provided for clinical diagnosis and therapy. In addition, since the study on these nano-carriers is in its infancy, many problems still remain unclear. The main challenge is how to solve the biocompatibility of nano-drug-loaded particles themselves or their degradation products, which is need to be solved in the field of nano-biomedicine in the future.

AUTHOR CONTRIBUTIONS

WL proposed and developed the research outline, MY contributed to the concept and content framework, YD wrote the first draft and XZ prepared the drawings and contributed to improving the draft. HS and QH polished the article. ZW modified the format.

REFERENCES

Afsharzadeh, M., Hashemi, M., Mokhtarzadeh, A., Abnous, K., and Ramezani, M. (2018). Recent advances in co-delivery systems based on polymeric nanoparticle for cancer treatment. *Artif. Cells Nanomed. Biotechnol.* 46, 1095–1110. doi: 10.1080/21691401.2017.1376675

Ahad, A., Aqil, M., Kohli, K., Sultana, Y., and Mujeeb, M. (2016). Nano vesicular lipid carriers of angiotensin II receptor blocker: anti-hypertensive and skin toxicity study in focus. *Artif. Cells Nanomed. Biotechnol.* 44, 1002–1007. doi: 10.3109/21691401.2015.1008509

Alam, S. R., Stirrat, C., Richards, J., Mirsadraee, S., Semple, S. I., Tse, G., et al. (2015). Vascular and plaque imaging with ultrasmall superparamagnetic particles of iron oxide. *J. Cardiovasc. Magn. Reson.* 17:83. doi: 10.1186/s12968-015-0183-4

Alam, T., Khan, S., Gaba, B., Haider, M. F., Baboota, S., and Ali, J. (2017). Nanocarriers as treatment modalities for hypertension. *Drug Deliv.* 24, 358–369. doi: 10.1080/10717544.2016.1255999

Alie, N., Eldib, M., Fayad, Z. A., and Mani, V. (2015). Inflammation, atherosclerosis, and coronary artery disease: PET/CT for the evaluation of atherosclerosis and inflammation. *Clin. Med. Insights Cardiol.* 8, 13–21. doi: 10.4137/CMC.S17063

Anselmo, A. C., Modery-Pawlowski, C. L., Menegatti, S., Kumar, S., Vogus, D. R., Tian, L. L., et al. (2014). Platelet-like nanoparticles: mimicking shape, flexibility, and surface biology of platelets to target vascular injuries. *ACS Nano* 8, 11243–11253. doi: 10.1021/nn503732m

Attia, M. F., Anton, N., Akasov, R., Chiper, M., Markvicheva, E., and Vandamme, T. F. (2016). Biodistribution and toxicity of X-ray iodinated contrast agent in nano-emulsions in function of their size. *Pharm. Res.* 33, 603–614. doi: 10.1007/s11095-015-1813-0

Baeza, A., Ruiz-Molina, D., and Vallet-Regi, M. (2017). Recent advances in porous nanoparticles for drug delivery in antitumoral applications: inorganic nanoparticles and nanoscale metal-organic frameworks. *Expert Opin. Drug Deliv.* 14, 783–796. doi: 10.1080/17425247.2016.1229298

Banai, S., Chorny, M., Gertz, S. D., Fishbein, I., Gao, J., Perez, L., et al. (2005). Locally delivered nanoencapsulated tyrphostin (AGL-2043) reduces neointima formation in balloon-injured rat carotid and stented porcine coronary arteries. *Biomaterials* 26, 451–461. doi: 10.1016/j.biomaterials.2004.02.040

Bao, A., Goins, B., Klipper, R., Negrete, G., and Phillips, W. T. (2003). 186Re-liposome labeling using 186Re-SNS/S complexes: *in vitro* stability, imaging, and biodistribution in rats. *J. Nucl. Med.* 44, 1992–1999. Available online at: http://apps.webofknowledge.com/full_record.do?product=UA&search_mode=GeneralSearch&qid=14&SID=5AxlSYBEVr5fqZXGOKg&page=1&doc=1

Bao, A., Goins, B., Klipper, R., Negrete, G., and Phillips, W. T. (2004). Direct 99mTc labeling of pegylated liposomal doxorubicin (Doxil) for pharmacokinetic and non-invasive imaging studies. *J. Pharmacol. Exp. Ther.* 308, 419–425. doi: 10.1124/jpet.103.059535

Barbieri, L. R., Lourenço-Filho, D. D., Tavares, E. R., Carvalho, P. O., Gutierrez, P. S., Maranhão, R. C., et al. (2017). Influence of drugs carried in lipid nanoparticles in coronary disease of rabbit transplanted heart. *Ann. Thorac. Surg.* 104, 577–583. doi: 10.1016/j.athoracsur.2016.12.044

Beck-Broichsitter, M., Kleimann, P., Gessler, T., Seeger, W., Kissel, T., and Schmehl, T. (2012). Nebulization performance of biodegradable sildenafil-loaded nanoparticles using the Aeroneb Pro: formulation aspects and nanoparticle stability to nebulization. *Int. J. Pharm.* 422, 398–408. doi: 10.1016/j.ijpharm.2011.10.012

Bejarano, J., Navarro-Marquez, M., Morales-Zavala, F., Morales, J. O., Garcia-Carvajal, I., Araya-Fuentes, E., et al. (2018). Nanoparticles for diagnosis and therapy of atherosclerosis and myocardial infarction: evolution toward prospective theranostic approaches. *Theranostics* 8, 4710–4732. doi: 10.7150/thno.26284

Braukmann, F., Jordan, D., and Miska, E. (2017). Artificial and natural RNA interactions between bacteria and *C. elegans*. *RNA Biol.* 14, 415–420. doi: 10.1080/15476286.2017.1297912

Cabrales, P., Han, G., Roche, C., Nacharaju, P., Friedman, A. J., and Friedman, J. M. (2010). Sustained release nitric oxide from long-lived circulating nanoparticles. *Free Radic. Biol Med.* 49, 530–538. doi: 10.1016/j.freeradbiomed.2010.04.034

Cagel, M., Tesan, F. C., Bernabeu, E., Salgueiro, M. J., Zubillaga, M. B., Moretton, M. A., et al. (2017). Polymeric mixed micelles as nanomedicines: achievements and perspectives. *Eur. J. Pharm. Biopharm.* 113, 211–228. doi: 10.1016/j.ejpb.2016.12.019

Chandramouli, S., Sanjana, S., and Swathi, S. (2015). Use of super paramagnetic iron-oxide nanoparticles in the treatment of atherosclerosis. *IFMBE Proc.* 46, 67–70. doi: 10.1007/978-3-319-11776-8_17

Chandrasekaran, S., and King, M. R. (2014). Microenvironment of tumor-draining lymph nodes: opportunities for liposome-based targeted therapy. *Int. J. Mol. Sci.* 15, 20209–20239. doi: 10.3390/ijms151120209

Chang, M. Y., Yang, Y. J., Chang, C. H., Tang, A. C., Liao, W. Y., Cheng, F. Y., et al. (2013). Functionalized nanoparticles provide early cardioprotection after acute myocardial infarction. *J. Control Release* 170, 287–294. doi: 10.1016/j.jconrel.2013.04.022

Chapoy-Villanueva, H., Martinez-Carlin, I., Lopez-Berestein, G., and Chavez-Reyes, A. (2015). Therapeutic silencing of HPV 16 E7 by systemic administration of siRNA-neutral DOPC nanoliposome in a murine cervical cancer model with obesity. *J. Buon.* 20, 1471–1479. Available online at: http://apps.webofknowledge.com/full_record.doproduct=UA&search_mode=GeneralSearch&qid=3&SID=5AxlSYBEVr5fqZXGOKg&page=1&doc=1

Charoenphol, P., Mocherla, S., Bouis, D., Namdee, K., Pinsky, D. J., and Eniola-Adefeso, O. (2011). Targeting therapeutics to the vascular wall in atherosclerosis–carrier size matters. *Atherosclerosis* 217, 364–370. doi: 10.1016/j.atherosclerosis.2011.04.016

Chen, J., Sun, Y., Chen, Q., Wang, L., Wang, S. H., Tang, Y., et al. (2016). Multifunctional gold nanocomposites designed for targeted CT/MR/optical trimodal imaging of human non-small cell lung cancer cells. *Nanoscale* 8, 13568–13573. doi: 10.1039/c6nr03143a

Chen, M., and Von, M. A. (2005). Formation of nucleoplasmic protein aggregates impairs nuclear function in response to SiO_2 nanoparticles. *Exp. Cell Res.* 305, 51–62. doi: 10.1016/j.yexcr.2004.12.021

Chetprayoon, P., Matsusaki, M., and Akashi, M. (2015). Three-dimensional human arterial wall models for *in vitro* permeability assessment of drug and nanocarriers. *Biochem. Biophys. Res. Commun.* 456, 392–397. doi: 10.1016/j.bbrc.2014.11.094

Chhour, P., Naha, P. C., O'Neill, S. M., Litt, H. I., Reilly, M. P., Ferrari, V. A., et al. (2016). Labeling monocytes with gold nanoparticles to track their recruitment in atherosclerosis with computed tomography. *Biomaterials* 87, 93–103. doi: 10.1016/j.biomaterials.2016.02.009

Cooke, J. P., and Atkins, J. (2016). Nanotherapeutic solutions for cardiovascular disease. *Methodist. Debakey Cardiovasc. J.* 12, 132–133. doi: 10.14797/mdcj-12-3-132.

Corot, C., Robert, P., Idee, J. M., and Port, M. (2006). Recent advances in iron oxide nanocrystal technology for medical imaging. *Adv. Drug Deliv. Rev.* 58, 1471–1504. doi: 10.1016/j.addr.2006.09.013

Cotten, M., Wagner, E., Zatloukal, K., Phillips, S., Curiel, D. T., and Birnstiel, M. L. (1992). High-efficiency receptor-mediated delivery of small and large (48 kilobase gene constructs using the endosome-disruption activity of defective or chemically inactivated adenovirus particles. *Proc. Natl. Acad. Sci. U.S.A.* 89, 6094–6098. doi: 10.1073/pnas.89.13.6094

Danhier, F., Ansorena, E., Silva, J. M., Coco, R., Le Breton, A., and Preat, V. (2012). PLGA-based nanoparticles: an overview of biomedical applications. *J. Control Release* 161, 505–522. doi: 10.1016/j.jconrel.2012.01.043

Dinarvand, R., Sepehri, N., Manoochehri, S., Rouhani, H., and Atyabi, F. (2011). Polylactide-co-glycolide nanoparticles for controlled delivery of anticancer agents. *Int. J. Nanomedicine* 6, 877–895. doi: 10.2147/IJN.S18905

Ding, J., Zhuang, X., Xiao, C., Cheng, Y., Li, Z., He, C., et al. (2011). Preparation of photo-cross-linked pH-responsive polypeptide nanogels as potential carriers for controlled drug delivery. *J. Mater. Chem.* 21, 11383–11391. doi: 10.1039/C1JM10391A

Dongkyu, K., Jueun, H., Hyung-Ho, M., Hye Yeong, N., Hyejung, M., Hoon, J. J., et al. (2013). Anti-apoptotic cardioprotective effects of SHP-1 gene silencing against ischemia-reperfusion injury: use of deoxycholic acid-modified low molecular weight polyethyleneimine as a cardiac siRNA-carrier. *J. Control Release* 168, 125–134. doi: 10.1016/j.jconrel.2013.02.031

Donnini, D., Perrella, G., Stel, G., Ambesi-Impiombato, F. S., and Curcio, F. (2000). A new model of human aortic endothelial cells *in vitro*. *Biochimie* 82, 1107–1114. doi: 10.1016/s0300-9084(00)01195-0

Dou, Y., Chen, Y., Zhang, X., Xu, X., Chen, Y., Guo, J., et al. (2017). Non-proinflammatory and responsive nanoplatforms for targeted treatment of atherosclerosis. *Biomaterials* 143, 93–108. doi: 10.1016/j.biomaterials.2017.07.035

Dou, Y., Guo, J., Chen, Y., Han, S., Xu, X., Shi, Q., et al. (2016). Sustained delivery by a cyclodextrin material-based nanocarrier potentiates antiatherosclerotic activity of rapamycin via selectively inhibiting mTORC1 in mice. *J. Control Release* 235, 48–62. doi: 10.1016/j.jconrel.2016.05.049

Duner, P., Goncalves, I., Grufman, H., Edsfeldt, A., To, F., Nitulescu, M., et al. (2015). Increased aldehyde-modification of collagen type IV in symptomatic plaques–a possible cause of endothelial dysfunction. *Atherosclerosis* 240, 26–32. doi: 10.1016/j.atherosclerosis.2015.02.043

Duong, H. T., Dong, Z., Su, L., Boyer, C., George, J., Davis, T. P., et al. (2015). The use of nanoparticles to deliver nitric oxide to hepatic stellate cells for treating liver fibrosis and portal hypertension. *Small* 11, 2291–2304. doi: 10.1002/smll.201402870

Dvir, T., Bauer, M., Schroeder, A., Tsui, J. H., Anderson, D. G., Langer, R., et al. (2011). Nanoparticles targeting the infarcted heart. *Nano. Lett.* 11, 4411–4414. doi: 10.1021/nl2025882

Elsabahy, M., and Wooley, K. L. (2012). Design of polymeric nanoparticles for biomedical delivery applications. *Chem. Soc. Rev.* 41, 2545–2561. doi: 10.1039/c2cs15327k

Fan, Y., Chen, C., Huang, Y., Zhang, F., and Lin, G. (2017). Study of the pH-sensitive mechanism of tumor-targeting liposomes. *Colloids Surf. B Biointerfaces* 151, 19–25. doi: 10.1016/j.colsurfb.2016.11.042

Fitzgerald, K., Frank-Kamenetsky, M., Shulga-Morskaya, S., Liebow, A., Bettencourt, B. R., Sutherland, J. E., et al. (2014). Effect of an RNA interference drug on the synthesis of proprotein convertase subtilisin/kexin type 9 (PCSK9) and the concentration of serum LDL cholesterol in healthy volunteers: a randomised, single-blind, placebo-controlled, phase 1 trial. *Lancet* 383, 60–68. doi: 10.1016/S0140-6736(13)61914-5

Flaht-Zabost, A., Gula, G., Ciszek, B., Czarnowska, E., Jankowska-Steifer, E., Madej, M., et al. (2014). Cardiac mouse lymphatics: developmental and anatomical update. *Anat. Rec. (Hoboken)* 297, 1115–1130. doi: 10.1002/ar.22912

Flogel, U., Ding, Z., Hardung, H., Jander, S., Reichmann, G., Jacoby, C., et al. (2008). *In vivo* monitoring of inflammation after cardiac and cerebral ischemia by fluorine magnetic resonance imaging. *Circulation* 118, 140–148. doi: 10.1161/CIRCULATIONAHA.107.737890

Freund, J. B., and Shapiro, B. (2012). Transport of particles by magnetic forces and cellular blood flow in a model microvessel. *Phys. Fluids* 24:51904. doi: 10.1063/1.4718752

Galperin, A., Margel, D., Baniel, J., Dank, G., Biton, H., and Margel, S. (2007). Radiopaque iodinated polymeric nanoparticles for X-ray imaging applications. *Biomaterials* 28, 4461–4468. doi: 10.1016/j.biomaterials.2007.06.032

Gao, W., Hu, Y., Xu, L., Liu, M., Wu, H., and He, B. (2018). Dual pH and glucose sensitive gel gated mesoporous silica nanoparticles for drug delivery. *Chin. Chem. Lett.* 12, 1795–1798. doi: 10.1016/j.cclet.2018.05.022.

Gatoo, M. A., Naseem, S., Arfat, M. Y., Dar, A. M., Qasim, K., and Zubair, S. (2014). Physicochemical properties of nanomaterials: implication in associated toxic manifestations. *Biomed. Res. Int.* 2014:498420. doi: 10.1155/2014/498420

Gaurav, C., Saurav, B., Goutam, R., and Goyal, A. K. (2015). Nano-systems for advanced therapeutics and diagnosis of atherosclerosis. *Curr. Pharm. Des.* 21, 4498–4508. doi: 10.2174/1381612821666150917094215

Ghasemian, E., Motaghian, P., and Vatanara, A. (2016). D-optimal design for preparation and optimization of fast dissolving Bosentan nanosuspension. *Adv. Pharm. Bull.* 6:211. doi: 10.15171/apb.2016.029

Glass, C. K., and Witztum, J. L. (2001). Atherosclerosis. the road ahead. *Cell* 104, 503–516. doi: 10.1016/s0092-8674(01)00238-0

Gullotti, E., and Yeo, Y. (2009). Extracellularly activated nanocarriers: a new paradigm of tumor targeted drug delivery. *Mol. Pharm.* 6, 1041–1051. doi: 10.1021/mp900090z

Guo, T., Wang, J., Yang, J., Chen, W., An, G., Fan, L., et al. (2013). Lentivirus-mediated RNA interference of chymase increases the plaque stability in atherosclerosis *in vivo*. *Exp. Mol. Pathol.* 95, 51–56. doi: 10.1016/j.yexmp.2013.05.005

Gupta, N., Al-Saikhan, F. I., Patel, B., Rashid, J., and Ahsan, F. (2015). Fasudil and SOD packaged in peptide-studded-liposomes: properties, pharmacokinetics and *ex-vivo* targeting to isolated perfused rat lungs. *Int. J. Pharm.* 488, 33–43. doi: 10.1016/j.ijpharm.2015.04.031

Gupta, P., Garcia, E., Sarkar, A., Kapoor, S., Rafiq, K., Chand, H. S., et al. (2019). Nanoparticle based treatment for cardiovascular diseases. *Cardiovasc. Hematol. Disord. Drug Targets* 19, 33–44. doi: 10.2174/1871529X18666180508113253

Hausenloy, D. J., and Yellon, D. M. (2013). Myocardial ischemia-reperfusion injury: a neglected therapeutic target. *J. Clin. Invest.* 123, 92–100. doi: 10.1172/JCI62874

Hauser, A. K., Mitov, M. I., Daley, E. F., McGarry, R. C., Anderson, K. W., and Hilt, J. Z. (2016). Targeted iron oxide nanoparticles for the enhancement of radiation therapy. *Biomaterials* 105, 127–135. doi: 10.1016/j.biomaterials.2016.07.032

Hayden, E. C. (2014). RNA interference rebooted. *Nature* 508:443. doi: 10.1038/508443a

He, H., Yuan, Q., Bie, J., Wallace, R. L., Yannie, P. J., Wang, J., et al. (2018). Development of mannose functionalized dendrimeric nanoparticles for targeted delivery to macrophages: use of this platform to modulate atherosclerosis. *Transl. Res.* 193, 13–30. doi: 10.1016/j.trsl.2017.10.008

Hemmati, K., and Ghaemy, M. (2016). Synthesis of new thermo/pH sensitive drug delivery systems based on tragacanth gum polysaccharide. *Int. J. Biol. Macromol.* 87, 415–425. doi: 10.1016/j.ijbiomac.2016.03.005

Hoelscher, S. C., Doppler, S. A., Dreßen, M., Lahm, H., Lange, R., and Krane, M. (2017). MicroRNAs: pleiotropic players in congenital heart disease and regeneration. *J. Thorac. Dis.* 9, S64–S81. doi: 10.21037/jtd.2017.03.149

Holback, H., and Yeo, Y. (2011). Intratumoral drug delivery with nanoparticulate carriers. *Pharm. Res.* 28, 1819–1830. doi: 10.1007/s11095-010-0360-y

Holme, M. N., Fedotenko, I. A., Abegg, D., Althaus, J., Babel, L., Favarger, F., et al. (2012). Shear-stress sensitive lenticular vesicles for targeted drug delivery. *Nat. Nanotechnol.* 7, 536–543. doi: 10.1038/nnano.2012.84

Hood, E. D., Greineder, C. F., Shuvaeva, T., Walsh, L., Villa, C. H., and Muzykantov, V. R. (2018). Vascular targeting of radiolabeled liposomes with bio-orthogonally conjugated ligands: single chain fragments provide higher specificity than antibodies. *Bioconjug. Chem.* 29, 3626–3637. doi: 10.1021/acs.bioconjchem.8b00564

Hu, J., Sheng, Y., Shi, J., Yu, B., Yu, Z., and Liao, G. (2018). Long circulating polymeric nanoparticles for gene/drug delivery. *Curr. Drug Metab.* 19, 723–738. doi: 10.2174/1389200219666171207120643

Huang, M., and Wu, J. C. (2011). Molecular imaging of RNA interference therapy targeting PHD2 for treatment of myocardial ischemia. *Methods Mol. Biol.* 709, 211–221. doi: 10.1007/978-1-61737-982-6_13

Jain, A., and Jain, S. K. (2018). Stimuli-responsive smart liposomes in cancer targeting. *Curr. Drug Targets* 19, 259–270. doi: 10.2174/1389450117666160208144143

James, N. R., Philip, J., and Jayakrishnan, A. (2006). Polyurethanes with radiopaque properties. *Biomaterials* 27, 160–166. doi: 10.1016/j.biomaterials.2005.05.099

Jayagopal, A., Su, Y. R., Blakemore, J. L., Linton, M. F., Fazio, S., and Haselton, F. R. (2009). Quantum dot mediated imaging of atherosclerosis. *Nanotechnology* 20:165102. doi: 10.1088/0957-4484/20/16/165102

Jokerst, J. V., Lobovkina, T., Zare, R. N., and Gambhir, S. S. (2011). Nanoparticle PEGylation for imaging and therapy. *Nanomedicine (Lond).* 6, 715–728. doi: 10.2217/nnm.11.19

Kamaly, N., Fredman, G., Fojas, J. J., Subramanian, M., Choi, W. I., Zepeda, K., et al. (2016). Targeted interleukin-10 nanotherapeutics developed with a microfluidic chip enhance resolution of inflammation in advanced atherosclerosis. *ACS Nano* 10, 5280–5292. doi: 10.1021/acsnano.6b01114

Kamaly, N., Fredman, G., Subramanian, M., Gadde, S., and Farokhzad, O. C. (2013). Development and *in vivo* efficacy of targeted polymeric inflammation-resolving nanoparticles. *Proc. Natl. Acad. Sci. U.S.A.* 110, 6506–6511. doi: 10.1073/pnas.1303377110

Kamath, K. R., Barry, J. J., and Miller, K. M. (2006). The Taxus^{TM} drug-eluting stent: a new paradigm in controlled drug delivery. *Adv. Drug Deliver. Rev.* 58, 412–436. doi: 10.1016/j.addr.2006.01.023

Kasner, M., Gast, M., Galuszka, O., Stroux, A., Rutschow, S., Wang, X., et al. (2016). Circulating exosomal microRNAs predict functional recovery after MitraClip repair of severe mitral regurgitation. *Int. J. Cardiol.* 215, 402–405. doi: 10.1016/j.ijcard.2016.04.018

Katyayani, T., Samaresh, S., Sushil, K., and Arun, I. (2017). siRNA delivery strategies: a comprehensive review of recent developments. *Nanomaterials (Basel)* 7:77. doi: 10.3390/nano7040077

Kesharwani, P., Gajbhiye, V., and Jain, N. K. (2012). A review of nanocarriers for the delivery of small interfering RNA. *Biomaterials* 33, 7138–7150. doi: 10.1016/j.biomaterials.2012.06.068

Khafaji, M., Zamani, M., Golizadeh, M., and Bavi, O. (2019). Inorganic nanomaterials for chemo/photothermal therapy: a promising horizon on effective cancer treatment. *Biophys. Rev.* 11, 335–352. doi: 10.1007/s12551-019-00532-3

Kim, E. H., Ahn, Y., and Lee, H. S. (2007). Biomedical applications of superparamagnetic iron oxide nanoparticles encapsulated within chitosan. *J. Alloys Comp.* 434–435:636. doi: 10.1016/j.jallcom.2006.08.311

Kimura, S., Egashira, K., Chen, L., Nakano, K., Iwata, E., Miyagawa, M., et al. (2009). Nanoparticle-mediated delivery of nuclear factor kappaB decoy into lungs ameliorates monocrotaline-induced pulmonary arterial hypertension. *Hypertension* 53, 877–883. doi: 10.1161/HYPERTENSIONAHA.108.121418

Korin, N., Kanapathipillai, M., Matthews, B. D., Crescente, M., Brill, A., Mammoto, T., et al. (2012). Shear-activated nanotherapeutics for drug targeting to obstructed blood vessels. *Science* 337, 738–742. doi: 10.1126/science.1217815

Kwekkeboom, R. F. J., Lei, Z., Doevendans, P. A., Musters, R. J. P., and Sluijter, J. P. G. (2014). Targeted delivery of miRNA therapeutics for cardiovascular diseases: opportunities and challenges. *Clin. Sci.* 127, 351–365. doi: 10.1042/CS20140005

Landesman-Milo, D., Goldsmith, M., Leviatan, B. S., Witenberg, B., Brown, E., Leibovitch, S., et al. (2013). Hyaluronan grafted lipid-based nanoparticles as RNAi carriers for cancer cells. *Cancer Lett.* 334, 221–227. doi: 10.1016/j.canlet.2012.08.024

Lee, D., Lockey, R., and Mohapatra, S. (2006). Folate receptor-mediated cancer cell specific gene delivery using folic acid-conjugated oligochitosans. *J. Nanosci. Nanotechnol.* 6, 2860–2866. doi: 10.1166/jnn.2006.465

Lee, G. Y., Kim, J. H., Choi, K. Y., Yoon, H. Y., Kim, K., Kwon, I. C., et al. (2015). Hyaluronic acid nanoparticles for active targeting atherosclerosis. *Biomaterials* 53, 341–348. doi: 10.1016/j.biomaterials.2015.02.089

Lee, Y., Pai, S. B., Bellamkonda, R. V., Thompson, D. H., and Singh, J. (2018). Cerivastatin nanoliposome as a potential disease modifying approach for the treatment of pulmonary arterial hypertension. *J. Pharmacol. Exp. Ther.* 366, 66–74. doi: 10.1124/jpet.118.247643

Lendeckel, W., Tuschl, T., Harborth, J., Weber, J. K., Yalçin, A. S., Elbashir, L. M., et al. (2001). Duplexes of 21-nucleotide RNAs mediate RNA interference in cultured mammalian cells. *Nature* 411, 494–498. doi: 10.1038/35078107

Li, Z., Ding, J., Xiao, C., Pan, H., Tang, Z., Xuan, P., et al. (2012). Glucose-sensitive polypeptide micelles for self-regulated insulin release at physiological pH. *J. Mater. Chem.* 22, 12319–12328. doi: 10.1039/c2jm31040f

Liang, J. J., Zhou, Y. Y., Wu, J., and Ding, Y. (2014). Gold nanoparticle-based drug delivery platform for antineoplastic chemotherapy. *Curr. Drug Metab.* 15, 620–631. doi: 10.2174/1389200215666140605131427

Lin, X., Wang, Z., Sun, G., Shen, L., Xu, D., and Feng, Y. (2010). A sensitive and specific HPGPC-FD method for the study of pharmacokinetics and tissue distribution of radix ophiopogonis polysaccharide in rats. *Biomed. Chromatogr.* 24, 820–825. doi: 10.1002/bmc.1369

Lobatto, M. E., Fayad, Z. A., Silvera, S., Vucic, E., Calcagno, C., Mani, V., et al. (2010). Multimodal clinical imaging to longitudinally assess a nanomedical anti-inflammatory treatment in experimental atherosclerosis. *Mol. Pharm.* 7, 2020–2029. doi: 10.1021/mp100309y

Ma, S., Tian, X. Y., Zhang, Y., Mu, C., Shen, H., Bismuth, J., et al. (2016). E-selectin-targeting delivery of microRNAs by microparticles ameliorates endothelial inflammation and atherosclerosis. *Sci. Rep.* 6:22910. doi: 10.1038/srep22910

Maeda, H., Nakamura, H., and Fang, J. (2013). The EPR effect for macromolecular drug delivery to solid tumors: improvement of tumor uptake, lowering of systemic toxicity, and distinct tumor imaging *in vivo*. *Adv. Drug Deliv. Rev.* 65, 71–79. doi: 10.1016/j.addr.2012.10.002

Majmudar, M. D., Keliher, E. J., Heidt, T., Leuschner, F., Truelove, J., Sena, B. F., et al. (2013). Monocyte-directed RNAi targeting CCR2 improves infarct healing in atherosclerosis-prone mice. *Circulation* 127, 2038–2046. doi: 10.1161/circulationaha.112.000116

Mansukhani, N. A., Peters, E. B., So, M. M., Albaghdadi, M. S., Wang, Z., Karver, M. R., et al. (2019). Peptide amphiphile supramolecular nanostructures as a targeted therapy for atherosclerosis. *Macromol. Biosci.* 19:e1900066. doi: 10.1002/mabi.201900066

Maranhao, R. C., Guido, M. C., de Lima, A. D., Tavares, E. R., Marques, A. F., Tavares, D. M. M., et al. (2017). Methotrexate carried in lipid core nanoparticles reduces myocardial infarction size and improves cardiac function in rats. *Int. J. Nanomedicine* 12, 3767–3784. doi: 10.2147/IJN.S129324

Marsh, J. N., Senpan, A., Hu, G., Scott, M. J., Gaffney, P. J., Wickline, S. A., et al. (2007). Fibrin-targeted perfluorocarbon nanoparticles for targeted thrombolysis. *Nanomedicine (Lond).* 2, 533–543. doi: 10.2217/17435889.2.4.533

Martin, G. V., Kassuha, D. E., and Manucha, W. (2017). Nanomedicine applied to cardiovascular diseases: latest developments. *Ther. Adv. Cardiovasc. Dis.* 11, 133–142. doi: 10.1177/1753944717692293

Matoba, T., and Egashira, K. (2014). Nanoparticle-mediated drug delivery system for cardiovascular disease. *Int. Heart J.* 55, 281–286. doi: 10.1536/ihj.14-150

Matoba, T., Koga, J. I., Nakano, K., Egashira, K., and Tsutsui, H. (2017). Nanoparticle-mediated drug delivery system for atherosclerotic cardiovascular disease. *J. Cardiol.* 70, 206–211. doi: 10.1016/j.jjcc.2017.03.005

McCarthy, J. R., Jaffer, F. A., and Weissleder, R. (2006). A macrophage-targeted theranostic nanoparticle for biomedical applications. *Small* 2, 983–987. doi: 10.1002/smll.200600139

Morachis, J. M., Mahmoud, E. A., and Almutairi, A. (2012). Physical and chemical strategies for therapeutic delivery by using polymeric nanoparticles. *Pharmacol. Rev.* 64, 505–519. doi: 10.1124/pr.111.005363

Mottu, F., Rufenacht, D. A., and Doelker, E. (1999). Radiopaque polymeric materials for medical applications. Current aspects of biomaterial research. *Invest. Radiol.* 34, 323–335. doi: 10.1097/00004424-199905000-00001

Mottu, F., Rüfenacht, D. A., Laurent, A., and Doelker, E. (2002). Iodine-containing cellulose mixed esters as radiopaque polymers for direct embolization of cerebral aneurysms and arteriovenous malformations. *Biomaterials* 23, 121–131. doi: 10.1016/s0142-9612(01)00087-4

Nabel, E. G., and Braunwald, E. (2012). A tale of coronary artery disease and myocardial infarction. *N. Engl. J. Med.* 366, 54–63. doi: 10.1056/NEJMra1112570

Nafee, N., Makled, S., and Boraie, N. (2018). Nanostructured lipid carriers versus solid lipid nanoparticles for the potential treatment of pulmonary hypertension via nebulization. *Eur. J. Pharm. Sci.* 125, 151–162. doi: 10.1016/j.ejps.2018.10.003

Nakano, K., Egashira, K., Masuda, S., Funakoshi, K., Zhao, G., Kimura, S., et al. (2009). Formulation of nanoparticle-eluting stents by a cationic electrodeposition coating technology: efficient nano-drug delivery via bioabsorbable polymeric nanoparticle-eluting stents in porcine coronary arteries. *JACC Cardiovasc. Interv.* 2, 277–283. doi: 10.1016/j.jcin.2008.08.023

Navickas, R., Gal, D., Laucevi Ius, A., Taparauskait, A., Zdanyt, M., and Holvoet, P. (2016). Identifying circulating microRNAs as biomarkers of cardiovascular disease: a systematic review. *Cardiovasc. Res.* 111, 322–337. doi: 10.1093/cvr/cvw174

Niaz, T., Hafeez, Z., and Imran, M. (2017). Prospectives of antihypertensive nano-ceuticals as alternative therapeutics. *Curr. Drug Targets* 18, 1269–1280. doi: 10.2174/1389450117666160711163119

Niaz, T., Shabbir, S., Manzoor, S., Rehman, A., Rahman, A., Nasir, H., et al. (2016). Antihypertensive nano-ceuticales based on chitosan biopolymer: physico-chemical evaluation and release kinetics. *Carbohydr. Polym.* 142, 268–274. doi: 10.1016/j.carbpol.2016.01.047

Oduk, Y., Zhu, W., Kannappan, R., Zhao, M., Borovjagin, A. V., Oparil, S., et al. (2018). VEGF nanoparticles repair the heart after myocardial infarction. *Am. J. Physiol. Heart Circ. Physiol.* 314, H278–H284. doi: 10.1152/ajpheart.00471.2017

Okamura, M., Yamanobe, T., Arai, T., Uehara, H., Komoto, T., Hosoi, S., et al. (2002). Synthesis and properties of radiopaque polymer hydrogels II: copolymers of 2,4,6-triiodophenyl- or N-(3-carboxy-2,4,6-triiodophenyl)- acrylamide and p-styrene sulfonate. *J. Mol. Struct.* 602, 17–28. doi: 10.1016/S0022-2860(01)00710-4

Park, K., Hong, H., Moon, H. J., Lee, B., Kim, I., Kwon, I. C., et al. (2008). A new atherosclerotic lesion probe based on hydrophobically modified chitosan nanoparticles functionalized by the atherosclerotic plaque targeted peptides. *J. Control Release* 128, 217–223. doi: 10.1016/j.jconrel.2008.03.019

Paulis, L. E., Jacobs, I., and van den Akker, N. M. (2012). Targeting of ICAM-1 on vascular endothelium under static and shear stress conditions using a liposomal Gd-based MRI contrast agent. *J. Nanobiotechnol.* 10:25. doi: 10.1186/1477-3155-10-25

Pechanova, O., Barta, A., Koneracka, M., Zavisova, V., Kubovcikova, M., Klimentova, J., et al. (2019). Protective effects of nanoparticle-loaded aliskiren on cardiovascular system in spontaneously hypertensive rats. *Molecules* 24:2710. doi: 10.3390/molecules24152710

Perioli, L., Pagano, C., and Ceccarini, M. R. (2019). Current highlights about the safety of inorganic nanomaterials in healthcare. *Curr. Med. Chem.* 26, 2147–2165. doi: 10.2174/0929867325666180723121804

Pietro, P. D., Strano, G., Zuccarello, L., and Satriano, C. (2016). Gold and silver nanoparticles for applications in theranostics. *Curr. Top Med. Chem.* 16, 3069–3102. doi: 10.2174/1568026616666160715163346

Ping, S., Wei, H., Lin, K., Mingji, J., Bo, F., Hongyan, J., et al. (2017). siRNA-loaded poly(histidine-arginine)6-modified chitosan nanoparticle with enhanced cell-penetrating and endosomal escape capacities for suppressing breast tumor metastasis. *Int. J. Nanomed.* 12, 3221–3234. doi: 10.2147/IJN.S129436

Prijic, S., and Sersa, G. (2011). Magnetic nanoparticles as targeted delivery systems in oncology. *Radiol. Oncol.* 45, 1–16. doi: 10.2478/v10019-011-0001-z

Qinghua, S., Aixia, W., Ximei, J., Alex, N., Damon, D., Brook, R. D., et al. (2005). Long-term air pollution exposure and acceleration of atherosclerosis and vascular inflammation in an animal model. *JAMA.* 294:3003. doi: 10.1001/jama.294.23.3003

Quan, X., Rang, L., Yin, X., Jin, Z., and Gao, Z. (2015). Synthesis of PEGylated hyaluronic acid for loading dichloro(1,2-diaminocyclohexane)platinum(II) (DACHPt) in nanoparticles for cancer treatment. *Chin. Chem. Lett.* 26, 695–699. doi: 10.1016/j.cclet.2015.04.024

Qumbar, M., Ameeduzzafar., Imam, S. S., Ali, J., Ahmad, J., and Ali, A. (2017). Formulation and optimization of lacidipine loaded niosomal gel for transdermal delivery: *in-vitro* characterization and *in-vivo* activity. *Biomed. Pharmacother.* 93, 255–266. doi: 10.1016/j.biopha.2017.06.043

Rana, S., Datta, K., Reddy, T. L., Chatterjee, E., Sen, P., Pal-Bhadra, M., et al. (2015). A spatio-temporal cardiomyocyte targeted vector system for efficient delivery of therapeutic payloads to regress cardiac hypertrophy abating bystander effect. *J. Control Release* 200, 167–178. doi: 10.1016/j.jconrel.2015.01.008

Rojas, J. D., Fanglue, L., Yun-Chen, C., Anna, C., Chong, C. D., Bautch, V. L., et al. (2018). Ultrasound molecular imaging of VEGFR-2 in clear-cell renal cell carcinoma tracks disease response to antiangiogenic and notch-inhibition therapy. *Theranostics* 8, 141–155. doi: 10.7150/thno.19658

Savic, R., Luo, L., Eisenberg, A., and Maysinger, D. (2003). Micellar nanocontainers distribute to defined cytoplasmic organelles. *Science* 300, 615–618. doi: 10.1126/science.1078192

Schröder, J., Vogt, F., Burgmaier, M., Reith, S., and Almalla, M. (2018). Long-term clinical outcomes after treatment of stent restenosis with two drug-coated balloons. *Coronary Artery Dis.* 29:1. doi: 10.1097/MCA.0000000000000664

Scott, R. C., Rosano, J. M., Ivanov, Z., Wang, B., Chong, P. L., Issekutz, A. C., et al. (2009). Targeting VEGF-encapsulated immunoliposomes to MI heart improves vascularity and cardiac function. *FASEB J.* 23, 3361–3367. doi: 10.1096/fj.08-127373

Setua, S., Menon, D., Asok, A., Nair, S., and Koyakutty, M. (2010). Folate receptor targeted, rare-earth oxide nanocrystals for bi-modal fluorescence and magnetic imaging of cancer cells. *Biomaterials* 31, 714–729. doi: 10.1016/j.biomaterials.2009.09.090

Sevick-Muraca, M. E. (2012). Translation of near-infrared fluorescence imaging technologies: emerging clinical applications. *Annu. Rev. Med.* 63, 217–231. doi: 10.1146/annurev-med-070910-083323

Sharma, M., Sharma, R., and Jain, D. K. (2016). Nanotechnology based approaches for enhançing oral bioavailability of poorly water soluble antihypertensive drugs. *Scientifica (Cairo)* 2016:8525679. doi: 10.1155/2016/8525679

Shi, C., He, Y., Ding, M., Wang, Y., and Zhong, J. (2019a). Nanoimaging of food proteins by atomic force microscopy. Part I: Components, imaging modes, observation ways, and research types. *Trends Food Sci. Tech.* 87, 3–13. doi: 10.1016/j.tifs.2018.11.028

Shi, C., He, Y., Ding, M., Wang, Y., and Zhong, J. (2019b). Nanoimaging of food proteins by atomic force microscopy. Part II: Application for food proteins from different sources. *Trends Food Sci. Tech.* 87, 14–25. doi: 10.1016/j.tifs.2018.11.027

Sioud, M. (2015). RNA interference: mechanisms, technical challenges, and therapeutic opportunities. *Methods Mol. Biol.* 1218, 1–15. doi: 10.1007/978-1-4939-1538-5_1

Somasuntharam, I., Boopathy, A. V., Khan, R. S., Martinez, M. D., Brown, M. E., Murthy, N., et al. (2013). Delivery of Nox2-NADPH oxidase siRNA with polyketal nanoparticles for improving cardiac function following myocardial infarction. *Biomaterials* 34, 7790–7798. doi: 10.1016/j.biomaterials.2013.06.051

Su, X., Chan, C., Shi, J., Tsang, M. K., Pan, Y., Cheng, C., et al. (2017). A graphene quantum dot@Fe_3O_4@SiO_2 based nanoprobe for drug delivery sensing and dual-modal fluorescence and MRI imaging in cancer cells. *Biosens. Bioelectron.* 92, 489–495. doi: 10.1016/j.bios.2016.10.076

Suckau, L., Fechner, H., Chemaly, E., Krohn, S., Hadri, L., Kockskamper, J., et al. (2009). Long-term cardiac-targeted RNA interference for the treatment of heart failure restores cardiac function and reduces pathological hypertrophy. *Circulation* 119, 1241–1252. doi: 10.1161/CIRCULATIONAHA.108.783852

Suwa, T., Hogg, J. C., Quinlan, K. B., Ohgami, A., Vincent, R., and van Eeden, S. F. (2002). Particulate air pollution induces progression of atherosclerosis. *J. Am. Coll. Cardiol.* 39, 935–942. doi: 10.1016/s0735-1097(02)01715-1

Tadin-Strapps, M., Robinson, M., Le Voci, L., Andrews, L., Yendluri, S., Williams, S., et al. (2015). Development of lipoprotein(a) siRNAs for mechanism of action studies in non-human primate models of atherosclerosis. *J. Cardiovasc. Transl.* 8, 44–53. doi: 10.1007/s12265-014-9605-1

Tan, J., Thomas, A., and Liu, Y. (2011). Influence of red blood cells on nanoparticle targeted delivery in microcirculation. *Soft Matter* 8, 1934–1946. doi: 10.1039/C2SM06391C

Torchilin, V. (2011). Tumor delivery of macromolecular drugs based on the EPR effect. *Adv. Drug Deliv. Rev.* 63, 131–135. doi: 10.1016/j.addr.2010.03.011

Torchilin, V. P. (2002). PEG-based micelles as carriers of contrast agents for different imaging modalities. *Adv. Drug Deliv. Rev.* 54, 235–252. doi: 10.1016/S0169-409X(02)00019-4

Vimbela, G. V., Ngo, S. M., Fraze, C., Yang, L., and Stout, D. A. (2017). Antibacterial properties and toxicity from metallic nanomaterials. *Int. J. Nanomedicine* 12, 3941–3965. doi: 10.2147/IJN.S134526

Wall, E. E. V. D. (2013). Molecular imaging of coronary atherosclerosis; predictive of an acute myocardial infarction? *Neth. Heart J.* 22, 1–2. doi: 10.1007/s12471-013-0500-1

Wang, J., Jin, X., Huang, Y., Ran, X., Luo, D., Yang, D., et al. (2018). Endovascular stent-induced alterations in host artery mechanical environments and their roles in stent restenosis and late thrombosis. *Regen. Biomater.* 5, 177–187. doi: 10.1093/rb/rby006

Wang, W., Ding, J., Xiao, C., Tang, Z., Li, D., Chen, J., et al. (2011). Synthesis of amphiphilic alternating polyesters with oligo(ethylene glycol) side chains and potential use for sustained release drug delivery. *Biomacromolecules* 12, 2466–2474. doi: 10.1021/bm200668n

Wang, W., Sun, X., Zhang, H., Yang, C., Liu, Y., Yang, W., et al. (2016). Controlled release hydrogen sulfide delivery system based on mesoporous silica nanoparticles protects graft endothelium from ischemia-reperfusion injury. *Int. J. Nanomedicine* 11, 3255–3263. doi: 10.2147/IJN.S104604

Wang, Y., Chen, J., Yang, B., Qiao, H., Gao, L., Su, T., et al. (2016). *In vivo* MR and fluorescence dual-modality imaging of atherosclerosis characteristics in mice using profilin-1 targeted magnetic nanoparticles. *Theranostics* 6, 272–286. doi: 10.7150/thno.13350

Wang, Z., Cuddigan, J. L., Gupta, S. K., and Meenach, S. A. (2016). Nanocomposite microparticles (nCmP) for the delivery of tacrolimus in the treatment of pulmonary arterial hypertension. *Int. J. Pharm.* 512, 305–313. doi: 10.1016/j.ijpharm.2016.08.047

Wei, D., Qiao, R., Dao, J., Su, J., Jiang, C., Wang, X., et al. (2018). Soybean lecithin-mediated nanoporous PLGA microspheres with highly entrapped and controlled released BMP-2 as a stem cell platform. *Small* 14:1800063. doi: 10.1002/smll.201800063.

Wei, H., Bruns, O. T., Kaul, M. G., Hansen, E. C., Barch, M., Wisniowska, A., et al. (2017). Exceedingly small iron oxide nanoparticles as positive MRI contrast agents. *Proc. Natl. Acad. Sci. U.S.A.* 114, 2325–2330. doi: 10.1073/pnas.1620145114

Wei, L., Chen, J., Zhao, S., Ding, J., and Chen, X. (2017). Thermo-sensitive polypeptide hydrogel for locally sequential delivery of two-pronged antitumor drugs. *Acta Biomater.* 58, 44–53. doi: 10.1016/j.actbio.2017.05.053

Weissleder, R., and Ntziachristos, V. (2003). Shedding light onto live molecular targets. *Nat. Med.* 9, 123–128. doi: 10.1038/nm0103-123

Winter, P. M., Caruthers, S. D., Zhang, H., Williams, T. A., Wickline, S. A., and Lanza, G. M. (2008). Antiangiogenic synergism of integrin-targeted fumagillin nanoparticles and atorvastatin in atherosclerosis. *JACC Cardiovasc. Imaging* 1, 624–634. doi: 10.1016/j.jcmg.2008.06.003

Wu, T., Ding, M., Shi, C., Qiao, Y., Wang, P., Qiao, R., et al. (2019). Resorbable polymer electrospun nanofibers: history, shapes and application for tissue engineering. *Chin. Chem. Lett.* doi: 10.1016/j.cclet.2019.07.033. [Epub ahead of print].

Xi, X., Trost, D. W., and Sista, A. K. (2018). Successful management of drug-coated balloon (DCB) for recurrent iliofemoral venous in-stent restenosis (ISR). *Clin. Imaging* 49, 184–186. doi: 10.1016/j.clinimag.2018.03.018

Xia, H., Jun, J., Wen-ping, L., Yi-feng, P., and Xiao-ling, C. (2013). Chitosan nanoparticle carrying small interfering RNA to platelet-derived growth factor B mRNA inhibits proliferation of smooth muscle cells in rabbit injured arteries. *Vascular* 21, 301–306. doi: 10.1177/1708538113478737

Yang, C., Gao, S., Dagn S-Hansen, F., Jakobsen, M., and Kjems, J. R. (2017). Impact of PEG chain length on the physical properties and bioactivity of PEGylated chitosan/siRNA nanoparticles *in vitro* and *in vivo*. *ACS Appl. Mater. Interfaces* 9, 12203–12216. doi: 10.1021/acsami.6b16556

Yang, H., Zhao, F., Li, Y., Xu, M., Li, L., Wu, C., et al. (2013). VCAM-1-targeted core/shell nanoparticles for selective adhesion and delivery to endothelial cells with lipopolysaccharide-induced inflammation under shear flow and cellular magnetic resonance imaging *in vitro*. *Int. J. Nanomedicine* 8, 1897–1906. doi: 10.2147/IJN.S44997

Yang, X., Hong, H., Grailer, J. J., Rowland, I. J., Javadi, A., Hurley, S. A., et al. (2011). cRGD-functionalized, DOX-conjugated, and 64Cu-labeled superparamagnetic iron oxide nanoparticles for targeted anticancer drug delivery and PET/MR imaging. *Biomaterials* 32, 4151–4160. doi: 10.1016/j.biomaterials.2011.02.006

Yi, Z., Cai, L., Di, L., Lao, Y. H., Liu, D., Li, M., et al. (2018). Tumor microenvironment-responsive hyaluronate-calcium carbonate hybrid nanoparticle enables effective chemotherapy for primary and advanced osteosarcomas. *Nano Res.* 11, 1–17. doi: 10.1007/s12274-018-2066-0

Yingchoncharoen, P., Kalinowski, D. S., and Richardson, D. R. (2016). Lipid-based drug delivery systems in cancer therapy: what is available and what is yet to come. *Pharmacol. Rev.* 68, 701–787. doi: 10.1124/pr.115.012070

Yoo, S. P., Pineda, F., Barrett, J. C., Poon, C., Tirrell, M., and Chung, E. J. (2016). Gadolinium-functionalized peptide amphiphile micelles for multimodal imaging of atherosclerotic lesions. *ACS Omega* 1, 996–1003. doi: 10.1021/acsomega.6b00210

Yu, F., Wu, H., Tang, Y., Xu, Y., Qian, X., and Zhu, W. (2018). Temperature-sensitive copolymer-coated fluorescent mesoporous silica nanoparticles as a reactive oxygen species activated drug delivery system. *Int. J. Pharm.* 536, 11–20. doi: 10.1016/j.ijpharm.2017.11.025

Yu, J., Li, W., and Yu, D. (2018). Atrial natriuretic peptide modified oleate adenosine prodrug lipid nanocarriers for the treatment of myocardial infarction: *in vitro* and *in vivo* evaluation. *Drug Des. Dev. Ther.* 12, 1697–1706. doi: 10.2147/DDDT.S166749

Yue, X., and Dai, Z. (2018). Liposomal nanotechnology for cancer theranostics. *Curr. Med. Chem.* 25, 1397–1408. doi: 10.2174/0929867324666170306105350

Zhang, M., He, J., Jiang, C., Zhang, W., Yang, Y., Wang, Z., et al. (2017). Plaque-hyaluronidase-responsive high-density- lipoprotein-mimetic nanoparticles for multistage intimal-macrophage-targeted drug delivery and enhanced anti-atherosclerotic therapy. *Int. J. Nanomedicine* 12, 533–558. doi: 10.2147/IJN.S124252

Zhang, X., Beduhn, M., Zheng, X., Lian, D., Chen, D., Li, R., et al. (2012). Induction of alloimmune tolerance in heart transplantation through gene silencing of TLR adaptors. *Am. J. Transplant.* 12, 2675–2688. doi: 10.1111/j.1600-6143.2012.04196.x

Zhang, Z., Runa, A., Wu, J., Zhang, H., Li, X., and He, Z. (2019). Bioresponsive nanogated ensemble based on structure-switchable aptamer directed assembly and disassembly of gold nanoparticles from mesoporous silica supports. *Chin. Chem. Lett.* 30, 267–270. doi: 10.1016/j.cclet.2018.10.019.

Zhou, F., Jia, X., Yang, Q., Yang, Y., Zhao, Y., Fan, Y., et al. (2016). Targeted delivery of microRNA-126 to vascular endothelial cells via REDV peptide modified PEG-trimethyl chitosan. *Biomater. Sci.* 4, 849–856. doi: 10.1039/C5BM00629E

Zhou, X., Hao, Y., Yuan, L., Pradhan, S., Shrestha, K., Pradhan, O., et al. (2018). Nano-formulations for transdermal drug delivery: a review. *Chin. Chem. Lett.* 29, 1713–1724. doi: 10.1016/j.cclet.2018.10.037

Zhou, X., Luo, Y. C., Ji, W. J., Zhang, L., Dong, Y., Ge, L., et al. (2013). Modulation of mononuclear phagocyte inflammatory response by liposome-encapsulated voltage gated sodium channel inhibitor ameliorates myocardial ischemia/reperfusion injury in rats. *PLoS ONE* 8:e0074390. doi: 10.1371/journal.pone.0074390

Zimmermann, T. S., Lee, A. C. H., Akinc, A., Bramlage, B., Bumcrot, D., Fedoruk, M. N., et al. (2006). RNAi-mediated gene silencing in non-human primates. *Nature* 441, 111–114. doi: 10.1038/nature04688

5

An Injectable Hydrogel Platform for Sustained Delivery of Anti-Inflammatory Nanocarriers and Induction of Regulatory T Cells in Atherosclerosis

*Sijia Yi, Nicholas B. Karabin, Jennifer Zhu, Sharan Bobbala, Huijue Lyu, Sophia Li, Yugang Liu, Molly Frey, Michael Vincent and Evan A. Scott**

Department of Biomedical Engineering, Northwestern University, Evanston, IL, United States

Correspondence:
Evan A. Scott
evan.scott@northwestern.edu

Chronic unresolved vascular inflammation is a critical factor in the development of atherosclerosis. Cardiovascular immunotherapy has therefore become a recent focus for treatment, with the objective to develop approaches that can suppress excessive inflammatory responses by modulating specific immune cell populations. A benefit of such immunomodulatory strategies is that low dosage stimulation of key immune cell populations, like antigen presenting cells, can subsequently propagate strong proliferation and therapeutic responses from effector cells. We have previously demonstrated that intravenous injections of anti-inflammatory nanocarriers provided atheroprotection that was mediated by regulatory T cells (Tregs) upregulated in lymphoid organs and atherosclerotic lesions. Here, we demonstrate an injectable filamentous hydrogel depot (FM-depot) engineered for low dosage, sustained delivery of anti-inflammatory nanocarriers. The bioactive form of vitamin D (aVD; 1, 25-Dihydroxyvitamin D3), which inhibits pro-inflammatory transcription factor NF-κB via the intracellular nuclear hormone receptor vitamin D receptor (VDR), was stably loaded into poly(ethylene glycol)-block-poly(propylene sulfide) (PEG-*b*-PPS) filomicelles. These aVD-loaded filaments underwent morphological transitions to release monodisperse drug-loaded micelles upon oxidation. This cylinder-to-micelle transition was characterized *in vitro* by cryogenic transmission electron microscopy (CryoTEM) and small angle X-ray scattering (SAXS). Following crosslinking with multi-arm PEG for *in situ* gelation, aVD-loaded FM-depots maintained high levels of Foxp3$^+$ Tregs in both lymphoid organs and atherosclerotic lesions for weeks following a single subcutaneous injection into ApoE$^{-/-}$ mice. FM-depots therefore present a customizable delivery platform to both develop and test nanomedicine-based approaches for anti-inflammatory cardiovascular immunotherapy.

Keywords: hydrogel, atherosclerosis, sustained delivery, regulatory T cells, immunotherapy, nanoparticle, filament

INTRODUCTION

Atherosclerosis is a chronic inflammatory disorder and a major source of cardiovascular disease (CVD) that involves the accumulation of fatty deposits and inflammatory cells within the intimal walls of arterial vessels (Virani et al., 2020). Lipid-lowering drugs, such as statins, have been widely used in the treatment of CVD. Statins inhibit HMG-CoA reductase and reduce cholesterol levels risk of coronary heart disease and stroke. However, numerous undesired side effects discourage patients from continuing statin treatment, such as stain-associated muscle symptoms, diabetes mellitus, and central nervous system complaints (Thompson et al., 2016). Many patients with reduced low-density lipoprotein (LDL) cholesterol levels still have a high risk of heart attack and stroke (Hu et al., 2003; Sampson et al., 2012; Fernández-Friera et al., 2017). Furthermore, systemic and plaque inflammation are not resolved by statin treatment (Sansbury and Spite, 2016). Recently, attention has shifted from focusing on lipids toward addressing the immune cell-mediated inflammation contributing to CVD. In particular, an imbalance between effector T cells and regulatory T cells (Tregs) can trigger a cascade of inflammatory responses leading to atherosclerosis progression and plaque vulnerability (Ou et al., 2018). Effector type 1 helper T (Th1) cells have been demonstrated to promote the migration of monocytes and T cells into plaques and activate antigen-presenting cells (APCs) by secreting interferon-γ (IFN-γ) and IL-6 (Dietel et al., 2013; Tabas and Lichtman, 2017). However, as an essential immunoregulatory cell population, Tregs induce and maintain systemic immune homeostasis and tolerance by suppressing diverse immune cells, including effector T cells (Th1 and Th17 cells), monocytes, dendritic cells, and natural killer cells, as well as by secreting anti-inflammatory cytokines (IL-10, TGF-β, and IL-35) (George et al., 2012; Chistiakov et al., 2013; Dietel et al., 2013). In the clinic, decreased numbers and dysfunction of Tregs are suggested to be involved in atherosclerosis pathogenesis as evidenced by low levels of circulating and lesional Tregs in patients with vulnerable plaques and acute coronary syndrome (George et al., 2012; Dietel et al., 2013; Jia et al., 2013). Strategies to controllably elicit Tregs *in vivo* are therefore needed to better investigate, develop, and harness their atheroprotective mechanisms.

As essential mediators of immunity and tolerance, APCs play a pivotal role in the induction of Tregs. A variety of approaches to modulate APCs and increase Tregs have yielded promising results in the treatment of atherosclerosis, such as oral administration of anti-inflammatory immunomodulators (Chistiakov et al., 2013), anti-inflammatory cytokine treatment (Ji et al., 2017), and adoptive transfer of tolerogenic dendritic cells (DCs) (Hermansson et al., 2011). Despite these major advances, the clinical use of immunotherapies faces several challenges in both efficacy and safety due to off-target effects. Biomaterials and nanotechnology have been shown to improve the efficacy and safety of immunomodulatory molecules through controlling the colocalization, biodistribution, and release kinetics of drugs (Kim et al., 2011; Shao et al., 2015; Allen et al., 2016). We have previously developed multiple strategies to inhibit inflammation and the progression of atherosclerosis by nanocarrier-enhanced immunomodulation of APCs (Allen et al., 2019; Yi et al., 2019). The nanocarriers were composed of poly(ethylene glycol)-block-poly(propylene sulfide) (PEG-*b*-PPS) and are both non-inflammatory and non-toxic in non-human primates (Allen et al., 2018), humanized mice (Dowling et al., 2017), or mouse models of atherosclerosis (Yi et al., 2016). By adjusting the hydrophilic PEG fraction (F_{PEG}) relative to the hydrophobic PPS blocks, PEG-*b*-PPS can self-assemble into diverse nanostructure morphologies that are highly stable *in vivo* due to their lyotropic mesophases and low critical micelle concentration of $\sim 10^{-7}$ M (Napoli et al., 2002, 2004). Using vesicular polymersomes, we selectively targeted DCs in atherosclerotic mice for intracellular delivery of 1, 25-Dihydroxyvitamin D3 (aVD) (Yi et al., 2019). 1, 25-Dihydroxyvitamin D3 is the active metabolite of vitamin D and has been shown to induce a tolerogenic DC phenotype via interaction with the vitamin D nuclear receptor (VDR) (Mathieu and Adorini, 2002). With a logP of 7.6, aVD stably partitioned into the hydrophobic domains of PEG-*b*-PPS assemblies. Indeed, weekly intravenous administration of these DC-targeted anti-inflammatory polymersomes induced tolerogenic DCs, promoted the proliferation of Tregs and significantly inhibited atherosclerosis in $ApoE^{-/-}$ mice (Yi et al., 2019). Although effective in mice, weekly intravenous administration is not a clinically practical option for human patients, which would instead be better served by a long-term delivery platform to sustain Treg levels after a single injection.

Recently, we reported an injectable filamentous (FM) PEG-*b*-PPS hydrogel, which can be employed for the sustainable delivery of drug-loaded nanocarriers in response to physiological levels of oxidation (Karabin et al., 2018). We found that subcutaneously injected FM hydrogel depots (FM-depots) can sustainably deliver monodisperse micelles (MC) to APC and lymphoid organs such as spleen and lymph nodes *in vivo* for months. We therefore hypothesized that FM-depots might serve as an excellent platform to maintain therapeutic immunomodulation of chronic inflammatory diseases. Although thoroughly characterized for *in vivo* sustained release of diagnostic micelles, FM-depots have never before been employed for the delivery of micelles transporting a bioactive or therapeutic molecule. Here, we demonstrate a controllable anti-inflammatory FM-depot, which can sustainably release aVD-loaded PEG-*b*-PPS MC for months following subcutaneous (s.c.) injection. In this proof of concept work, we aimed to verify that delivery of the immunomodulator aVD in a controlled spatiotemporal manner using FM-depots exhibits the superior capacity to induce $Foxp3^+$ Tregs compared to free aVD after 2 months of treatment. This nanocarrier delivery system may therefore serve as an excellent tool to investigate and optimize strategies employing Tregs for CVD immunotherapy and presents new opportunities for long-term, low dosage anti-inflammatory treatment regiments.

MATERIALS AND METHODS

Materials

All chemical solvents and reagents were purchased from Sigma-Aldrich (St. Louis, MO, USA) unless indicated. All antibodies and reagents used for flow cytometry were purchased from BioLegend (San Diego, CA, USA).

PEG-*b*-PPS Polymer Synthesis

Poly(ethylene glycol)-block-poly(propylene sulfide) copolymers PEG_{45}-*b*-PPS_{44} and vinyl sulfone functionalized PEG_{45}-*b*-PPS_{44} (VS-PEG_{45}-*b*-PPS_{44}) were synthesized as described previously (Karabin et al., 2018). Briefly, benzyl mercaptan initiated the living anionic ring-opening polymerization of propylene sulfide. The thiolate was then end-capped with either monomethoxy poly (ethylene glycol)-mesylate to form PEG_{45}-*b*-PPS_{44} or α-tosyl-ω-hydroxyl PEG to form OH-PEG_{45}-*b*-PPS_{44}. The vinyl sulfone functionalized PEG_{45}-*b*-PPS_{44} was obtained from converting the hydroxyl group to a vinyl sulfone group. The obtained polymers (PEG_{45}-*b*-PPS_{44} and VS-PEG_{45}-*b*-PPS_{44}) were purified by precipitation in cold diethyl ether, dried under vacuum and characterized by ^1H NMR ($CDCl_3$) and gel permeation chromatography (GPC) (ThermoFisher Scientific) using Waters Styragel THF columns with refractive index and UV-Vis detectors in a tetrahydrofuran (THF) mobile phase.

Preparation of Filomicelle (FM) Depots

Filomicelles were self-assembled from PEG_{45}-*b*-PPS_{44} and VS-PEG_{45}-*b*-PPS_{44} polymers via thin-film rehydration method in PBS as described previously (Karabin et al., 2018). Briefly, the mixture of PEG_{45}-*b*-PPS_{44} (40 mg) and VS- PEG_{45}-*b*-PPS_{44} (10 mg) polymers were dissolved in 1 ml dichloromethane within 1.8 ml glass vials (ThermoFisher Scientific) and placed under vacuum to remove the solvent. The resulting thin films were hydrated with 493 μl of phosphate-buffered saline (PBS) and gently mixed using a Stuart SB3 rotator for at least 36 h. To prepare FM-depots, eight-arm PEG-thiol (10% w/v in PBS solution, Creative PEGWorks) was added to FM solution corresponding to a 1.1:1 molar ratio of thiol:vinyl sulfone. The obtained mixture was vortexed and a Teflon mold (6 mm) was filled with 55 μl of the mixture. The FM-depots were formed after incubation at 37°C in a humidified environment for 30 min.

Material Characterization

The morphology of nanostructures was determined using cryogenic transmission electron microscopy (CryoTEM). Prior to plunge-freezing, 200 mesh Cu grids with a lacey carbon membrane (EMS Cat# LC200-CU-100) were glow-discharged in a Pelco easiGlow glow discharger (Ted Pella Inc., Redding, CA, USA) using an atmosphere plasma generated at 15 mA for 15 s with a pressure of 0.24 mbar. This treatment created a negative charge on the carbon membrane, allowing liquid samples to spread evenly over the grid. 4 μL of FM samples (10 mg/ml in PBS) was pipetted onto the grid and blotted for 5 s with a blot offset of +0.5 mm, followed by immediate plunging into liquid ethane within a FEI Vitrobot Mark III plunge freezing instrument (Thermo Fisher Scientific, Waltham, MA, USA). Grids were then transferred to liquid nitrogen for storage. The plunge-frozen grids were kept vitreous at−180°C in a Gatan Cryo Transfer Holder model 626.6 (Gatan Inc., Pleasanton, CA, USA) while viewing in a JEOL JEM1230 LaB6 emission TEM (JEOL USA, Inc., Peabody, MA,) at 100 keV. Image data were collected by a Gatan Orius SC1000 CCD camera Model 831 (Gatan Inc., Pleasanton, CA, USA). The images were processed and analyzed using ImageJ.

Small angle X-ray scattering (SAXS) experiments were completed at the DuPont-Northwestern-Dow Collaborative Access Team (DND-CAT) beamline at Argonne National Laboratory's Advanced Photon Source (Argonne, IL, USA) with 10 keV (wavelength $\lambda = 1.24$ Å) collimated X-rays. The q-range calibration was performed using a diffraction standard, silver behenate. All the sample measurements were in the q-range 0.001 to 0.5 $Å^{-1}$. The data reduction procedure including subtraction of solvent buffer scattering to obtain a final scattering curve was made using PRIMUS 2.8.2 software. The filomicelle and micelle samples were confirmed using flexible cylinder and polymer micelle model fits, respectively, using SasView.

In vitro Release Study

To determine the release kinetics of payload from FM-depots, lipophilic dye DiIC18(3) (DiI) (ThermoFisher Scientific) was loaded into the polymer mixture at a final fluorophore concentration of 0.067% w/w. The DiI-loaded polymers were mixed with eight-arm PEG-thiol (10% w/v in PBS solution, Creative PEGWorks) to form a DiI-loaded scaffold in Teflon molds. The DiI-loaded FM-depots were incubated in 1 ml DI water with different concentrations of hydrogen peroxide (0, 1, 100 and 500 mM). At different time points (from 1 h to 30 days), 0.5 ml of supernatant was collected and replaced with 0.5 ml fresh DI water. The amount of payload that had been released was then determined using a fluorescence plate reader (SpectraMax M3, Molecular Devices) at an excitation of 549 nm and an emission of 565 nm.

Zetasizer Nano (Malvern Instruments) equipped with a 4mW He-Ne 633 laser was performed to characterize the size distribution of released nanostructures in the supernatant under different oxidation conditions at different time points. Given that the size of micelles in CryoTEM aligned very well with the number average in DLS (Karabin et al., 2018), the number average was used for the representation of the released nanostructure population. The polydispersity index (PDI) was calculated using a two-parameter fit to the DLS correlation data.

Animals

The apolipoprotein E-deficient ($ApoE^{-/-}$) female mice with C57BL/6 background were purchased from The Jackson Laboratory at 4–6 weeks old. The mice were fed a high-fat diet (HFD, Harlan Teklad TD.88137, 42% kcal from fat) starting at 7 weeks old for 18 weeks until sacrifice. All mice were housed and maintained in the Center for Comparative Medicine at Northwestern University. All experimental animal procedures were performed according to protocols approved by the Northwestern University Institutional Animal Care and Use Committee (IACUC). For each experiment, mice were allocated randomly to each group.

Treatment

Seven weeks old female $ApoE^{-/-}$ were fed a high-fat diet (HFD, Harlan Teklad TD.88137, 42% kcal from fat) for 3 months before

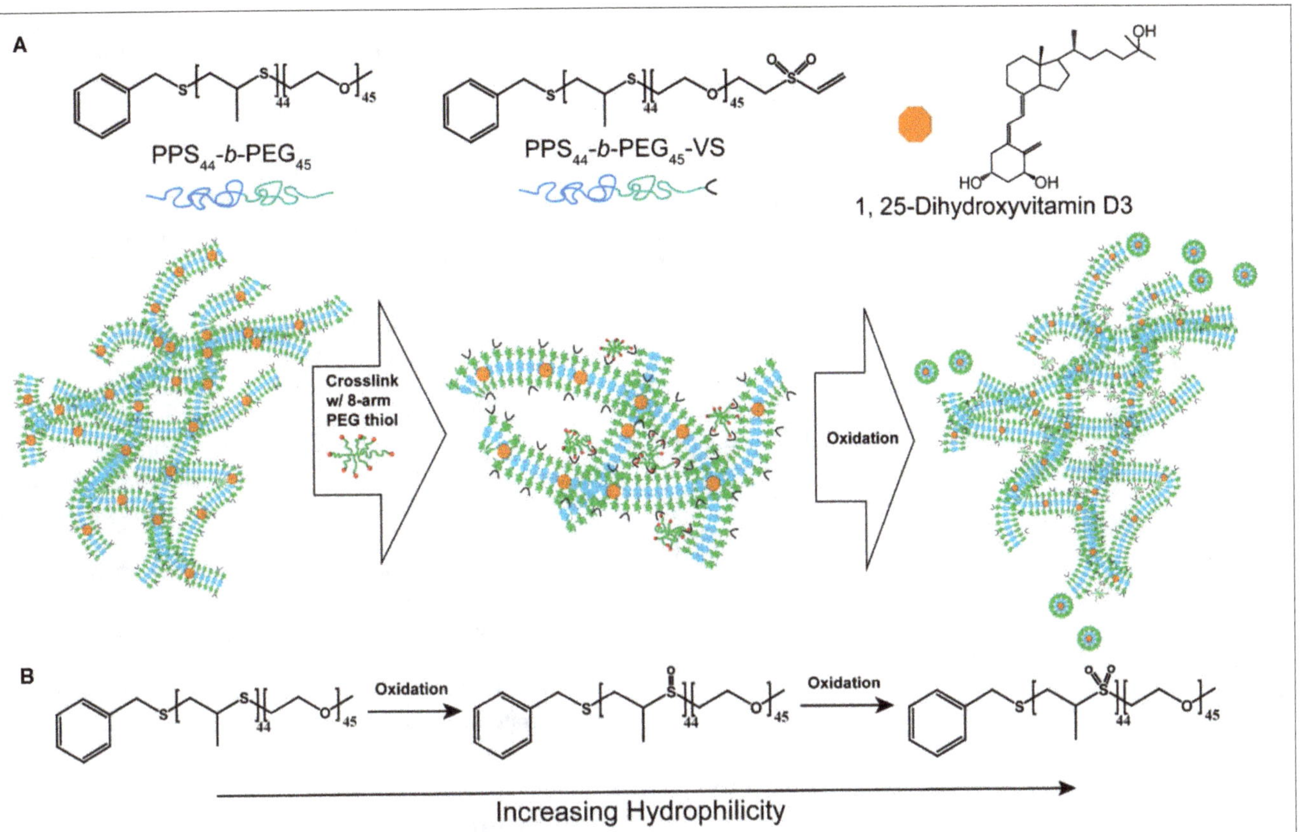

FIGURE 1 | The strategy for sustainably delivering aVD-loaded nanostructures from FM-depots. **(A)** Schematic of the PEG-*b*-PPS copolymers and 1,25-Dihyroxyvitamin D3 (aVD) structures and aVD-loaded filomicelle hydrogel formation. aVD was loaded in filomicelles assembled from PEG-*b*-PPS polymers with 20% vinyl sulfone (VS) functionalization. aVD-loaded FM-depots were formed following crosslinking of VS moieties with 8-arm PEG thiol. aVD-loaded micelles (MC) release from aVD-FM-depots in response to physiological oxidation at the site of injection. **(B)** This thermodynamically driven cylinder-to-sphere transition occurs due to modulation of the hydrophilic/hydrophobic ratio within the filomicelles as the PPS hydrophobic block oxidizes into polypropylene sulfoxide and sulfone derivatives.

treatment. To prepare the 1,25-Dihydroxyvitamin D3 (aVD)-loaded FM scaffold, 1,25-Dihydroxyvitamin D3 (0.0067% w/w) (Sigma) was loaded into the polymers (PEG_{45}-*b*-PPS_{44} and 20% VS-PEG_{45}-*b*-PPS_{44}) to form aVD-loaded FMs. The aVD-loaded FMs in PBS were then quickly vortexed with eight-arm PEG-thiol (10% w/v in PBS solution) before use. After 4 months on a high fat diet, 50 μl of various treatment groups were injected s.c. into the mid-scapular region of $ApoE^{-/-}$ mice every month for 2 months: 1, PBS control; 2, free aVD; 3, aVD-FM-depots. The same amount of aVD (8 μg/kg/month) was used in groups 2 and 3. Mice were kept maintaining on a high-fat diet, and their activities were monitored during treatment.

Flow Cytometry Analysis

After 2 months of treatment, spleen and lymph nodes (two brachial and two axillary from both sides of the mouse) were collected from all groups. Single-cell suspensions from spleen and LNs were prepared as described previously. RBC lysis buffer was used to eliminate red blood cells in spleen samples. Anti-mouse CD16/CD32 was used to block FcRs and Zombie Aqua fixable viability dye was used to determine live/dead cells. For flow cytometric analysis, cells were stained using cocktails of fluorophore-conjugated anti-mouse antibodies: BUV396 anti-CD45, FTIC anti-CD3, PerCP/Cy5.5 anti-CD4, PE anti-CD25, and Alex Fluor 647 anti-Foxp3. After washes, cells were suspended in cell staining buffer and then fixed by IC cell fixation buffer. Intracellular staining of Foxp3 was performed using Foxp3 Fix/Perm Buffer Set following the instruction (Biolegend). At least 200,000 events were recorded per tube on a BD LSRFortessa 6-Laser flow cytometer (BD Biosciences) and data were analyzed with FlowJo software.

Immunohistochemistry

For immunohistochemical analysis, mice were anesthetized and aortas were carefully harvested after perfusion with PBS under a microscope. The heart with aorta was fixed with 4% paraformaldehyde (PFA)/5% sucrose in PBS solution 12 h at 4°C. The tissue samples were immersed in 15% sucrose solution for 12 h and then 30% sucrose solution for 24 h. The resulting specimens were embedded in Tissue-Tek OCT and frozen at −80°C and then sectioned with a cryostat as described previously (Yi et al., 2019). Briefly, serial sections (10 μm thick) of the aortic roots were collected (10–12 sections per mouse) starting at the appearance of aortic valves. The distance between each section was 150 μm, and totally of 100–120 serial cross-sections were obtained. To determine the immune cell populations in aortic lesions, the slides with multiple frozen aortic root sections were fixed in acetone and washed twice with PBS. Antibodies were performed on consecutive cross-sections for Treg cells (anti-Foxp3, 1:500, Abcam). Slides were stained using the Tyramide Signal Amplification kits in MHPL core facility of Northwestern University. All slides containing the cross-sections were digitally imaged with Leica DM6B widefield fluorescent microscope. An in-house software written in Python was used for automated and quantitative image analysis (Yi et al., 2019).

Statistical Analysis

The sample sizes were determined based on the results of pilot experiments so that relevant statistical tests would reveal significant differences. For animal studies, 5–8 mice per group were selected in each experiment. GraphPad Prism software (version 8) was used for data analysis. Data are presented as means ± SD. The two-tailed unpaired *t*-test was performed to determine statistical significance.

RESULTS AND DISCUSSION

Preparation and Characterization of aVD-FM Hydrogel

To achieve sustainable delivery of micellar nanocarriers *in vivo*, an injectable filamentous hydrogel drug depot has been applied. FM-depots allow the sustained delivery of nanocarriers to APC via the cylinder-to-sphere transition at the injection site, wherein the synthetic FM that comprise the depot reassemble into nanocarrier vehicles. In contrast to alternative sustained delivery platforms that employ more stable porous scaffolds to retain nanocarriers for diffusion-based release, FM-depots efficiently degrade into monodisperse nanocarriers to both minimize the amount of administered polymer and avoid chronic inflammation (Yi et al., 2016; Karabin et al., 2018). Cylindrical filomicelles composed of PEG_{45}-*b*-PPS_{44} (F_{PEG} ~0.38) and 20% (w/w%) vinyl sulfone (VS)-functionalized PEG_{45}-*b*-PPS_{44} were assembled and loaded with aVD using the thin-film hydration method (**Figure 1A**), as previously described (Yi et al., 2016; Karabin et al., 2018). The crosslinking density can significantly affect the hydrogel stability, degradation, and the rate of nanostructure release. We have previously investigated the physicochemical properties of the crosslinked hydrogels composed of 10, 20, and 30% (w/w%) VS-PEG_{45}-*b*-PPS_{44}. Mixed filomicelles containing 20% (w/w%) VS-PEG_{45}-*b*-PPS_{44} were found to achieve optimal hydrogel stability and degradation rate while releasing monodisperse nanocarriers following crosslinking with 8-arm PEG-thiol. We, therefore, used 20% VS-PEG_{45}-*b*-PPS_{44} to form the FM-depots in this study. Given the filamentous structure is critical to the hydrogel formation, the structure of aVD-loaded filomicelles (aVD-FM) was verified using both cryogenic transmission electron microscopy (CryoTEM) and small angle x-ray scattering (SAXS). Furthermore, CryoTEM confirmed that loading of hydrophobic immunomodulator aVD into filomicelles does not change the filamentous structure (**Figures 2A,B**). aVD-FM showed micron-scale length, which was comparable with the unloaded filomicelles. SAXS scattering profiles of both unloaded and aVD-FM were fitted using a flexible cylinder model with a cylinder length of 2.1 μm and a core radius of 16 nm (**Figures 2D,F**). Suspensions of filomicelles were simply mixed with the 8-arm PEG thiol, which can be spontaneously crosslinked with VS-functionalized filomicelles. The aVD-FM-depot stably formed within minutes. Due to the oxidation sensitivity of PPS blocks, photo- or physiological oxidation converts the hydrophobic poly(propylene sulfide) into more hydrophilic poly(propylene sulfoxide) and ultimately poly(propylene sulfone) derivatives (**Figure 1B**). Changing the hydrophilic/hydrophobic ratio can trigger a cylinder-to-sphere transition in filomicelles, which we have previously demonstrated via thermodynamic modeling and interfacial measurements to be driven by interfacial tension (Karabin et al., 2018). This morphological transition at the end of the PEG-*b*-PPS filaments into spherical MC, highlighted by white arrows, was clearly observed for aVD-FM using CryoTEM (**Figure 2C**). Moreover, the SAXS analysis showed that the scattering of the oxidized aVD-FM in 500 mM H_2O_2 was fitted well to a MC model with a diameter of 18.4 nm, which is consistent with the oxidized filomicelles without aVD (**Figures 2E,G**). These data suggested that the aVD-FM demonstrated a similar morphological transition with blank FMs upon oxidation.

Sustained Release of Drug-Loaded Micelles From the FM-Depots Upon Oxidation

Excessive ROS is widely acknowledged in atherosclerosis, and high levels of ROS induce systemic oxidative stress, leading to cell apoptosis and redox-dependent signaling disruption (Goncharov et al., 2015). Given the continuous and dynamic production of ROS in the progress of atherosclerosis, it is difficult to accurately quantify the dynamic ROS concentrations in mice. We have previously demonstrated that PEG-*b*-PPS nanostructure morphology is sensitive to physiologic levels of ROS (Du et al., 2017; Karabin et al., 2018), and here we further verified the oxidative responses of FM-depots under various degrees of oxidation *in vitro*. To investigate the release of drug-loaded MC from FM-depots, we chose lipophilic indocarbocyanine dye DiI as a model for hydrophobic drugs. The DiI-loaded FM-depots were immersed in PBS solution with a variety of H_2O_2 concentrations (0, 1, 100, and 500 mM). The poor water solubility of DiI induces its aggregation and precipitation in aqueous environments, allowing fluorescence in the supernatant to be attributed solely to DiI-loaded MC released from FM-depots in response to oxidation. The degradation rate of the hydrogels was found to be dependent on the degree of oxidation (**Figure 3A**), as increasing the H_2O_2 concentration accelerated the disassembly of FM-depots. The supernatants were collected and the release of DiI-loaded MC was then quantified for up to 30 days using a fluorescence plate reader. The *in vitro* release kinetics suggested that the release rate of DiI-loaded MC was correlated with the concentration of H_2O_2 (**Figure 3B**), with a rapid release of >90% after only 1 day in the highest concentration solution of

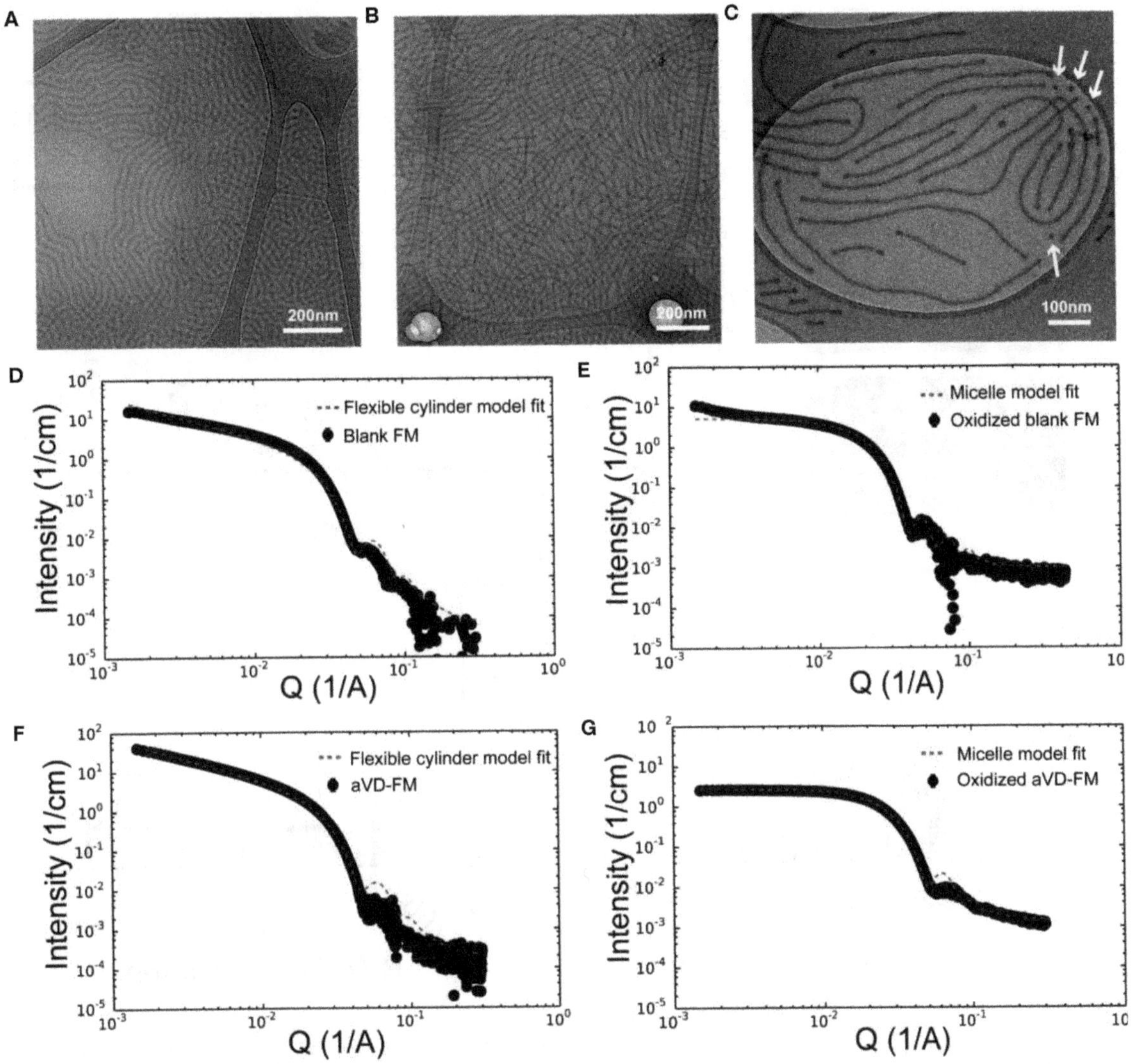

FIGURE 2 | Characterization of aVD-loaded filomicelles. CryoTEM images of filomicelles (FM) **(A)** and aVD-loaded FM **(B,C)**. The white arrows identify the morphological transition from filaments to spherical micelles. Small angle X-ray scattering (SAXS) results are shown for blank FM **(D,E)** and aVD-loaded FM **(F,G)** in PBS solution **(D,F)** or 500 mM H_2O_2 oxidizer **(E,G)**.

500 mM H_2O_2. However, the release rate significantly decreased with decreasing H_2O_2 levels, and excellent stability was observed for the 0% H_2O_2 sample over the course of 30 days. These data are consistent with oxidation induced reassembly of the filomicelle network within the hydrogel into DiI-loaded MC. The DLS data confirmed the morphology transition from FM to MC with an average diameter ranging from 16 to 30 nm (**Figure 3C**). It is noticeable that smaller MC diameters were observed in higher concentrations of H_2O_2 (500 mM) compared to a low H_2O_2 (1 mM) or the PBS control (**Figure 3C**). These data further indicate that the lower interfacial tension of the oxidized PPS drives the disassembly of FM and reassembly into more thermodynamically stable MCs. In addition, more oxidation may lead to a higher hydrophilic/hydrophobic balance and the formation of smaller MC, as the increased steric repulsion within the thicker hydrophilic corona would induce higher MC curvature. It's noteworthy that the released MC are highly uniform with a polydispersity index (PDI) < 0.1 (**Figure 3D**). These results verify that FM-depots can serve as controllable delivery systems for the sustainable release of drug-loaded MC under a wide range of oxidative conditions.

aVD-Loaded FM-Depots Elicit Treg Responses in Atherosclerotic Mice

Although typically associated with modulating bone metabolism, aVD also has potent effects on the regulation of immune responses. Of note, many patients with chronic inflammation like CVD have low levels of the precursor to aVD, 25(OH)VD3, suggesting a potential role for vitamin D in inflammation (Kassi et al., 2013; Yin and Agrawal, 2014). However, clinical

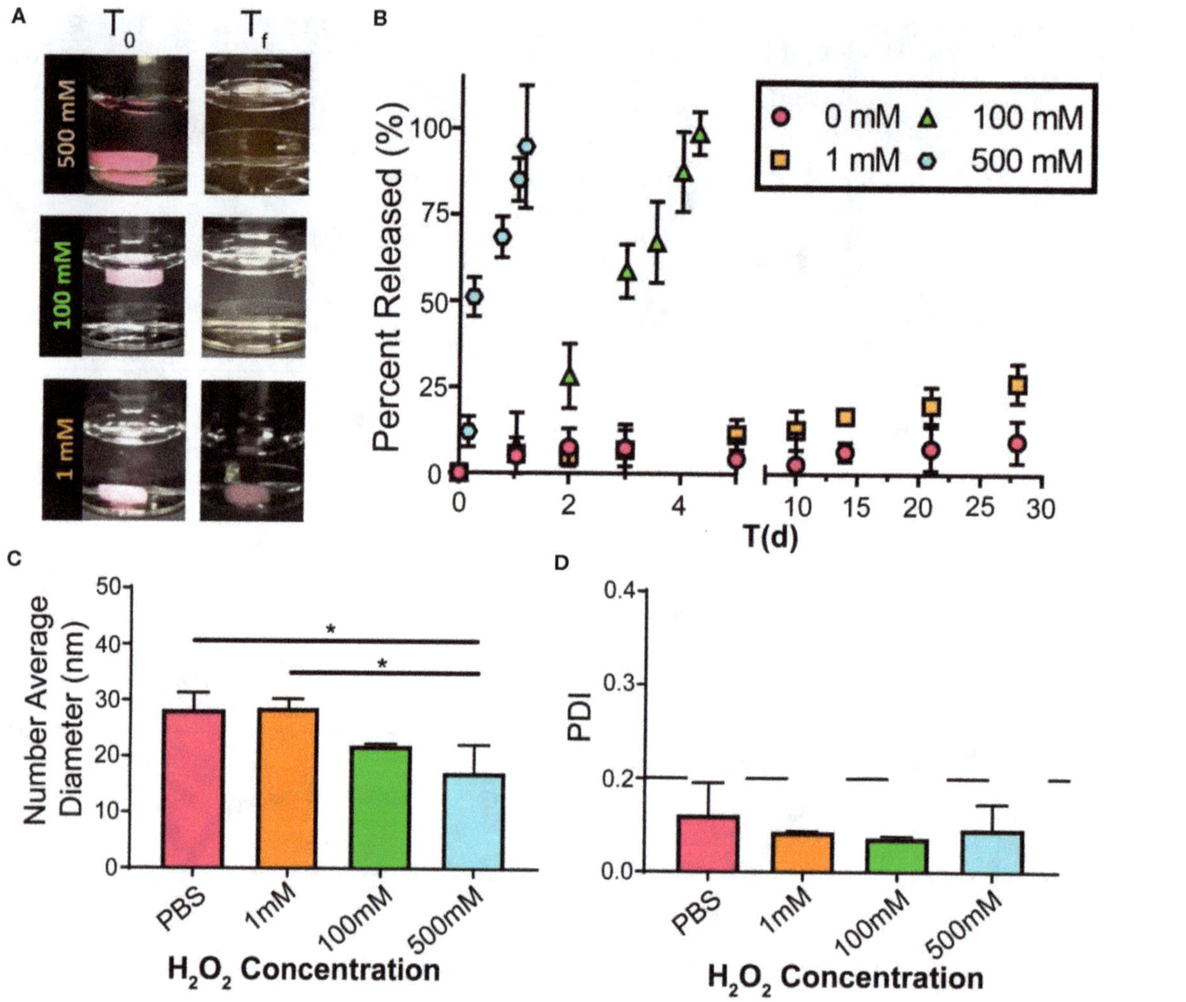

FIGURE 3 | Drug release from FM-depots dependent on the concentration of the oxidizer. **(A)** Pictures of DiI-loaded FM-depots in PBS before and after adding different concentrations of H_2O_2 (1, 100, and 500 mM). **(B)** *in vitro* release kinetics of DiI-loaded MC from the hydrogels upon oxidation with different H_2O_2 concentrations over 30 days. **(C,D)** Average diameters and PDI of DiI-loaded nanostructures in the supernatant released from DiI-loaded FM-depots. $N = 3$. Two-tailed *t*-tests were used for statistical significance: $^*p < 0.05$.

studies showed that oral supplementation of vitamin D has very limited effects on systemic inflammation, likely due to the low bioavailability and the broad distribution of the vitamin D receptor (VDR) (Anderson et al., 2010; Carvalho and Sposito, 2015). Intravenous administration of vitamin D in the form of calcitriol is associated with extensive side effects (Goodman et al., 1994), most notably hypercalcemia (Andress, 2001). We have previously demonstrated that encapsulation of aVD in PEG-*b*-PPS nanostructures significantly enhances the efficacy of aVD without side effects and induces tolerogenic DCs, Foxp3$^+$ Tregs, and anti-inflammatory effects in atherosclerotic mice (Yi et al., 2019). Building upon this work, an injectable hydrogel delivery system may present a more practical option for the administration of aVD-loaded nanocarriers and provide a means for sustained, low-dosage delivery (Li and Mooney, 2016). It is noteworthy that the monodisperse MC released from FM-depots were within the optimal size range for efficient lymphatic drug delivery following subcutaneous injection (Reddy et al., 2006, 2007). As a proof of concept, we loaded aVD at half the dosage employed in our previous work into FM-depots, sustained the delivery over the course of 2 months and assessed the increased levels of Tregs in the lymph nodes and spleen of ApoE$^{-/-}$ mice.

We evaluated the *in vivo* generation of Tregs by aVD loaded FM-depots in 8–10 weeks old female ApoE$^{-/-}$ mice. After receiving a high-fat diet for 3 months, mice were injected s.c. once per month with a PBS control, free aVD (8 μg/kg/month), or an aVD-loaded FM-depot (8 μg aVD/kg/month) (**Figure 4A**). After 2 months of administration, the mice were euthanized and no inflammation (swelling or irritation) was observed at the injection site. Activation of antigen-presenting cells (APCs) has been demonstrated to occur within atherosclerotic lesions and in peripheral lymphoid organs, especially draining lymph

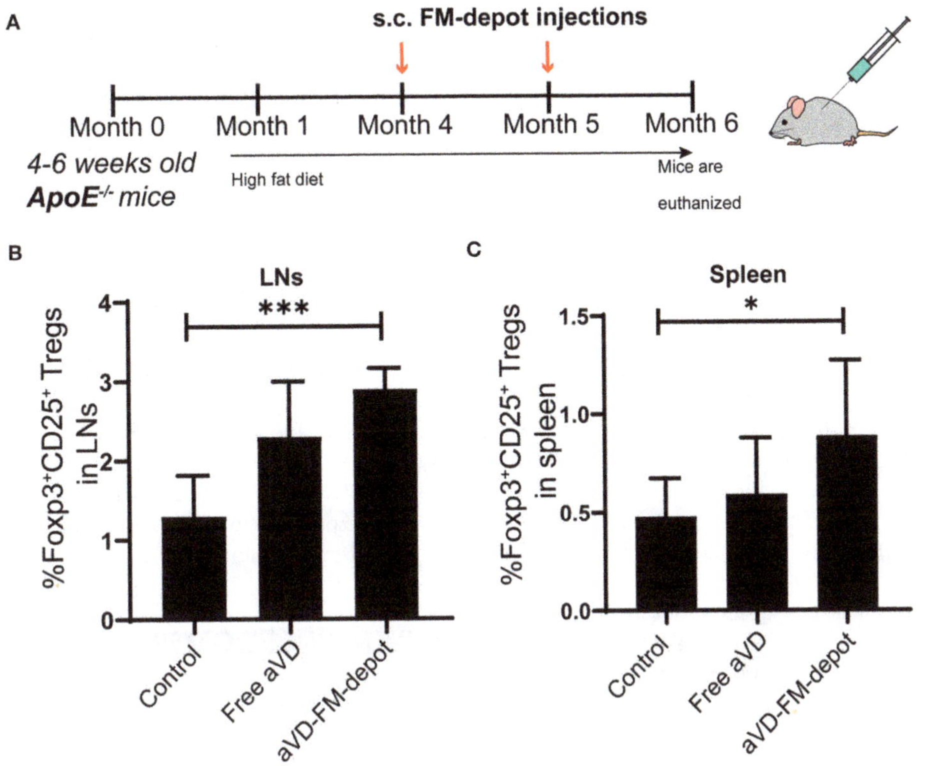

FIGURE 4 | aVD-loaded FM-depots elicit Treg responses in lymph nodes and spleen of ApoE$^{-/-}$ mice. **(A)** Schematic diagram outlining the experimental design for inducing Tregs in ApoE$^{-/-}$ mice. Ten-week old mice were fed with high fat diet for 3 months and then s.c. injected with PBS, free aVD, and aVD-loaded FM-depots monthly. Flow cytometric analysis showed the percentages of Foxp3$^+$ Tregs (Foxp3$^+$CD25$^+$CD4$^+$) gated on CD45$^+$CD3$^+$ live cells in the spleen **(B)** and lymph nodes (LNs) **(C)** of ApoE$^{-/-}$ mice. $N = 5$–8 mice per group. Two-tailed t-tests were used for statistical significance: $^*p < 0.05$, $^{***}p < 0.001$.

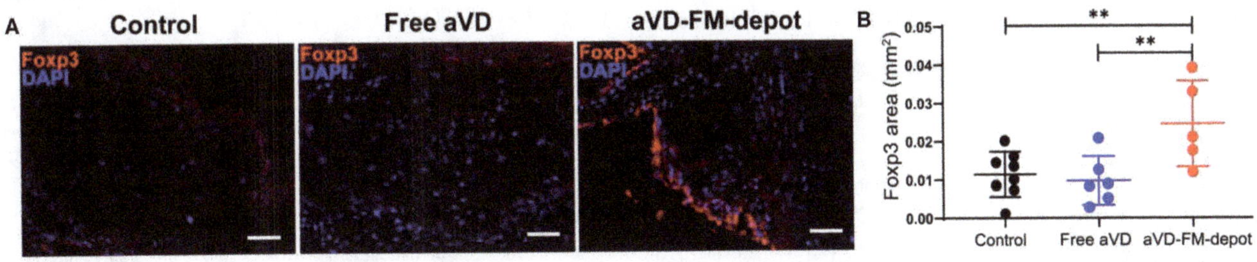

FIGURE 5 | Tregs elicited by aVD-loaded FM-depots migrate to aorta of ApoE$^{-/-}$ mice. **(A)** The expression of Foxp3 (red) was detected by immunofluorescence staining in aortic sinus of ApoE$^{-/-}$ mice. Nuclei were counterstained with DAPI (blue). Scale bar=200 μm. **(B)** Foxp3$^+$ Treg content in aorta was quantified in a serial of cross sections using an in-house developed software. $N = 5$–8 mice per group. Two-tailed t-tests were used for statistical significance: $^{**}p < 0.01$.

nodes and spleen, where T cells migrate back to lesions to manipulate local immune responses (Weber et al., 2008; Zhu et al., 2016). The released MC from s.c. FM-depots have been demonstrated to strongly associate with APCs (macrophages and DCs) in both spleen and lymph nodes (Karabin et al., 2018). We hypothesized that our aVD-FM-depots would deliver aVD-loaded MC to APCs and elicit Treg generation in spleen and migration to vascular lesions. We, therefore, characterized Tregs in lymphoid organs of ApoE$^{-/-}$ mice after a 2-month treatment using flow cytometry. The number of Foxp3$^+$CD25$^+$ Treg cells was significantly increased in CD4$^+$ T cell populations in both lymph nodes ($p < 0.001$) (**Figure 4B**) and spleen ($p < 0.05$) (**Figure 4C**) for the aVD-FM-depot treatments compared to PBS control. However, no statistical difference was observed in the free aVD group compared to the PBS control group. The T cell responses were further evaluated using immunohistochemistry analysis in serial cross-sections of the aortic root. The levels of Foxp3$^+$ Tregs were significantly higher in mice receiving aVD-FM-depots compared to both the free aVD ($p < 0.01$) and PBS controls ($p < 0.01$) (**Figure 5**). Our results indicated that our FM-depots could sustainably deliver aVD-loaded MC and induce accumulation of Tregs responses for at least 2 months in atherosclerotic mice.

CONCLUSIONS

An injectable s.c. hydrogel delivery system for sustained release of aVD-loaded nanocarriers was characterized and validated *in vivo* to elicit Treg responses in a mouse model of atherosclerosis. As a proof of concept, we used a simple system that delivered solely non-targeted, aVD-loaded MC monthly at low dosages. We verified that aVD could be stably loaded into PEG-*b*-PPS filomicelles without modulating the filamentous structure or inhibiting the crosslinking of filomicelles into hydrogels. Both CryoTEM and SAXS showed these aVD-loaded filaments to undergo cylinder-to-sphere transitions as expected under oxidative conditions to release monodisperse MC. In $ApoE^{-/-}$ mice fed a high-fat diet, significantly increased levels of Tregs were found in the lymph nodes, spleen and atheroma following monthly s.c. injections of aVD-loaded FM-depots. Thus, our work indicated that even at low doses and with less frequent administration, the sustained delivery of aVD via FM-depots could significantly induce the proliferation, expansion and homing of $Foxp3^+$ Tregs. This capability may prove to be a promising strategy for clinical translation by offering a practical monthly drug administration regimen and decreased systemic side effects. Although we previously demonstrated that PEG-*b*-PPS filamentous hydrogels could deliver a model fluorescent dye as a payload (Karabin et al., 2018), this is the first demonstration of the sustained delivery of a therapeutic molecule using the cylinder-to-sphere transition to modulate cell function. In future work, we will investigate the therapeutic efficacy of these sustained released FM-depots for inhibition of atherosclerotic plaque development by employing our previously developed nanomedicine-based anti-inflammatory strategies, which include cell-specific targeting (Yi et al., 2019) and alternative atheroprotective immunomodulators (Allen et al., 2019). In summary, this work demonstrates that FM-depots can serve as an effective sustainable delivery platform for the development of combinatorial and sustained delivery approaches to CVD immunotherapy.

AUTHOR CONTRIBUTIONS

SY designed experiments, synthesized and characterized the materials and performed the mouse experiments, wrote the manuscript, and discussed the results. NK, SB, SL, and MF synthesized and characterized the materials and discussed the results. JZ, HL, MV, and YL assisted with the animal experiments. ES was responsible for conceptualization, designing experiments, results discussion, and revising the manuscript.

ACKNOWLEDGMENTS

The authors would like to thank Dr. Eric W. Roth for CryoTEM assistance. The CryoTEM made use of the BioCryo facility of Northwestern University's NUANCE Center, which has received support from the Soft and Hybrid Nanotechnology Experimental (SHyNE) Resource (NSF ECCS-1542205); the MRSEC program (NSF DMR-1720139) at the Materials Research Center; the International Institute for Nanotechnology (IIN); and the State of Illinois, through the IIN. It also made use of the CryoCluster equipment, which has received support from the MRI program (NSF DMR-1229693).

REFERENCES

Allen, S., Liu, Y.-G., and Scott, E. (2016). Engineering nanomaterials to address cell-mediated inflammation in atherosclerosis. *Regen. Eng. Transl. Med.* 2, 37–50. doi: 10.1007/s40883-016-0012-9

Allen, S. D., Liu, Y.-G., Bobbala, S., Cai, L., Hecker, P. I., Temel, R., et al. (2018). Polymersomes scalably fabricated via flash nanoprecipitation are non-toxic in non-human primates and associate with leukocytes in the spleen and kidney following intravenous administration. *Nano Res.* 11, 5689–5703. doi: 10.1007/s12274-018-2069-x

Allen, S. D., Liu, Y.-G., Kim, T., Bobbala, S., Yi, S., Zhang, X., et al. (2019). Celastrol-loaded PEG-b-PPS nanocarriers as an anti-inflammatory treatment for atherosclerosis. *Biomater. Sci.* 7, 657–668. doi: 10.1039/C8BM01224E

Anderson, J. L., May, H. T., Horne, B. D., Bair, T. L., Hall, N. L., Carlquist, J. F., et al. (2010). Relation of vitamin D deficiency to cardiovascular risk factors, disease status, and incident events in a general healthcare population. *Am. J. Cardiol.* 106, 963–968. doi: 10.1016/j.amjcard.2010.05.027

Andress, D. L. (2001). Intravenous versus oral vitamin d therapy in dialysis patients: what is the question? *Am. J. Kidney Dis.* 38, S41–44. doi: 10.1053/ajkd.2001.28108

Carvalho, L. S. F., and Sposito, A. C. (2015). Vitamin D for the prevention of cardiovascular disease: are we ready for that? *Atherosclerosis* 241, 729–740. doi: 10.1016/j.atherosclerosis.2015.06.034

Chistiakov, D. A., Sobenin, I. A., and Orekhov, A. N. (2013). Regulatory T cells in atherosclerosis and strategies to induce the endogenous atheroprotective immune response. *Immunol. Letters* 151, 10–22. doi: 10.1016/j.imlet.2013.01.014

Dietel, B., Cicha, I., Voskens, C. J., Verhoeven, E., Achenbach, S., and Garlichs, C. D. (2013). Decreased numbers of regulatory T cells are associated with human atherosclerotic lesion vulnerability and inversely correlate with infiltrated mature dendritic cells. *Atherosclerosis* 230, 92–99. doi: 10.1016/j.atherosclerosis.2013.06.014

Dowling, D. J., Scott, E. A., Scheid, A., Bergelson, I., Joshi, S., Pietrasanta, C., et al. (2017). Toll-like receptor 8 agonist nanoparticles mimic immunomodulating effects of the live BCG vaccine and enhance neonatal innate and adaptive immune responses. *J. Allergy Clin. Immunol.* 140, 1339–1350. doi: 10.1016/j.jaci.2016.12.985

Du, F., Liu, Y. G., and Scott, E. A. (2017). Immunotheranostic polymersomes modularly assembled from tetrablock and diblock copolymers with oxidation-responsive fluorescence. *Cell Mol. Bioeng.* 10, 357–370. doi: 10.1007/s12195-017-0486-7

Fernández-Friera, L., Fuster, V., López-Melgar, B., Oliva, B., García-Ruiz, J. M., Mendiguren, J., et al. (2017). Normal LDL-cholesterol levels are associated with subclinical atherosclerosis in the absence of risk factors. *J. Am. College Cardiol.* 70, 2979–2991. doi: 10.1016/j.jacc.2017.10.024

George, J., Schwartzenberg, S., Medvedovsky, D., Jonas, M., Charach, G., Afek, A., et al. (2012). Regulatory T cells and IL-10 levels are reduced in patients with vulnerable coronary plaques. *Atherosclerosis* 222, 519–523. doi: 10.1016/j.atherosclerosis.2012.03.016

Goncharov, N., V., Avdonin, P., D., Nadeev, A., Zharkikh, I. L., and Jenkins, R. O. (2015). Reactive oxygen species in pathogenesis of atherosclerosis. *Curr. Pharm. Des.* 21, 1134–1146. doi: 10.2174/1381612820666141014142557

Goodman, W. G., Ramirez, J. A., Belin, T. R., Chon, Y., Gales, B., Segre, G. V., et al. (1994). Development of adynamic bone in patients with secondary hyperparathyroidism after intermittent calcitriol therapy. *Kidney Int.* 46, 1160–1166. doi: 10.1038/ki.1994.380

Hermansson, A., Johansson, D. K., Ketelhuth, D. F. J., Andersson, J., Zhou, X., and Hansson, G. K. (2011). Immunotherapy with tolerogenic apolipoprotein B-100–loaded dendritic cells attenuates atherosclerosis in hypercholesterolemic mice. *Circulation* 123, 1083–1091. doi: 10.1161/CIRCULATIONAHA.110.973222

Hu, P., Seeman, T. E., Harris, T. B., and Reuben, D. B. (2003). Does inflammation or undernutrition explain the low cholesterol–mortality association in high-functioning older persons? MacArthur studies of successful aging. *J. Am. Geriatr. Soc.* 51, 80–84. doi: 10.1034/j.1601-5215.2002.51014.x

Ji, Q., Meng, K., Yu, K., Huang, S., Huang, Y., Min, X., et al. (2017). Exogenous interleukin 37 ameliorates atherosclerosis via inducing the Treg response in ApoE-deficient mice. *Sci. Reports* 7:3310. doi: 10.1038/s41598-017-02987-4

Jia, L., Zhu, L., Wang, J. Z., Wang, X. J., Chen, J. Z., Song, L., et al. (2013). Methylation of FOXP3 in regulatory T cells is related to the severity of coronary artery disease. *Atherosclerosis* 228, 346–352. doi: 10.1016/j.atherosclerosis.2013.01.027

Karabin, N. B., Allen, S., Kwon, H.-K., Bobbala, S., Firlar, E., Shokuhfar, T., et al. (2018). Sustained micellar delivery via inducible transitions in nanostructure morphology. *Nature Commun.* 9:624. doi: 10.1038/s41467-018-03001-9

Kassi, E., Adamopoulos, C., Basdra, E. K., and Papavassiliou, A. G. (2013). Role of vitamin D in atherosclerosis. *Circulation* 128, 2517–2531. doi: 10.1161/CIRCULATIONAHA.113.002654

Kim, J., Cao, L., Shvartsman, D., Silva, E. A., and Mooney, D. J. (2011). Targeted delivery of nanoparticles to ischemic muscle for imaging and therapeutic angiogenesis. *Nano Letters* 11, 694–700. doi: 10.1021/nl103812a

Li, J., and Mooney, D. J. (2016). Designing hydrogels for controlled drug delivery. *Nature Rev. Mater.* 1:16071. doi: 10.1038/natrevmats.2016.71

Mathieu, C., and Adorini, L. (2002). The coming of age of 1,25-dihydroxyvitamin D3 analogs as immunomodulatory agents. *Trends in Molecular Medicine* 8, 174–179. doi: 10.1016/S1471-4914(02)02294-3

Napoli, A., Tirelli, N., Wehrli, E., and Hubbell, J. A. (2002). Lyotropic behavior in water of amphiphilic ABA triblock copolymers based on poly(propylene sulfide) and poly(ethylene glycol). *Langmuir* 18, 8324–8329. doi: 10.1021/la025897n

Napoli, A., Valentini, M., Tirelli, N., Muller, M., and Hubbell, J. A. (2004). Oxidation-responsive polymeric vesicles. *Nat. Mater.* 3, 183–189. doi: 10.1038/nmat1081

Ou, H.-X., Guo, B.-B., Liu, Q., Li, Y.-K., Yang, Z., Feng, W.-J., et al. (2018). Regulatory T cells as a new therapeutic target for atherosclerosis. *Acta Pharmacol. Sinica* 39, 1249–1258. doi: 10.1038/aps.2017.140

Reddy, S. T., Rehor, A., Schmoekel, H. G., Hubbell, J. A., and Swartz, M. A. (2006). *In vivo* targeting of dendritic cells in lymph nodes with poly(propylene sulfide) nanoparticles. *J. Control. Release* 112, 26–34. doi: 10.1016/j.jconrel.2006.01.006

Reddy, S. T., Van Der Vlies, A. J., Simeoni, E., Angeli, V., Randolph, G. J., O'neil, C. P., et al. (2007). Exploiting lymphatic transport and complement activation in nanoparticle vaccines. *Nature Biotechnol.* 25, 1159–1164. doi: 10.1038/nbt1332

Sampson, U. K., Fazio, S., and Linton, M. F. (2012). Residual cardiovascular risk despite optimal LDL cholesterol reduction with statins: the evidence, etiology, and therapeutic challenges. *Curr. Atheroscler. Rep.* 14, 1–10. doi: 10.1007/s11883-011-0219-7

Sansbury, B. E., and Spite, M. (2016). Resolution of acute inflammation and the role of resolvins in immunity, thrombosis, and vascular biology. *Circ. Res.* 119, 113–130. doi: 10.1161/CIRCRESAHA.116.307308

Shao, K., Singha, S., Clemente-Casares, X., Tsai, S., Yang, Y., and Santamaria, P. (2015). Nanoparticle-based immunotherapy for cancer. *ACS Nano* 9, 16–30. doi: 10.1021/nn5062029

Tabas, I., and Lichtman, A. H. (2017). Monocyte-macrophages and T cells in atherosclerosis. *Immunity* 47, 621–634. doi: 10.1016/j.immuni.2017.09.008

Thompson, P. D., Panza, G., Zaleski, A., and Taylor, B. (2016). Statin-associated side effects. *J. Am. College Cardiol.* 67, 2395–2410. doi: 10.1016/j.jacc.2016.02.071

Virani, S. S., Alonso, A., Benjamin, E. J., Bittencourt, M. S., Callaway, C. W., Carson, A. P. (2020). Heart disease and stroke statistics-2020 update: a report from the american heart association. *Circulation* 141, e139–e596. doi: 10.1161/CIR.0000000000000757

Weber, C., Zernecke, A., and Libby, P. (2008). The multifaceted contributions of leukocyte subsets to atherosclerosis: lessons from mouse models. *Nature Rev. Immunol.* 8:802. doi: 10.1038/nri2415

Yi, S., Allen, S. D., Liu, Y.-G., Ouyang, B. Z., Li, X., Augsornworawat, P., et al. (2016). Tailoring nanostructure morphology for enhanced targeting of dendritic cells in atherosclerosis. *ACS Nano* 10, 11290–11303. doi: 10.1021/acsnano.6b06451

Yi, S., Zhang, X., Sangji, M. H., Liu, Y., Allen, S. D., Xiao, B., et al. (2019). Surface engineered polymersomes for enhanced modulation of dendritic cells during cardiovascular immunotherapy. *Adv. Functional Mater.* 29:1904399. doi: 10.1002/adfm.201904399

Yin, K., and Agrawal, D. K. (2014). Vitamin D and inflammatory diseases. *J. Inflamm. Res.* 7, 69–87. doi: 10.2147/JIR.S63898

Zhu, L., Giunzioni, I., Tavori, H., Covarrubias, R., Ding, L., Zhang, Y., et al. (2016). Loss of macrophage LDL receptor related protein 1 (LRP1) confers resistance to the anti-atherogenic effects of TNFα inhibition. *Arterioscler. Thromb. Vasc. Biol.* 36, 1483–1495. doi: 10.1161/ATVBAHA.116.307736

6

Nitric Oxide-Producing Cardiovascular Stent Coatings for Prevention of Thrombosis and Restenosis

Jingdong Rao [1,2], Ho Pan Bei [1], Yuhe Yang [1], Yu Liu [1], Haodong Lin [3] and Xin Zhao [1]**

[1] Department of Biomedical Engineering, The Hong Kong Polytechnic University, Hong Kong, China, [2] State Key Laboratory of Molecular Engineering of Polymers, Department of Orthopedic Surgery, Fudan University, Shanghai, China, [3] General Hospital, Shanghai Jiaotong University School of Medicine, Shanghai, China

***Correspondence:**
Haodong Lin
haodonglin@hotmail.com
Xin Zhao
xin.zhao@polyu.edu.hk

Cardiovascular stenting is an effective method for treating cardiovascular diseases (CVDs), yet thrombosis and restenosis are the two major clinical complications that often lead to device failure. Nitric oxide (NO) has been proposed as a promising small molecule in improving the clinical performance of cardiovascular stents thanks to its anti-thrombosis and anti-restenosis ability, but its short half-life limits the full use of NO. To produce NO at lesion site with sufficient amount, NO-producing coatings (including NO-releasing and NO-generating coatings) are fashioned. Its releasing strategy is achieved by introducing exogenous NO storage materials like NO donors, while the generating strategy utilizes the *in vivo* substances such as *S*-nitrosothiols (RSNOs) to generate NO flux. NO-producing stents are particularly promising in future clinical use due to their ability to store NO resources or to generate large NO flux in a controlled and efficient manner. In this review, we first introduce NO-releasing and -generating coatings for prevention of thrombosis and restenosis. We then discuss the advantages and drawbacks on releasing and generating aspects, where possible further developments are suggested.

Keywords: cardiovascular stents, surface coating, nitric oxide, restenosis, thrombosis

INTRODUCTION

Cardiovascular diseases (CVDs) are a common cause of morbidity worldwide, accounting for 18 million deaths per year, and serve as a third of all global deaths (Frieden and Jaffe, 2018; Yusuf et al., 2020). To treat CVDs, surgical interventions including heart valve replacements (Saito et al., 2003), angioplasty (Stone et al., 2002), and intravascular stents (Zhu et al., 2014) are employed. Among these surgical procedures, cardiovascular stent is most commonly used in coronary heart disease, myocardial infarction, and stenocardia due to its effectiveness at dilating blood vessels and maintaining the circulation of blood (Kubo et al., 2008; Geng et al., 2013; Wei et al., 2013). In the United States alone, ~2 million patients undergo stent implantation each year (Cicha et al., 2016). However, stenting has a high tendency to cause thrombosis and restenosis. Intravascular injuries during surgical implantation stimulate coagulation pathways to facilitate platelet adhesion (Furie and Furie, 2008), and the production of thrombin further contributes to platelet activation and converses fibrinogen into fibrin-formed thrombus (Zhao et al., 2014). The accumulation of platelets and leucocytes causes acute inflammatory response and results in endothelial malfunction, which can lead to excessive proliferation of smooth muscle cells (SMCs) (Naghavi et al., 2013). The extracellular matrix (ECM) produced by SMCs then induces thickening of the vessel wall, contributing to neointimal hyperplasia and restenosis (Scott and Panitch, 2014). As a result, thrombosis and restenosis hamper the long-term effectiveness of cardiovascular devices and induce other related symptoms.

To ease the risk of thrombosis and restenosis, cardiovascular stents are modified with different polymers, biomolecules, or coatings. Compared to the traditional bare metal stents (BMSs) with unacceptable levels of thrombosis and restenosis (Nakamura et al., 2016), drug-eluting stents (DESs) can reduce neointimal hyperplasia and preserve vessel patency by releasing drugs from surface polymers (Joner et al., 2006). However, DESs may induce late thrombosis, which can be attributed to the depletion of drug reservoir, off-target effect of drugs, and the inflammatory response (Mcfadden et al., 2004; Ma et al., 2010). The most recent DES technology fabricates dual-therapy stents (DTSs) that combine two therapeutic regents like aspirin and adenosine diphosphate-receptor blockade for anti-platelet therapy (Ohkubo et al., 2011). Meanwhile, bioresorbable vascular scaffolds (BVSs) can decrease the propensity for thrombosis, since BVSs allow implants to degrade over time and leave an intact vessel (Stone, 2016). Furthermore, bio-engineered stents (BESs) adopt biocompatible materials, cell capture technology, or autologous venous tissue for better therapeutic effects (Stone et al., 2002; Hara et al., 2006; Colombo et al., 2019). In addition to material innovation, novel stent designs also employ coatings to improve the surface properties and clinical behaviors (Yang et al., 2020a). The coating materials possess the feasibility to directly attach or deposit onto the stents' surface and the ability to maintain a high local therapeutic concentration at specific site (Yang et al., 2017). Drugs and biomolecules such as paclitaxel (Palmerini et al., 2015), adhesive peptides (Wei et al., 2013), anti-CD 34 antibodies (Yoon et al., 2002), and nitric oxide (NO)-producing moieties (Gunasekera et al., 2018) are employed to improve the clinical behaviors of stents (see **Table 1** for details). Although these molecules achieved good therapeutic effects, they still present some limitations. For example, high toxicity and non-selective function of paclitaxel raises safety concerns about its side effects while high cost and potential complications of antibodies and adhesive peptides may hinder treatment efficacy (Pacelli et al., 2017). Among all therapeutic molecules, while NO still possesses some drawbacks such as low diffusion distance in blood, it remains highly effective because of its anti-thrombosis and anti-restenosis ability. As an endogenous substance, its pro-proliferative activity to endothelium and anti-adhesion/aggregation effect on platelets additionally allow NO to serve as a guardian of cardiovascular implants (Winther et al., 2018). As reported by the ClinicalTrials.gov website, there are 678 NO-related clinical studies in CVD treatment by April 2020, which reveals the highly promising research and clinical application prospects of NO.

In a healthy vasculature, endothelial cells (ECs) produce NO to achieve thrombotic homeostasis by preventing platelet activation (Seabra et al., 2015). The mechanism of NO inhibition of platelet activity is multifaceted. The main way is to activate the soluble guanylate cyclase (sGC), thereby increasing

TABLE 1 | Typical drugs and biomolecules for anti-thrombosis and anti-restenosis treatment.

Type	Therapeutic substance	Mechanism of action	Therapeutic ability	Drawbacks	References
Drugs	Paclitaxel	Inhibit cell proliferation, adhesion, and migration	Reduce intimal hyperplasia	Indiscriminate cell suppression, delayed re-endothelialization and impaired endothelial functions	(Lundberg et al., 2015; Palmerini et al., 2015)
	Sirolimus/zotarolimus	Interfere cell cycle by inhibiting the mammalian target of rapamycin	Promote re-endothelialization	Long-term safety concerns, late stent thrombosis	(Joner et al., 2006; Park et al., 2010)
Biomolecules	NO and NO-producing materials	Activate soluble guanylate cyclase related signal pathway	Vasodilatation, stimulate EC growth, inhibit SMC proliferation and platelet activation/aggregation	Short-lived, limited diffusion distance, by-products during NO-producing process	De (Mel et al., 2011; Carpenter and Schoenfisch, 2012)
	Antibodies (e.g., CD34 antibody)	Selectively recruit endothelial progenitor cells	Enhance growth of neointimal layer and prevent adhesion of thrombotic tissues	Complex preparation process, high cost, immune response	(Hristov et al., 2003; De Visscher et al., 2012)
	Cell-adhesive peptides (e.g., Arg-Glu-Asp-Val)	Mediate the adsorption and migration of targeted cells	Enhance re-endothelialization and anti-restenosis	Immune response, concerns on complications or undesired tissue growth	(Wei et al., 2013; Mahara et al., 2015)
	Growth factors (e.g., endothelial growth factor)	Promotes EC recruitment, adhesion, migration, and proliferation	Facilitate re-endothelialization	Short half-life, high dose with high cost	(Poh et al., 2010; Shin et al., 2012)
	Heparin	Inhibit the activation of thrombin	Possess anti-coagulant effect and reduce platelet aggregation	Hemorrhage and thrombocytopenia	(Gurbel and Bliden, 2003; Chuang and Masters, 2009)

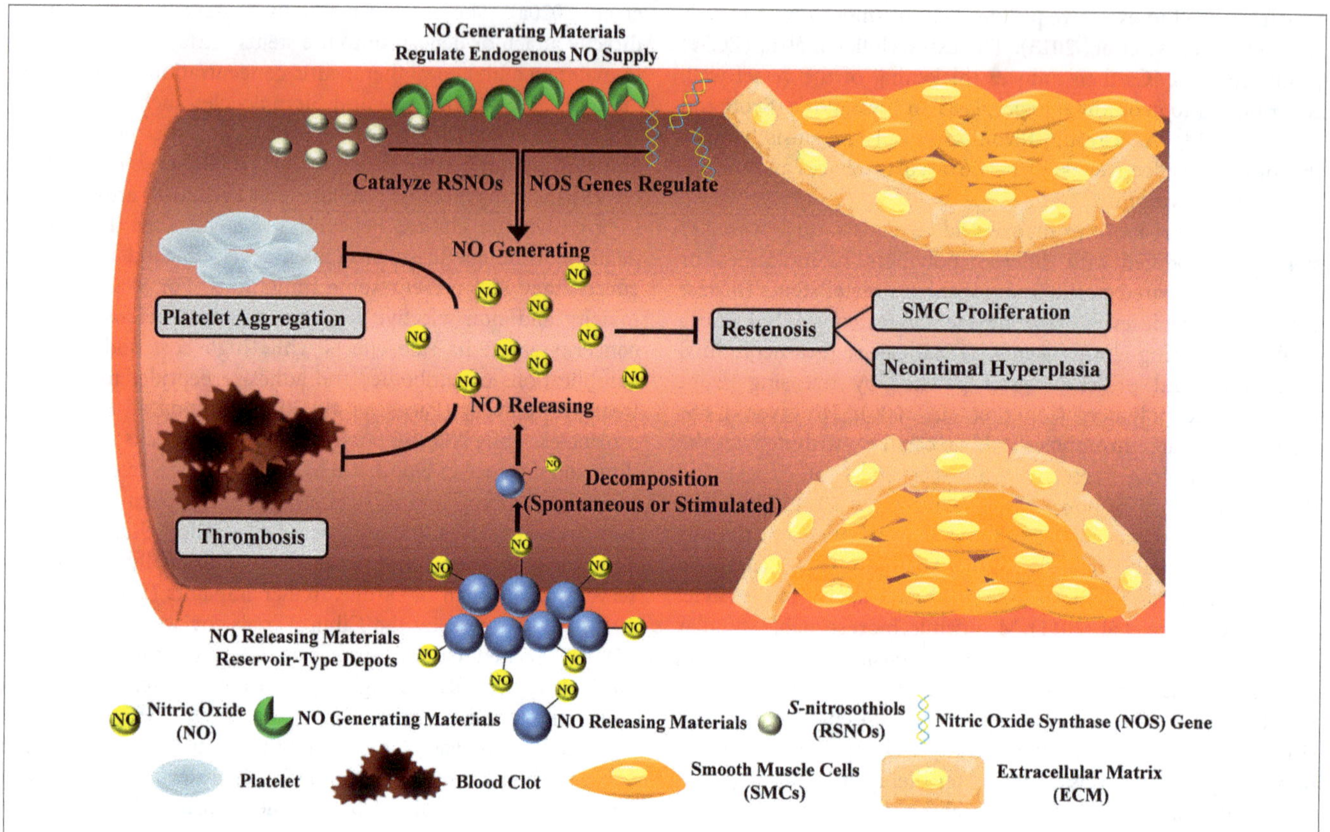

FIGURE 1 | NO-producing strategies for prevention of thrombosis and restenosis. NO-releasing materials such as NO donors and peptides work as a finite reservoir, while NO-generating materials utilize catalytic substances or genes to achieve endogenous NO supply. The NO flux inhibits platelet activation and SMC proliferation, thereby preventing thrombosis and restenosis.

concentrations of cyclic guanosine monophosphate (cGMP) and stimulating the downstream platelet inhibition molecule—Protein Kinase G (PKG) (Francis et al., 2010; Kraehling and Sessa, 2017). The other anti-platelet activity of NO is to inhibit the thromboxane receptor on platelet membranes (Fuentes and Palomo, 2016). Meanwhile, NO is also closely related to cardiovascular homeostasis. In the cardiovascular system, NO can relax the surrounding smooth muscle, lead to vasodilation, and increase blood flow (Jon O Lundberg et al., 2015). Moreover, NO stimulates EC migration and suppresses SMC proliferation (Mel et al., 2011). It also influences angiogenesis and vascular remodeling as well as kills various pathogens (Devine et al., 2019).

Under physical condition, NO can only diffuse around 100 μm and degrades within seconds in blood, so NO must be administered or produced at the diseased site (Thomas, 2015). Hence, incorporating NO production moieties with stent coatings will work as a functional platform to achieve the anti-thrombosis and anti-restenosis purpose. In this review, we will discuss NO-producing coatings, with the emphasis on the NO-releasing and -generating strategies (**Figure 1** and **Table 2**). NO-releasing materials such as NO donors or peptides work as a finite reservoir, while NO-generating strategies utilize catalytic substances or genes to achieve endogenous NO supply. These coatings overcome the challenges of NO administration, and serve as great delivery platforms since they can maintain the physiologically relevant concentrations of NO at a specific site.

NO-RELEASING COATINGS

In NO-releasing strategies, the potential NO can be stored in small molecules or biomolecules, and through connecting, dispersing, or encapsulating those functional molecules as a part of delivery system, the platform will act as a reservoir for conditional and spontaneous release of NO.

NO Donors

NO donors [e.g., N-diazeniumdiolates (NONOates), *S*-nitroso-*N*-acetylpenicillamine (SNAP)] are pharmacologically active substances that carry NO for localized release (Major et al., 2010; Midgley et al., 2019). NONOates can be synthesized by reacting gaseous NO with secondary amines under high pressure (5 atm) and spontaneously decomposed to release two moles of NO per mole of donor at physiological condition (Midgley et al., 2019), while SNAP, a kind of synthetic *S*-nitrosothiols (RSNOs), requires reactions between nitrosating agents and thiols, and NO can be exhausted from SNAP by heat, light (340 and 590 nm), or copper ions (Naghavi et al., 2013).

TABLE 2 | NO-producing strategies in anti-thrombosis and anti-restenosis treatment.

Category	Functional substance	Mechanism of NO production	Advantages	Drawbacks
NO-releasing materials	NO donors (e.g., NONOates, SNAP)	Release NO at physiological condition by heat, light, copper ions	Store NO molecules	Limited releasing period, instability of the NO donors, finite reservoir of NO
	NO prodrugs (e.g., Gal-NONOates)	Release NO upon enzyme-triggering	Keep NO donors stable, prolong the releasing time	Drug waste and side effects by systemic delivery, finite reservoir of NO
	Peptide amphiphiles	Spontaneously release NO from NO donating residues	Mimic biochemical properties, prolong the releasing time	High cost, difficulties in peptide activity control, finite reservoir of NO
NO-generating materials	Gene therapy	Initiate NOS production	Achieve durable regulation by long-term expression	Instability, deliverability, release kinetics, off-target transduction, and high cost
	Catalytic approaches (e.g., Se, Cu^{II})	Catalyze decomposition of RSNOs by GPx-like catalytic substances	Exhibit significant long-lasting NO production with relative high NO flux	Lack of smart control in different disease stages
Combination strategy	Integration of NO release and generation (e.g., SNAP with copper nanoparticles, EPT with ZnO particles)	Ensure the supply of both exogenous and endogenous of NO	Achieve flexible, extended and controllable NO supply, be suitable in various therapeutic needs	Raise excessive NO production concerns

For example, Joung et al. fabricated NONOates containing liposome stent coatings via layer-by-layer (LBL) method to control the release of NO (Elnaggar et al., 2016). The NO release profiles showed that the release rate sustained up to 5 days with good thrombo-resistant effect. As thrombus involves the formation of fibrin and activation of platelets, Yang et al. proposed a novel concept to integrate anti-coagulant agent bivalirudin (BVLD) and NO as a bulk synergetic modification on surface coating (Yang et al., 2020b). BVLD was covalently connected with the primary amine groups on plasma polymerized allylamine (PPAm)-coated surface, and then the coating was immersed in basic solution under high-pressure NO gas to form a NONOate-like bulk depot. For circumventing NO burst release, hydrophobic hexafluoroethane was introduced into this system, which prolonged the release time of NO to more than 8 h. Compared to 316L SS, the occlusion rate and thrombus weight in BVLD/NO-PPAmF were reduced from $58.7 \pm 3.9\%$ to $3.3 \pm 1.2\%$ and 64.1 ± 3.9 mg to 1.7 ± 1.2 mg after 2 h of extracorporeal circulation (ECC), respectively. Since the complexity of thrombogenic process requires multi-therapy procedures, the combination of anti-platelet and anti-coagulant dual functions is a promising strategy to integrate into cardiovascular coatings.

However, the NO release period in these studies was limited. To extend the NO release time, Hopkins et al. designed a highly stable NO-releasing coating by covalently attaching SNAP with poly(dimethylsiloxane) (PDMS) (Hopkins et al., 2018). Previous studies demonstrated that SNAP-based polymers have exhibited significant leaching of SNAP, which will result in non-localized NO release (Brisbois et al., 2016). Through tethering to PDMS, SNAP leaching into surrounding environment was prevented and allowed for lengthened potency. The NO flux formation of SNAP-PDMS reached up to 125 days *in vitro* and maintained at 0.1×10^{-10} mol $\times$ cm^{-2} $\times$ min^{-1} till the end of the testing period. The SNAP-PDMS showed long-duration anti-bacterial efficacy, and it exhibited 78% thrombus reduction (compared with blank control) after testing by ECC over 4 h. Although this strategy achieved long-term NO release, the low NO levels in the later release stages limited the long-lasting anti-thrombotic effect.

Despite these efforts on NO donor applications, the long-term therapeutic effect after implantation was unsatisfying. Integrating NO-donor loaded liposomes with stents faces the risk of low loading capacity, carrier detachment from the stents and delayed NO release. Chemical covalent bond offers bulk NO donor storage, but it also brings extra reaction regents and shows relative low NO flux. Besides, the instability of the NO donors is a big obstacle that cannot be solved by simple connection or encapsulation. Hence, many other coatings have been developed for better application.

NO Prodrugs

Since NO donors are unstable under thermal, acidic, or physiological conditions, researchers use enzyme prodrug therapy (EPT) to maintain the stability of donors and control the release (Chandrawati et al., 2017). By fabricating NO donors (e.g., NONOates) with enzyme-sensitive linkers, the formed prodrugs remain stable and inactive in non-enzymatic environment and only release NO upon enzyme-triggering.

In a study of NO EPT, Wang et al. designed a galactosidase (Gal) immobilized surface coating and prepared glycosylated NONOate (Gal-NONOate) as NO prodrug (Wang et al., 2015). After the *in vivo* implantation of enzyme-functional platform, Gal-NONOate was administrated by tail vein injection, it then circulated until contact with the coating and the enzyme would catalyze the decomposition of the prodrug to release NO locally. The *in situ* release of NO was verified using a fluorescent probe to trace the NO flux. The immobilized enzyme retained the catalytic property up to 1 month *in vivo* and the results revealed effective inhibition of thrombosis and enhancement of vascular tissue regeneration and remodeling in EPT group. To engineer EPT for diverse medicinal implants, Zelikin et al. optimized EPT coating by adopting LBL method to fabricate multilayered polyelectrolyte coating with immobilized β-Gal enzyme (Winther et al., 2018). This method was all-aqueous and solution-based, which could accommodate modification of any substrate with no restriction on surface topography and geometry.

In addition to maintaining NO donors' stability, through using different concentrations of prodrugs or regulating administration time to adjust physiological effect, EPT can achieve personalized, fine-tuned therapeutic delivery of NO (Pan et al., 2015). Nevertheless, EPT requires systemic delivery of NO prodrugs, which only has effect at the enzyme-modified lesion site. This means that even with a bulky administration, only a small portion of drugs would work, which causes drug waste and side effects due to the high cytotoxicity of the drug. Scientists thus have developed other biomolecules to achieve NO release.

NO-Releasing Peptide Amphiphiles

Peptide amphiphiles (PAs) consist of hydrophobic tails coupled to hydrophilic functional peptide sequences that are attractive in biomimetic scaffolds, since enzyme-mediated degradable sites and cell adhesion ligands can be incorporated into PAs to mimic some biochemical properties (Jun et al., 2005; Cheng et al., 2015).

In a report by Matson et al., a NO-releasing PA coating was designed (Kushwaha et al., 2010). The functional peptide sequences involved a matrix metalloprotease-2 (MMP2) mediated cleavage site Gly-Thr-Ala-Gly-Leu-Ile-Gly-Gln (GTAGLIGQ), coupled to an EC-adhesive ligand Tyr-Ile-Gly-Ser-Arg (YIGSR) or a polylysine (KKKKK) group to form NO donating residue peptide. Burst release of NO occurred within 48 h, followed by sustained release for 30 days. This functional peptide increased initial adhesion of ECs from $51 \pm 3\%$ to $67 \pm 2\%$, while the proliferation of SMCs were inhibited from $35 \pm 2\%$ to $16 \pm 3\%$ after 48 h of incubation. Additionally, compared with the positive control collagen group, the peptide group showed 150-fold decrease in platelet attachment, suggesting the potential of such coating for modification of various cardiovascular implants. Similarly, Alexander et al. used the same PAs to form a nanomatrix coating (Alexander et al., 2016), and they proved the vasodilatory effects *ex vivo* and the anti-inflammatory ability *in vitro*. This coating could address the shortcomings of the implanted stents and had the potential to be developed in animal models with cardiovascular stents. However, it is difficult to popularize peptide clinical application due to the high cost of peptides and the lack of control over their activity.

NO-releasing strategies have showed appropriate therapeutic effects on thrombosis and restenosis, but they still possess some shortcomings. In addition to the problems of different NO-releasing materials discussed above, all these strategies have to face the biggest obstacle—the finite reservoir of NO. With the NO release reaction proceeding, the elements will be exhausted within a short time frame. Therefore, reliable long-term and sufficient NO supplies need to be achieved.

NO-GENERATING COATINGS

Radical NO species are short-lived. To overcome this drawback, NO-generating materials were developed, which utilize genes and catalytic substances such as selenium (Se) or copper ions to stimulate NO production. These strategies can achieve sufficient and long-term NO release depending on the endogenous regulation and continuous supply of NO resources.

NOS Gene Therapy

In the cardiovascular system, nitric oxide synthase (NOS) especially endothelial NOS (eNOS) and inducible NOS (iNOS) play a very important role. eNOS is highly related to the function of the endothelium, which can catalyze the production of NO via enzymatic effect (Zhao et al., 2013). iNOS is normally absent in the vasculature under physiological conditions, but it expresses in blood vessels under pathological situations (Sessa, 2004), and it can generate large amounts of NO over long periods of time (Kleinert et al., 2005). Since NOS has emerged as an active player in NO generation, a lot of therapeutic strategies have been developed around it. Gene therapy in CVDs can improve the selectivity of exerted effects toward certain cells and has the potential for combination therapy. Many researchers have thus investigated the therapeutic effect of NOS genes (Forstermann et al., 2017). In a study, DiMuzio et al. developed a natural vascular tissue mimetic stent by seeding it with autologous adipose-derived stem cells (ASCs) differentiated endothelial-like cells, and they used the eNOS gene to transfect these ASCs (McIlhenny et al., 2013). The transfection initiated eNOS production, yielding eNOS to generate functional NO gas. They found that the transfected ASCs produced NO (247 ± 10 nM) at a similar level to EC controls (288 ± 29 nM) *in vitro*, and exhibited a non-thrombogenic surface compared to unseeded controls *in vivo*.

In addition to *in vitro* gene transfection therapy, gene delivery is another approach to achieve targeted protein expression. To deliver NOS gene, Levy et al. described a gene delivery platform that provided local arterial gene transfer via iNOS-encoding adeno-associated virus serotype 2 (AAV2) vectors (Fishbein et al., 2017). Through affinity effect, the iNOS-cDNA sequence loaded AAV2 vectors could be immobilized onto stent surfaces. Compared to the non-gene group, $AAV2_{iNOS}$ showed a 16-fold higher NO production *in vitro*. $AAV2_{iNOS}$ demonstrated escalating expression of encoded transgene for 12 weeks and showed the anti-restenosis efficacy with 95% inhibition rate *in vivo*.

Although there are many attempts in using NOS gene strategies, the instability, deliverability, release kinetics, off-target transduction, and high cost of gene limit the clinical application. Researchers are hence working hard on more effective NO-generating pathways.

Endogenous NO Catalytic Approaches

RSNOs, a kind of endogenous NO donors in the blood, has highly promising opportunities to achieve localized synthesis of NO for continuous supply (Li et al., 2018). It was found that glutathione peroxidase (GPx) and Se or copper ions with GPx-like catalytic

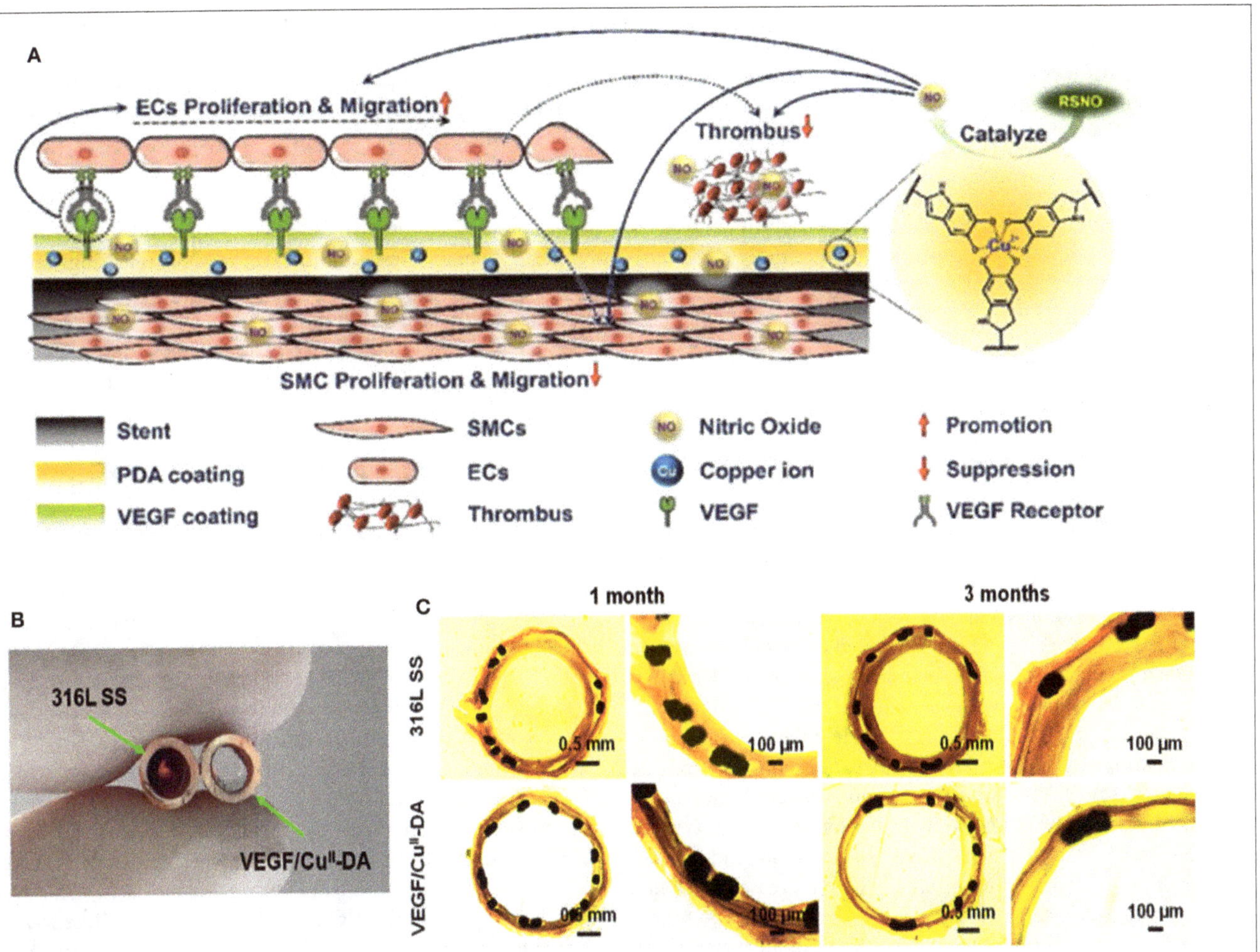

FIGURE 2 | Cardiovascular stents with VEGF/Cu^{II}-DA coatings for enhanced re-endothelialization and reduced thrombosis. **(A)** Mechanism of thrombosis and restenosis prevention of VEGF/Cu^{II}-DA-coated stents. The spatiotemporal dual delivery of VEGF and NO enabled the fast re-endothelialization of stents and prevented thrombosis and restenosis. **(B)** Images of cross-sectioned tubing containing uncoated and VEGF/Cu^{II}-DA-coated 316L SS foils exposed for 1.5 h to blood flow in a rabbit arteriovenous shunt model. **(C)** Histomorphometric analysis on restenosis at bare 316L SS and VEGF/Cu^{II}-DA-coated stents using Van Gieson's staining. Image source: Tu et al. (2020).

activity can catalyze the decomposition of RSNOs into NO *in vivo* (Weng et al., 2011; McCarthy et al., 2016).

Recently, our group developed one-pot approach to incorporate selenocystamine (SeCA) in the framework of dopamine (DA) via co-immobilization (Yang et al., 2018). The NO release rates could be controlled (from 0.5 to 2.2 $\times$ 10^{-10} mol $\times$ cm^{-2} $\times$ min^{-1}) by regulating the SeCA–DA molar ratio. The study showed that the SeCA/DA coating could release NO for more than 60 days, which achieved long-lasting prevention of thrombosis and restenosis. Additionally, the simple operation avoided the tedious process and toxic chemicals. This coating is believed to be universally formed on diverse types of materials with great clinical potential. We further improved the NO production ability by employing Cu^{II} instead of SeCA, since Cu^{II} possesses superior NO catalytic efficacy (Zhang et al., 2019). The NO release rates could reach to natural endothelium rates (0.5 to 4 $\times$ 10^{-10} mol $\times$ cm^{-2} $\times$ min^{-1}) by adjusting the dose of Cu^{II} with NO flux ranging from 0.4 to 6.5 $\times$ 10^{-10} mol $\times$ cm^{-2} $\times$ min^{-1}. After implantation for 3 months, the DA-Cu^{II}-coated stents not only inhibited thrombosis, but also promoted re-endothelialization and reduced neointimal formation. We then additionally endowed our stents with anti-bacterial properties (Tu et al., 2019). In this system, cystamine (CySA) was chosen to fabricate the metal-phenolic-amine-based coatings with gallic acid (GA) and Cu^{II}. GA was added as chelating agent with anti-bacterial properties, which worked synergistically with Cu^{II} in bacterial inhabitation. The integrated coating showed 99% anti-bacterial rate *in vitro* and 3.4 $\pm$ 0.2% occlusion rate *in vivo* after implantation for 30 days. In our most recent study, we further immobilized vascular endothelial growth factor (VEGF) with DA-Cu^{II} coating (**Figure 2A**) (Tu et al., 2020). The introduction of VEGF was found to accelerate the early-stage EC adhesion, migration, and growth, forming a new and complete endothelium on the stents. The NO flux generated by the DA-Cu^{II} coatings successfully suppressed thrombosis (**Figure 2B**). Scanning electron microscope images showed that after 1 and 3 months of implantation, VEGF/Cu^{II}-DA coating demonstrated greater re-endothelialization compared to 316L SS (**Figure 2C**). Altogether, the multiple programmed therapeutic strategies for spatiotemporal dual delivery of NO and VEGF significantly prevented thrombosis and restenosis.

Nevertheless, these RSNO catalytic stents face difficulty in smart control of NO production. Additionally, different stages of disease and therapeutic purposes require different amounts of NO, a flexible, extended, and controllable NO supply is therefore highly sought after.

NO-RELEASING AND -GENERATING INTEGRATING COATINGS

There are substantial achievements of the anti-thrombosis and anti-restenosis therapeutic effects of NO-releasing and -generating strategies, but limitations still exist. Researchers thus make effort to combine those two strategies to supplement NO delivery. Maintaining NO release within the physiological region (0.5 to 4×10^{-10} mol $\times$ cm^{-2} $\times$ min^{-1}, and preferably at the up end) can be more efficient for biomedical applications, but the NO donors such as SNAP have been shown to release NO near the low end of the physiological levels. Based on this, Handa et al. incorporated SNAP in a medical grade polymer coated with copper nanoparticles to achieve better regulation of NO release (Pant et al., 2017). This strategy not only ensured the supply of exogenous NO by SNAP, but also provided the enzymatic NO release via the reaction of copper ions on endogenous RSNOs in the blood. The Cu-SNAP had increased NO flux values to around 4.48 or 4.84×10^{-10} mol $\times$ cm^{-2} $\times$ min^{-1} when using different dosage of Cu. Additionally, significant reduction in bacterial growth and effective prevention of platelet adhesion has been achieved. Similarly, Brisbois et al. developed a multi-layered SNAP-doped polymer with a blended Se interface, and they focused on the different needs during the therapy process (Mondal et al., 2019). The first few hours after device implantation are crucial in preventing infection, since biofilm formation can occur rapidly after insertion (<24 h). The initial NO flux of generating materials may, however, be inadequate in preventing platelet activation or infection at early onslaught. Hence, in this strategy, SNAP offered initial NO release and Se interface could continuously generate NO in the presence of RSNOs. The results showed that there was a burst NO release on day 1, then the coating maintained a high and continuous NO release in the subsequent days. As a result, the enhanced initial NO flux would provide a potent anti-microbial activity acutely at the time of surgical placement, while the continuous NO generation contributed to inhibiting blood clot formation and protecting chronic or late device infections.

In addition to the above strategies to regulate the NO flux by using different coating compositions, Chandrawati et al. incorporated zinc oxide (ZnO) particles with EPT (Yang et al., 2020c). ZnO possess innate glutathione peroxidase and glycosidase activities, which allowed ZnO to catalytically decompose both endogenous (RSNOs) and exogenous (β-Gal-NONOate) donors to produce NO at physiological conditions. This strategy could solve problems such as finite pool of NO donors, short shelf life and low stability of natural enzymes in EPT. ZnO preserved its catalytic property for at least 6 months and the activity in producing NO was demonstrated. By tuning ZnO and NO prodrugs, physiologically NO levels were achieved. This method will be beneficial in long-term NO production and extra NO supplement can be achieved by on-demand NO prodrug administration, which has promising development in diverse blood-contacting devices.

In a word, the combination of NO-releasing and NO-generating chemistries within a single platform allows for a release profile that achieves the best of both worlds. However, further studies should effectively control the amount of NO flux to avoid excessive NO production and related potential toxicity.

CONCLUSION AND FUTURE WORK

The progress of the NO-producing stent coatings are highly inspiring in the prevention of thrombosis and restenosis, and researchers have also attempted to improve the fabrication process and committed to developing simple materials for future clinical application. However, the immune reaction, inflammation, anaphylaxis, and biocompatibility of the coatings need to be further investigated. Although these problems cannot be solved temporarily, in the long term, what can be done is to promote the development of NO production strategies from those achievable directions: (1) Combination strategies of NO and other pathway regulation need to be carefully considered about the dosage ratio between the drugs to avoid the antagonism effect and ensure synergistic effect. (2) The toxicity and metabolism of the NO reaction, by-products [like N-Acetyl-D-penicillamine (NAP) and disulfide] should be taken into account. (3) Scientists should develop precise methods of NO quantitative detection *in vivo* to meet different needs. (4) Smart NO production system can be further developed to respond to the microenvironment changes and to produce NO flux on-demand during different pathologic process. (5) Most researchers use healthy animals to evaluate the effect of NO; however, differences between the healthy and the CVD individuals should be assessed. Researchers should also combine the effects of NO-producing coatings and the implanted materials as a whole to investigate the therapeutic effect in their corresponding disease models, which will have much more clinical significance.

In summary, NO-releasing and NO-generating strategies still have significant room for improvement, and a thorough understanding of NO production and solutions for the corresponding pathological reaction will ensure the safe clinical practices for the next generation of technological devices. We hope that this review can be helpful for the further development in this research field.

AUTHOR CONTRIBUTIONS

XZ and HL supervised the whole review. JR and HP wrote the manuscript. YY and YL performed literature search and revised the manuscript. All the authors approved the review for publication.

ACKNOWLEDGMENTS

The authors acknowledge the financial support from the seed projects of the Hong Kong Innovation and Technology Support Programme (ITS/065/19), the Program of Outstanding Medical Talent of Shanghai Municipal Health Bureau (grant number 2017BR034), and the State Key Laboratory of Molecular Engineering of Polymers of Fudan University (K2019-20).

REFERENCES

Alexander, G. C., Vines, J. B., Hwang, P. T. J., Kim, T., Kim, J., Brott, B. C., et al. (2016). Novel multifunctional nanomatrix reduces inflammation in dynamic conditions *in vitro* and dilates arteries *ex vivo*. *ACS Appl. Mater. Inter.* 8, 5178–5187. doi: 10.1021/acsami.6b00565

Brisbois, E. J., Kim, M., Wang, X., Mohammed, A., Major, T. C., Wu, J., et al. (2016). Improved hemocompatibility of multilumen catheters via nitric oxide (NO) release from S-Nitroso-N-acetylpenicillamine (SNAP) composite filled lumen. *ACS Appl. Mater. Interfaces* 8, 29270–29279. doi: 10.1021/acsami.6b08707

Carpenter, A. W., and Schoenfisch, M. H. (2012). Nitric oxide release: part II. Therapeutic applications. *Chem. Soc. Rev.* 41, 3742–3752. doi: 10.1039/c2cs15273h

Chandrawati, R., Chang, J. Y., Reinatorres, E., Jumeaux, C., Sherwood, J. M., Stamer, W. D., et al. (2017). Localized and controlled delivery of nitric oxide to the conventional outflow pathway via enzyme biocatalysis: toward therapy for glaucoma. *Adv. Mater.* 29:1604932. doi: 10.1002/adma.201604932

Cheng, Y., Cheng, H., Zhao, X., Xu, X., Zhuo, R., and He, F. (2015). Self-assembled micelles of a multi-functional amphiphilic fusion (MFAF) peptide for targeted cancer therapy. *Polym. Chem.* 6, 3512–3520. doi: 10.1039/C5PY00125K

Chuang, T., and Masters, K. S. (2009). Regulation of polyurethane hemocompatibility and endothelialization by tethered hyaluronic acid oligosaccharides. *Biomaterials* 30, 5341–5351. doi: 10.1016/j.biomaterials.2009.06.029

Cicha, I., Singh, R., Garlichs, C. D., and Alexiou, C. (2016). Nano-biomaterials for cardiovascular applications: clinical perspective. *J. Control. Release* 229, 23–36. doi: 10.1016/j.jconrel.2016.03.015

Colombo, A., Chandrasekhar, J., Aquino, M., Ong, T. K., Sartori, S., Baber, U., et al. (2019). Safety and efficacy of the COMBO bio-engineered stent in an all-comer PCI cohort: 1-year final clinical outcomes from the MASCOT post-marketing registry. *Int. J. Cardiol.* 283, 67–72. doi: 10.1016/j.ijcard.2019.01.053

De Visscher, G., Mesure, L., Meuris, B., Ivanova, A., and Flameng, W. (2012). Improved endothelialization and reduced thrombosis by coating a synthetic vascular graft with fibronectin and stem cell homing factor SDF-1α. *Acta Biomater.* 8, 1330–1338. doi: 10.1016/j.actbio.2011.09.016

Devine, R., Singha, P., and Handa, H. (2019). Versatile biomimetic medical device surface: hydrophobin coated, nitric oxide-releasing polymer for antimicrobial and hemocompatible applications. *Biomater. Sci.* 7, 3438–3449. doi: 10.1039/C9BM00469F

Elnaggar, M. A., Seo, S., Gobaa, S., Lim, K. S., Bae, I., Jeong, M. H., et al. (2016). Nitric oxide releasing coronary stent: a new approach using layer-by-layer coating and liposomal encapsulation. *Small* 12, 6012–6023. doi: 10.1002/smll.201600337

Fishbein, I., Guerrero, D. T., Alferiev, I. S., Foster, J. B., Minutolo, N. G., Chorny, M., et al. (2017). Stent-based delivery of adeno-associated viral vectors with sustained vascular transduction and iNOS-mediated inhibition of in-stent restenosis. *Gene Ther.* 24, 717–726. doi: 10.1038/gt.2017.82

Forstermann, U., Xia, N., and Li, H. (2017). Roles of vascular oxidative stress and nitric oxide in the pathogenesis of atherosclerosis. *Circ. Res.* 120, 713–735. doi: 10.1161/CIRCRESAHA.116.309326

Francis, S. H., Busch, J. L., and Corbin, J. D. (2010). cGMP-dependent protein kinases and cGMP phosphodiesterases in nitric oxide and cGMP action. *Pharmacol. Rev.* 62, 525–563. doi: 10.1124/pr.110.002907

Frieden, T. R., and Jaffe, M. (2018). Saving 100 million lives by improving global treatment of hypertension and reducing cardiovascular disease risk factors. *J. Clin. Hypertens.* 20, 208–211. doi: 10.1111/jch.13195

Fuentes, E., and Palomo, I. (2016). Role of oxidative stress on platelet hyperreactivity during aging. *Life Sci.* 148, 17–23. doi: 10.1016/j.lfs.2016.02.026

Furie, B., and Furie, B. C. (2008). Mechanisms of thrombus formation. *N. Engl. J. Med.* 359, 938–949. doi: 10.1056/NEJMra0801082

Geng, W., Zhang, T., Yang, Y., Song, D., Meng, H., Liu, Q., et al. (2013). GW24-e0802 The study of polymer-free paclitaxel-eluting stent in treatment of coronary heart disease. *Heart* 99:A169. doi: 10.1136/heartjnl-2013-304613.468

Gunasekera, B., Diwan, C. A., Altawallbeh, G., Kalil, H. F., Maher, S., Xu, S., et al. (2018). Functional layer-by-layer thin films of inducible nitric oxide (NO) synthase oxygenase and polyethylenimine: modulation of enzyme loading and NO-release activity. *ACS Appl. Mater. Inter.* 10, 7745–7755. doi: 10.1021/acsami.7b17575

Gurbel, P. A., and Bliden, K. P. (2003). Platelet activation after stenting with heparin-coated versus noncoated stents. *Am. Heart J.* 146:E10. doi: 10.1016/S0002-8703(03)00317-X

Hara, H., Nakamura, M., Palmaz, J. C., and Schwartz, R. S. (2006). Role of stent design and coatings on restenosis and thrombosis. *Adv. Drug Deliver. Rev.* 58, 377–386. doi: 10.1016/j.addr.2006.01.022

Hopkins, S. P., Pant, J., Goudie, M. J., Schmiedt, C. W., and Handa, H. (2018). Achieving long-term biocompatible silicone via covalently immobilized S-Nitroso- N-acetylpenicillamine (SNAP) that exhibits 4 months of sustained nitric oxide release. *ACS Appl. Mater. Interfaces* 10, 27316–27325. doi: 10.1021/acsami.8b08647

Hristov, M., Erl, W., and Weber, P. (2003). Endothelial progenitor cells mobilization, differentiation, and homing. *Arterioscl. Throm. Vas.* 23, 1185–1189. doi: 10.1161/01.ATV.0000073832.49290.B5

Joner, M., Finn, A. V., Farb, A., Mont, E., Kolodgie, F. D., Ladich, E., et al. (2006). Pathology of drug-eluting stents in humans: delayed healing and late thrombotic risk. *J. Am. Coll. Cardiol.* 48, 193–202. doi: 10.1016/j.jacc.2006.03.042

Jun, H., Yuwono, V. M., Paramonov, S. E., and Hartgerink, J. D. (2005). Enzyme-mediated degradation of peptide-amphiphile nanofiber networks. *Adv. Mater.* 17, 2612–2617. doi: 10.1002/adma.200500855

Kleinert, H., Pautz, A., Linker, K., and Schwarz, P. M. (2005). Regulation of the expression of inducible nitric oxide synthase. *Nitric Oxide* 384, 75–93. doi: 10.1016/j.niox.2010.04.007

Kraehling, J. R., and Sessa, W. C. (2017). Contemporary approaches to modulating the nitric oxide-cGMP pathway in cardiovascular disease. *Circ. Res.* 120, 1174–1182. doi: 10.1161/CIRCRESAHA.117.303776

Kubo, T., Imanishi, T., Kitabata, H., Kuroi, A., Ueno, S., Yamano, T., et al. (2008). Comparison of vascular response after sirolimus-eluting stent implantation between patients with unstable and stable angina pectoris: a serial optical coherence tomography study. *Cardiovasc. Imaging* 1, 475–484. doi: 10.1016/j.jcmg.2008.03.012

Kushwaha, M., Anderson, J. M., Bosworth, C. A., Andukuri, A., Minor, W. P., Lancaster, J. R., et al. (2010). A nitric oxide releasing, self assembled peptide amphiphile matrix that mimics native endothelium for coating implantable cardiovascular devices. *Biomaterials* 31, 1502–1508. doi: 10.1016/j.biomaterials.2009.10.051

Li, X., Qiu, H., Gao, P., Yang, Y., Yang, Z., and Huang, N. (2018). Synergetic coordination and catecholamine chemistry for catalytic generation of nitric oxide on vascular stents. *NPG Asia Mater.* 10, 482–496. doi: 10.1038/s41427-018-0052-3

Lundberg, J. O., Gladwin, M. T., and Weitzberg, E. (2015). Strategies to increase nitric oxide signalling in cardiovascular disease. *Nat. Rev. Drug Discov.* 14, 623–641. doi: 10.1038/nrd4623

Ma, X., Hibbert, B., Dhaliwal, B., Seibert, T., Chen, Y., Zhao, X., et al. (2010). Delayed re-endothelialization with rapamycin-coated stents is rescued by the addition of a glycogen synthase kinase-3β inhibitor. *Cardiovasc. Res.* 86, 338–345. doi: 10.1093/cvr/cvq047

Mahara, A., Somekawa, S., Kobayashi, N., Hirano, Y., Kimura, Y., Fujisato, T., et al. (2015). Tissue-engineered acellular small diameter long-bypass grafts with neointima-inducing activity. *Biomaterials* 58, 54–62. doi: 10.1016/j.biomaterials.2015.04.031

Major, T. C., Brant, D. O., Reynolds, M. M., Bartlett, R. H., Meyerhoff, M. E., Handa, H., et al. (2010). The attenuation of platelet and monocyte activation in a rabbit model of extracorporeal circulation by a nitric oxide releasing polymer. *Biomaterials* 31, 2736–2745. doi: 10.1016/j.biomaterials.2009.12.028

McCarthy, C. W., Guillory, R. J., Goldman, J., and Frost, M. C. (2016). Transition metal mediated release of nitric oxide (NO) from S-Nitroso-N-acetylpenicillamine (SNAP): potential applications for endogenous release of NO on the surface of stents via corrosion products. *Acs Appl. Mater. Interfaces* 16, 10128–10135. doi: 10.1021/acsami.6b00145

Mcfadden, E. P., Stabile, E., Regar, E., Cheneau, E., Ong, A. T. L., Kinnaird, T., et al. (2004). Late thrombosis in drug-eluting coronary stents after discontinuation of antiplatelet therapy. *Lancet* 364, 1519–1521. doi: 10.1016/S0140-6736(04)17275-9

McIlhenny, S., Zhang, P., Tulenko, T., Comeau, J., Fernandez, S., Policha, A., et al. (2013). eNOS transfection of adipose-derived stem cells yields bioactive nitric oxide production and improved results in vascular tissue engineering. *J. Tissue Eng. Regenerat. Med.* 9, 1277–1285. doi: 10.1002/term.1645

Mel, A. D., Murad, F., and Seifalian, A. M. (2011). Nitric oxide: a guardian for vascular grafts? *Chem. Rev.* 111, 5742–5767. doi: 10.1021/cr200008n

Midgley, A. C., Wei, Y., Li, Z., Kong, D., and Zhao, Q. (2019). Nitric-oxide-releasing biomaterial regulation of the stem cell microenvironment in regenerative medicine. *Adv. Mater.* 32:1805818. doi: 10.1002/adma.201805818

Mondal, A., Douglass, M., Hopkins, S. P., Singha, P., Tran, M., Handa, H., et al. (2019). Multifunctional S-Nitroso-N-acetylpenicillamine-incorporated medical-grade polymer with selenium interface for biomedical applications. *ACS Appl. Mater. Interfaces* 11, 34652–34662. doi: 10.1021/acsami.9b10610

Naghavi, N., De Mel, A., Alavijeh, O. S., Cousins, B. G., and Seifalian, A. M. (2013). Nitric oxide donors for cardiovascular implant applications. *Small* 9, 22–35. doi: 10.1002/smll.201200458

Nakamura, K., Keating, J., and Edelman, E. R. (2016). Pathology of endovascular stents. *Interv. Cardiol. Clin.* 5, 391–403. doi: 10.1016/j.iccl.2016.02.006

Ohkubo, K., Kobayashi, Y., Nakamura, Y., and Miyazaki, A. (2011). Incidence of side-effects of dual antiplatelet therapy with clopidogrel and aspirin after coronary stent implantation. *Cardiovasc. Interv. Ther.* 26, 33–37. doi: 10.1007/s12928-010-0031-2

Pacelli, S., Basu, S., Whitlow, J., Chakravarti, A. R., Acosta, F. M., Varshney, A., et al. (2017). Strategies to develop endogenous stem cell recruiting bioactive materials for tissue repair and regeneration. *Adv. Drug Deliv. Rev.* 120, 50–70. doi: 10.1016/j.addr.2017.07.011

Palmerini, T., Benedetto, U., Biondizoccai, G., Riva, D. D., Bacchireggiani, L., Smits, P. C., et al. (2015). Long-term safety of drug-eluting and bare-metal stents: evidence from a comprehensive network meta-analysis. *J. Am. Coll. Cardiol.* 65, 2496–2507. doi: 10.1016/j.jacc.2015.04.017

Pan, G., Liu, S., Zhao, X., Zhao, J., Fan, C., and Cui, W. (2015). Full-course inhibition of biodegradation-induced inflammation in fibrous scaffold by loading enzyme-sensitive prodrug. *Biomaterials* 53, 202–210. doi: 10.1016/j.biomaterials.2015.02.078

Pant, J., Goudie, M. J., Hopkins, S. P., Brisbois, E. J., and Handa, H. (2017). Tunable nitric oxide release from S-Nitroso-N-acetylpenicillamine via catalytic copper nanoparticles for biomedical applications. *ACS Appl. Mater. Inter.* 11, 15254–15264. doi: 10.1021/acsami.7b01408

Park, D. W., Kim, Y. H., Yun, S. C., Kang, S. J., Lee, S. W., Lee, C. W., et al. (2010). Comparison of zotarolimus-eluting stents with sirolimus- and paclitaxel-eluting stents for coronary revascularization: the ZEST (comparison of the efficacy and safety of zotarolimus-eluting stent with sirolimus-eluting and paclitaxel-eluting stent for coronary lesions) randomized trial. *J. Am. Coll. Cardiol.* 56, 1187–1195. doi: 10.1016/j.jacc.2010.03.086

Poh, C. K., Shi, Z., Lim, T. Y., Neoh, K. G., and Wang, W. (2010). The effect of VEGF functionalization of titanium on endothelial cells *in vitro*. *Biomaterials* 31, 1578–1585. doi: 10.1016/j.biomaterials.2009.11.042

Saito, G., Swanson, J. A., and Lee, K. D. (2003). Drug delivery strategy utilizing conjugation via reversible disulfide linkages: role and site of cellular reducing activities. *Adv. Drug Deliver. Rev.* 55, 199–215. doi: 10.1016/S0169-409X(02)00179-5

Scott, R. A., and Panitch, A. (2014). Macromolecular approaches to prevent thrombosis and intimal hyperplasia following percutaneous coronary intervention. *Biomacromolecules* 15, 2825–2832. doi: 10.1021/bm5007757

Seabra, A. B., Justo, G. Z., and Haddad, P. S. (2015). State of the art, challenges and perspectives in the design of nitric oxide-releasing polymeric nanomaterials for biomedical applications. *Biotechnol. Adv.* 33, 1370–1379. doi: 10.1016/j.biotechadv.2015.01.005

Sessa, W. C. (2004). eNOS at a glance. *J. Cell Sci.* 117, 2427–2429. doi: 10.1242/jcs.01165

Shin, Y. M., Lee, Y. B., Kim, S. J., Kang, J. K., Park, J., Jang, W., et al. (2012). Mussel-inspired immobilization of vascular endothelial growth factor (VEGF) for enhanced endothelialization of vascular grafts. *Biomacromolecules* 13, 2020–2028. doi: 10.1021/bm300194b

Stone, G. W. (2016). Bioresorbable vascular scaffolds. *JACC Cardiovasc. Inte.* 9:575. doi: 10.1016/j.jcin.2016.01.012

Stone, G. W., Grines, C. L., Cox, D. A., Garcia, E., Tcheng, J. E., Griffin, J. J., et al. (2002). Comparison of angioplasty with stenting, with or without abciximab, in acute myocardial *infarction. N. Engl. J. Med.* 346, 957–966. doi: 10.1056/NEJMoa013404

Thomas, D. D. (2015). Breathing new life into nitric oxide signaling: a brief overview of the interplay between oxygen and nitric oxide. *Redox Biol.* 5, 225–233. doi: 10.1016/j.redox.2015.05.002

Tu, Q., Shen, X., Liu, Y., Zhang, Q., Zhao, X., Maitz, M. F., et al. (2019). A facile metal–phenolic–amine strategy for dual-functionalization of blood-contacting devices with antibacterial and anticoagulant properties. *Mater. Chem. Front.* 3, 265–275. doi: 10.1039/C8QM00458G

Tu, Q., Zhao, X., Liu, S., Li, X., Zhang, Q., Yu, H., et al. (2020). Spatiotemporal dual-delivery of therapeutic gas and growth factor for prevention of vascular stent thrombosis and restenosis. *Appl. Mater. Today.* 19:100546. doi: 10.1016/j.apmt.2019.100546

Wang, Z., Lu, Y., Qin, K., Wu, Y., Tian, Y., Wang, J., et al. (2015). Enzyme-functionalized vascular grafts catalyze in-situ release of nitric oxide from exogenous NO prodrug. *J. Control. Release* 210, 179–188. doi: 10.1016/j.jconrel.2015.05.283

Wei, Y., Ji, Y., Xiao, L., Lin, Q., Xu, J., Ren, K., et al. (2013). Surface engineering of cardiovascular stent with endothelial cell selectivity for *in vivo* re-endothelialisation. *Biomaterials* 34, 2588–2599. doi: 10.1016/j.biomaterials.2012.12.036

Weng, Y., Song, Q., Zhou, Y., Zhang, L., Wang, J., Chen, J., et al. (2011). Immobilization of selenocystamine on TiO_2 surfaces for in situ catalytic generation of nitric oxide and potential application in intravascular stents. *Biomaterials* 32, 1253–1263. doi: 10.1016/j.biomaterials.2010.10.039

Winther, A. K., Fejerskov, B., Ter Meer, M., Jensen, N. B. S., Dillion, R., Schaffer, J. E., et al. (2018). Enzyme prodrug therapy achieves site-specific, personalized physiological responses to the locally produced nitric oxide. *ACS Appl. Mater. Inter.* 10, 10741–10751. doi: 10.1021/acsami.8b01658

Yang, T., Du, Z., Qiu, H., Gao, P., Zhao, X., Wang, H., et al. (2020a). From surface to bulk modification: plasma polymerization of amine-bearing coating by synergic strategy of biomolecule grafting and nitric oxide loading. *Bioac. Mater.* 5, 17–25. doi: 10.1016/j.bioactmat.2019.12.006

Yang, T., Fruergaard, A. S., Winther, A. K., Zelikin, A. N., and Chandrawati, R. (2020b). Zinc oxide particles catalytically generate nitric oxide from endogenous and exogenous prodrugs. *Small* 5:1906744. doi: 10.1002/smll.201906744

Yang, T., Zelikin, A. N., and Chandrawati, R. (2017). Progress and promise of nitric oxide-releasing platforms. *Adv. Sci.* 5:1701043. doi: 10.1002/advs.201701043

Yang, Y., Gao, P., Wang, J., Tu, Q., Bai, L., Xiong, K., et al. (2020c). Endothelium-mimicking multifunctional coating on cardiovascular stents via a stepwise metal-catechol-(amine) surface engineering strategy. *Research* 2020:9203906. doi: 10.34133/2020/9203906

Yang, Z., Yang, Y., Zhang, L., Xiong, K., Li, X., Zhang, F., et al. (2018). Mussel-inspired catalytic selenocystamine-dopamine coatings for long-term generation of therapeutic gas on cardiovascular stents. *Biomaterials* 178, 1–10. doi: 10.1016/j.biomaterials.2018.06.008

Yoon, J. H., Wu, C. J., Homme, J., Tuch, R. J., Wolff, R. G., Topol, E. J., et al. (2002). Local delivery of nitric oxide from an eluting stent to inhibit neointimal thickening in a porcine coronary injury model. *Yonsei Med. J.* 43, 242–251. doi: 10.3349/ymj.2002.43.2.242

Yusuf, S., Joseph, P., Rangarajan, S., Islam, S., Mente, A., Hystad, P., et al. (2020). Modifiable risk factors, cardiovascular disease, and mortality in 155 722 individuals from 21 high-income, middle-income, and low-income countries (PURE): a prospective cohort study. *Lancet* 395, 795–808. doi: 10.1016/S0140-6736(19)32008-2

Zhang, F., Zhang, Q., Li, X., Huang, N., Zhao, X., and Yang, Z. (2019). Mussel-inspired dopamine-CuII coatings for sustained *in situ* generation of nitric oxide for prevention of stent thrombosis and restenosis. *Biomaterials* 194, 117–129. doi: 10.1016/j.biomaterials.2018.12.020

Zhao, P., Metcalf, M., and Bunnett, N. W. (2014). Biased signaling of protease-activated receptors. *Front. Endocrinol.* 5:67. doi: 10.3389/fendo.2014.00067

Zhao, Q., Zhang, J., Song, L., Ji, Q., Yao, Y., Cui, Y., et al. (2013). Polysaccharide-based biomaterials with on-demand nitric oxide releasing property regulated by enzyme *catalysis*. 34, 8450–8458. doi: 10.1016/j.biomaterials.2013.07.045

Zhu, Y., Edmonds, L., Zhao, X., Chen, X., Hu, C., Cheng, Y., et al. (2014). *In vitro* and *in vivo* evaluation of rapamycin-eluting nanofibers coated on cardia stents. *RSC Adv.* 4, 34405–34411. doi: 10.1039/C4RA04771K

7

Interactions of Alginate-Deferoxamine Conjugates with Blood Components and their Antioxidation in the Hemoglobin Oxidation Model

*Tong Sun[1,2], Xi Guo[1,2], Rui Zhong[3], Chengwei Wang[1,4], Hao Liu[1,2], Hao Li[2], Lu Ma[2], Junwen Guan[2], Chao You[1,2,5] and Meng Tian[1,2,5]**

[1] Neurosurgery Research Laboratory, National Clinical Research Center for Geriatrics, West China Hospital, Sichuan University, Chengdu, China, [2] Department of Neurosurgery, West China Hospital, Sichuan University, Chengdu, China, [3] Institute of Blood Transfusion, Chinese Academy of Medical Sciences and Peking Union Medical College, Chengdu, China, [4] Department of Integrated Traditional Chinese and Western Medicine, West China Hospital, Sichuan University, Chengdu, China, [5] West China Brain Research Centre, West China Hospital, Sichuan University, Chengdu, China

***Correspondence:**
Meng Tian
tianmong007@gmail.com;
6744710@qq.com

While deferoxamine (DFO) has long been used as an FDA-approved iron chelator, its proangiogenesis ability attracts increasing number of research interests. To address its drawbacks such as short plasma half-life and toxicity, polymeric conjugated strategy has been proposed and shown superiority. Owing to intravenous injection and application in blood-related conditions, however, the blood interactions and antioxidation of the DFO-conjugates and the mechanisms underlying these outcomes remain to be elucidated. In this regard, incubating with three different molecular-weight (MW) alginate-DFO conjugates (ADs) red blood cells (RBCs), coagulation system, complement and platelet were investigated. To prove the antioxidant activity of ADs, we used hemoglobin oxidation model *in vitro*. ADs did not cause RBCs hemolysis while reversible aggregation and normal deformability ability were observed. However, the coagulation time, particularly APTT and TT, were significantly prolonged in a dose-dependent manner, and fibrinogen was dramatically decreased, suggesting ADs could dominantly inhibit the intrinsic pathways in the process of coagulation. The dose-dependent anticoagulation might be related with the functional groups along the alginate chains. The complements, C3a and C5a, were activated by ADs in a dose-dependent manner through alternative pathway. For platelet, ADs slightly suppressed the activation and aggregation at low concentration. Based on above results, the cross-talking among coagulation, complement and platelet induced by ADs was proposed. The antioxidation of ADs through iron chelation was proved and the antioxidant activity was shown in a MW-dependent manner.

Keywords: deferoxamine, blood components, antioxidation, alginate, conjugates

INTRODUCTION

Deferoxamine (DFO) has long been used as an FDA-approved intravenously injected iron chelator in clinic for half a century in the treatment of iron overload diseases, while in the recent years, a great deal of attention was given to the important applications of DFO in the growing field of tissue regeneration as a result of its unique properties to inhibit inflammation and promote vascularization (Guo et al., 2019; Holden and Nair, 2019). In the early studies, DFO was proved to stimulate angiogenesis and neovascularization in the ischemia model of sheep and rabbit, and since then, increasing number of studies attempt to elucidate the related mechanisms (Chekanov et al., 2003). To date, it is widely accepted that DFO is contributed to the prevention of degradation of hypoxia-inducible factor-1 alpha (HIF-1α), an oxygen-sensitive molecule to upregulate the expression of vascular endothelial growth factor (VEGF) (Wu et al., 2010). In the meanwhile, some studies indicated that angiogenesis induced by DFO was closely associated with the property of antioxidation, as a secondary effect (Jiang et al., 2014). Despite the dispute, the ability of angiogenesis in addition to the antioxidation make it serve as a promising candidate for various biomedical use.

However, the application of DFO is still of much limitation owing to its drawbacks, like other small molecular drugs, including short plasma half-life and toxicity (Cassinerio et al., 2014). In this regard, polymer-drug conjugation strategy is appropriate for DFO to overcome these obstacles (Yan et al., 2016). Polymer-drug conjugates belonging to nano-sized drug delivery system attracts great research interest and are becoming established as a shining platform for drug delivery due to the reasons that the conjugation strategy deeply changes the behavior of the corresponding parent drugs and offers them many benefits, including high drug-loading, prolonged circulatory half-life, and reduced toxicity (Zhou et al., 2015; Ding et al., 2019a; Jesus et al., 2019; Macha et al., 2019; Qi et al., 2019). However, the therapeutic efficiency in clinic is not as expected, e.g., less than 10% of a systemically administered dose accumulates within the lesion, and in some cases there is no significant improvement for patient survival rate such as FDA approved doxorubicin HCl liposome (DOXIL) for anticancer (Zhang et al., 2013). Hence, the reasons why these conjugates with fine-tuned structures do not function as intended need to be elucidated in order to advance the therapy in clinic (Feng et al., 2019).

One of the most factors that contributes to this discrepancy is the interactions that exist between intravenously injected conjugates and the blood, since these interactions may change the target and transport capabilities of conjugates, thus determining the fate and the final therapeutic efficiency of conjugates in body (Lazarovits et al., 2015; Ding et al., 2019b). To develop solutions to these barriers, it is crucial to study the blood-conjugates interactions, e.g., RBCs, coagulation function, protein adsorption, complement system and platelets, which depended on the properties of conjugates such as structure, molecular weight (MW), and the functional groups along the chains (Wu et al., 2017). Besides, several pathways and mechanisms underlying these interactions suggest that some cross-talking among them has to be involved (Fornaguera et al., 2015). For instance, protein adsorption is deemed as the initial event in blood-conjugates interactions (Kenry et al., 2016), leading to the activation of coagulation cascade that can contribute significantly to both of complement system and platelet through certain coagulation enzymes (Liu et al., 2014). Nevertheless, the interplay among coagulation, platelet and complement is still of much limitation to be fully understood in the process of thrombus formation and inflammation response (Speth et al., 2015).

Actually, some studies had proven that conjugation of DFO into polymer carriers, such as hydroxyethyl starch, dextran, dialdehyde cellulose, nanoparticles, and polyethylene glycol copolymer, significantly prolonged the half-life comparing to the free of DFO (Tian et al., 2016a). To better of our knowledge, there is no report on systematic study of the DFO-based blood-conjugates interactions. Alginate, consisting of α-L-guluronate (G unit) and β-D-mannuronate (M unit), has long been used in delivery systems and in terms of the interactions with blood, alginate could induce aggregation of RBCs, allowing it be used as a viscosity modifier for blood substitutes. Contributing to the versatile functional groups, e.g., carboxyl and hydroxyl, along the molecular chains, alginate is also suggested to have effects on the protein adsorption and complement activation (Zhao et al., 2010; Şen, 2011). In this light, the interactions of alginate-DFO conjugates is rather crucial to quest the potential mechanism. On the other hand, alginate has its intrinsic antioxidant activity due to the reductive ability of residues along the molecular chains, which may benefit to protect hemoglobin from oxidation in a different manner comparable to DFO. However, the polymer drug carrier also leads to steric hindrance for DFO cheating, resulting in iron binding occurring at a slower rate, depending on the density and location of conjugated DFO molecules.

In this work, alginate was chosen as a polymer carrier to prepare a series of alginate-DFO conjugates (ADs) with various MW and study their interactions with blood. We hypothesize that the molecular weight and functional groups along the alginate chains have specific interactions with blood. To address this hypothesis, a series of ADs with different MW were synthesized (**Figure 1A**). Incubating with ADs, RBCs, coagulation system, complement, and platelet, were investigated (**Figure 1B**). Specifically, the RBCs' properties including hemolysis, aggregation and deformability, were determined. Blood coagulation time including prothrombin time (PT), activated partial thromboplastin time (APTT) and thrombin time (TT), and the concentration of fibrinogen (Fib), were tested. The concentration of completement 3a (C3a) and completement 5a (C5a) were investigated. In terms of platelet, the activation and aggregation of platelet were determined. Based on above results, the interplay among coagulation system, complement and platelet incubating with ADs was proposed. Finally, the antioxidation of ADs was determined using the hemoglobin oxidation model, in which the effect of MW on iron chelation was discussed (**Figure 1C**).

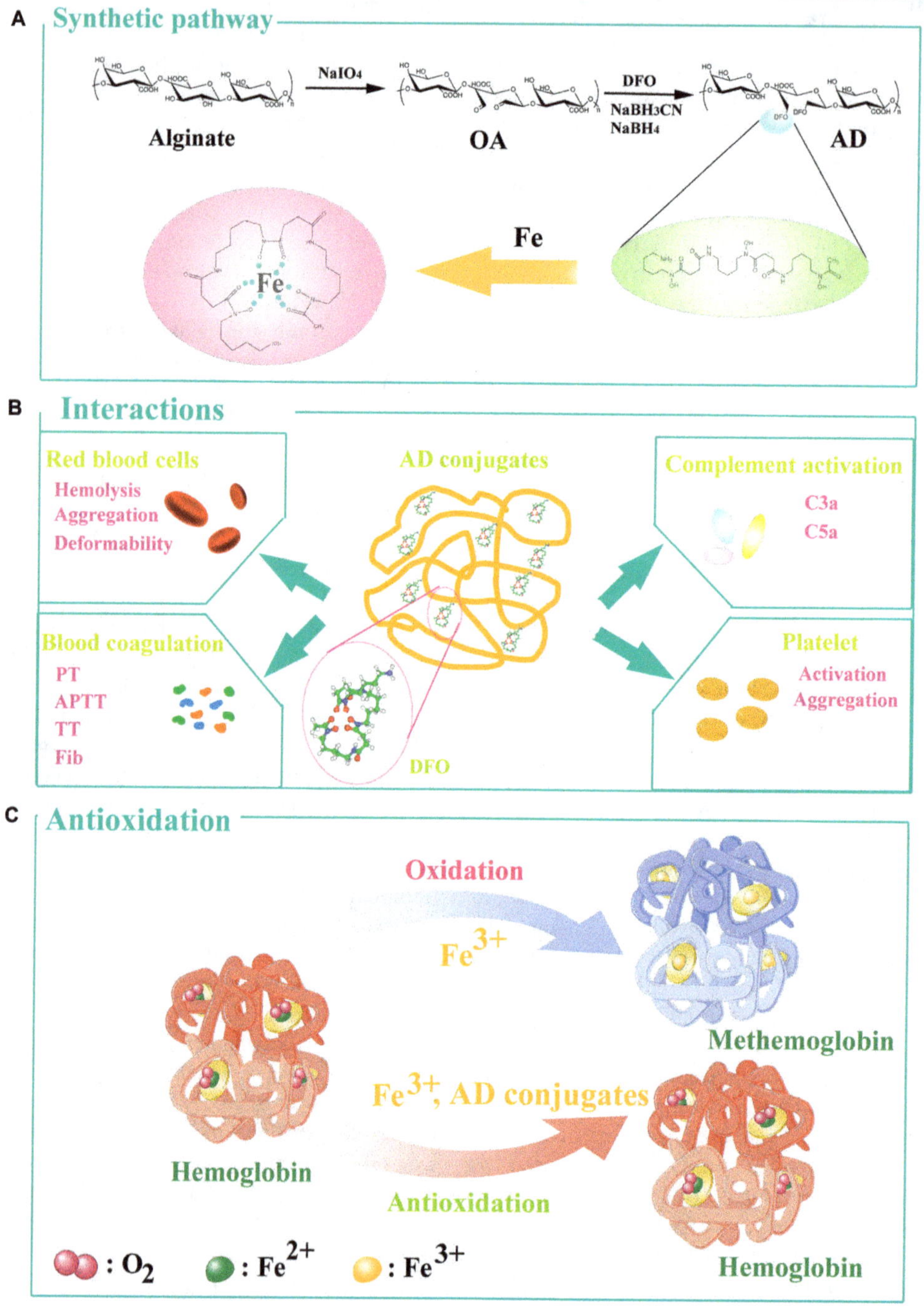

FIGURE 1 | (A) The synthesis of conjugates. **(B)** The interactions of ADs with blood in vitro. **(C)** Hemoglobin oxidation model. Under normal circumstance, the hemoglobin converts to oxyhemoglobin in ferrous state (Fe^{2+}), able to bind and transport oxygen, and methemoglobin in the presence of ferric iron (Fe^{3+}). AD conjugates can bind to Fe^{3+} so that oxyhemoglobin was generated to transport oxygen.

MATERIALS AND METHODS

Materials

Deferoxamine and sodium alginate were purchased from Sigma-Aldrich (St. Louis, MO, United States). $NaBH_3$-CN and $NaBH_4$ were obtained from AAD-50din Co. (Shanghai, China). Normal saline (NS), phosphate buffer saline (PBS), sodium periodate, peroxide hydrogen, polyetherimide and ferric sulfate, were obtained from Kelong Co., Ltd. (Chengdu, China). Heparin sodium was purchased from Alading Co., Ltd. (Chengdu, China). Blood was collected from Chengdu Blood Center. Coagulation-related kits were purchased from Union Bio-tech Co., Ltd. (Chengdu, China). The ELISA Kit II was purchased from Becton-Dickinson Co., Ltd. (United States). Flow cytometry-related agents, anti-CD61-fluorecein isothiocyanate (FITC), anti-CD62p-phycoerythrin (PE) and IgG1 (mouse) – PE, were purchased from BD Pharmingen, BD Bioscience Co., Ltd. (San Jose', CA, United States). Platelet aggregation-inducers, adenosine-disphosphate and epinephrine, were obtained from Kelong Co., Ltd. (Chengdu, China).

Synthesis of the ADs

The ADs were synthesized by Schiff-base reaction through the terminal amine groups in DFO and reactive aldehyde groups in oxidized alginate (OA) and followed by reduction as our previous report (Tian et al., 2016b). In brief, 10.0 g of sodium alginate was dissolved with 700 mL deionized water (DW) and 100 mL ethanol followed by different ratios of sodium periodate to uronate units (15, 30, 50 mol%) were used. The mixture was stirred in dark for 6 h and then mixed with 20 mL ethylene glycol before stirred for another 2 h. After that, to separate and purify each prepared ADA, the precipitant, presented by adding 10 g of NaCl and 2000 mL ethanol, was redissolved in 400 mL DW and 2000 mL ethanol again, and the progress was repeated three times. The products prepared from 15, 30, and 50 mol % of periodate/uronate units are corresponding to OA-15, OA-30, and OA-50 respectively. To obtain AD conjugates, 1 g of each OA was incubated with 2.5 g of DFO under stirring in room temperature. After 2 h, $NaBH_3CN$ (125 mg/mL) was slowly added to the solution under stirring for 4 h and then $NaBH_4$ was added to the mixture for another 24 h. It respectively takes 3 days to dialyze against 1 M NaCl and DW using a dialysis tube (MWCO, 3500), totally 6 days. The conjugates were synthesized by OA-15, OA-30, and OA-50 named AD-15, AD-30, and AD-50 respectively. The structure of the synthesized conjugates was characterized as our previous report and shown in **Table 1**. The degree of DFO (% DFO) incorporation was calculated and described as moles of DFO attached per uronate residue.

Blood Collection and Preparation of AD Solutions

The study was approved by Ethical Committee of Institute of Blood Transfusion, Chinese Academy of Medical Sciences and Peking Union Medical College. We collected blood samples at Chengdu Blood Center from three healthy donors. The whole blood was obtained through venipuncture and then mixed with 3.8% sodium citrate at radio of 9:1(blood/sodium citrate) to obtain citrated whole blood (CWB). To prepare 10% hematocrit of RBCs suspension, CWB was used to mix with the same volume of NS and centrifuged at 5000 r/min for 4 min, and then removed the supernatant. Repeated wash three times by NS for a total of four washes. While the supernatant was clear, removed it out and then added corresponding volume of NS to ensure the hematocrit of RBC suspension was 10%. CWB was centrifuged at 1200 *g* for 20 min to obtain platelet-rich plasma (PRP). Serum was prepared by centrifuging CWB he citrated at 1200 *g* for 30 min. The fresh frozen plasma (FFP) supplied by Chengdu blood center has anticoagulated with citrate-phosphate-adenine. ADs were dissolved in normal saline (NS) to obtain solutions with different concentration.

TABLE 1 | The structure characteristics of the conjugates.

Conjugate	Mw (x 10^5Da)	Mn (x 10^4 Da)	PDI	DFO content (mol %)
AD-15	2.5	4.9	5.0	8.7
AD-30	1.3	3.6	3.6	14.7
AD-50	0.6	1.8	3.5	20.4

Red Blood Cells

Hemolysis

The percent of RBC lysis was measured by the Free Hemoglobin Colorimetric Assay Kit using. Two hundred and seventy µl of RBC suspension (hematocrit: 10%) was respectively incubated with 30 µl of three ADs solutions with different concentrations for 1 h at 37°C to obtain a final concentration of 1, 5, and 10 mg/ml. We investigated the concentration of free hemoglobin by the method of ortho-tolidine to determine the hemolysis of incubated RBCs according to previous study (Lin et al., 2019). The absorbance was obtained by spectrophotometer (EON, Bio-Tech CO., Ltd., United States) at 435 nm. The percent of hemolysis was calculated by the following eq. (1). The RBCs suspension incubated with distilled water (DW) was used as a positive control.

$$\text{Hemolysis (\%)} = \frac{A(1)}{A(0)} \times \frac{100 - \text{Hct (\%)}}{\text{Hb (g/l)} \times 1000} \times 100\% \quad (1)$$

$A_{(1)}$: the absorbance of sample. $A_{(0)}$: the absorbance of standard sample. Hct, hematocrit. Hb, 100 mg/L

Aggregation

Two hundred and seventy µl of CWB was respectively incubated with 30 µl of three ADs solutions with different concentrations for 1 h at 37°C to obtain a final concentration of 1, 5, and 10 mg/ml followed by centrifuging at 1000 *g* for 3 min. Three µl of RBCs sediment and 40 µl of supernatant were mixed and examined by optical microscopy. We captured the imagines by a digital microscope camera. CWB incubated with NS and polyetherimide (PEI) were respectively used as a normal control and positive control.

Deformability

Two hundred and seventy µl of CWB was respectively incubated with 30 µl of three ADs solutions with different concentrations for 1 h at 37°C to obtain a final concentration of 1, 5, and 10 mg/ml After incubation, the mixture (20 µl) was suspended in PBS (1 mL) containing 15% polyvinylpyrrolidone and then was tested by a Laser-diffraction Ektacytometer (LBYBX, Beijing Pencil Instrument CO., Ltd., China) according to the manufacture's manual. Four shear stress, 0.39, 0.77, 1.54, and 7.7 Pa, were used, corresponding to the shear rate 50, 100, 200, and 1000 respectively. CWB incubated with NS was used as a normal control.

Blood Coagulation

Sixty µl of three ADs solutions at 10 and 50 mg/ml were respectively incubated with 540 µl of FFP at 37°C for 3 min.

After incubation, we used Prothrombin Time Diagnostic Kit to determine PT in the presence of Ca^{2+}, and Activated Partial Thromboplastin Time Diagnostic Kit to determine APTT by adding kaolin and encephalin. We tested TT using Thrombin Time Determination Kit and the concentration of Fib in the presence of thrombin using Fibrinogen Determination Reagent Kit respectively. The coagulation time of incubated FFP, including APTT, prothrombin time (PT), thrombin time (TT), and the concentration of fibrinogen (Fib) were determined by an automated coagulation analyzer (Instrumentation Laboratory ACL ELITE, United States). To be specific, FFP incubated with NS and heparin (HP, 2 IU/mL) were respectively used as normal control and negative control.

Complement Activation

The concentration of C3a and C5a were tested to prove the effect of ADs on complement system. Thirty μl of three ADs solutions at 10 and 50 mg/ml were respectively incubated with 270 μl of serum at 37°C for 3 min followed by analysis of complement activation using ELISA Kit II (Becton-Dickinson Co., Ltd., United States). The standards and samples were finally read by spectrophotometer (EON, Bio-Tech Co., Ltd., United States) at 450 nm and the concentration of C3a and C5a were calculated by utilizing standard curve. Serum incubated with zymosan (7 mg/ml) was used as a positive control.

Platelet

Platelet Activation

Thirty μl of three ADs solutions at 10 and 50 mg/ml were respectively incubated with 270 μl of PRP at 37°C for 1 h. Five μl of incubated PRP, 5 μl of CD61, 5 μl of CD62p and 40 μl of PBS buffer (10 mM) were mixed in dark at 15 min and then added to 400 μl PBS (10 mM) for flow cytometric analysis. The activation of platelet was defined as the percentage of marker CD62p detected in 10000 total events counted by flow cytometry (Becton-Dickinson) using anti-CD61-fluorecein isothiocyanate (FITC), anti-CD62p-phycoerythrin (PE) and IgG1 (mouse)-PE (BD Pharmingen, BD Bioscience, San Jose̕, CA, United States). The data was analyzed by BD FACSD via Software (Version 8.0.1.1). Human thrombin (10 IU/mL) and NS were respectively used as positive and normal control.

Platelet Aggregation

Thirty μl of three ADs solutions at 10 and 50 mg/ml were respectively incubated with 270 μl of PRP at 37°C for 1 h. Incubated PRP (225 μl) were mixed with two aggregation-inducers, adinosinedisphosphate (0.1 mM, 12.5 μl) and epinephrine (0.15 mM, 12.5 μl), and then we used platelet aggregometer (MODEL700, Chrono-Log Co., Ltd., United States) to determine the platelet aggregation.

Antioxidation

To prove the effect of ADs on prevention of iron-mediated oxidation in the presence of hemoglobin (Hb), we observed the dynamic changes of oxyhemoglobin (oxyHb) while mixing ADs with ferric solutions containing Hb. Briefly, washed RBCs were frozen and thawed and then mixed with NS to obtain hemolysate (22 μM). To guarantee each sample, except for Hb control, contains 0.4 mM of DFO equivalent and 0.4 mM of ferric ion, ADs or DFO solutions (10 μl) and ferric sulfate solution (50 μl) were mixed with hemolysate solution (440 μl). The full wavelength scanning of each group was immediately performed by spectrophotometer (EON, Bio-Tech Co., Ltd., United States). In addition, the absorbance at 560, 576, 630, and 700 nm was respectively measured again every 30 s, in total of 5 min. The containing of oxyHbA was respectively calculated using the method of Winterbourn in different times, shown as the following eq. (2) (Winterbourn, 1985). The percent of oxyHbA was the ratio of oxyHbA to the primary containing of oxyHbA in blood samples.

$$oxyHbA(\%) = \frac{1.013 \times (A1-A4) - 0.3269 \times (A3-A4) - 0.7353 \times (A2-A4)}{10000} \times 100\% \quad (2)$$

A1 means the absorbance at 560 nm; A2 means the absorbance at 570 nm; A3 means the absorbance at 630 nm; A4 means the absorbance at 700 nm.

Further assessing the antioxidation activity of three AD conjugates and DFO, the degree of ADs and DFO chelating to iron was investigated. Fifty μl ferric sulfate solution (0.11 mM) was mixed with 50 μl AD conjugates or DFO solutions (DFO equivalent, 0.2 mM), and then the absorbance at 430 nm was respectively measured every 5 s, in total of 1 min.

Statistical Analysis

We use analysis of variance and paired t-test to perform the statistical analysis. The probability (P) values less than 0.05 was considered to have significant difference and was calculated with the software assistance of Excel 2007 and SPSS 19.0. The results are presented as mean ± SD (n = 3).

RESULTS AND DISCUSSION

Synthesis of ADs

ADs were synthesized through a two-step process in which alginate was oxidized to ADA firstly, and then the conjugates were prepared by Schiff-base reaction through the terminal amine groups in DFO and reactive aldehyde groups in ADA and followed by reduction with $NaBH_3CN$ and $NaBH_4$ (**Figure 1A**). To prepare a series of conjugates with different molecular weight, alginate was oxidized to different oxidation degree by adjusting the mol ratio of periodate/uronate units, since oxidation of alginate with sodium periodate results not only cleavage of the C2-C3 bond, but also main chain scission as a simultaneous reaction. The structure characteristics of the prepared conjugates are summarized in **Table 1**. As expected, the Mw of the conjugates are 245, 128, and 62.7 kDa, respectively. The DFO contents in the conjugates were increased with the decrease of the Mw due to the coupling of the oxidation and Mw, with 8.7, 14.7, and 20.4% by molar and corresponding to around one DFO per eleven, seven, and five uronate units for AD-15, AD-30, and AD-50, respectively.

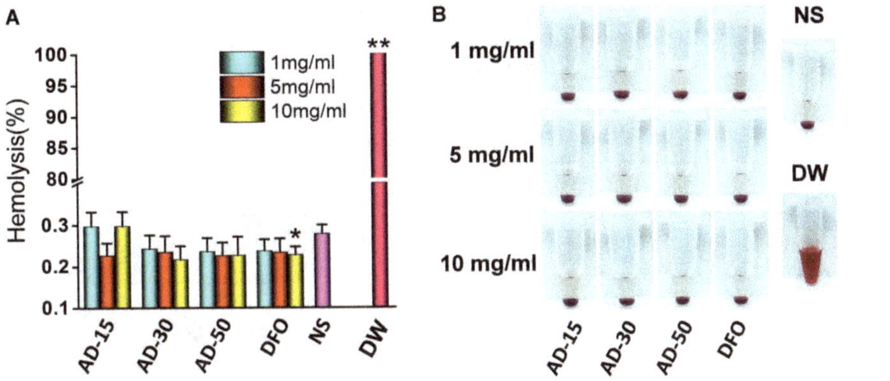

FIGURE 2 | Effect of ADs on hemolysis. Three ADs and DFO were incubated with 10% hematocrit RBCs suspension at 1, 5, and 10 mg/mL. **(A)** The percent of hemolysis, **(B)** the visual appearance of AD, DFO and controls. $^{*}P < 0.05$ versus NS; **DW has significant differences with the others, $P < 0.05$.

Red Blood Cells

Hemolysis is characterized as the rupture of RBCs and the release of the cytoplasm, and the evaluation of hemolysis is essential regarding the biosafety of exogenous materials. To investigate the device-associated hemolysis, static or semi-static testing *in vitro* was widely used (Haishima et al., 2014). Based on ISO10993-5, ISO10993-4 and ASTMF756-00, the percent less than 5% will be considered as a very low risk of hemolysis (Zhen et al., 2015). According to the results as shown in **Figure 2**, the percent of hemolysis in AD-15, AD-30, AD-50 and DFO at any concentration fluctuated around 0.2%, while the hemolysis of DW group is approximately 90%. Except for the DFO in 10 mg/mL, the others rarely showed any significant difference compared with normal saline (NS), indicating ADs had a quite low risk of hemolysis.

The property of RBCs to aggregate is one of the typical features that plays a vital role in the blood circulation (Claveria et al., 2016). The aggregation of RBCs has been proved to affect their viscosity ability owing to the non-Newtonian behavior of blood in the body and reversible aggregation may physiologically occur in the presence of macromolecules and calcium ion, serving as the bridge among RBCs (Mehri et al., 2014). However, irreversible RBCs aggregation, induced by some chemicals, such as phosphodiesterase and polyethyleneimine (PEI), could damage RBCs and even potentially disrupt capillaries (Muravyov and Tikhomirova, 2014). Herein, photomicrographs of RBCs incubated with PEI, used as positive control, and ADs at 1, 5, and 10 mg/mL were shown in **Figure 3**. Compared with PEI, neither ADs nor DFO showed any irreversible aggregation. The likely aggregation in ADs group as well as NS control was contributed to rouleau formation, as a typical result of reversible aggregation (Flormann et al., 2015). According to the previous study, it has long been known that alginate increased whole blood viscosity and induced aggregation of RBCs thus being used as a viscosity modifier for blood substitutes (Xu et al., 2017). In this work, ADs showed negative response to RBCs aggregation, which could be ascribed to the possibly low content of alginate in the reaction system (Zhao et al., 2010).

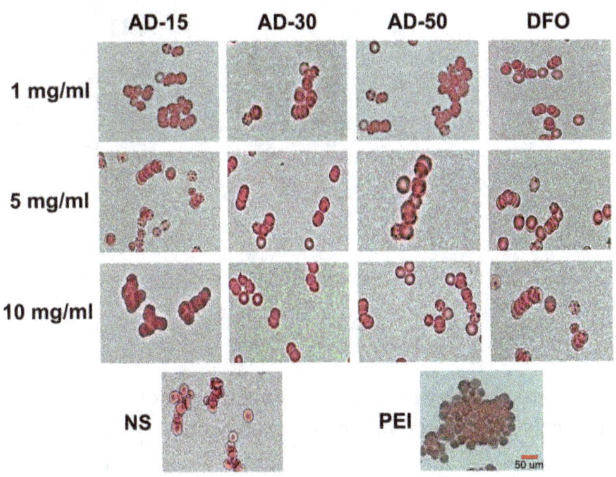

FIGURE 3 | Red blood cells aggregation. Three ADs and DFO were incubated with whole blood at 1, 5, and 10 mg/mL. The RBCs in plasma was observed by a digital microscopy followed by capturing the imagines.

The property of allows them to change their shape according to the diameter of blood vessel as a result of natural shape of RBCs. The regulation of RBCs deformability depends on three aspects, cytoplasm viscosity, membrane mechanical properties and surface area and volume of RBCs (Uhl et al., 2018). Malfunction of RBCs deformability is contributed to the occurrence of several diseases, such as sickle cell anemia, malaria and hereditary spherocytosis (Zhao et al., 2010). **Figures 4A–D** showed the deformability of incubated RBCs at various shear stress. The results indicated there is no significant difference among three ADs and NS at any concentration or shear stress. The deformability of DW group was significantly lower than three ADs at the shear rate 100, 200, and 1000 while at 50, DW group was slightly lower than AD-15 at 5 mg/ml (P = 0.046) and AD-30 at 1 mg/ml (P = 0.038). Generally, the elongation index (EI) significantly increased while being exposed to a higher shear stress. For DW group, the EI stayed a low level as the shear

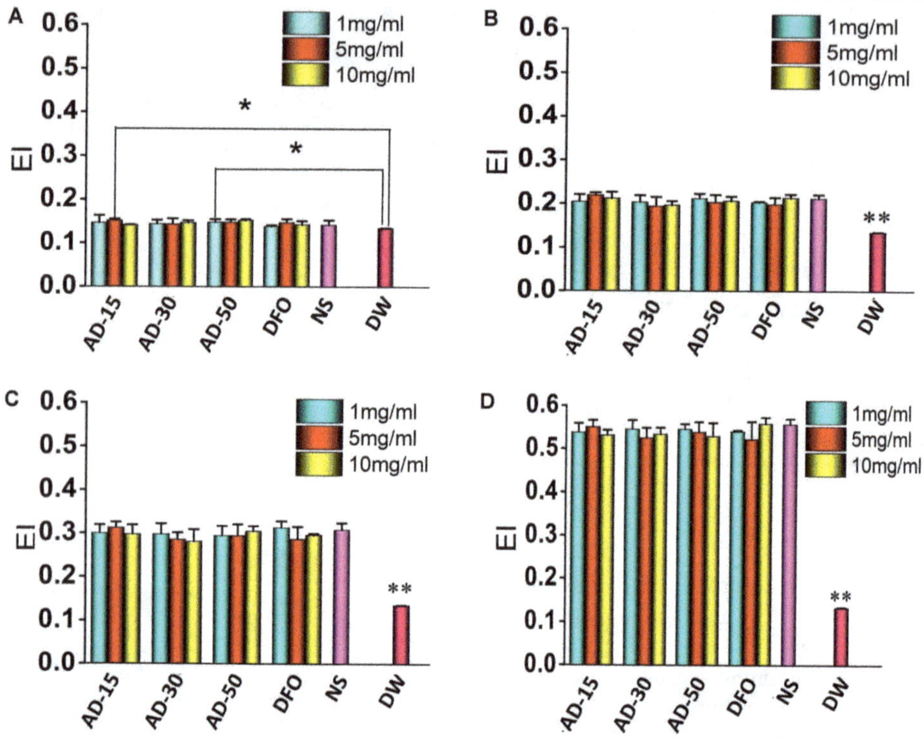

FIGURE 4 | Red blood cells deformability. Three ADs and DFO were incubated with whole blood at 1, 5, and 10 mg/mL and then, incubated RBCs were tested by a Laser-diffraction Ektacytometer at different shear stress, **(A)** 0.39, **(B)** 0.77, **(C)** 1.54, and **(D)** 7.7 Pa. *$P < 0.05$ versus DW; **DW has significant differences with the others, $P < 0.05$.

rate changed, suggesting that the deformability of RBCs could be significantly suppressed in the presence of hemolysis.

Coagulation Function

To determine the effect of ADs on coagulation system, we tested the coagulation time, including PT, APTT, and TT, together along with the concentration of Fib. The results of blood coagulation were shown in **Figure 5**. Comparing with DFO or NS group, the PT of three ADs, on behalf of extrinsic coagulation pathway, were simultaneously lengthened to some extent. Unlike AD-15 and AD-30, the PT of AD-50 presented a dose-dependent effect. For APTT and TT, reflecting the intrinsic coagulation pathway and common coagulation pathway respectively, three ADs significantly prolonged APTT and TT compared with DFO or NS in a dose-dependent manner and at the concentration of 5 mg/mL, the values of APTT and TT were too high to be tested by analyzer (the detection range for APTT is 6–245 s, for TT is from 3–169 s). In terms of Fib, the concentration of Fib of three ADs was approximately 1.2 g/L while DFO or NS group was approximately 1.6 g/L. Additionally, ADs could decrease the concentration of Fib in a dose-dependent manner since the concentration of Fib ADs at 5 mg/mL was approximately 0.6 g/L with statistical difference.

To the best of our knowledge, this is the first study demonstrated that polymer-drug conjugate using alginate as drug carrier was capable of anticoagulant activity. ADs significantly prolonged the coagulation time, particularly APTT, indicating that the intrinsic pathway was dominantly blocked in the process of anticoagulation. To explain this phenomenon, two main mechanisms were proposed to involve in anticoagulation pathway. Firstly, interacting with the coagulation factors, such as factor I (Fib), II, V, and X, ADs can significantly inhibit their activity, thus preventing them from participating in coagulation cascade reaction (Zou et al., 2014; Xin et al., 2016). Secondly, the anticoagulative activity relates with the negative functional groups along the chains of the polysaccharides since the negative functional group would form a complex interaction with antithrombin in plasma (Li et al., 2017). Alginate is the only polysaccharide that naturally contains negative carboxyl groups along the chains, indicating that anticoagulant activity probably has to be involved. Besides carboxyl groups, there are many hydroxyl groups along the chains of alginate, both of which have been suggested to have significant effect on the coagulation function (Shiu et al., 2014; Guo et al., 2018). The anticoagulation induced by carboxyl groups and hydroxyl groups is supported by the work of Sperling et al. (2005), who studied the influence of different content of carboxyl groups or hydroxyl groups on coagulation function and indicated that pure-carboxyl groups showed a strong anticoagulative effect while the effect of pure-hydroxyl groups was milder.

Among three ADs, AD-50, with the lowest MW, showed a weaker anticoagulative activity than that of AD-15 and 30, indicating that ADs-induced anticoagulation was partially depended on the MW, which was consistent with previous

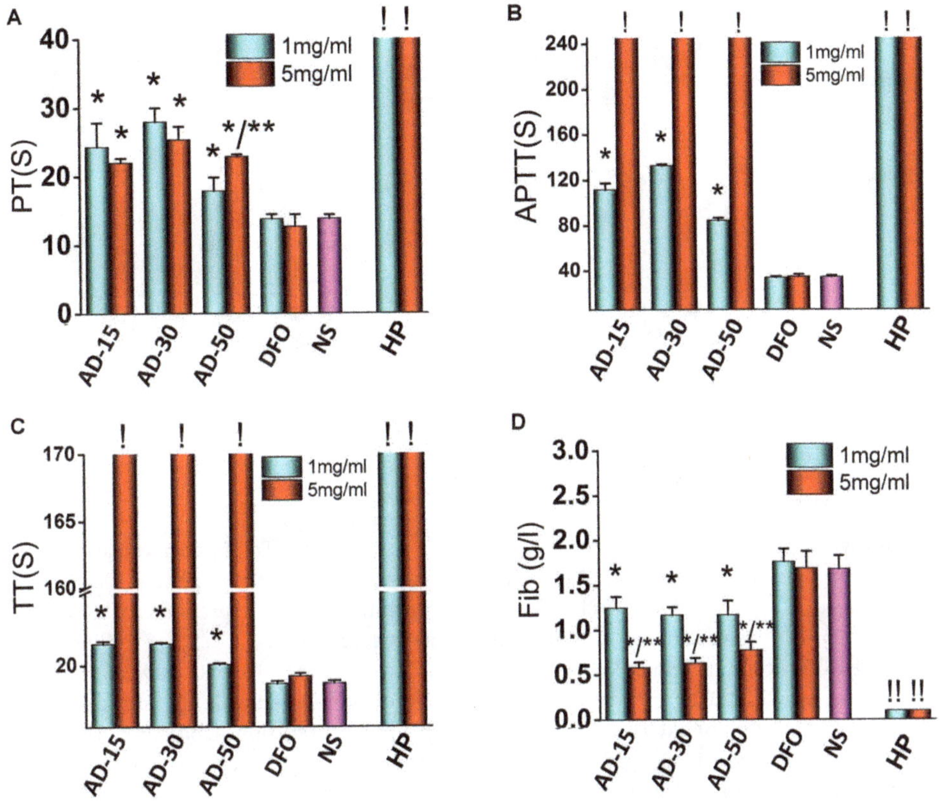

FIGURE 5 | Effect of ADs on blood coagulation. Three ADs and DFO were incubated with fresh frozen plasma (FFP) at 1 and 5 mg/mL. **(A)** PT, **(B)** APTT, **(C)** TT, and **(D)** Fib, were tested by an automated coagulation analyzer. $^*P < 0.05$ versus NS or DFO; **means 5 mg/mL has significant differences with 1 mg/mL, $P < 0.05$. **!** : The values are too high that cannot be determined by the analyzer (APTT > 245 s, TT > 169 s). **! !**: The values are too low that cannot be determined by the analyzer. HP, heparin.

studies. For instance, Xu et al. (2017) studied the blood compatibility of alginate with different MW (1170–50075 kDa) prepared by heterogeneous phase acid degradation and the results indicated that the blood clotting time was prolonged with increasing of MW of alginate. Similarly, the anticoagulation of sulfated polysaccharides depends not only on the substituted functional groups along main chains, but also the MW. Xin et al. (2016) investigated the anticoagulative properties of a series of low MW propylene glycol alginate sodium sulfate (2.99–8.91 KDa) and they found it could prolong the APTT and clotting time and the anticoagulative activity declined with the decrease in MW. Besides, Fan et al. (2011) aimed at prove the correlation between MW and anticoagulative activity and indicated that the clotting time induced by sodium alginate sulfate (14900–35300 KDa) initially increased as the MW decreased but fall with the further decrease in MW. Therefore, based on the previous study, it is suggested that within a certain MW range, the degree of anticoagulative activity through absorption coagulation factors through negative charged groups along the chains has a main dependence on MW, and with the reduction of MW, the anticoagulation activity is much weaker probably ascribing to the decrease of negative groups.

In addition, it should be noted that the anticoagulative effect induced by ADs were weaker than HP, a widely used anticoagulant in clinic. Besides, the mild anticoagulative activity of ADs would rather extend the application in the treatment of iron-overload diseases. For instance, in some iron-overload diseases like thalassanemia and sideroblastic anaemia, long-term repeated-transfusion is needed to improve the content of hemoglobin while transfusion-associated thrombosis is unacceptably common in clinic as well (Xenos et al., 2012). To simultaneously overcome iron-overload and hypocoagulability state, ADs show superiorities contributing to their anticoagulative effect. Additionally, hemorrhage is another concern in clinic following the application of anticoagulant and some research indicated that the concentration of Fib had a closely link with the incidence of hemorrhage and there is a much higher risk of bleeding as Fib concentration is less than 0.5 g/L (Lunde et al., 2014). In this light, our results showed that the concentration of Fib of three ADs at 1 or 5 mg/mL were higher than HP group, indicating that ADs had a quite lower risk of hemorrhage than HP.

Complement Activation

Complement can be activated by cascade reaction in three pathway, classic pathway, alternative pathway and mannose binding lectin pathway (Koscielska-Kasprzak et al., 2014). It has long been known that exogenous biomaterials mainly

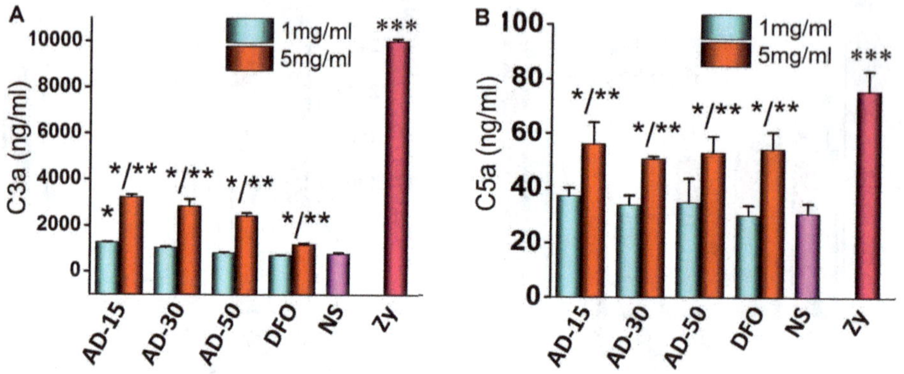

FIGURE 6 | Effect of ADs on complement activation. Three ADs and DFO were incubated with serum at 1 and 5 mg/mL and then, **(A)** C3a and **(B)** C5a were investigated by ELISA KIT II. *$P < 0.05$ for NS; **5 mg/mL has significant differences with 1 mg/mL, $P < 0.05$; ***$P < 0.05$ for the others. zy, zymosan.

activate alternative pathway, which could cause severe side-effects, such as inflammation (Liu et al., 2013). In alternative pathway, C3, directly activated by biomaterials, cleaves to produce C3a and C3b. C3b can regulate the function of monocytes and macrophages. C3a is component of C3ADesArg, and make up C5 convertase, which causes change of C5 to C5a and C5b. C5a and C5b are component of C5ADesArg and membrane attack complex respectively. In a word, concentrations of C3a and C5a are canonical indexes to access the activation of complement pathway (Nesargikar et al., 2012). Serum incubated with 1 and 5mg/mL AD conjugates or DFO were adopted to measure the concentrations of C3a and C5a. The results of incubated complement were shown in **Figures 6A,B**. At the concentration of 1 mg/mL, except for the mild activation of C3 induced by AD-15, C3 and C5 were rarely activated by AD-30 or AD-50. At the concentration of 5 mg/mL, C3a and C5a of three ADs sharply increased almost two times than low concentration suggesting high-dose of ADs could activate complement system through alternative pathway. The activation of C3a and C5a induced by ADs, however, were significantly lower than that of positive control, zymosan. The dose-dependent complement activation is closely dependent on the content of hydroxyl groups along the chains, one of negative groups that can trigger the complement cascade response (Zhong et al., 2013). Besides binding to complement directly, hydroxyl group also interact with complement through absorption numerous complement-related proteins (Wetterö et al., 2002).

Platelet

Platelets, derived from megakaryocytes in the bone marrow with plasmolemma, usually maintain the integrity of blood vessel and participate in the process of hemostasis following vascular injury (Sun et al., 2019). CD62P (platelet surface *P*-selectin) has long been used as markers to determine the activation of platelet since its considerable stability (Lu and Malinauskas, 2011). In this work, CD62P was used to determine the effect of ADs on platelet activation using flow cytometry. To further measure platelet function, the aggregation of incubated platelet was investigated using platelet aggregometer. The expression of CD62P and the percent of platelet aggregation were shown in **Figure 7**. At the concentration of 1 mg/mL, AD-15 and AD-30 slightly suppressed platelet activation compared with NS, which is accordant with the results of platelet aggregation. Compared with ADs at 1 mg/mL, mild activation of platelet can be observed at the concentration of 5 mg/mL. Based on the results, AD-50 rarely influenced the platelet function.

Platelet activation, in which fib has been reported one of requisite stimulating factors, involving in a complicated multistep process including adhesion, release and aggregation for hemostatic plug formation and thrombosis, has been reported that could be influenced by coagulation function and complement system in the blood (Khanbeigi et al., 2015). For instance, coagulants, like thrombin, can significantly activate platelet and inhibit the coagulation process while some complement inhibitors can similarly inhibit the platelet function (Speth et al., 2015). However, few studies fully revealed the interplay of coagulation and complement in platelet function *in vitro*. Therefore, according to our findings, it is proposed that AD conjugates can inhibit the platelet by the means of inhibition of Fib through functional groups along the chains and in the meantime, the inhibition can be antagonized by complement activation to some extent. However, few studies fully revealed the interplay of coagulation and complement in platelet function *in vitro*. According to the results of coagulation, complement, and platelet function, it is proposed that ADs can inhibit the platelet by the means of inhibition of Fib through functional groups along the chains, which could be antagonized by complement-associated activation to some extent. As shown in **Figure 8**, ADs, as mild anticoagulants, can absorb Fib to make them be absence of the process of platelet activation through the functional groups along the chains, like hydroxyl and carboxyl group. However, with the elimination of anticoagulative activity, the anticoagulation-associated platelet inhibition is negligible since AD-50 barely influenced the platelet activation. On the

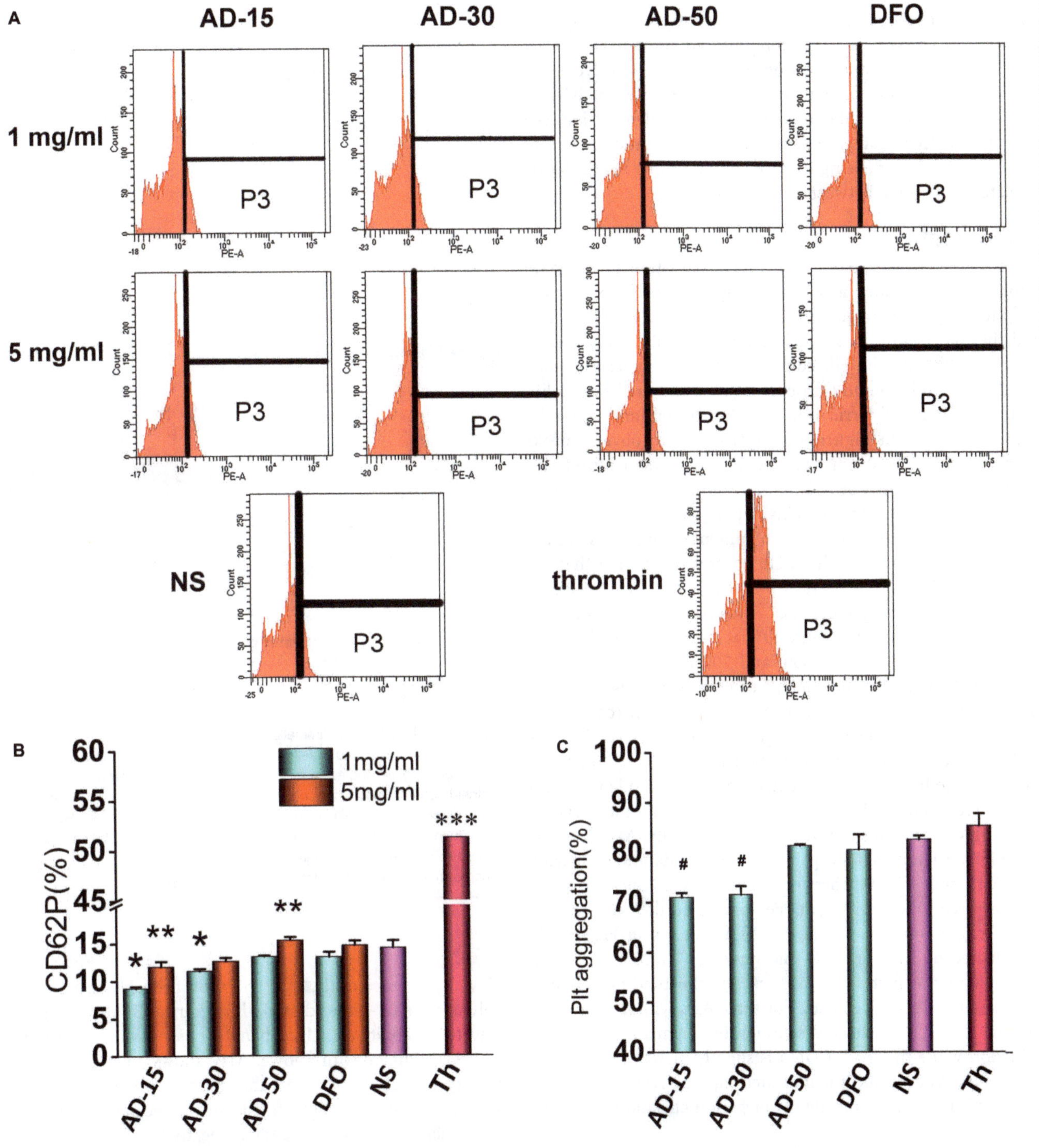

FIGURE 7 | Effect of ADs on platelet. **(A)** Flow cytometry data profiles from platelet activation analysis. The part of P3 means the percent of CD62P. **(B)** Platelet activation. Three ADs and DFO were incubated with platelet-fresh plasma (PFP) at 1 and 5 mg/mL for and the expression of CD62P was determined using anti-CD62P antibody by flow cytometry. **(C)** Platelet aggregation. Three ADs and DFO were incubated with platelet-fresh plasma (PFP) at 1 mg/mL and then, the aggregation was determined by aggregometer. *$P < 0.05$ for NS; **5 mg/mL has significant differences with 1 mg/mL, $P < 0.05$; ***$P < 0.05$ for the others; #$P < 0.05$ versus NS and thrombin. Th, thrombin.

other hand, it has been reported that platelets express many complement molecules, including some complement receptors and complement regulatory molecules that can generate C3a and C5a and as a return, the complement system and its activation products can also stimulate platelets by several complement factors, such as the anaphylatoxins C3a and C5a

(Speth et al., 2015). Herein, at the concentration of 1 mg/mL, comparing to the platelet inhibition through absorbing Fib, complement-associated activation induced by ADs is milder as a result of slight reduction on platelet activation. However, at the concentration of 5 mg/mL, with the raised activity in both anticoagulation and complement, the complement-induced activation is significantly enhanced against the anticoagulation-associated inhibition, being balanced and resulting in equal level of platelet activation between ADs and NS.

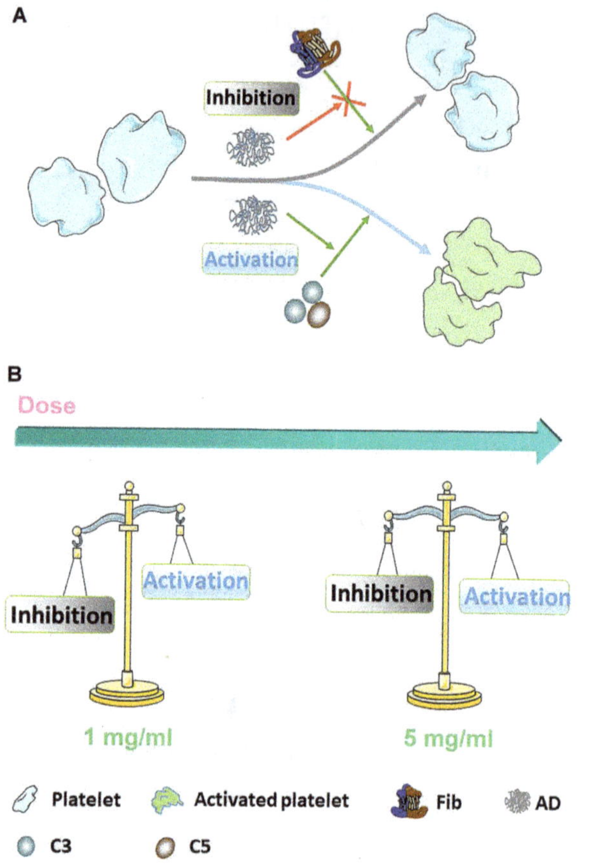

FIGURE 8 | (A) The diagrammatic sketch of coagulation- and complement-associated platelet activation. ADs can inhibit platelet through absorbing Fib, serving as an important stimulator for platelet activation. On the other hand, AD conjugates can also stimulate platelet through activating complement system. **(B)** In 1 mg/mL, coagulation-associated inhibition is dominant leading to a reduction of platelet activation for AD-50 and AD-30 while in 5 mg/mL, the coagulation-associated inhibition and complement-associated activation keep in balance.

Antioxidation

To prove the prevention of iron-mediated oxidation, hemoglobin (Hb) oxidation model, in which mimic the process underlying the pathology of hemoglobinopathies such as sickle cell anemia and the thalassemia, was widely used (Xu et al., 2014). Under normal condition, the Hb converts to oxyHb in ferrous state (Fe^{2+}), able to bind and transport oxygen, and methemoglobin in the presence of ferric iron (Fe^{3+}) (Pichert and Arnhold, 2015). As shown in **Figure 9A**, oxyHb has two obvious peaks between 500 and 600 nm while methemoglobin (oxidized Hb) has another new peak at 630 nm, a feature that can be utilized to distinguish these two proteins. Upon addition of DFO, the absorption spectrum that refers to content of oxyHb is similar to oxyHb rather than oxidized Hb control, suggesting that the conjugates can bind to ferric iron to protect Hb from being oxidized to methemoglobin in Fe^{3+}-rich condition. To detail the prevention, the percent of oxyHb was calculated on the basis of absorbance at 560, 576, 630, and 700 nm. The results are shown in **Figure 9B**. The content of oxyHb in ADs and DFO are dramatically higher than oxidized Hb control (containing Hb and Fe^{3+}) all the time, suggesting that ADs or DFO as a chelator for ferric iron prevents Hb from being oxidized. However, the binding to iron could be time-dependent since a sharply reduction is observed in the first 30 s, and then reaches a stable lever. In terms of three ADs, additionally, AD-50 seems to exhibit a slightly better capability on antioxidation comparing to AD-15 and AD-30. Therefore, the ability of the conjugates and the free DFO binding to Fe^{3+} were further determined by spectrophotometer and the results are shown in **Figure 9C**. The degree of ADs or DFO chelating Fe^{3+} rapidly reach to the peak in the first 5 s, which means the binding to Fe^{3+} occurs as soon as they contact. For three ADs with similar DFO content, the level of chelates significantly augment as the MW reduction while the free of DFO is slightly higher than that of conjugates. As a result, it is indicated that the ADs are capable of antioxidant activity mainly through iron chelation in a MW dependence manner.

Although there are several reports attempt to reveal the links between MW and antioxidative property, that found biomaterials with a lower MW have a higher antioxidant activity, the mechanism remains controversial. Alginate has its intrinsic antioxidant activity due to the reductive ability of residues along the molecular chains and its antioxidant activity is increased with the decrease of the MW (Xu et al., 2017), which may benefit to protect Hb from oxidation in a different manner comparing to the free of DFO. However, the conjugates did not show superior antioxidant activity as the expected. The reasons for the MW dependence of the iron chelation probably relate with the polymer carrier-induced steric hinderance. By determining the scavenging ability of 1, 1-diphenyl-2- picrylhydrazyl free radical (DPPH), alginate with a lower MW shows a better antioxidant activity probably ascribe to the increase in the a-L-guluronic acids (G) content of alginate and in the meanwhile, the nature of alginate chain was extended due to the diaxial linkage in G-blocks, which may hind the rotation around glycosidic acid as the MW increase (Şen, 2011). Nevertheless, the polymer drug carrier also leads to steric hinderance for DFO chelating, resulting in iron binding occurring at a slower rate, depending on the density and location of conjugated DFO molecules (Banerjee, 2009; Yu et al., 2019). As shown in **Figure 9D**, iron chelation results in a locally ordered molecular configuration which is a process of losses of entropy. The higher MW and longer molecular chains, the higher losses of entropy, which in turn makes it more difficult for iron chelation.

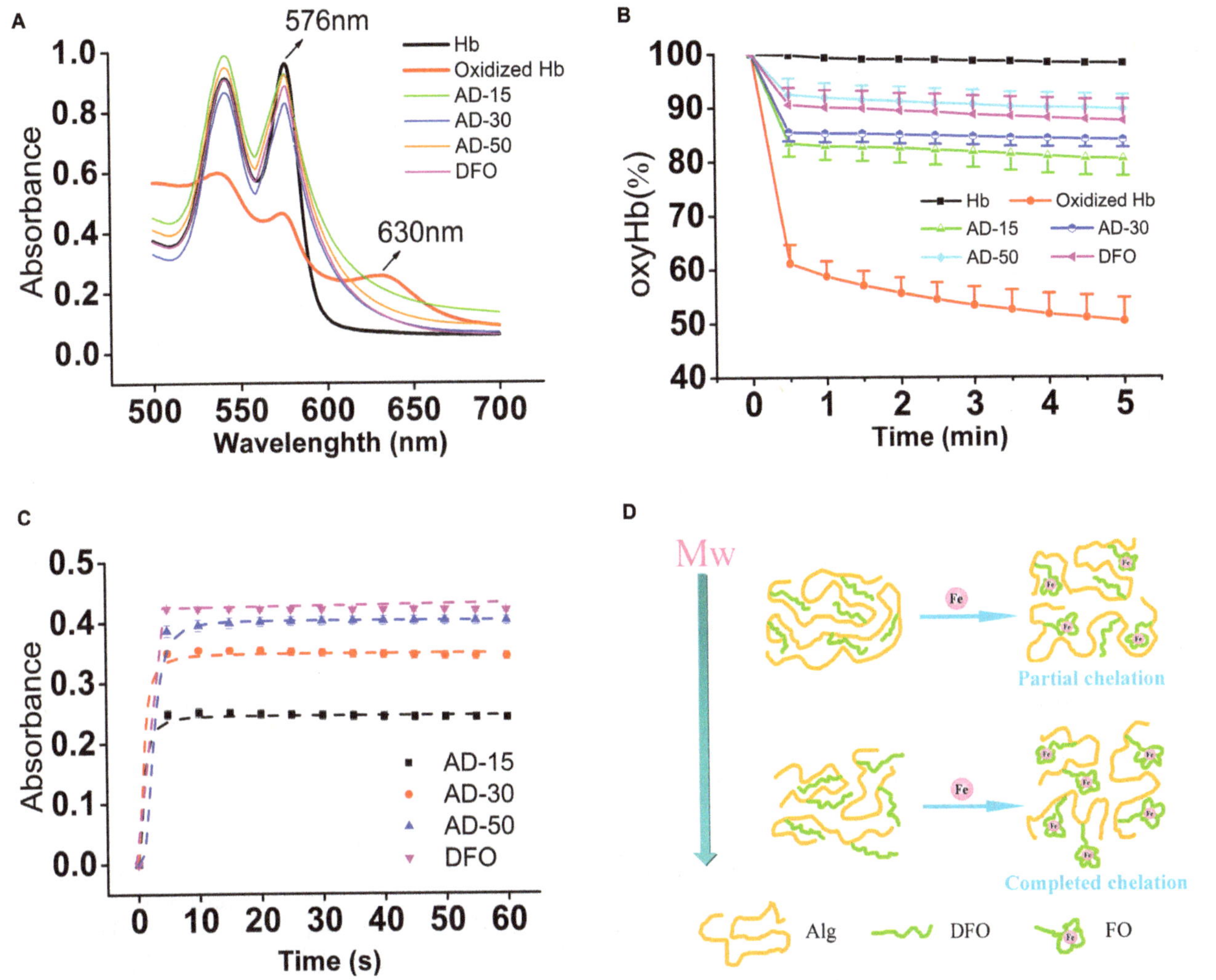

FIGURE 9 | Protection against iron-mediated oxidation in hemolysate. Each group, except for the hemolysate (Hb) and oxyHb (containing Hb and Fe^{3+}) control, similarly contains 0.4 mM of DFO equivalent (AD or DFO) and Fe^{3+}, dissolving in Hb solution (22 μM). **(A)** The full wavelength scanning. **(B)** The tendency of the percent of oxyHb in each group, scanning every 30 s in total of 5 min. **(C)** The lever of DFO-Fe^{3+} chelates. The absorbance was obtained at 430 nm, which means the degree of ADs or DFO chelating to iron. **(D)** The diagrammatic sketch of different MW ADs to Fe^{3+}. With the Mw of AD conjugates increasing, the ability to chelating to iron will be repressed ascribing to the steric hinderance effect.

CONCLUSION

In conclusion, we successfully synthesized a series of ADs with various MW and the interactions with RBCs, coagulation, complement, and platelet had been studied for the conjugates as a function of their dose and MW. Interactions of ADs with RBCs did not reveal any hemolysis and showed reversible aggregation contributing to rouleau formation of RBCs and normal deformability ability. On the contrary, ADs significantly prolonged the coagulation time in a dose-dependent manner, particularly APTT and TT, suggesting ADs could dominantly inhibit the intrinsic and common pathways in the process of coagulation. The results of complement and platelet tests showed ADs could activate complements C3a and C5a, presenting dose-dependence while AD-15 and AD-30 slightly inhibit the platelet activation and aggregation in low concentration. Besides, the interplay among coagulation, complement, and platelet activation was proposed. Finally, the antioxidant activity of ADs was demonstrated in a MW-dependent manner.

AUTHOR CONTRIBUTIONS

TS performed the blood evaluation, wrote the manuscript, and discussed the results. XG performed the blood evaluation. RZ performed the other experiments. CW, HLiu, HLi, LM, JG, and CY were involved in the results discussion. MT was responsible for conceptualization, results discussion, and revising the manuscript.

REFERENCES

Banerjee, R. (2009). Nanoparticles for intravesical therapy in bladder cancer. *Nanomedicine* 4, 261–264.

Cassinerio, E., Orofino, N., Roghi, A., Duca, L., Poggiali, E., Fraquelli, M., et al. (2014). Combination of deferasirox and deferoxamine in clinical practice: an alternative scheme of chelation in thalassemia major patients. *Blood Cells Mol. Dis.* 53, 164–167. doi: 10.1016/j.bcmd.2014.04.006

Chekanov, V. S., Nikolaychik, V., Maternowski, M. A., Mehran, R., and Akhtar, M. (2003). Deferoxamine enhances neovascularization and recovery of ischemic skeletal muscle in an experimental sheep model. *Ann. Thorac. Surgery* 75, 184–189. doi: 10.1016/s0003-4975(02)04122-x

Claveria, V., Aouane, O., Thiebaud, M., Abkarian, M., Coupier, G., Misbah, C., et al. (2016). Clusters of red blood cells in microcapillary flow: hydrodynamic versus macromolecule induced interaction. *Soft Matter* 12, 8235–8245. doi: 10.1039/c6sm01165a

Ding, J., Chen, J., Gao, L., Jiang, Z., Zhang, Y., Li, M., et al. (2019a). Engineered nanomedicines with enhanced tumor penetration. *Nano Today* 29:100800. doi: 10.1016/j.nantod.2019.100800

Ding, J., Feng, X., Jiang, Z., Xu, W., Guo, H., Zhuang, X., et al. (2019b). Polymer-mediated penetration-independent cancer therapy. *Biomacromolecules* 20, 4258–4271. doi: 10.1021/acs.biomac.9b01263

Fan, L., Jiang, L., Xu, Y., Zhou, Y., Shen, Y., Xie, W., et al. (2011). Synthesis and anticoagulant activity of sodium alginate sulfates. *Carbohydr. Polym.* 83, 1797–1803. doi: 10.1016/j.carbpol.2010.10.038

Feng, X., Xu, W., Li, Z., Song, W., Ding, J., and Chen, X. (2019). Immunomodulatory Nanosystems. *Adv. Sci.* 6:1900101. doi: 10.1002/advs.201900101

Flormann, D., Kuder, E., Lipp, P., Wagner, C., and Kaestner, L. (2015). Is there a role of C-reactive protein in red blood cell aggregation? *Int. J. Lab. Hematol.* 37, 474–482. doi: 10.1111/ijlh.12313

Fornaguera, C., Caldero, G., Mitjans, M., Vinardell, M. P., Solans, C., and Vauthier, C. (2015). Interactions of PLGA nanoparticles with blood components: protein adsorption, coagulation, activation of the complement system and hemolysis studies. *Nanoscale* 7, 6045–6058. doi: 10.1039/c5nr00733j

Guo, X., Qi, X., Li, H., Duan, Z., Wei, Y., Zhang, F., et al. (2019). Deferoxamine alleviates iron overload and brain injury in a rat model of brainstem hemorrhage. *World Neurosurg* 128, e895–e904. doi: 10.1016/j.wneu.2019.05.024

Guo, X., Sun, T., Zhong, R., Ma, L., You, C., Tian, M., et al. (2018). Effects of chitosan oligosaccharides on human blood components. *Front. Pharmacol.* 9:1412. doi: 10.3389/fphar.2018.01412

Haishima, Y., Hasegawa, C., Nomura, Y., Kawakami, T., Yuba, T., Shindo, T., et al. (2014). Development and performance evaluation of a positive reference material for hemolysis testing. *J. Biomed. Mater. Res. B Appl. Biomater.* 102, 1809–1816. doi: 10.1002/jbm.b.33169

Holden, P., and Nair, L. S. (2019). Deferoxamine: an angiogenic and antioxidant molecule for tissue regeneration. *Tissue Eng. Part B Rev.* 25, 461–470. doi: 10.1089/ten.TEB.2019.0111

Jesus, S., Schmutz, M., Som, C., Borchard, G., Wick, P., and Borges, O. (2019). Hazard assessment of polymeric nanobiomaterials for drug delivery: what can we learn from literature so far. *Front. Bioeng Biotechnol.* 7:261. doi: 10.3389/fbioe.2019.00261

Jiang, X., Malkovskiy, A. V., Tian, W., Sung, Y. K., Sun, W., Hsu, J. L., et al. (2014). Promotion of airway anastomotic microvascular regeneration and alleviation of airway ischemia by deferoxamine nanoparticles. *Biomaterials* 35, 803–813. doi: 10.1016/j.biomaterials.2013.09.092

Kenry, K., Loh, K. P., and Lim, C. T. (2016). Molecular interactions of graphene oxide with human blood plasma proteins. *Nanoscale* 8, 9425–9441. doi: 10.1039/c6nr01697a

Khanbeigi, R. A., Hashim, Z., Abelha, T. F., Pitchford, S., Collins, H., Green, M., et al. (2015). Interactions of stealth conjugated polymer nanoparticles with human whole blood. *J. Mater. Chem. B* 3, 2463–2471. doi: 10.1039/c4tb01822b

Koscielska-Kasprzak, K., Bartoszek, D., Myszka, M., Zabinska, M., and Klinger, M. (2014). The complement cascade and renal disease. *Arch. Immunol .Ther. Exp.* 62, 47–57. doi: 10.1007/s00005-013-0254-x

Lazarovits, J., Chen, Y. Y., Sykes, E. A., and Chan, W. C. (2015). Nanoparticle-blood interactions: the implications on solid tumour targeting. *Chem. Commun.* 51, 2756–2767. doi: 10.1039/c4cc07644c

Li, Q., Zeng, Y., Wang, L., Guan, H., Li, C., and Zhang, L. (2017). The heparin-like activities of negatively charged derivatives of low-molecular-weight polymannuronate and polyguluronate. *Carbohydr. Polym.* 155, 313–320. doi: 10.1016/j.carbpol.2016.08.084

Lin, H., Wang, Q., Zhong, R., Li, Z., Zhao, W., Chen, Y., et al. (2019). Biomimetic phosphorylcholine strategy to improve the hemocompatibility of pH-responsive micelles containing tertiary amino groups. *Collo. Surf B Biointerfaces* 184:110545. doi: 10.1016/j.colsurfb.2019.110545

Liu, X., Yuan, L., Li, D., Tang, Z., Wang, Y., Chen, G., et al. (2014). Blood compatible materials: state of the art. *J. f Mater. Chem. B* 2, 5718–5738. doi: 10.1039/c4tb00881b

Liu, Y., Yin, Y., Wang, L., Zhang, W., Chen, X., Yang, X., et al. (2013). Engineering biomaterial-associated complement activation to improve vaccine efficacy. *Biomacromolecules* 14, 3321–3328. doi: 10.1021/bm400930k

Lu, Q., and Malinauskas, R. A. (2011). Comparison of two platelet activation markers using flow cytometry after in vitro shear stress exposure of whole human blood. *Artif Organs* 35, 137–144. doi: 10.1111/j.1525-1594.2010.01051.x

Lunde, J., Stensballe, J., Wikkelso, A., Johansen, M., and Afshari, A. (2014). Fibrinogen concentrate for bleeding–a systematic review. *Acta Anaesthesiol. Scand.* 58, 1061–1074. doi: 10.1111/aas.12370

Macha, I. J., Ben-Nissan, B., Vilchevskaya, E. N., Morozova, A. S., Abali, B. E., Muller, W. H., et al. (2019). Drug delivery from polymer-based nanopharmaceuticals-an experimental study complemented by simulations of selected diffusion processes. *Front. Bioeng Biotechnol.* 7:37. doi: 10.3389/fbioe.2019.00037

Mehri, R., Mavriplis, C., and Fenech, M. (2014). Design of a microfluidic system for red blood cell aggregation investigation. *J. Biomech. Eng.* 136:064501. doi: 10.1115/1.4027351

Muravyov, A., and Tikhomirova, I. (2014). Signaling pathways regulating red blood cell aggregation. *Biorheology* 51, 135–145. doi: 10.3233/BIR-140664

Nesargikar, P. N., Spiller, B., and Chavez, R. (2012). The complement system: history, pathways, cascade and inhibitors. *Eur. J. Microbiol. Immunol.* 2, 103–111. doi: 10.1556/EuJMI.2.2012.2.2

Pichert, A., and Arnhold, J. (2015). Interaction of the chlorite-based drug WF10 and chlorite with hemoglobin, methemoglobin and ferryl hemoglobin. *Arch. Biochem. Biophys.* 585, 82–89. doi: 10.1016/j.abb.2015.09.009

Qi, B., Wang, C., Ding, J., and Tao, W. (2019). Editorial: applications of Nanobiotechnology in Pharmacology. *Front,. Pharmacol.* 10:1451. doi: 10.3389/fphar.2019.01451

Şen, M. (2011). Effects of molecular weight and ratio of guluronic acid to mannuronic acid on the antioxidant properties of sodium alginate fractions prepared by radiation-induced degradation. *Appl. Radiat. Isot.* 69, 126–129. doi: 10.1016/j.apradiso.2010.08.017

Shiu, H. T., Goss, B., Lutton, C., Crawford, R., and Xiao, Y. (2014). Controlling whole blood activation and resultant clot properties by carboxyl and alkyl functional groups on material surfaces: a possible therapeutic approach for enhancing bone healing. *J. Mater. Chem. B* 2, 3009–3021. doi: 10.1039/c4tb00009a

Sperling, C., Schweiss, R. B., Streller, U., and Werner, C. (2005). In vitro hemocompatibility of self-assembled monolayers displaying various functional groups. *Biomaterials* 26, 6547–6557. doi: 10.1016/j.biomaterials.2005.04.042

Speth, C., Rambach, G., Wurzner, R., Lass-Florl, C., Kozarcanin, H., Hamad, O. A., et al. (2015). Complement and platelets: mutual interference in the immune network. *Mol. Immunol.* 67, 108–118. doi: 10.1016/j.molimm.2015.03.244

Sun, T., Guo, X., Zhong, R., Ma, L., Li, H., Gu, Z., et al. (2019). Interactions of oligochitosan with blood components. *Int. J. Bio.l Macromol.* 124, 304–313. doi: 10.1016/j.ijbiomac.2018.11.109

Tian, M., Chen, X., Gu, Z., Li, H., Ma, L., Qi, X., et al. (2016a). Synthesis and evaluation of oxidation-responsive alginate-deferoxamine conjugates with increased stability and low toxicity. *Carbohydr. Polym.* 144, 522–530. doi: 10.1016/j.carbpol.2016.03.014

Tian, M., Chen, X., Li, H., Ma, L., Gu, Z., Qi, X., et al. (2016b). Long-term and oxidative-responsive alginate–deferoxamine conjugates with a low toxicity for iron overload. *RSC Adv.* 6, 32471–32479. doi: 10.1039/c6ra02674e

Uhl, C. G., Gao, Y., Zhou, S., and Liu, Y. (2018). The shape effect on polymer nanoparticle transport in a blood vessel. *RSC Adv.* 8, 8089–8100. doi: 10.1039/c8ra00033f

Wetterö, J., Askendal, A., Bengtsson, T., and Tenvall, P. (2002). On the binding of complement to solid artificial surfaces in vitro. *Biomaterials* 23, 981–991. doi: 10.1016/s0142-9612(01)00203-4

Winterbourn, C. C. (1985). Free-radical production and oxidative reactions of hemoglobin. *Environ. Health Perspect.* 64, 321–330. doi: 10.1289/ehp.856 4321

Wu, S., Duan, B., Zeng, X., Lu, A., Xu, X., Wang, Y., et al. (2017). Construction of blood compatible lysine-immobilized chitin/carbon nanotube microspheres and potential applications for blood purified therapy. *J. Mater. Chem. B* 5, 2952–2963. doi: 10.1039/c7tb00101k

Wu, Y., Li, X., Xie, W., Jankovic, J., and Pan, T. (2010). Neuroprotection of deferoxamine on rotenone-induced injury via accumulation of HIF-1α and induction of autophagy in SH-SY5Y cells. *Neurochem. Int.* 57, 198–205. doi: 10.1016/j.neuint.2010.05.008

Xenos, E. S., Vargas, H. D., and Davenport, D. L. (2012). Association of blood transfusion and venous thromboembolism after colorectal cancer resection. *Thromb. Res.* 129, 568–572. doi: 10.1016/j.thromres.2011.07.047

Xin, M., Ren, L., Sun, Y., Li, H. H., Guan, H. S., He, X. X., et al. (2016). Anticoagulant and antithrombotic activities of low-molecular-weight propylene glycol alginate sodium sulfate (PSS). *Eur. J. Med. Chem.* 114, 33–40. doi: 10.1016/j.ejmech.2016.02.063

Xu, M., Feng, C., Wang, J., Lang, X., Xia, G., Yu, X., et al. (2017). In vitro heterogeneous degradation of alginate and its validation of different molecular weight on blood bio-compatibility. *J. Biomater. Sci. Polym. Ed.* 28, 380–393. doi: 10.1080/09205063.2016.1277624

Xu, X., He, J., Liu, G., Diao, X., Cao, Y., Ye, Q., et al. (2014). Hemolysis assessment and antioxidant activity evaluation modified in an oxidized erythrocyte model. *J. Agric. Food Chem.* 62, 2056–2061. doi: 10.1021/jf4049935

Yan, J., Ji, Y., Zhang, P., Lu, X., Fan, Q., Pan, D., et al. (2016). Melanin nanoparticles as an endogenous agent for efficient iron overload therapy. *J. Mater. Chemi. B* 4, 7233–7240. doi: 10.1039/c6tb01558a

Yu, Y., Xu, Q., He, S., Xiong, H., Zhang, Q., Xu, W., et al. (2019). Recent advances in delivery of photosensitive metal-based drugs. *Coord. Chem. Rev.* 387, 154–179. doi: 10.1016/j.ccr.2019.01.020

Zhang, Q., Zhu, J., Song, L., Zhang, J., Kong, D., Zhao, Y., et al. (2013). Engineering magnetic-molecular sequential targeting nanoparticles for anti-cancer therapy. *J. Mater. Chem. B* 1:6402. doi: 10.1039/c3tb20715c

Zhao, L., You, G., Liao, F., Kan, X., Wang, B., Sun, Q., et al. (2010). Sodium alginate as viscosity modifier may induce aggregation of red blood cells. *Artif. Cells Blood Substit. Immobil Biotechnol.* 38, 267–276. doi: 10.3109/10731191003776736

Zhen, Z., Liu, X., Huang, T., Xi, T., and Zheng, Y. (2015). Hemolysis and cytotoxicity mechanisms of biodegradable magnesium and its alloys. *Mater Sci. Eng. C Mater. Biol. Appl.* 46, 202–206. doi: 10.1016/j.msec.2014.08.038

Zhong, R., Wang, H., Wu, X., Cao, Y., He, Z., He, Y., et al. (2013). In vitro investigation of the effect of plasticizers on the blood compatibility of medical grade plasticized poly (vinyl chloride). *J. Mater. Sci. Mater. Med.* 24, 1985–1992. doi: 10.1007/s10856-013-4950-1

Zhou, D., He, S., Cong, Y., Xie, Z., Chen, X., Jing, X., et al. (2015). A polymer-(multifunctional single-drug) conjugate for combination therapy. *J. Mater. Chem. B* 3, 4913–4921. doi: 10.1039/c5tb00576k

Zou, W., Qin, H., Shi, W., Sun, S., and Zhao, C. (2014). Surface modification of poly(ether sulfone) membrane with a synthesized negatively charged copolymer. *Langmuir* 30, 13622–13630. doi: 10.1021/la502343c

8

Developing an Injectable Nanofibrous Extracellular Matrix Hydrogel with an Integrin αvβ3 Ligand to Improve Endothelial Cell Survival, Engraftment and Vascularization

*Dake Hao[1,2], Ruiwu Liu[3], Kewa Gao[1,2], Chuanchao He[1], Siqi He[1,2], Cunyi Zhao[4], Gang Sun[4], Diana L. Farmer[1,2], Alyssa Panitch[1,5], Kit S. Lam[3] and Aijun Wang[1,2,5]**

[1] Department of Surgery, School of Medicine, University of California, Davis, Sacramento, CA, United States, [2] Institute for Pediatric Regenerative Medicine, Shriners Hospitals for Children, Sacramento, CA, United States, [3] Department of Biochemistry and Molecular Medicine, School of Medicine, University of California, Davis, Sacramento, CA, United States, [4] Department of Biological and Agricultural Engineering, University of California, Davis, Davis, CA, United States, [5] Department of Biomedical Engineering, University of California, Davis, Davis, CA, United States

***Correspondence:**
Aijun Wang
aawang@ucdavis.edu

Endothelial cell (EC) transplantation via injectable collagen hydrogel has received much attention as a potential treatment for various vascular diseases. However, the therapeutic effect of transplanted ECs is limited by their poor viability, which partially occurs as a result of cellular apoptosis triggered by the insufficient cell-extracellular matrix (ECM) engagement. Integrin binding to the ECM is crucial for cell anchorage to the surrounding matrix, cell spreading and migration, and further activation of intracellular signaling pathways. Although collagen contains several different types of integrin binding sites, it still lacks sufficient specific binding sites for ECs. Previously, using one-bead one-compound (OBOC) combinatorial technology, we identified LXW7, an integrin αvβ3 ligand, which possessed a strong binding affinity to and enhanced functionality of ECs. In this study, to improve the EC-matrix interaction, we developed an approach to molecularly conjugate LXW7 to the collagen backbone, via a collagen binding peptide SILY, in order to increase EC specific integrin binding sites on the collagen hydrogel. Results showed that in the *in vitro* 2-dimensional (2D) culture model, the LXW7-treated collagen surface significantly improved EC attachment and survival and decreased caspase 3 activity in an ischemic-mimicking environment. In the *in vitro* 3-dimensional (3D) culture model, LXW7-modified collagen hydrogel significantly improved EC spreading, proliferation, and survival. In a mouse subcutaneous implantation model, LXW7-modified collagen hydrogel improved the engraftment of transplanted ECs and supported ECs to form vascular network structures. Therefore, LXW7-functionalized collagen hydrogel has shown promising potential to improve vascularization in tissue regeneration and may be used as a novel tool for EC delivery and the treatment of vascular diseases.

Keywords: collagen hydrogel, endothelial cell, integrin-based ligand, cell engraftment, tissue regeneration

INTRODUCTION

Endothelial cell (EC) transplantation has been widely used for the treatment of various types of vascular diseases, such as myocardial ischemia, cerebrovascular disease, and peripheral vascular disease (Fadini et al., 2005; Singhal et al., 2010; Blum et al., 2012). However, exploration and tracking of EC behavior and fate after transplantation has indicated that ECs exhibit poor survival and engraftment rates, which proves to be the crucial limitation of EC transplantation (Hall and Jevnikar, 2003). To overcome this limitation, different approaches, such as cell pre-conditioning, genetic modification and co-transplantation (Penn and Mangi, 2008; Yu et al., 2013; Sun et al., 2016; Shafiee et al., 2017; Hao et al., 2019), have been used to improve EC engraftment after transplantation. However, these approaches have raised safety concerns and have complicated regulatory pathways. Thus, there is still an urgent need to develop safe and easy-for-translation approaches for EC transplantation that allow for improved cell engraftment rates.

Biomaterial carriers are attractive tools for improving cell delivery and survival (Qi et al., 2015). Hydrogel systems are currently widely studied in the field of stem cell transplantation, due to their 3-dimensional (3D) cross-linked networks, cytocompatibility, injectability, and biocompatibility (Mulyasasmita et al., 2014; Robinson et al., 2016; Hao et al., 2020b). Collagen is the main structural protein in natural extracellular matrix (ECM), which can mimic the physical characteristics of ECM (Di Lullo et al., 2002). Particularly, type I collagen has great potential as a cell delivery medium, because it is ubiquitous and can self-assemble under physiological conditions (Glowacki and Mizuno, 2008; Copes et al., 2019). Integrins are heterodimeric transmembrane receptors present on the cell surface (Giancotti and Ruoslahti, 1999). Upon ligand binding, integrins facilitate cell-cell and cell-ECM adhesion, activate signal transduction pathways, and regulate cell functions (Caiado and Dias, 2012; Malinin et al., 2012). Integrins have been shown to play critical roles in cartilage (Liang et al., 2015), bone (Kundu et al., 2009), neuronal (Chen et al., 2018), pancreatic (Krishnamurthy and Wang, 2009) and vascular (Li et al., 2017) regeneration. Consequently, increasing specific integrin binding sites will be significant in advancing the development of an engineered hydrogel cell delivery system for use in tissue regeneration applications. Although collagen has several integrin binding sites (Xu et al., 2000; Znoyko et al., 2006; Zeltz and Gullberg, 2016), such as α1β1, α2β1, α10β1, and α11β1, it lacks sufficient EC specific integrin binding sites. According to previous studies, αvβ3 integrin expressed on ECs has been shown to be crucial for EC adhesion and for advancing angiogenic development (Tzima et al., 2001; Sheppard, 2002; Avraamides et al., 2008). Therefore, identifying an integrin αvβ3 ligand specifically bound to ECs and using it to engineer the collagen hydrogel will be valuable for EC transplantation in tissue regeneration applications.

One-bead one-compound (OBOC) combinatorial technology is an ultra-high throughput chemical library synthesis and screening method, which is suitable for integrin-based ligand discovery (Lam et al., 1991). Previously, we have identified various potent ligands, such as LXY30, LXW7, and LLP2A targeting integrins α3β1, αvβ3, and α4β1, respectively, by employing the OBOC combinatorial technology (Peng et al., 2006; Yao et al., 2009; Xiao et al., 2010). We have also found that LXW7 had specific binding to ECs via αvβ3 integrin and biomaterial scaffolds decorated with LXW7 was found to improve EC adhesion and functions *in vitro* and promoted vascularization in a rat carotid artery bypass vascular graft model (Hao et al., 2017, 2020a). Thus, LXW7 will be an ideal choice to modify collagen hydrogel for increasing the number of EC specific integrin binding sites. SILY peptide, RRANAALKAGELYKSILY, is a high-affinity collagen binding ligand derived from platelet membrane receptors that bind to α1 chains in collagen (Paderi and Panitch, 2008; Goldbloom-Helzner et al., 2019). SILY has also been conjugated to other functional molecules and used in medical applications related to collagen (Paderi et al., 2011; Scott et al., 2013). Therefore, in this study, we propose to molecularly immobilize LXW7 onto collagen backbone by using SILY as the junction to increase the EC specific integrin binding sites of collagen hydrogel to improve EC binding, survival and ultimately engraftment after transplantation.

MATERIALS AND METHODS

Cell Culture

We used endothelial colony forming cell (ECFC) banks as described in our previous study (Hao et al., 2017, 2020a). ECFCs were expanded and cultured in Endothelial Cell Growth Medium-2 BulletKit medium (EGM-2, Lonza). ECFCs between P3 and P6 were used for all experiments.

ECFC Attachment on LXW7-Treated Collagen Surface

To facilitate the LXW7 modification on 2-dimensional (2D) collagen culture surface and 3-dimensional (3D) collagen hydrogel, we synthesized $(SILY)_2$-LXW7 and SILY-$(LXW7)_2$ (**Figure 1**) through three steps: 1) standard solid phase peptide synthesis (SPPS) of LXW7-$2N_3$ or SILY-$2N_3$, 2) SPPS synthesis of SILY-DBCO or LXW7-DBCO, 3) DBCO-azido copper-free Click conjugation by mixing LXW7-$2N_3$ with 2 eq. of SILY-DBCO or SILY-$2N_3$ with 2 eq. of LXW7-DBCO, respectively. Detailed synthesis was described in **Supplementary Figure S1**. To modify the collagen culture surface with LXW7, target culture wells in a 24-well plate were coated with 500 μL of 100 ng/mL collagen type I (PureCol) and incubated for 1 h at 37 °C. Collagen coated wells were rinsed three times with PBS (HyClone) and were treated with 500 μL 20 μM of $(SILY)_2$-LXW7 or SILY-$(LXW7)_2$. After 1 h, the wells were washed three times with PBS and blocked with 1% BSA (Thermo Fisher Scientific) for 1 h. After, the wells were rinsed three times with PBS. For the cell attachment assay, 5×10^3 ECFCs were added to the wells and incubated for 5 min at 37°C and 5% CO_2. The wells were washed three times with PBS, and the adhered cells were fixed in 10% formalin (Azer Scientific) for 20 min. The wells were washed, and then nuclei were stained with 4′, 6-diamidino-2-phenylindole (DAPI, Sigma). After three washings with PBS,

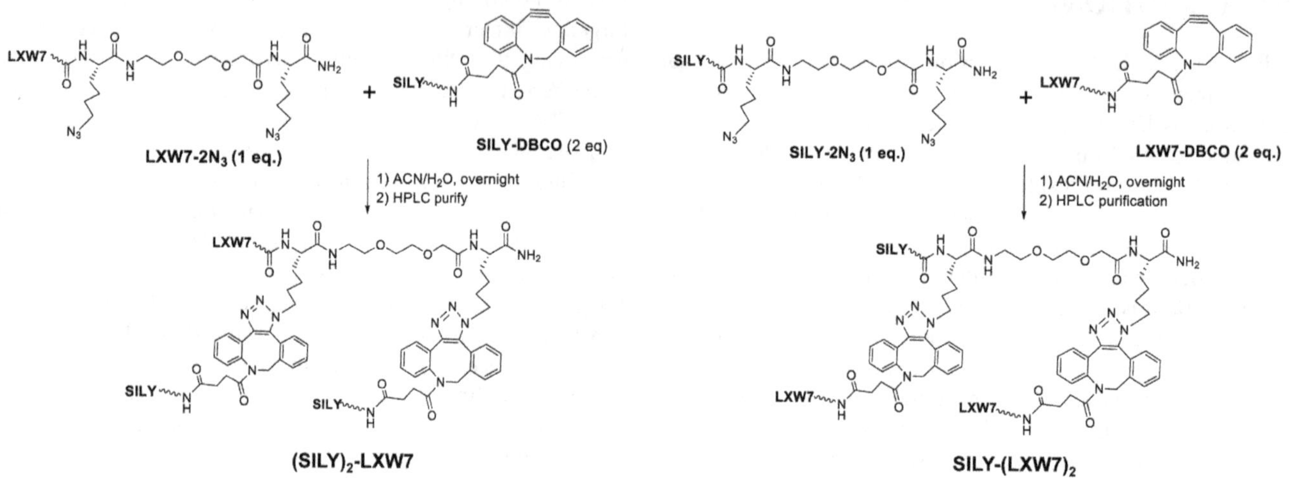

FIGURE 1 | Chemical synthesis of $(SILY)_2$-LXW7 or SILY-$(LXW7)_2$.

the ECFCs were imaged using a Carl Zeiss Axio Observer D1 inverted microscope. Image quantification was performed using the ImageJ software (NIH).

ECFC Apoptosis and Survival on LXW7-Treated Collagen Surface Under Ischemic-Mimicking Hypoxic Environment

The ischemic-mimicking hypoxic environment was set up as cells cultured in EGM-2 with 1% fetal bovine serum (FBS) and low concentration growth factors (1/10 of the original bulk in the EGM-2 bullet kit) at 1% O_2, 37°C and 5% CO_2. ECFCs were seeded in 96-well plates treated with collagen, collagen and $(SILY)_2$-LXW7, or collagen and SILY-$(LXW7)_2$. For caspase 3 assay, the cells were cultured in ischemic-mimicking hypoxic environment for 6 h, then lysed and analyzed by using a Caspase 3 Assay Kit (Cell Signaling Technology) according to the manufacturer's instruction. Fluorescence (ex 380 nm/em 450 nm) was measured using a SpectraMax i3x Multi-Mode Detection Platform (Molecular Devices). For the cell survival assay, the ECFCs were cultured for 5 d and determined using a CellTiter 96® AQueous One Solution Cell Proliferation Assay (MTS, Promega) according to the manufacturer's instruction. The amount of soluble formazan product produced by the reduction of MTS by metabolically active cells was measured at the 490 nm absorbance using the SpectraMax i3x Multi-Mode Detection Platform.

Preparation and Characterization of LXW7-Modified Collagen Hydrogel

For optimization of collagen hydrogel concentration, the original 10 mg/mL collage type I was diluted to 1, 2, 4, and 8 mg/mL with PBS, respectively. The same number of ECFCs was loaded into the collagen hydrogel with different concentration and cultured at 37°C, 5% CO_2 for 5 days, then the number of cells was determined using MTS as described above. For the preparation and evaluation of LXW7-modified collagen hydrogel, the diluted 2 mg/mL collagen was mixed with SILY-$(LXW7)_2$ at the different concentration of SILY-$(LXW7)_2$/collagen (nmol/mg), such as 0, 0.005, 0.05, 0.25, 0.5, 2.5, 5, 12.5, or 25 nmol/mg. The LXW7-modified collagen (0.1 mL) was then put in 48-well plates and incubated at 37°C for 1 h, then 100 μL PBS was added into the wells. After 24 h, the PBS was collected for High-performance liquid chromatography (HPLC) analysis to quantify the amount of unbound free SILY-$(LXW7)_2$ that was eluted to the solution. Briefly, HPLC analysis was performed on the Waters 2996 HPLC system equipped with a Waters XTerra® MS column (5 μm, C18, 150 × 4.6 mm). A linear gradient was run from 100% solution A (water/0.1% trifluoroacetic acid) to 100% solution B (acetonitrile/0.1% trifluoroacetic acid) within 20 min with a flow rate at 1.0 mL/min. The UV detection wavelength was 214 nm. The compressive modulus of the untreated collagen hydrogel and the LXW7-modified collagen hydrogel were determined using the Instron 5566 Universal Testing Machine.

Lentiviral Vector Transduction

All lentiviral constructs were generated at the UC Davis Institute for Regenerative Cures (IRC) Vector Core. To track the cell fate and behavior *in vitro* and *in vivo*, ECFCs were transduced with the pCCLc-MNDU3-LUC-PGK-EGFP-WPRE vector as previously described (Kumar et al., 2018; Gao et al., 2019, 2020; Rose et al., 2020). Transduction was performed in transduction medium consisting of DMEM high glucose (HyClone), 10% FBS (HyClone), and 8 μg/mL protamine sulfate (MP Biomedicals) for 6 h. The vectors were transduced at a multiplicity of infection (MOI) of 10. After that, ECFCs were cultured in EGM-2 medium for 72 h. After 72 h, ECFCs were screened for neomycin resistance for 7 days cultured in medium containing 2 μg/mL of G418 (EMD, Millipore). Successfully transduced ECFCs were then cultured and expanded in EGM-2 medium.

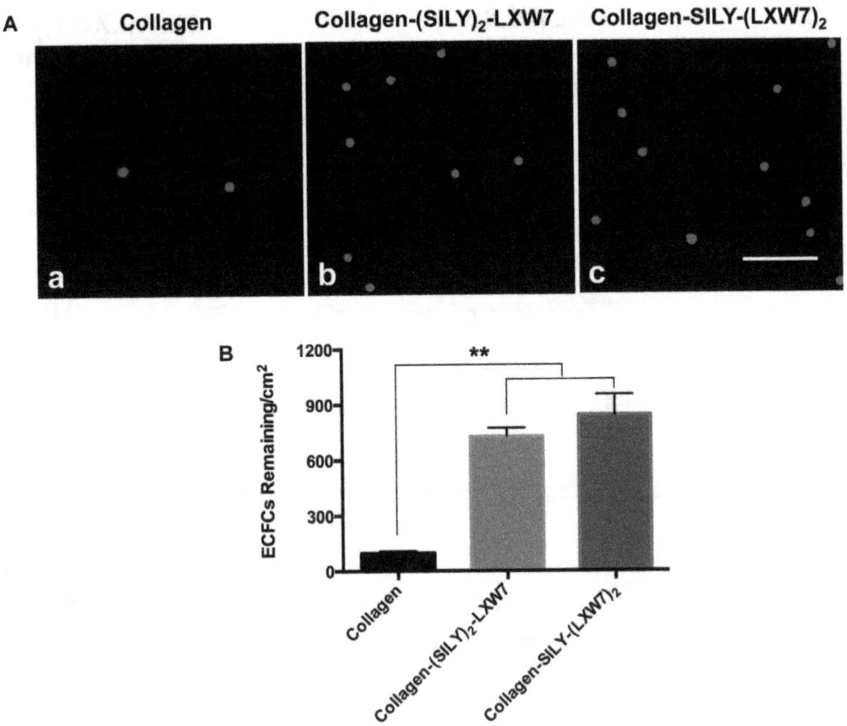

FIGURE 2 | Attachment of ECFCs on LXW7-treated collagen surface. **(A)** Images of ECFC attachment on untreated collagen surface **(a)**, $(SILY)_2$-LXW7 treated collagen surface **(b)** and SILY-$(LXW7)_2$ treated collagen surface **(c)**. Scale bar = 100 μm. **(B)** Quantification of the number of ECFCs attached on the different treated surfaces. Data were expressed as mean ± standard deviation: $^{**}p < 0.01$ ($n = 5$).

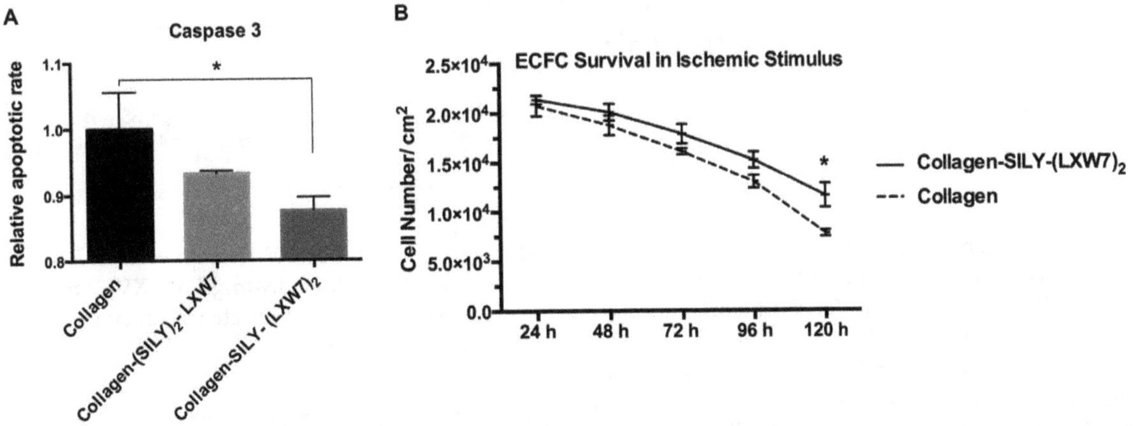

FIGURE 3 | Apoptosis and survival of ECFCs on LXW7-treated collagen surface. **(A)** Quantification of caspase 3 expression of ECFCs cultured on different treated surfaces under ischemic-mimicking hypoxic environment. **(B)** Quantification of survival of ECFCs cultured on the different treated surfaces under ischemic-mimicking hypoxic environment. Data were expressed as mean ± standard deviation: $^{*}p < 0.05$ ($n = 5$).

ECFC Behavior in LXW7-Modified Collagen Hydrogel

For cell sprouting assay, ECFCs were loaded in the untreated collagen hydrogel, or LXW7-modified collagen hydrogel, respectively, and cultured in EGM-2 for 3 d. Images were taken at day 1 and day 3 by using the Carl Zeiss Axio Observer D1 inverted microscope. Image quantification was performed using the ImageJ software. For capillary network formation, three groups were set up: (1) ECFCs cultured in untreated collagen hydrogel, (2) ECFCs cultured in LXW7-modified collagen hydrogel, (3) ECFCs incubated with a monoclonal anti-αvβ3 integrin blocking antibody (MAB1876, Millipore) first to block the integrin αvβ3 expressed on the ECFCs, then cultured in the LXW7-modified collagen hydrogel. Images were taken at day 5 by using the Carl Zeiss Axio Observer D1 inverted

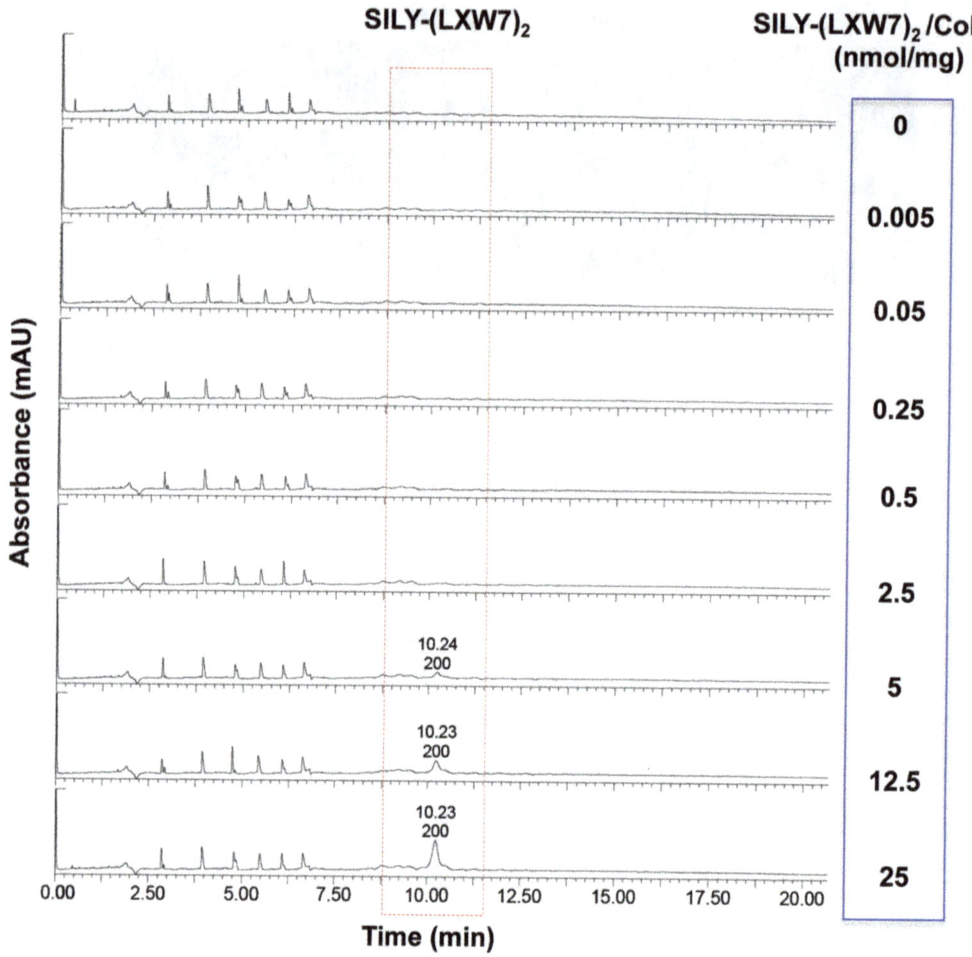

FIGURE 4 | HPLC evaluation of LXW7 conjugation on collagen hydrogel. The elution of unbound free SILY-(LXW7)$_2$ into the incubating PBS was quantified using HPLC. The peak of SILY-(LXW7)$_2$ was not shown until the amount of SILY-(LXW7)$_2$ used to modify collagen hydrogel was up to 5 nmol/mg, and the peaks increased as the amount of SILY-(LXW7)$_2$ increased.

microscope. Image quantification was performed using the ImageJ software. For cell proliferation, ECFCs were loaded in the untreated collagen hydrogel or LXW7-modified collagen hydrogel, respectively, and cultured in EGM-2 at 37°C, 20% O_2 and 5% CO_2 for 5 days. Cell metabolic activity and proliferation was quantified every 24 h using MTS as described above. For cell survival, ECFCs were loaded in the untreated collagen hydrogel or LXW7-modified collagen hydrogel, respectively, and cultured under ischemic-mimicking hypoxic environment for 5 days. Cell metabolic activity was quantified every 24 h using MTS, as described above.

In vivo Cell Transplantation

All animal procedures were approved by the Institutional Animal Care and Use Committee at the University of California, Davis. All facilities used during the study period were accredited by the Association for the Assessment and Accreditation of Laboratory Animal Care International (AAALAC). NSG (NOD/SCID/ IL2R$\gamma^{-/-}$) immunodeficient mice were purchased from The Jackson Laboratory. 5×10^5 transduced ECFCs were loaded in 500 μL untreated collagen hydrogel or LXW7-modified collagen hydrogel, respectively, and injected subcutaneously to the groin at both sides of each mouse.

Bioluminescence Imaging

Cells transplanted in NSG mice were monitored via the *In Vivo* Imaging Spectrum (IVIS) system (PerkinElmer) as previously described (Kumar et al., 2018; Gao et al., 2019; Rose et al., 2020). Briefly, animals were injected intraperitoneally with luciferase substrate D-luciferin (Gold Biotechnology) at 100 mg/kg body weight and maintained under anesthesia with 2% inhaled isoflurane for 5 min before imaging. The transplanted NSG mice were imaged at the day of transplantation (week 0) and weekly thereafter for up to 10 weeks after transplantation. Images were analyzed by using Living Image®2.50 (Perkin Elmer). Total intensity was measured within a defined area of the signal. Baseline intensity was determined by using the same defined area where there is no positive signal in the same animal.

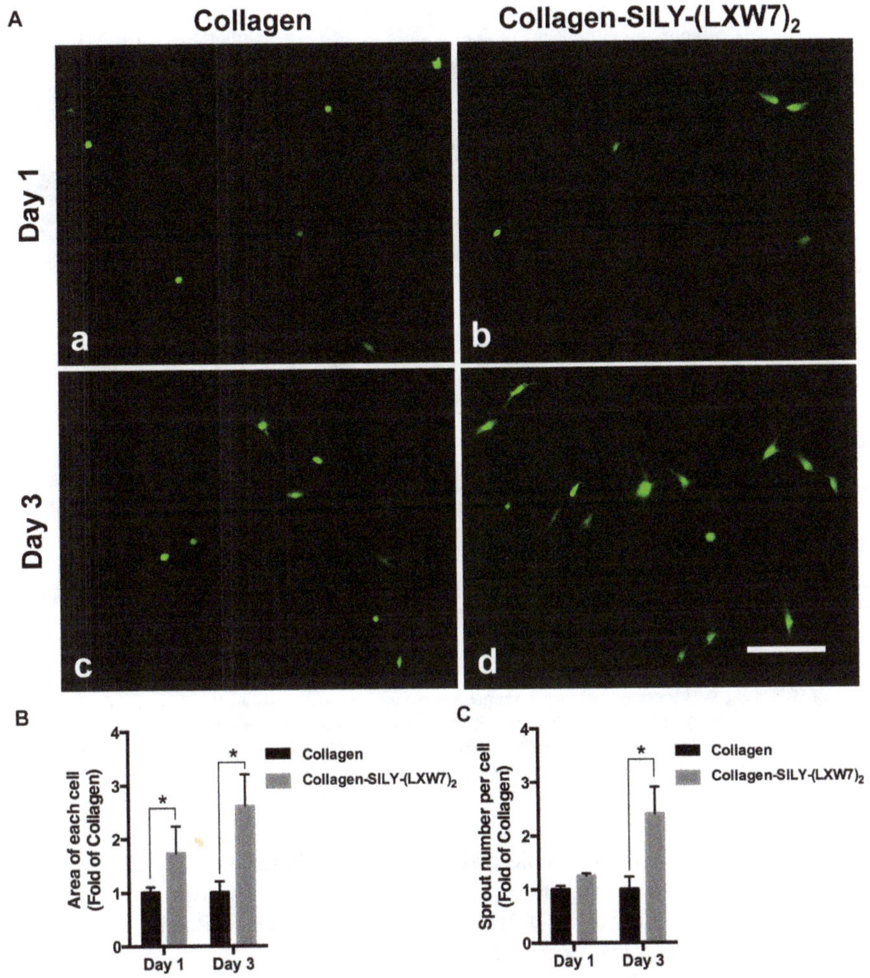

FIGURE 5 | ECFC spreading and spouting in LXW7-modified collagen hydrogel. **(A)** Images of ECFC morphology in untreated collagen hydrogel **(a)** and LXW7-modified collagen hydrogel **(b)** after 1 day culture and ECFC morphology in untreated collagen hydrogel **(c)** and LXW7-modified collagen hydrogel **(d)** after 3 day culture. Scale bar = 100 nm. **(B)** Quantification of the cell area of ECFCs cultured in collagen hydrogel with different modification. **(C)** Quantification of the number of sprouts of ECFCs cultured in collagen hydrogel with different modification. Data were expressed as mean ± standard deviation: $^*p < 0.05$ ($n = 5$).

Immunohistochemistry

Samples were collected, fixed with 4% paraformaldehyde for 24 h, protected by 30% sucrose dehydration for 48 h, and embedded in the O.C.T compound (Sakura Finetek USA, Inc). Serial sections were made at the thickness of 15 μm using a Cryostat (Leica CM3050S) and collected onto microscope slides (Matsunami Glass). Tissue sections were extensively washed with PBS, blocked with 5% BSA in PBS at room temperature for 1 h, and stained with primary antibody at 4°C overnight. The dilution of primary antibody was goat anti-GFP (Novus Biologicals) at 1:100. Sections were incubated with secondary antibodies diluted at 1:500 for 1 h at room temperature. The secondary antibody was donkey anti-goat (Thermo Fisher Scientific) conjugated with Alexa488. The slides were counterstained with 1:5000 dilution of DAPI for 5 min, mounted with Prolong Diamond Antifade Mountant (Invitrogen), and imaged with the Zeiss Observer Z1 microscope.

Statistical Analysis

For two-sample comparison, a student's t-test was used. For multiple-sample comparison, analysis of variance (ANOVA) was performed to detect whether a significant difference existed between groups with different treatments. A p-value of 0.05 or less indicates a significant difference between samples in comparison.

RESULTS AND DISCUSSION

LXW7-Treated Collagen Surface Improved ECFC Attachment

Natural ECM displays numerous copies of several cell binding sites to support cell-matrix adhesion that is crucial for cell functions (Werb, 1997; Yue, 2014). Cell-matrix adhesion is formed through the utilization of cell adhesion molecules that bind to the cell surface (Zhong and Rescorla, 2012). Integrins are

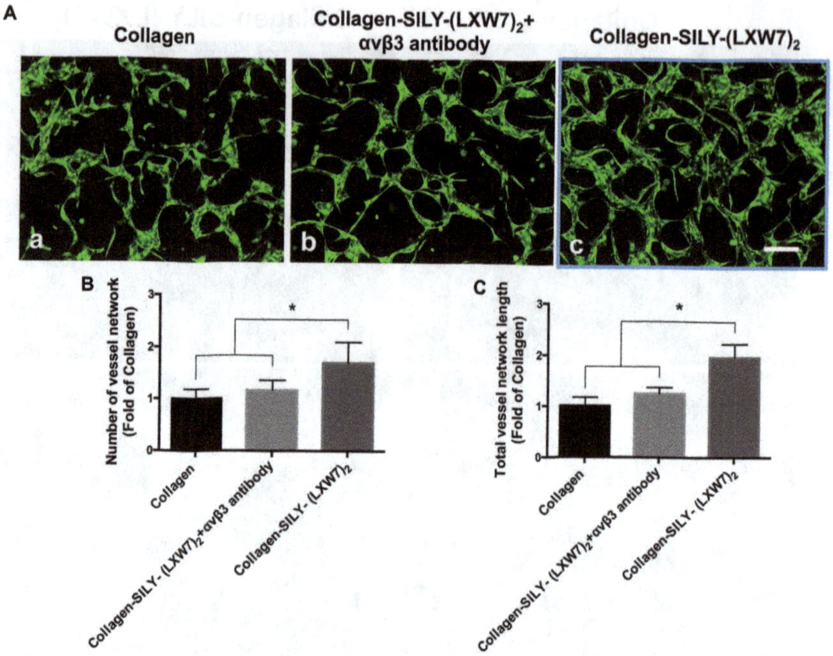

FIGURE 6 | Network formation of ECFCs in LXW7-modified collagen hydrogel was blocked by an anti-$\alpha v\beta 3$ integrin blocking antibody. **(A)** Network formation of ECFCs cultured in untreated collagen hydrogel **(a)**, network formation of ECFCs pretreated with an anti-$\alpha v\beta 3$ integrin blocking antibody cultured in LXW7-modified collagen hydrogel **(b)** and network formation of ECFCs cultured in LXW7-modified collagen hydrogel **(c)**. Scale bar = 200 μm. **(B)** Quantification of the numbers of vessel network. **(C)** Quantification of the total vessel network length. Data were expressed as mean $\pm$ standard deviation: $^*p < 0.05$ ($n = 5$).

a very important class of cell adhesion heterodimer molecules, comprised of two subunits that facilitate attachments between the cell surface and the ECM, and can greatly influence cell behavior (Gumbiner, 1996). Although collagen is the main component of natural ECM, it still lacks specific EC adhesion sites. Our previous study demonstrated an integrin $\alpha v\beta 3$ ligand LXW7 possessed specific binding to ECs (Hao et al., 2017). Thus, to increase ECFC binding sites that facilitate ECFC attachment on the collagen surface and evaluate density effects of binding sites on ECFC functions, we synthesized two different types of SILY-LXW7 derived compounds, (SILY)$_2$-LXW7 and SILY-(LXW7)$_2$, that can be used conveniently to conjugate LXW7 onto the collagen backbone. The results showed that cell culture surface treated with both (SILY)$_2$-LXW7 and SILY-(LXW7)$_2$ significantly improved ECFC attachment compared to the untreated collagen surface (**Figure 2**). The SILY-(LXW7)$_2$ treated collagen surface supported more ECFC attachment, compared to the (SILY)$_2$-LXW7 treated collagen surface indicating that a higher density of LXW7 was more beneficial for ECFC attachment (**Figure 2**).

LXW7-Treated Collagen Surface Suppressed ECFC Apoptosis and Improved ECFC Survival Under Ischemic-Mimicking Hypoxic Environment

Cell-matrix interaction regulates cellular homeostasis in multiple ways (Almeida et al., 2000; Niit et al., 2015). Disruption of this connection has deleterious effects on cell binding and survival, which leads to a specific type of apoptosis known as anoikis in most cell types (Reddig and Juliano, 2005). Caspase-3 is

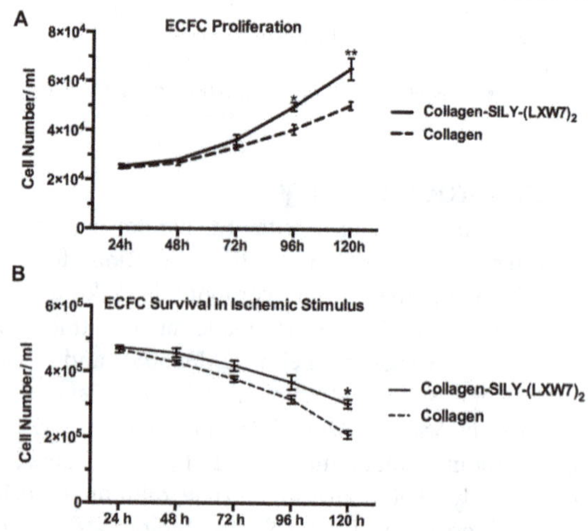

FIGURE 7 | ECFC proliferation and survival in LXW7-modified collagen hydrogel. **(A)** Quantification of cell metabolic activity and proliferation of ECFCs cultured in collagen hydrogel with or without LXW7 modification for 5 days. **(B)** Quantification of survival of ECFCs cultured in collagen hydrogel with or without LXW7 modification under ischemic-mimicking hypoxic environment for 5 days. Data were expressed as mean $\pm$ standard deviation: $^*p < 0.05$, $^{**}p < 0.01$ ($n = 5$).

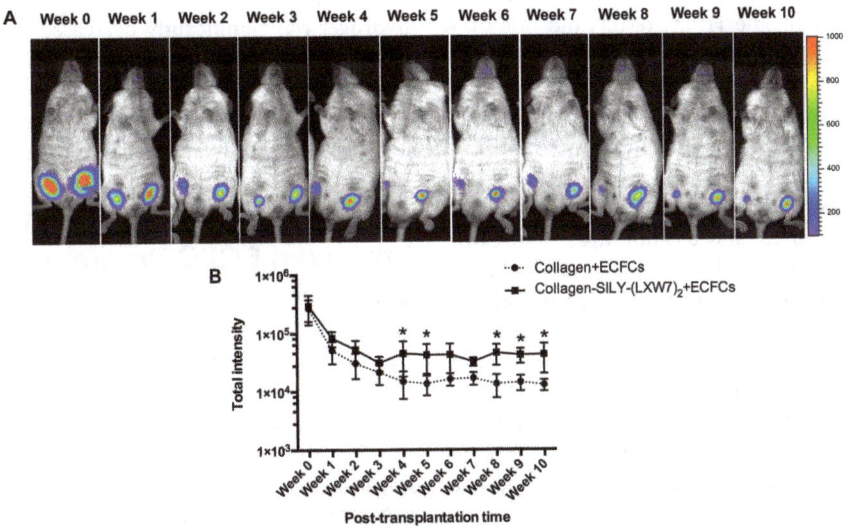

FIGURE 8 | ECFC engraftment in LXW7-modified collagen hydrogel after implantation. **(A)** IVIS imaging of implanted ECFC engraftment in untreated collagen hydrogel (right side on animal) and LXW7-modified collagen hydrogel (left side on animal) at different time points. The belly of animal was facing you in the image. **(B)** Quantification of the luciferase intensity of the engrafted ECFCs in collagen hydrogel with or without LXW7 modification at different time points. Data were expressed as mean ± standard deviation: $^*p < 0.05$ ($n = 4$).

responsible for chromatin condensation and DNA fragmentation that is necessary in apoptosis (Porter and Janicke, 1999). The results showed both $(SILY)_2$-LXW7 and SILY-$(LXW7)_2$ treated collagen surfaces suppressed expression of caspase 3 in ECFCs, compared to the collagen surface under the ischemic-mimicking hypoxic environment, and only SILY-$(LXW7)_2$ treated collagen surface significantly decreased the expression of caspase 3 in ECFCs, compared to the collagen surface (**Figure 3A**). These results may be caused by the different binding sites provided by $(SILY)_2$-LXW7 or SILY-$(LXW7)_2$. Stoichiometrically, the LXW7 binding sites provided by SILY-$(LXW7)_2$ was four times greater compared to the LXW7 binding sites provided by $(SILY)_2$-LXW7. Subsequently, the results showed that the SILY-$(LXW7)_2$ treated collagen surface significantly improved ECFC survival under the ischemic-mimicking hypoxic environment (**Figure 3B**), indicating that the LXW7-treated collagen surface was beneficial for ECFC survival by increasing the number of ECFC specific integrin binding sites.

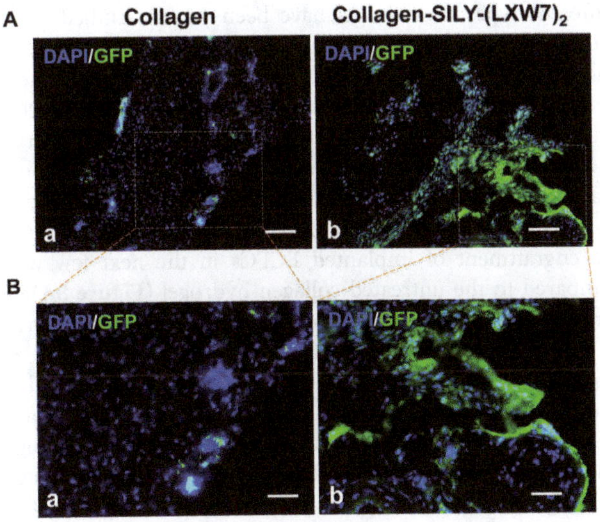

FIGURE 9 | Immunohistological analysis of ECFC survival and engraftment after *in vivo* transplantation. **(A)** GFP staining of implanted ECFCs in untreated collagen hydrogel **(a)** and LXW7-modified collagen hydrogel **(b)** at week 10. **(B)** High magnification imaging of the boxed area of **(A)**.

Evaluation of LXW7 Conjugation on Collagen Hydrogel

The effect of ECM stiffness on cell biology, signaling and response has been well-established, which has significant implications for tissue regeneration (Antoine et al., 2014). Particularly, ECM stiffness has also been linked with endothelial integrity and consequently regulation of angiogenesis (Sieminski et al., 2004). The concentrations of hydrogel could significantly influence cell behavior and growth, due to their physical properties such as stiffness (Banerjee et al., 2009; Ahearne, 2014). Before LXW7 modification, we identified the optimal concentration of collagen hydrogel for ECFC growth. The results showed that both 1 mg/mL and 2 mg/mL collagen hydrogel significantly improved ECFC growth, compared to 4 mg/mL and 8 mg/mL collagen hydrogel. There was no significant difference between the 1 mg/mL and 2 mg/mL collagen hydrogel (**Supplementary Figure S2**). In addition, to consider the difference in solidification time, we chose 2 mg/mL as the optimal concentration of collagen hydrogel for the following tests. For the LXW7 modification on collagen hydrogel, different concentration of SILY-$(LXW7)_2$ were used to modify the collagen hydrogel. HPLC has been widely used to separate and analyze the sample mixture in a discrete small volume (Gerber et al., 2004). The HPLC results did not show any peak of SILY-$(LXW7)_2$ until the amount of SILY-$(LXW7)_2$ used to modify collagen hydrogel was up to 5 nmol/mg, and the peaks increased as the amount of SILY-$(LXW7)_2$ increased (**Figure 4**). These results demonstrated that LXW7 had been successfully conjugated onto the collagen hydrogel via the "SILY-collagen" binding approach, and the saturation concentration of modification was between 2.5 and 5 nmol/mg. Compressive modulus of the collagen hydrogel before and after LXW7 modification showed no significant difference (**Supplementary Figure S3**) indicating the SILY-$(LXW7)_2$ modification approach did not significantly change the stiffness of the collagen hydrogel. This was probably because only one end of the SILY-$(LXW7)_2$ molecule carried the –SILY group that could bind to collagen, and the –$(LXW7)_2$ end could not bind to collagen, therefore the SILY-$(LXW7)_2$ modification approach did not induce molecular cross-linking of collagen.

LXW7-Modified Collagen Hydrogel Improved ECFC Sprouting and Promoted ECFC Vascular Network Formation by Increasing Integrin αvβ3 Binding Sites

Endothelial cell sprouting is important for the EC migration and vascular network formation, which are essential for angiogenesis and vascularization (Blanco and Gerhardt, 2013). Improving EC binding in the hydrogel, by increasing integrin-based binding sites, is vital to promote EC sprouting and branching (Li et al., 2017). The results of ECFC sprouting showed that most of the ECFCs cultured in LXW7-modified collagen hydrogel exhibited long spindle morphology after 1 day culture (**Figure 5A,b**), but the ECFCs cultured in untreated collagen hydrogel still displayed a round morphology (**Figure 5A,a**). After 3-day culture, the ECFCs cultured in LXW7-modified collagen hydrogel exhibited obvious sprouting (**Figure 5A,d**), but only few ECFCs cultured in untreated collagen hydrogel exhibited sprouting (**Figure 5A,c**). Quantification of cell area (**Figure 5B**) and number of sprouts (**Figure 5C**) showed that LXW7 modification significantly improved ECFC spreading and sprouting in collagen hydrogel, indicating that the LXW7-modified collagen hydrogel could promote EC migration and new vascular network formation in vascular tissue regeneration. Capillary morphogenesis is a reliable *in vitro* analog of *in vivo* angiogenesis. Also, it is know that cell-matrix interaction could generate cellular force that can impact capillary network formation. The results of network formation showed the ECFCs cultured in LXW7-modified collagen hydrogel for 5 days formed uniform and integrated network (**Figure 6A,c**), but the ECFCs cultured in untreated collagen hydrogel (**Figure 6A,a**) and the anti-αvβ3 integrin antibody blocked ECFCs cultured in LXW7-modified collagen hydrogel (**Figure 6A,b**) for 5 days only formed few intermittent network and some branches. Quantification of the number of vessel network (**Figure 6B**) and total vessel network length (**Figure 6C**) showed the LXW7-modified collagen hydrogel significantly improved the network formation of ECFCs compared to the untreated collagen hydrogel, and the network formation of the ECFCs cultured in LXW7-modified collagen hydrogel was significantly decreased by blocking the anti-αvβ3 integrins using a monoclonal anti-αvβ3 integrin antibody, which indicated that LXW7-modified collagen hydrogel promotes the vascular network formation of ECFCs compared to the untreated collagen hydrogel by increasing integrin αvβ3 binding sites.

LXW7-Modified Collagen Hydrogel Improved ECFC Proliferation and Survival

Cell proliferation and survival play key roles in stem cell therapy and tissue regeneration (Lambrou and Remboutsika, 2014; Soteriou and Fuchs, 2018). Integrin-mediated cell binding to the ECM strictly regulates cell cycle progression in mammalian cells, which is crucial for cell proliferation and survival (Schwartz and Assoian, 2001; Vachon, 2011). For ECFC metabolic activity and proliferation evaluation, MTS results showed that the number of ECFCs cultured in LXW7-modified collagen hydrogel was higher, compared to the number of ECFCs cultured in untreated collagen hydrogel, and showed the significant difference after day 4 (**Figure 7A**). For ECFC survival evaluation, results showed that the number of ECFCs cultured in LXW7-modified collagen hydrogel under the ischemic-mimicking hypoxic environment was significantly higher, compared to the number of ECFCs cultured in untreated collagen hydrogel at day 5 (**Figure 7B**). Thus, LXW7-modified collagen hydrogel can promote ECFC proliferation and survival and therefore will be beneficial to vascular tissue regeneration.

LXW7-Modified Collagen Hydrogel Improved ECFC Survival and Engraftment in a Mouse Subcutaneous Implantation Model

Different types of hydrogel have been widely studied for cell transplantation (Drury and Mooney, 2003), however, cell survival and engraftment after transplantation remains as one of the key limiting factors for translational applications (Cao et al., 2001). Integrin-ECM interaction is important to regulate cell survival and engraftment (Kumaran et al., 2005). IVIS results showed that LXW7-modified collagen hydrogel prevented the decline in the number of implanted ECFCs at week 1 and improved the engraftment of implanted ECFCs in the next few weeks, compared to the untreated collagen hydrogel (**Figure 8A**), and further showed the significant difference from week 4, according to the luciferase intensity quantification results (**Figure 8B**). Because the implanted ECFCs have also been transduced with GFP before implantation, the engraftment of implanted ECFCs was further evaluated using immunohistological staining with anti-GFP antibody. The immunohistological staining results showed that LXW7-modified collagen hydrogel promoted the ECFC survival and engraftment, compared to the untreated collagen hydrogel, and some ECFCs formed vascular network structures in the LXW7-modified collagen hydrogel construct (**Figure 9**). Thus, LXW7-modified collagen hydrogel represents a good candidate for promoting ECFC engraftment and holds promise for improving vascularization and tissue regeneration. It is known that neovascularization plays the key role in many different kinds of tissue regeneration, therefore, the LXW7-functionalized collagen hydrogel developed in this study could be widely used as a novel injectable EC delivery biomaterial tool for a variety of tissue regeneration applications, including hindlimb ischemia, myocardial ischemia and so on. Therefore, in this proof-of-concept study, we chose to use a more generic but widely applicable subcutaneous implantation model to evaluate the function of the novel LXW7-modified collagen hydrogel on neovascularization. Data obtained from this model have broad implications for a wide range of tissue regeneration applications. Further detailed evaluation of the functions of LXW7-modified collagen hydrogel in specific disease models is warranted in future studies.

CONCLUSION

This study sought to engineer collagen hydrogel, a widely used ECM biomaterial hydrogel, to improve its function for EC transplantation and tissue regeneration. To improve the EC-matrix interaction, we engineered the collagen hydrogel by increasing EC specific integrin binding sites. We successfully developed a technology to molecularly conjugate an integrin αvβ3 ligand LXW7 onto the collagen backbone via "SILY-collagen" binding approach. The LXW7-modified collagen hydrogel exhibited the capacities for promoting EC survival in an ischemic-mimicking environment *in vitro* and improved the engraftment of transplanted ECs and supported ECs to form functional vascular network structures *in vivo*. The LXW7-functionalized collagen hydrogel holds the promise to be used as a novel EC delivery tool and injectable biomaterial for tissue engineering and regenerative medicine.

AUTHOR CONTRIBUTIONS

DH performed the construction and the *in vitro* and *in vivo* evaluation of LXW7-modified collagen hydrogel, wrote the manuscript, and discussed the results. RL performed the synthesis of $(SILY)_2$-LXW7 and SILY-$(LXW7)_2$, performed the HPLC analysis, and discussed the results. KG assisted the *in vivo* evaluation. CH, SH, and CZ assisted the *in vitro* evaluation. GS, DF, AP, and KL were involved in the results discussion. AW was responsible for conceptualization, results, discussion, and revision of the manuscript. All authors contributed to the article and approved the submitted version.

ACKNOWLEDGMENTS

The authors would like to thank the Combinatorial Chemistry and Chemical Biology Shared Resource at University of California, Davis, for design and synthesis of $(SILY)_2$-LXW7 and SILY-$(LXW7)_2$. We acknowledge Alexandra Maria Iavorovschi and Olivia K. Vukcevich for their help with manuscript editing and submission.

REFERENCES

Ahearne, M. (2014). Introduction to cell-hydrogel mechanosensing. *Interface Focus* 4:20130038. doi: 10.1098/rsfs.2013.0038

Almeida, E. A., Ilic, D., Han, Q., Hauck, C. R., Jin, F., Kawakatsu, H., et al. (2000). Matrix survival signaling: from fibronectin via focal adhesion kinase to c-Jun NH(2)-terminal kinase. *J. Cell Biol.* 149, 741–754.

Antoine, E. E., Vlachos, P. P., and Rylander, M. N. (2014). Review of collagen I hydrogels for bioengineered tissue microenvironments: characterization of mechanics, structure, and transport. *Tissue Eng. B Rev.* 20, 683–696. doi: 10.1089/ten.teb.2014.0086

Avraamides, C. J., Garmy-Susini, B., and Varner, J. A. (2008). Integrins in angiogenesis and lymphangiogenesis. *Nat. Rev. Cancer* 8, 604–617. doi: 10.1038/nrc2353

Banerjee, A., Arha, M., Choudhary, S., Ashton, R. S., Bhatia, S. R., Schaffer, D. V., et al. (2009). The influence of hydrogel modulus on the proliferation and differentiation of encapsulated neural stem cells. *Biomaterials* 30, 4695–4699. doi: 10.1016/j.biomaterials.2009.05.050

Blanco, R., and Gerhardt, H. (2013). VEGF and Notch in tip and stalk cell selection. *Cold Spring Harb. Perspect. Med.* 3:a006569. doi: 10.1101/cshperspect.a006569

Blum, A., Balkan, W., and Hare, J. M. (2012). Advances in cell-based therapy for peripheral vascular disease. *Atherosclerosis* 223, 269–277. doi: 10.1016/j.atherosclerosis.2012.03.017

Caiado, F., and Dias, S. (2012). Endothelial progenitor cells and integrins: adhesive needs. *Fibrogenesis Tissue Repair* 5:4.

Cao, T. M., Kusnierz-Glaz, C., Valone, F., Hu, W. W., Johnston, L., Blume, K. G., et al. (2001). Rapid engraftment after allogeneic transplantation of density-enriched peripheral blood CD34+ cells in patients with advanced hematologic malignancies. *Cancer* 91, 2205–2213. doi: 10.1002/1097-0142(20010615)91:12<2205::aid-cncr1250>3.0.co;2-q

Chen, W. S., Guo, L. Y., Tang, C. C., Tsai, C. K., Huang, H. H., Chin, T. Y., et al. (2018). The effect of laminin surface modification of electrospun silica nanofiber substrate on neuronal tissue engineering. *Nanomaterials* 8:165. doi: 10.3390/nano8030165

Copes, F., Pien, N., Van Vlierberghe, S., Boccafoschi, F., and Mantovani, D. (2019). Collagen-based tissue engineering strategies for vascular medicine. *Front. Bioeng. Biotechnol.* 7:166. doi: 10.3389/fbioe.2019.00166

Di Lullo, G. A., Sweeney, S. M., Korkko, J., Ala-Kokko, L., and San Antonio, J. D. (2002). Mapping the ligand-binding sites and disease-associated mutations on the most abundant protein in the human, type I collagen. *J. Biol. Chem.* 277, 4223–4231. doi: 10.1074/jbc.m110709200

Drury, J. L., and Mooney, D. J. (2003). Hydrogels for tissue engineering: scaffold design variables and applications. *Biomaterials* 24, 4337–4351. doi: 10.1016/s0142-9612(03)00340-5

Fadini, G. P., Agostini, C., and Avogaro, A. (2005). Endothelial progenitor cells in cerebrovascular disease. *Stroke* 36, 1112–1113. doi: 10.1161/01.str.0000167418.29431.a8

Gao, K., He, S., Kumar, P., Farmer, D., Zhou, J., and Wang, A. (2020). Clonal isolation of endothelial colony-forming cells from early gestation chorionic villi of human placenta for fetal tissue regeneration. *World J. Stem Cells* 12, 123–138. doi: 10.4252/wjsc.v12.i2.123

Gao, K., Kumar, P., Cortez-Toledo, E., Hao, D., Reynaga, L., and Rose, M. (2019). Potential long-term treatment of hemophilia A by neonatal co-transplantation of cord blood-derived endothelial colony-forming cells and placental mesenchymal stromal cells. *Stem Cell Res. Ther.* 10:34.

Gerber, F., Krummen, M., Potgeter, H., Roth, A., Siffrin, C., and Spoendlin, C. (2004). Practical aspects of fast reversed-phase high-performance liquid chromatography using 3 microm particle packed columns and monolithic columns in pharmaceutical development and production working under current good manufacturing practice. *J. Chromatogr. A* 1036, 127–133. doi: 10.1016/j.chroma.2004.02.056

Giancotti, F. G., and Ruoslahti, E. (1999). Integrin signaling. *Science* 285, 1028–1032.

Glowacki, J., and Mizuno, S. (2008). Collagen scaffolds for tissue engineering. *Biopolymers* 89, 338–344.

Goldbloom-Helzner, L., Hao, D., and Wang, A. (2019). Developing regenerative treatments for developmental defects, injuries, and diseases using extracellular matrix collagen-targeting peptides. *Int. J. Mol. Sci.* 20:4072. doi: 10.3390/ijms20174072

Gumbiner, B. M. (1996). Cell adhesion: the molecular basis of tissue architecture and morphogenesis. *Cell* 84, 345–357. doi: 10.1016/s0092-8674(00)81279-9

Hall, A. V., and Jevnikar, A. M. (2003). Significance of endothelial cell survival programs for renal transplantation. *Am. J. Kidney Dis.* 41, 1140–1154. doi: 10.1016/s0272-6386(03)00345-7

Hao, D., Fan, Y., Xiao, W., Liu, R., Pivetti, C., and Walimbe, T. (2020a). Rapid endothelialization of small diameter vascular grafts by a bioactive integrin-binding ligand specifically targeting endothelial progenitor cells and endothelial cells. *Acta Biomater.* 108, 178–193. doi: 10.1016/j.actbio.2020.03.005

Hao, D., He, C., Ma, B., Lankford, L., Reynaga, L., Farmer, D. L., et al. (2019). Hypoxic preconditioning enhances survival and proangiogenic capacity of human first trimester chorionic villus-derived mesenchymal stem cells for fetal tissue engineering. *Stem Cells Int.* 2019:9695239.

Hao, D., Ma, B., He, C., Liu, R., Farmer, D. L., Lam, K. S., et al. (2020b). Surface modification of polymeric electrospun scaffolds via a potent and high-affinity integrin alpha4beta1 ligand improved the adhesion, spreading and survival of human chorionic villus-derived mesenchymal stem cells: a new insight for fetal tissue engineering. *J. Mater. Chem. B* 8, 1649–1659. doi: 10.1039/c9tb02309g

Hao, D., Xiao, W., Liu, R., Kumar, P., Li, Y., Zhou, P., et al. (2017). Discovery and characterization of a potent and specific peptide ligand targeting endothelial progenitor cells and endothelial cells for tissue regeneration. *ACS Chem. Biol.* 12, 1075–1086. doi: 10.1021/acschembio.7b00118

Krishnamurthy, M., and Wang, R. (2009). Integrins and extracellular matrices in pancreatic tissue engineering. *Front. Biosci.* 1, 477–491. doi: 10.2741/s39

Kumar, P., Gao, K., Wang, C., Pivetti, C., Lankford, L., and Farmer, D. (2018). In utero transplantation of placenta-derived mesenchymal stromal cells for potential fetal treatment of hemophilia A. *Cell Transplant* 27, 130–139. doi: 10.1177/0963689717728937

Kumaran, V., Joseph, B., Benten, D., and Gupta, S. (2005). Integrin and extracellular matrix interactions regulate engraftment of transplanted hepatocytes in the rat liver. *Gastroenterology* 129, 1643–1653. doi: 10.1053/j.gastro.2005.08.006

Kundu, A. K., Khatiwala, C. B., and Putnam, A. J. (2009). Extracellular matrix remodeling, integrin expression, and downstream signaling pathways influence the osteogenic differentiation of mesenchymal stem cells on poly(lactide-co-glycolide) substrates. *Tissue Eng. A* 15, 273–283. doi: 10.1089/ten.tea.2008.0055

Lam, K. S., Salmon, S. E., Hersh, E. M., Hruby, V. J., Kazmierski, W. M., and Knapp, R. J. (1991). A new type of synthetic peptide library for identifying ligand-binding activity. *Nature* 354, 82–84. doi: 10.1038/354082a0

Lambrou, G. I., and Remboutsika, E. (2014). Proliferation versus regeneration: the good, the bad and the ugly. *Front. Physiol.* 5:10. doi: 10.3389/fphys.2014.00010

Li, S., Nih, L. R., Bachman, H., Fei, P., Li, Y., Nam, E., et al. (2017). Hydrogels with precisely controlled integrin activation dictate vascular patterning and permeability. *Nat. Mater.* 16, 953–961. doi: 10.1038/nmat4954

Liang, W., Zhu, C., Liu, F., Cui, W., Wang, Q., Chen, Z., et al. (2015). Integrin beta1 gene therapy enhances in vitro creation of tissue-engineered cartilage under periodic mechanical stress. *Cell. Physiol. Biochem.* 37, 1301–1314. doi: 10.1159/000430253

Malinin, N. L., Pluskota, E., and Byzova, T. V. (2012). Integrin signaling in vascular function. *Curr. Opin. Hematol.* 19, 206–211. doi: 10.1097/moh.0b013e3283523df0

Mulyasasmita, W., Cai, L., Dewi, R. E., Jha, A., Ullmann, S. D., Luong, R. H., et al. (2014). Avidity-controlled hydrogels for injectable co-delivery of induced pluripotent stem cell-derived endothelial cells and growth factors. *J. Control. Release* 191, 71–81. doi: 10.1016/j.jconrel.2014.05.015

Niit, M., Hoskin, V., Carefoot, E., Geletu, M., Arulanandam, R., Elliott, B., et al. (2015). Cell-cell and cell-matrix adhesion in survival and metastasis: Stat3 versus Akt. *Biomol. Concepts* 6, 383–399. doi: 10.1515/bmc-2015-0022

Paderi, J. E., and Panitch, A. (2008). Design of a synthetic collagen-binding peptidoglycan that modulates collagen fibrillogenesis. *Biomacromolecules* 9, 2562–2566. doi: 10.1021/bm8006852

Paderi, J. E., Stuart, K., Sturek, M., Park, K., and Panitch, A. (2011). The inhibition of platelet adhesion and activation on collagen during balloon angioplasty by collagen-binding peptidoglycans. *Biomaterials* 32, 2516–2523. doi: 10.1016/j.biomaterials.2010.12.025

Peng, L., Liu, R., Marik, J., Wang, X., Takada, Y., and Lam, K. S. (2006). Combinatorial chemistry identifies high-affinity peptidomimetics against alpha4beta1 integrin for in vivo tumor imaging. *Nat. Chem. Biol.* 2, 381–389. doi: 10.1038/nchembio798

Penn, M. S., and Mangi, A. A. (2008). Genetic enhancement of stem cell engraftment, survival, and efficacy. *Circ. Res.* 102, 1471–1482. doi: 10.1161/circresaha.108.175174

Porter, A. G., and Janicke, R. U. (1999). Emerging roles of caspase-3 in apoptosis. *Cell Death Differ.* 6, 99–104. doi: 10.1038/sj.cdd.4400476

Qi, C., Yan, X., Huang, C., Melerzanov, A., and Du, Y. (2015). Biomaterials as carrier, barrier and reactor for cell-based regenerative medicine. *Protein Cell* 6, 638–653. doi: 10.1007/s13238-015-0179-8

Reddig, P. J., and Juliano, R. L. (2005). Clinging to life: cell to matrix adhesion and cell survival. *Cancer Metastasis Rev.* 24, 425–439. doi: 10.1007/s10555-005-5134-3

Robinson, S. T., Douglas, A. M., Chadid, T., Kuo, K., Rajabalan, A., Li, H., et al. (2016). A novel platelet lysate hydrogel for endothelial cell and mesenchymal stem cell-directed neovascularization. *Acta Biomater.* 36, 86–98. doi: 10.1016/j.actbio.2016.03.002

Rose, M., Gao, K., Cortez-Toledo, E., Agu, E., Hyllen, A. A., Conroy, K., et al. (2020). Endothelial cells derived from patients' induced pluripotent stem cells for sustained factor VIII delivery and the treatment of hemophilia A. *Stem Cells Transl. Med.* 9, 686–696. doi: 10.1002/sctm.19-0261

Schwartz, M. A., and Assoian, R. K. (2001). Integrins and cell proliferation: regulation of cyclin-dependent kinases via cytoplasmic signaling pathways. *J. Cell Sci.* 114(Pt 14), 2553–2560.

Scott, R. A., Paderi, J. E., Sturek, M., and Panitch, A. (2013). Decorin mimic inhibits vascular smooth muscle proliferation and migration. *PLoS One* 8:e82456. doi: 10.1371/journal.pone.0082456

Shafiee, A., Patel, J., Wong, H. Y., Donovan, P., Hutmacher, D. W., Fisk, N. M., et al. (2017). Priming of endothelial colony-forming cells in a mesenchymal niche improves engraftment and vasculogenic potential by initiating mesenchymal transition orchestrated by NOTCH signaling. *FASEB J.* 31, 610–624. doi: 10.1096/fj.201600937

Sheppard, D. (2002). Endothelial integrins and angiogenesis: not so simple anymore. *J. Clin. Investig.* 110, 913–914. doi: 10.1172/jci0216713

Sieminski, A. L., Hebbel, R. P., and Gooch, K. J. (2004). The relative magnitudes of endothelial force generation and matrix stiffness modulate capillary morphogenesis in vitro. *Exp. Cell Res.* 297, 574–584. doi: 10.1016/j.yexcr.2004.03.035

Singhal, A. K., Symons, J. D., Boudina, S., Jaishy, B., and Shiu, Y. T. (2010). Role of endothelial cells in myocardial ischemia-reperfusion injury. *Vasc. Dis. Prev.* 7, 1–14. doi: 10.2174/1874120701007010001

Soteriou, D., and Fuchs, Y. (2018). A matter of life and death: stem cell survival in tissue regeneration and tumour formation. *Nat. Rev. Cancer* 18, 187–201. doi: 10.1038/nrc.2017.122

Sun, K., Zhou, Z., Ju, X., Zhou, Y., Lan, J., Chen, D., et al. (2016). Combined transplantation of mesenchymal stem cells and endothelial progenitor cells for tissue engineering: a systematic review and meta-analysis. *Stem Cell Res. Ther.* 7:151.

Tzima, E., del Pozo, M. A., Shattil, S. J., Chien, S., and Schwartz, M. A. (2001). Activation of integrins in endothelial cells by fluid shear stress mediates Rho-dependent cytoskeletal alignment. *EMBO J.* 20, 4639–4647. doi: 10.1093/emboj/20.17.4639

Vachon, P. H. (2011). Integrin signaling, cell survival, and anoikis: distinctions, differences, and differentiation. *J. Signal. Transduct.* 2011:738137.

Werb, Z. (1997). ECM and cell surface proteolysis: regulating cellular ecology. *Cell* 91, 439–442. doi: 10.1016/s0092-8674(00)80429-8

Xiao, W., Wang, Y., Lau, E. Y., Luo, J., Yao, N., Shi, C., et al. (2010). The use of one-bead one-compound combinatorial library technology to discover high-affinity alphavbeta3 integrin and cancer targeting arginine-glycine-aspartic acid ligands with a built-in handle. *Mol. Cancer Ther.* 9, 2714–2723. doi: 10.1158/1535-7163.mct-10-0308

Xu, Y., Gurusiddappa, S., Rich, R. L., Owens, R. T., Keene, D. R., and Mayne, R. (2000). Multiple binding sites in collagen type I for the integrins alpha1beta1 and alpha2beta1. *J. Biol. Chem.* 275, 38981–38989. doi: 10.1074/jbc.m007668200

Yao, N., Xiao, W., Wang, X., Marik, J., Park, S. H., Takada, Y., et al. (2009). Discovery of targeting ligands for breast cancer cells using the one-bead one-compound combinatorial method. *J. Med. Chem.* 52, 126–133. doi: 10.1021/jm801062d

Yu, S. P., Wei, Z., and Wei, L. (2013). Preconditioning strategy in stem cell transplantation therapy. *Transl. Stroke Res.* 4, 76–88. doi: 10.1007/s12975-012-0251-0

Yue, B. (2014). Biology of the extracellular matrix: an overview. *J. Glaucoma* 23(8 Suppl. 1), S20–S23.

Zeltz, C., and Gullberg, D. (2016). The integrin-collagen connection - a glue for tissue repair? *J. Cell Sci.* 129:1284. doi: 10.1242/jcs.188672

Zhong, X., and Rescorla, F. J. (2012). Cell surface adhesion molecules and adhesion-initiated signaling: understanding of anoikis resistance mechanisms and therapeutic opportunities. *Cell. Signal.* 24, 393–401. doi: 10.1016/j.cellsig.2011.10.005

Znoyko, I., Trojanowska, M., and Reuben, A. (2006). Collagen binding alpha2beta1 and alpha1beta1 integrins play contrasting roles in regulation of Ets-1 expression in human liver myofibroblasts. *Mol. Cell. Biochem.* 282, 89–99. doi: 10.1007/s11010-006-1400-0

9

Endothelial Cell Morphology Regulates Inflammatory Cells Through MicroRNA Transferred by Extracellular Vesicles

*Jiaqi Liang[1], Shuangying Gu[1], Xiuli Mao[1], Yiling Tan[1], Huanli Wang[1], Song Li[2] and Yue Zhou[1]**

[1] *Shanghai Jiao Tong University Affiliated Sixth People's Hospital, School of Biomedical Engineering, Med-X Research Institution, Shanghai Jiao Tong University, Shanghai, China,* [2] *Department of Bioengineering, Department of Medicine, University of California, Los Angeles, Los Angeles, CA, United States*

***Correspondence:**
Yue Zhou
yzhou2009@sjtu.edu.cn

Vascular inflammation plays an important role in the pathogenesis and the development of cardiovascular diseases such as arteriosclerosis and restenosis, and the dysfunction of endothelial cells (ECs) may result in the activation of monocytes and other inflammatory cells. ECs exhibit an elongated morphology in the straight part of arteries but a cobblestone shape near the pro-atherogenic region such as branch bifurcation. Although the effects of hemodynamic forces on ECs have been widely studied, it is not clear whether the EC morphology affects its own function and thus the inflammatory response of monocytes. Here we showed that elongated ECs cultured on poly-(dimethyl siloxane) membrane surface with microgrooves significantly suppressed the activation of the monocytes in co-culture, in comparison to ECs with a cobblestone shape. The transfer of EC-conditioned medium to monocytes had the same effect, suggesting that soluble factors were involved in EC–monocyte communication. Further investigation demonstrated that elongated ECs upregulated the expression of anti-inflammatory microRNAs, especially miR-10a. Moreover, miR-10a was found in the extracellular vesicles (EVs) released by ECs and transferred to monocytes, and the inhibition of EV secretion from ECs repressed the upregulation of miR-10a. Consistently, the inhibition of miR-10a expression in ECs reduced their anti-inflammatory effect on monocytes. These results reveal that the EC morphology can regulate inflammatory response through EVs, which provides a basis for the design and the optimization of biomaterials for vascular tissue engineering.

Keywords: extracellular vesicles, microtopology, vascular inflammation, monocytes, miR-10a

INTRODUCTION

Atherosclerosis is the major cause of cardiovascular diseases (Momiyama et al., 2005). Although atherosclerosis develops through multiple discrete stages (Puri et al., 2011), vascular inflammation is involved in the whole process of disease progression (Ross, 1999; Davignon and Ganz, 2004). Healthy endothelial cells (ECs) control vascular tone, limit vascular smooth muscle cell (VSMC) proliferation, inhibit leukocyte adherence, and block thrombosis (Landmesser et al., 2004).

However, a variety of vascular injuries destroy the functions of the endothelium from protecting the vessel wall (Vanhoutte et al., 2009). Endothelial injury represents a major initiating step in the pathogenesis of vascular disease and atherosclerosis (Boos et al., 2007), followed by the activation and the recruitment of circulating monocytes to the region of vascular injury or infection (Ley et al., 2007). After their entry into the vessel wall, the monocytes differentiate into macrophages, which contributes to inflammatory response to neutralize invading pathogens, repair tissue damage, or activate other immune cells (Shi and Pamer, 2011). In addition to EC injury, there is evidence that the flow pattern also regulates EC morphology and activation. ECs in the straight part of an artery have an elongated morphology and align in the direction of laminar flow. In contrast, in the branched area and the curved part of artery, the formation of vortex and disturbed flow activated ECs and promoted inflammatory signaling (Li et al., 2005), and the ECs in these areas exhibit a cobblestone shape. However, whether the EC morphology *per se* has direct effects on inflammatory cells is not well-understood.

Monocyte activation contributes to the pathogenesis of various inflammatory conditions and atherosclerosis (Woollard and Geissmann, 2010). Such inflammatory response is regulated by various signals in the microenvironment, such as microbial products, cytokines, and microRNAs. It has been reported that circulating microRNAs exert great influence in modulating monocyte/macrophage phenotype and function in the process of vascular inflammation (O'Connell et al., 2007; Tili et al., 2007; Ono et al., 2011). Vascular inflammation is an important early event in atherogenesis, where many microRNAs are involved, including miR-10 (Fang et al., 2010), miR-17, miR-31 (Suarez et al., 2010), miR-92 (Wu et al., 2011), miR-155 (Zhu et al., 2011), miR-221, and miR-222 (Liu et al., 2012; Chen et al., 2019). Circulating miRNAs are not only biomarkers for disease but also serve as cell-to-cell messengers (Hergenreider et al., 2012; Yamakuchi, 2012).

Since naked RNAs are easy to be degraded by ribonuclease, microRNAs in circulation can exist either in protein binding form or enclosed in extracellular vesicles (EVs). The transfer of microRNAs in EVs mediating through interactions between the wide varieties of cell types in the cardiovascular system (Das and Halushka, 2015) has now been reported in cardiovascular systems and disease. ECs can modulate myeloid inflammatory responses through the secretion of EVs containing anti-inflammatory miRNAs (Njock et al., 2015).

In addition to biochemical signals, biophysical factors in the microenvironment may cause significant changes in the gene expression and the cellular behavior to execute regulatory function in diverse vascular events. For example, nano/micro-topographic cues can significantly affect the gene expression of human vascular ECs, which can also affect the progress of cardiovascular diseases (Biela et al., 2009; Gasiorowski et al., 2010). In addition, biophysical cues, in the form of parallel microgroove on the surface of cell-adhesive poly-(dimethyl siloxane) (PDMS) substrates, can replace the effects of small-molecule epigenetic modifiers and significantly improve cell reprogramming efficiency (Downing et al., 2013). However, it is not clear whether micro/nano-topography regulates cell–cell communications through EVs.

Here we investigated whether and how a specific pattern on culture substrates could induce pronounced changes in EC morphology and functions through microRNA-enclosing EVs to modulate inflammatory cells.

MATERIALS AND METHODS

Fabrication and Characterization of the Culture Substrate

Microfabrication technique was used to fabricate PDMS membranes with desired surface topography (10 μm in width, 3 μm in depth, and 10 μm spacing between each microgroove). PDMS was prepared according to the manufacturer's instruction (Dow Corning, United States), spin-coated onto the patterned silicon wafers to achieve the desired thickness, degassed under vacuum, and cured at 75°C for 1.5 h. The micropatterned membranes were removed from the template, cut to appropriate dimensions and thoroughly cleaned by sonication, treated with Plasma Prep III (11050Q-AX) to enhance the surface hydrophilicity, and coated with 2% gelatin for 1.5 h to promote cell attachment. The images of surface topography of the micropatterned PDMS membranes were collected by using scanning electron microscopy (SEM; JEOL JSM-5600, Japan).

Cell Culture

Human umbilical vein endothelial cells (Sciencell, United States) were cultured in ECM medium (Sciencell, United States) with 5% fetal bovine serum (FBS), 1% penicillin/streptomycin, and 1% endothelial cell growth supplement at 37°C in a humidified 5% CO_2 incubator. The cells were seeded on the PDMS membrane and cultured to reach confluence before proceeding

TABLE 1 | Primer sequences for mRNA quantitation in qRT-PCR.

Primers	Forward primer (5'–3')	Reverse primer (5'–3')
GAPDH	5' GGG AAG GTG AAG GTC GGA GT	5' GGG GTC ATT GAT GGC AAC A
MAP3K7	5' TGA CTC CTC CAT AGC ATT GT	5' CAT CAA GCC TTA GCA TTC AC
IL-6	5' GCA CCT CAG ATT GTT GTT G	5' AAA TAG TGT CCT AAC GCT CA
TNF-α	5' AGT CG GGC AGG TCT ACT TT	5' CGT TTG GGA AGG TTG GAT GT
IL-1β	5' GCT GGC AGA AAG GGA ACA GA	5' GCA GTT GGG CAT TGG TGT AG
IL-10	5' CCA AGA GAA AGG CAT CTA CA	5' GGG GGT TGA GGT ATC AGA G

TABLE 2 | Primer sequences for microRNA quantitation in qRT-PCR.

Primers	Forward primer
hsa-miR-10a-5p	5' CAC AAA UUC GGA UCU ACA GGG UA
hsa-miR-126-3p	5' CGC AUU AUU ACU CAC GGU ACG A

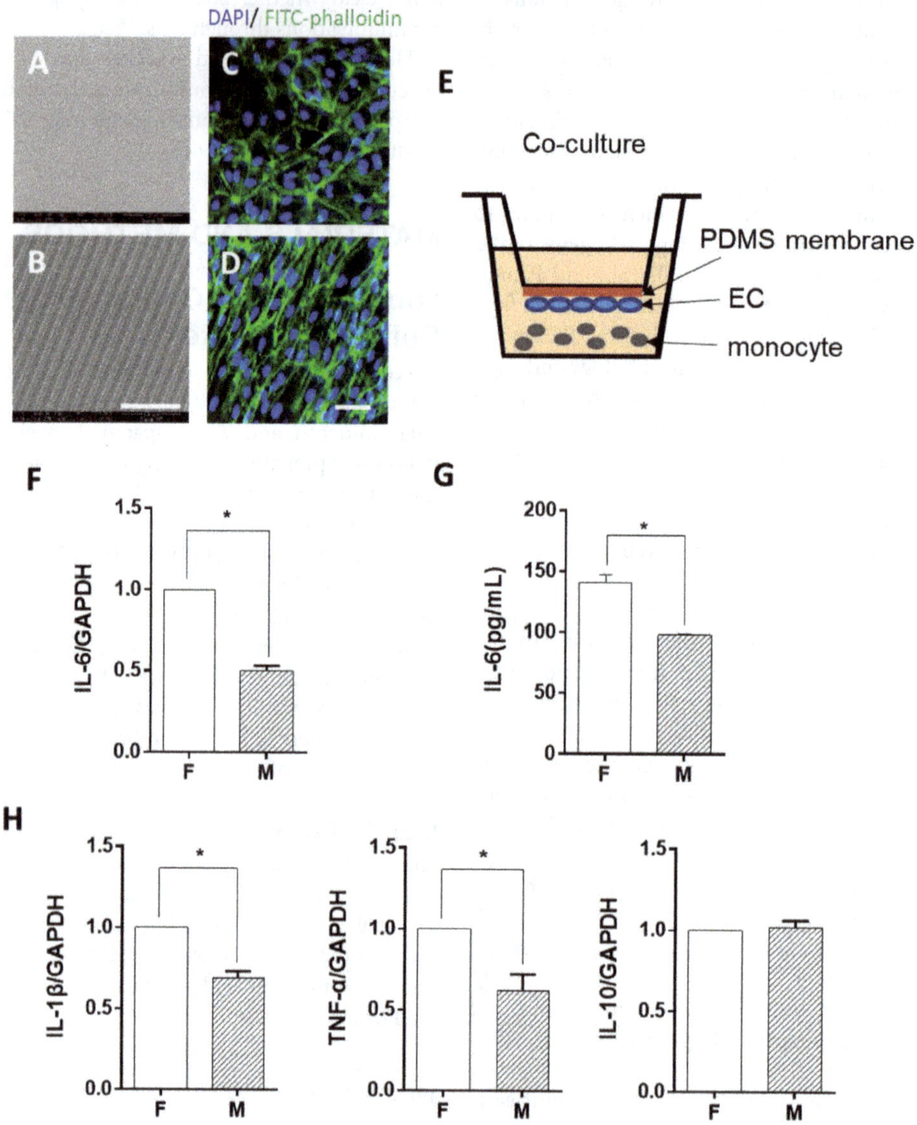

FIGURE 1 | Morphology-modified endothelial cells (ECs) inhibited the inflammatory cytokine expression in monocytes in the co-culture system. **(A,B)** Scanning electron micrograph image of the flat (F) and microgrooved (M) PDMS membranes, showing the parallel microgrooves with 10 μm in width and 3 μm in depth. Scale bar is 100 μm. ECs were seeded on flat **(C)** or microgrooved **(D)** poly-(dimethyl siloxane) (PDMS) membrane and cultured for 24 h. The F-actin was stained by FITC-phalloidin (green). The cell nucleus was stained by 4′,6-diamidino-2-phenylindole (blue). Scale bar is 75 μm. **(E)** Schematic of the EC–monocyte co-culture system using a transwell apparatus. **(F,H)** LPS-treated monocytes were co-cultured with ECs on either flat or microgrooved PDMS membrane for 24 h. The expression level of inflammatory cytokines (IL-6, IL-1β, TNF-α, and IL-10) in the monocytes was assessed by qRT-PCR. **(G)** The secreted protein level of IL-6 was determined by ELISA. Data were normalized to GAPDH expression. All the experiments were repeated for at least three times, $^{*}p < 0.05$.

to the experiments. Monocyte cell line THP-1 (human acute monocytic leukemia cell line) was obtained from the American Type Culture Collection and cultured in RPMI 1640 medium supplemented with 1% penicillin/streptomycin, 10% fetal bovine serum, L-glutamine, and 0.05 mM β-mercaptoethanol. The cells were grown to a density of 1×10^6cells/ml and treated with 50 ng/ml lipopolysaccharide (LPS) for 2 h for activation.

Co-culture

Monocytes and ECs co-culture was carried out in a Transwell^{TM} system purchased from Thermo (Cat# Nunc, 140660). The PDMS membrane was attached to the outer surface at the bottom of the Transwell insert, with the ECs facing down to the monocyte culture in the lower well, leaving an ~1-mm space in between. Before co-culturing with ECs, the monocytes were stimulated with LPS at a concentration of 50 ng/ml for 2 h and washed thoroughly to remove the additional LPS. The total volume of the medium in the co-culture system was 2 ml, comprising of 1 ml of EC medium and 1 ml of RPMI medium (for monocyte). To make sure that the EVs that we extracted were from ECs and not from the FBS, exosome-depleted FBS (System Biosciences,

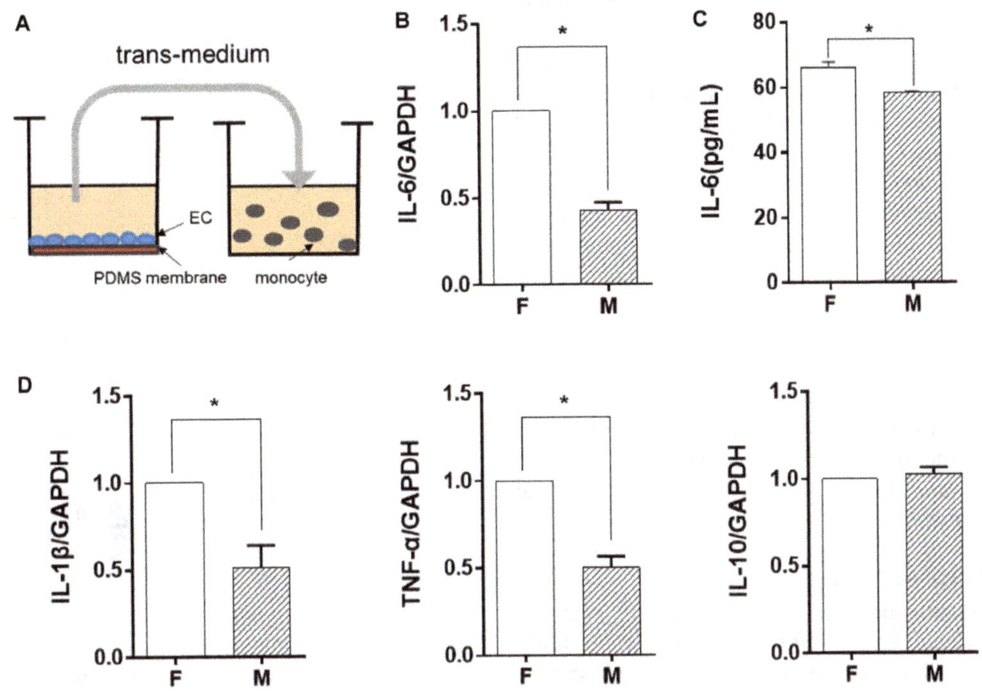

FIGURE 2 | Endothelial cells (EC) morphology-regulated monocytes in a trans-medium system. ECs were cultured on flat (F) or microgrooved (M) membrane for 24 h, and the conditioned medium was collected and transferred to treat lipopolysaccharide-activated monocytes for 24 h. **(A)** Schematic of the trans-medium system. **(B,D)** The expression level of inflammatory cytokines (IL-6, IL-1β, TNF-α, and IL-10) was assessed by qRT-PCR. Data were normalized to GAPDH expression. **(C)** The protein level of IL-6 was determined by ELISA. All the experiments were repeated at least three times, $^{*}p < 0.05$.

LLC, United States) was used in the co-culture and trans-medium system.

Immunofluorescence Staining

The cells were fixed with 4% paraformaldehyde (Electron Microscopy Sciences, United States) and blocked with 10% BSA-PBST (Merck, United States). For actin–cytoskeleton staining, the samples were incubated with fluorescein-isothiocyanate-conjugated phalloidin (FITC; AAT Bioquest, United States) for 1 h. For immunostaining, primary antibodies were incubated overnight at 4°C, followed by 1 h of incubation with proper secondary antibodies in the dark. The nuclei were stained with 4',6-diamidino-2-phenylindole (DAPI; Beyotime Biotechnology, China). The microscopic images were acquired with confocal laser scanning microscope TCS SP5II (Leica, Germany).

Nanoparticle Tracking Analysis

After culturing for 24 h, the EVs were isolated from the EC culture medium by ultracentrifugation. Briefly, cell culture medium was collected and centrifuged at 300 *g* for 10 min and at 2,000 *g* for 10 min to remove cell debris. Then, the supernatant was centrifuged at 100,000 *g* for 70 min (Beckman XE-90, United States) to separate the EVs and the EV-depleted medium. Finally, the EVs were resuspended in 1 ml Dulbecco's phosphate-buffered saline. The size of the EVs was analyzed by the manufacturer's default software of Zeta View 8.04.02 SP2 (Bachurski et al., 2019).

EV Uptaking

The EVs extracted from the conditioned medium of ECs by ultracentrifugation were labeled with I-135 according to a previously published method (Zhang et al., 2016) and added into the monocyte medium. After 2 h, the intensity of the radiation from the monocytes was measured with a scintillation counter and expressed as counts. Normal culture medium was used as blank for background reading.

RNA Isolation and qRT-PCR Analysis

The total RNA and microRNAs in the cells were isolated using TRIzol® plus RNA Purification (Invitrogen, United States) and miRcute miRNA isolation kit (Tiangen, China), respectively, following the manufacturer's instruction. For qRT-PCR, cDNA of mRNA synthesis was performed using the FastQuant RT kit (with gDNase) (Tiangen, China), and the mRNA level was measured using SuperReal PreMix Plus (SYBR Green) (Tiangen, China). Here the GAPDH was used as a normalization control. The sequences of the primers used for real-time PCR are listed in **Table 1**.

Total Exosome RNA and Protein Isolation Kit (Invitrogen, United States) was used for microRNA isolation from EVs. The EVs were dissolved in a 37°C pre-warmed denaturing solution. The microRNAs were extracted by a mixture of phenol/chloroform solution and precipitated from the aqueous phase by ethanol, followed by a series of wash and elution steps. The purified microRNAs were finally dissolved in the elution solution provided in the kit before the subsequent cDNA first-strand synthesis experiments. The cDNAs of the microRNAs were synthesized with miRcute miRNA First-Strand cDNA Synthesis Kit, and the quantitative real-time PCR was performed with miRcute miRNA qPCR Detection Kit (SYBR Green) (Tiangen, China) according to the manufacturer's instruction. RNU6-2 was used as a normalization control in all microRNA measurements. The relevant primers are listed in **Table 2**. The qRT-PCR was run on Applied Biosystems 7900HT Fast Real-Time PCR System (ABI, United States). The qRT-PCR data were analyzed using the comparative $2^{-\Delta\Delta CT}$ method.

Enzyme-Linked Immunosorbent Assay

The total of IL-6 protein in monocyte culture media was quantified by enzyme-linked immunosorbent assay (ELISA) (R&D, United States). The operating procedure follows the manufacturer's recommendations.

EV Secretion Inhibition

N-SMase Spiroepoxide inhibitor is a potent and selective irreversible inhibitor of neutral sphingomyelinase (N-SMase), and it has been used to inhibit exosome release (Devhare et al., 2017). To inhibit EV production, N-SMase Spiroepoxide inhibitor ($C_{20}H_{30}N_2O_5$, Santa Cruz, United States) was used at a concentration of 2.5 μm to treat the ECs for 24 h. Dimethyl sulfoxide (Invitrogen, United States) was used as the solvent control.

MicroRNA Inhibition

ECs were seeded on the flat or microgrooved PDMS membranes for 24 h, and then miR-10a inhibitor or negative control was added into the medium at a concentration of 100 nM, following the manufacturer's protocol. The trans-medium system was applied to culture monocytes for 24 h. The micrOFFTM hsa-miR-10a-5p inhibitor, the negative control of micrOFFTM inhibitor, and the FECT™ CP Transfection Kit (Ribobio, China) were used in this experiment.

Western Blotting

For Western blotting analysis of the exosome marker, the exosomes were isolated using Total Exosome Isolation Kit (Invitrogen, United States), according to the manufacturer's instruction. Exosome samples were directly denatured with the loading buffer, separated by sodium dodecyl sulfate-polyacrylamide gel electrophoresis (SDS-PAGE), and transferred to polyvinylidene fluoride membranes. The membrane was blocked in 5% non-fat milk and incubated with primary antibody against CD63 (Thermo Fisher Scientific, United States) at a concentration of 2 μg/ml and HRP conjugated goat anti-mouse IgG (Jackson immunoResearch Laboratories, Inc., United States) as secondary antibody. Then, blots were incubated using Immobilon Western Chemiluminescent HRP substrate (Merck Millipore, United States) and visualized and recorded on Tanon 5200 chemiluminescence imaging analysis system (Tanon Science & Technology Co Ltd., China).

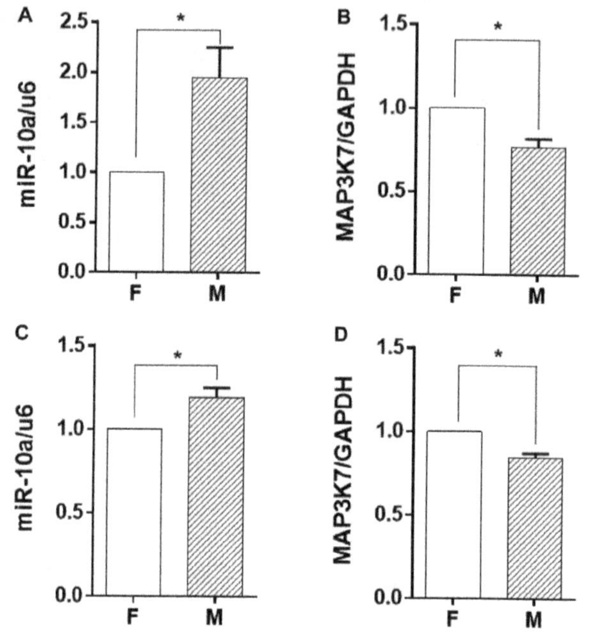

FIGURE 3 | The miR-10a expression in monocytes was affected by morphology-modified endothelial cells. In both co-culture (panels in the upper row) and trans-medium (panels in the lower row) systems, the expression level of miR-10a in monocytes **(A,C)** was analyzed. Data were normalized to U6 expression. **(B,D)** The mRNA expression level of MAP3K7 in monocytes was analyzed by qRT-PCR. Data were normalized to GAPDH expression. All the experiments were repeated three times, $^*p < 0.05$.

Statistical Analysis

Unless otherwise indicated, data represent the mean of at least three independent experiments and error bars represent the standard error of the mean. Pairwise comparisons were made using Student's *t*-test. A comparison of three or more groups was performed using ANOVA. Differences between groups were then determined using Tukey's *post-hoc* test. For all cases, $p < 0.05$ were considered as statistically significant. In all figures, the asterisks represent $P < 0.05$. GraphPad Prism 6.0 software was used for all the statistical evaluations.

RESULTS

Elongated ECs Suppressed Inflammatory Response in Co-cultured Monocytes

ECs were seeded on either flat PDMS membrane (**Figure 1A**) or micropatterned PDMS with 10-μm parallel microgrooves (**Figure 1B**), as shown in the SEM image. The morphology of the ECs was demonstrated by both FITC-phalloidin (green) and DAPI (blue) (**Figures 1C,D**) staining. Phalloidin staining of the stress fibers indicated that the microgrooved substrates had a pronounced effect on EC cytoskeleton and morphology. In general, cells grown on microgrooved PDMS membranes exhibited a more elongated morphology, following the guide of parallel microgrooves, compared to those cultured on flat PDMS

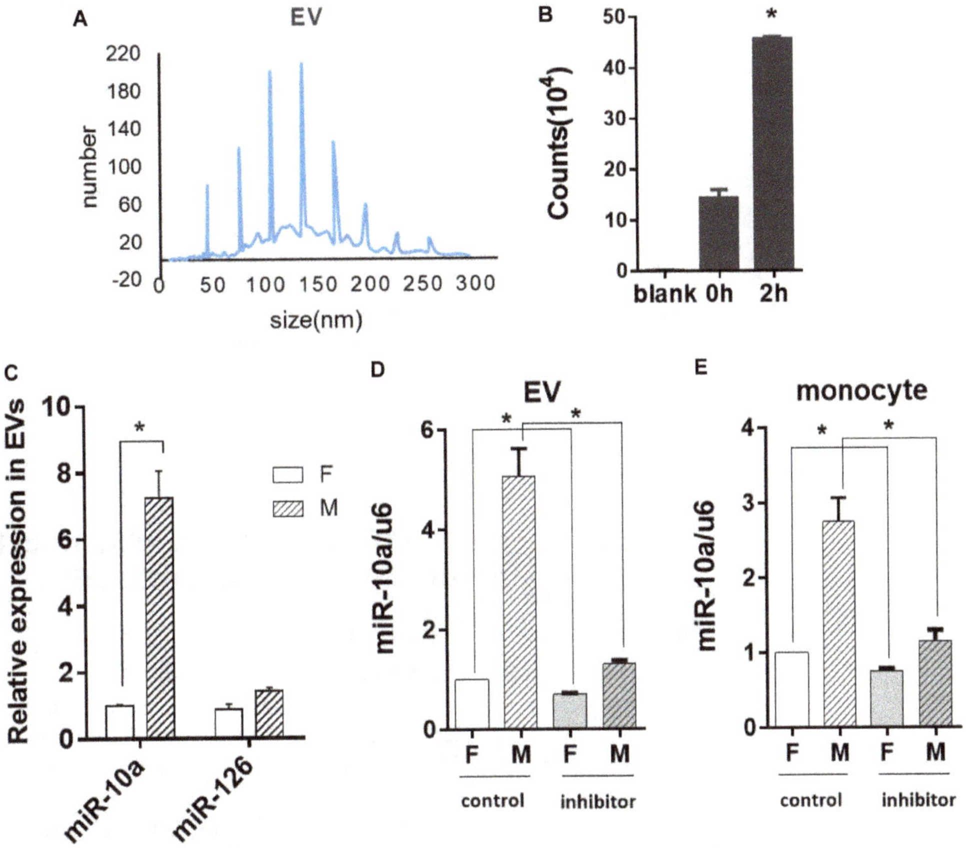

FIGURE 4 | Morphology-modified endothelial cells (ECs) altered the miR-10a expression in monocytes through extracellular vesicles (EVs). ECs were cultured on flat or microgrooved poly-(dimethyl siloxane) membranes, and the conditioned medium of ECs was collected to extract EVs. **(A)** Nanoparticle tracking analysis was applied to analyze the size of EVs. **(B)** EVs extracted from the conditioned medium of ECs were uptaken by monocytes. **(C)** The expression level of miR-10a and miR-126 in EVs was determined by qRT-PCR. **(D)** N-SMase Spiroepoxide inhibitor was added to the cell medium to treat the ECs for 24 h. The expression level of miR-10a in EVs from the conditioned medium of ECs was determined. **(E)** The conditioned medium of ECs was transferred to culture monocytes for 24 h. The expression level of miR-10a in monocytes was determined by qRT-PCR. Data were normalized to U6 expression. Dimethyl sulfoxide was used as control. Inhibitor refers to N-SMase Spiroepoxide inhibitor. All the experiments were repeated three times, $^*p < 0.05$.

membrane, and the stress fibers were also parallel to the axis of the microgrooves. LPS was used to treat the monocytes, which induced a robust expression of IL-6, IL-1β, and TNF-α. The EC co-culture (**Supplementary Figure S1**) significantly decreased the expression of these inflammatory genes. This is consistent with the precious findings that ECs suppress inflammatory responses. In addition, ECs on microgrooves showed more suppressive effects. Therefore, in the rest of the studies, we focused on the effects of EC morphology on monocytes following LPS stimulation.

To determine whether ECs cultured on microgrooved PDMS membranes could modulate the inflammatory cells, THP-1 cell line was used as a pro-inflammatory monocyte model in this study. The monocytes were treated with LPS for 2 h and were co-cultured with ECs in the system illustrated in **Figure 1E**. After 24 h, the expression level of the inflammatory cytokines IL-6, IL-1β, and TNF-α was assessed (**Figures 1F,H**). Compared with ECs on the flat PDMS membrane, the mRNA expression level of IL-6, IL-1β, and TNF-α was significantly decreased. In addition, the amount of the soluble IL-6 protein in the culture medium was further verified by ELISA (**Figure 1G**), showing the same trend as its mRNA expression level. The decrease in the inflammatory cytokine level suggested that the inflammatory response of the monocytes was significantly suppressed by ECs grown on the microgrooved PDMS membrane.

EC Morphology Regulated Monocytes Through Soluble Factors

In order to identify the possible regulator in the EC-conditioned medium, which altered the monocyte inflammatory response, we used a trans-medium system (as shown in **Figure 2A**). The purpose was to verify whether ECs could exert a unidirectional regulatory effect on monocyte inflammation. The EC-conditioned medium was transferred to LPS-activated monocytes. The monocytes were treated for 24 h and the mRNA expression level of the inflammatory cytokines IL-6, IL-1β, TNF-α, and IL-10 was assessed (**Figures 2B,D**). Similar to the results demonstrated in **Figure 1**, compared with ECs on the flat PDMS membrane, the level of IL-6, IL-1β, and TNF-α was significantly

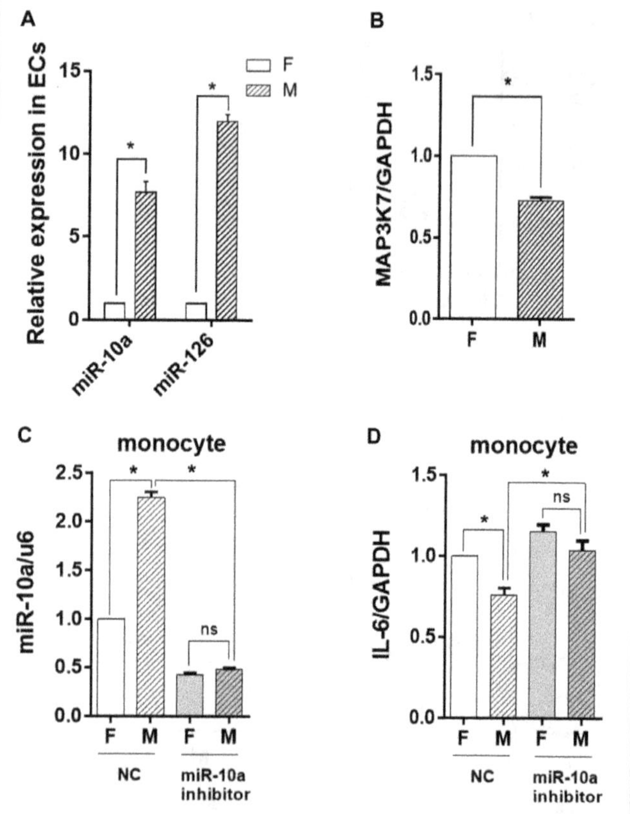

FIGURE 5 | The inflammatory response of the monocytes was inhibited by miR-10a from morphology-modified endothelial cells (ECs). **(A)** The expression level of miR-10a and miR-126 in ECs cultured on flat (F) or microgrooved (M) poly-(dimethyl siloxane) membranes was determined by qRT-PCR. **(B)** The expression level of MAP3K7 in ECs was determined by qRT-PCR. ECs were treated with miR-10a inhibitor for 24 h. The conditioned medium of ECs was transferred to culture the LPS-treated monocytes for 24 h. **(C)** The expressions level of miR-10a in monocytes was determined. **(D)** The expression level of IL-6 was determined. NC refers to negative control. All the experiments were repeated three times, $^{*}p < 0.05$ (ns, non-significant).

decreased, except for IL-10. Therefore, we focused on IL-6 expression in the studies thereafter. The level of soluble IL-6 protein in the culture medium determined by ELISA (**Figure 2C**) also showed a significant decrease, which was consistent with its mRNA expression level. The decrease in the inflammatory cytokine level indicated that the inflammatory response of the monocytes was significantly suppressed by the factors secreted from the ECs grown on the microgrooved PDMS membrane.

miR-10a Expression in Monocytes Was Affected by Morphology-Modified ECs

Among the soluble factors in the conditioned medium, microRNAs have been reported to have a great regulatory effect on cellular inflammatory response, and miR-10a has an inhibitory effect on IL-6 expression (Njock et al., 2015). Therefore, we explored further to determine whether miR-10a was the upstream regulator of the inflammation-suppressed status of the monocytes. The expression level of miR-10a in monocytes was analyzed in both co-culture and trans-medium systems. In the co-culture system, the miR-10a expression level in monocytes was elevated while they were co-cultured with ECs on the microgrooved PDMS membrane (**Figure 3A**). Consistently, the mRNA expression of MAP3K7, known as miR-10a direct target (Fang et al., 2010), was suppressed in monocytes (**Figure 3B**). Similarly, while only the EC-conditioned medium was used to treat the monocytes, the expression level of miR-10a in monocytes was elevated by the conditioned medium of ECs on the microgrooved PDMS membrane in comparison to that on the flat PDMS membrane (**Figure 3C**), and the mRNA expression of MAP3K7 in monocytes was suppressed accordingly (**Figure 3D**). Both the co-culture and the trans-medium experiments showed that miR-10a expression in monocytes was affected by morphology-modified ECs.

miR-10a Expression in Monocytes Was Affected by EC-Secreted EVs

Since miR-10a expression in the monocytes was affected by soluble factors in the conditioned medium, we further explored whether miRNA could be transferred by EVs. Thus, EVs from the culture medium of the ECs were isolated and analyzed. Nanoparticle tracking analysis demonstrated that the isolated EVs were 40–200 nm in diameter (**Figure 4A**), which is consistent with the size of small to medium EVs. Since EVs are heterogeneous and exosome is one of the major subpopulations in EVs, we performed exosome isolation and verified the presence of exosomes in isolated EVs by transmission electron microscopy and Western blotting analysis of CD63 expression (**Supplementary Figure S2**).

In order to confirm whether the EVs were uptaken by monocytes, the EVs extracted from the EC-conditioned medium were labeled with I-135 and added into the culture medium of the monocytes. Normal culture medium was used as blank control. The intensity of the radiation from the monocytes incubated with I-135-labeled EVs within 2 h was measured with a scintillation counter and expressed as counts. The result indicated that the EVs were uptaken by monocytes immediately and increased gradually (**Figure 4B**). Then, we analyzed the expression level of microRNAs in EVs. The miR-10a showed a robust increase in EVs (**Figure 4C**). In contrast, there was no significant change of another inflammatory-modulator miR-126.

If the anti-inflammatory effect of the morphology-modified ECs was indeed passed by EVs enclosing a specific microRNA, the inhibition of EV secretion from the ECs should block the change of miR-10a in monocytes. N-SMase Spiroepoxide inhibitor was used to block the formation and the release of the EVs from the ECs. To avoid the possible side effects of the inhibitor on the monocytes, a trans-medium system was used to culture the cells separately. The ECs were treated with the inhibitor for 24 h. Then, the conditioned medium was transferred to the monocytes for an additional 24 h. Upon the inhibition of EV secretion, the level of miR-10a was significantly decreased in EVs (**Figure 4D**) and monocytes (**Figure 4E**). In order to confirm that the monocyte response was affected by miR-10a in EVs, we used EVs only and EV-excluded medium (both from flat and microgrooved surfaces) to culture LPS-stimulated monocytes (**Supplementary Figure S3**). We found that EVs from ECs cultured on the microgrooved surface significantly inhibited the inflammatory response of the monocytes, while EV-excluded medium showed no significant change. These results confirmed that monocyte response was affected by miR-10a in EVs, not random miR-10a in trans-medium.

The Inflammatory Response of the Monocytes Was Inhibited by miR-10a Suppression in ECs

To determine whether the change of the EV-microRNA expression was sourced from ECs, we directly examined the level of miRNAs in ECs. The results in **Figure 5A** showed that the change of miRNA levels in ECs was consistent with those in EVs, i.e., miR-10a and miR-126 in ECs were also significantly induced. This result was confirmed by checking the mRNA level of MAP3K7, a miR-10a target gene, which had a significant decrease in ECs cultured on a microgrooved PDMS membrane (**Figure 5B**).

To investigate the effects of EC miRNA on miRNA and cytokine expression in monocytes, miR-10a inhibitor was applied to ECs cultured on a flat or a microgrooved surface. After 24 h, the EC-conditioned medium was transferred to culture the LPS-treated monocytes for additional 24 h. qRT-PCR analysis demonstrated that the expression level of miR-10a in monocytes decreased significantly and there was no more significant difference between ECs cultured on a flat surface and those cultured on a microgrooved membrane (**Figure 5C**). At the same time, the expression level of IL-6 in the monocytes was upregulated after inhibiting miR-10a, and also there was no more significant difference between ECs on a flat surface and those on a microgrooved surface (**Figure 5D**).

DISCUSSION AND CONCLUSION

The pathogenesis and the progression of a lot of cardiovascular diseases such as atherosclerosis and thrombosis are accompanied by an inflammation response (Gistera and Hansson, 2017). In the blood vessel, the athero-prone regions are usually near the bifurcation of the arteries, where the hemodynamic forces are different from those in the straight part of the artery due to the blood flow (Wang et al., 2016). In this athero-prone lesion area, ECs show a cobblestone morphology in contrast to the elongated ECs in the straight part of the artery. Our study provides a direct evidence that this EC morphology change in the athero-prone area may upregulate microRNAs that can be transferred to monocytes *via* EVs and thus induce inflammatory signals.

MicroRNAs have long been implicated as key regulators of inflammatory responses in monocytes or macrophages (Fish and Cybulsky, 2012; Sun et al., 2013). In addition, the fluctuations in shear stress contribute to microRNA-mediated epigenetic regulation on the function of ECs, which are essential for the maintenance of vascular homeostasis (Ando and Yamamoto, 2011). A recent study identified miR-10a as a flow-responsive microRNA in ECs *in vitro* (Davignon and Ganz, 2004), and miR-10a could be induced by high shear stress as an athero-protective mechanism (Neth et al., 2013). Another study revealed that the expression of endothelial miR-10a was lower in the athero-susceptible regions of the inner aortic arch and the aorta–renal branches than that in other regions (Fang et al., 2010). Interestingly, the physical effect of the microgroove surface on EC morphology is similar to laminar shear stress, and consistently, elongated ECs have a higher level of miR-10a, suggesting that EC morphology change is sufficient to induce miR-10a expression.

Previous studies have demonstrated that miR-10a acts as a post-transcriptional modulator of the IκB/NF-κB signaling pathway by inhibiting MAP3K7 and βTRC (Fang et al., 2010; Njock et al., 2015). The increased proteolysis of IκBα and nuclear p65 in atherosclerotic susceptible areas resulted in a significantly up-regulated expression of the inflammatory biomarkers including IL-6, IL-8, MCP-1, VCAM-1, etc. (Fang et al., 2010). This provides a possible mechanism of how miR-10a regulates inflammatory cytokines in monocytes.

Based on our investigation, miR-10a was not the only microRNA with a significant change in the expression level. However, the level of miR-10a in both ECs and EVs was increased significantly, while miR-126 was increased significantly only in ECs on microgrooved PDMS membranes. A previous report (Asgeirsdottir et al., 2012) shows that miR-126 targets VCAM-1 in ECs to regulate the adhesion of ECs to monocytes. Therefore, miR-126 mainly functions in ECs but not in extracellular vesicles.

Another significant finding is that miR-10a made by ECs could be transferred to monocytes through EVs to modulate the expression of IL-6 in monocytes, which was demonstrated by the inhibition of EV secretion and miR-10a inhibition in ECs. This contact-independent EV transfer mechanism suggests a novel EC–monocyte signaling in the vascular microenvironment. These findings provide another explanation of how elongated ECs in the straight part of the arteries are anti-inflammatory and athero-protective.

This study not only unravels a new mechanism of EC–monocyte communication through EVs but also provides an insight into the biophysical regulation of cell–cell signaling in a vascular microenvironment. Our findings provide a rational basis for the design and the fabrication of micro/nano-materials that can be used to regulate EC and monocyte functions for vascular tissue engineering.

AUTHOR CONTRIBUTIONS

SL and YZ: conception or design of the work. JL, SG, XM, YT, and HW: acquisition of the data. JL, SG, YZ, and SL: manuscript writing. All authors have made significant contributions to the work, including analysis and interpretation of data, have approved the submitted version, and have agreed both to be personally accountable for the author's own contributions and to ensure that questions related to the accuracy or integrity of any part of the work.

REFERENCES

Ando, J., and Yamamoto, K. (2011). Effects of shear stress and stretch on endothelial function. *Antioxid. Redox Signal.* 15, 1389–1403. doi: 10.1089/ars.2010.3361

Asgeirsdottir, S. A., Van Solingen, C., Kurniati, N. F., Zwiers, P. J., Heeringa, P., van Meurs, M., et al. (2012). Microrna-126 contributes to renal microvascular heterogeneity of Vcam-1 protein expression in acute inflammation. *Am. J. Physiol. Renal Physiol.* 302, F1630–F1639. doi: 10.1152/ajprenal.00400.2011

Bachurski, D., Schuldner, M., Nguyen, P. H., Malz, A., Reiners, K. S., Grenzi, P. C., et al. (2019). Extracellular vesicle measurements with nanoparticle tracking analysis - An accuracy and repeatability comparison between NanoSight Ns300 and ZetaView. *J. Extracell. Vesicles* 8:1596016. doi: 10.1080/20013078.2019.1596016

Biela, S. A., Su, Y., Spatz, J. P., and Kemkemer, R. (2009). Different sensitivity of human endothelial cells, smooth muscle cells and fibroblasts to topography in the nano-micro range. *Acta Biomater.* 5, 2460–2466. doi: 10.1016/j.actbio.2009.04.003

Boos, C. J., Blann, A. D., and Lip, G. Y. H. (2007). *Assessment of Endothelial Damage/Dysfunction: A Focus on Circulating Endothelial Cells.* Totowa: Humana Press.

Chen, W., Tian, B., Liang, J., Yu, S., Zhou, Y., and Li, S. (2019). Matrix stiffness regulates the interactions between endothelial cells and monocytes. *Biomaterials* 221:119362. doi: 10.1016/j.biomaterials.2019.119362

Das, S., and Halushka, M. K. (2015). Extracellular vesicle microrna transfer in cardiovascular disease. *Cardiovasc. Pathol.* 24, 199–206. doi: 10.1016/j.carpath.2015.04.007

Davignon, J., and Ganz, P. (2004). Role of endothelial dysfunction in atherosclerosis. *Circulation* 109, 27–32.

Devhare, P. B., Sasaki, R., Shrivastava, S., Di Bisceglie, A. M., Ray, R., Ray, R. B., et al. (2017). Exosome-mediated intercellular communication between hepatitis C virus-infected hepatocytes and hepatic stellate cells. *J. Virol.* 91:e02225-16. doi: 10.1128/JVI.00349-17

Downing, T. L., Soto, J., Morez, C., Houssin, T., Fritz, A., Yuan, F., et al. (2013). Biophysical regulation of epigenetic state and cell reprogramming. *Nat. Mater.* 12, 1154–1162. doi: 10.1038/nmat3777

Fang, Y., Shi, C., Manduchi, E., Civelek, M., and Davies, P. F. (2010). Microrna-10a regulation of proinflammatory phenotype in athero-susceptible endothelium in vivo and in vitro. *Proc. Natl. Acad. Sci. U.S.A.* 107, 13450–13455. doi: 10.1073/pnas.1002120107

Fish, J. E., and Cybulsky, M. I. (2012). Taming endothelial activation with a microrna. *J. Clin. Investig.* 122, 1967–1970. doi: 10.1172/JCI63818

Gasiorowski, J. Z., Liliensiek, S. J., Russell, P., Stephan, D. A., Nealey, P. F., Murphy, C. J., et al. (2010). Alterations in gene expression of human vascular endothelial cells associated with nanotopographic cues. *Biomaterials* 31, 8882–8888. doi: 10.1016/j.biomaterials.2010.08.026

Gistera, A., and Hansson, G. K. (2017). The immunology of atherosclerosis. *Nat. Rev. Nephrol.* 13, 368–380. doi: 10.1038/nrneph.2017.51

Hergenreider, E., Heydt, S., Treguer, K., Boettger, T., Horrevoets, A. J., Zeiher, A. M., et al. (2012). Atheroprotective communication between endothelial cells and smooth muscle cells through mirnas. *Nat. Cell Biol.* 14, 249–256. doi: 10.1038/ncb2441

Landmesser, U., Hornig, B., and Drexler, H. (2004). Endothelial function - A critical determinant in atherosclerosis. *Circulation* 109, 27–33. doi: 10.1161/01.CIR.0000129501.88485.1f

Ley, K., Laudanna, C., Cybulsky, M. I., and Nourshargh, S. (2007). Getting to the site of inflammation: the leukocyte adhesion cascade updated. *Nat. Rev. Immunol.* 7:678. doi: 10.1038/nri2156

Li, Y. S. J., Haga, J. H., and Chien, S. (2005). Molecular basis of the effects of shear stress on vascular endothelial cells. *J. Biomech.* 38, 1949–1971. doi: 10.1016/j.jbiomech.2004.09.030

Liu, X., Cheng, Y., Yang, J., Xu, L., and Zhang, C. (2012). Cell-specific effects of miR-221/222 in vessels: molecular mechanism and therapeutic application. *J. Mol. Cell. Cardiol.* 52, 245–255. doi: 10.1016/j.yjmcc.2011.11.008

Momiyama, Y., Adachi, H., Fairweather, D. L., Ishizaka, N., and Saita, E. (2005). Inflammation, atherosclerosis and coronary artery disease. *N. Engl. J. Med.* 352, 429–430.

Neth, P., Nazari-Jahantigh, M., Schober, A., and Weber, C. (2013). Micrornas in flow-dependent vascular remodelling. *Cardiovasc. Res.* 99, 294–303. doi: 10.1093/cvr/cvt096

Njock, M. S., Cheng, H. S., Dang, L. T., Nazari-Jahantigh, M., Lau, A. C., Boudreau, E., et al. (2015). Endothelial cells suppress monocyte activation through secretion of extracellular vesicles containing antiinflammatory micrornas. *Blood* 125, 3202–3212. doi: 10.1182/blood-2014-11-611046

O'Connell, R. M., Taganov, K. D., Boldin, M. P., Cheng, G., and Baltimore, D. (2007). Microrna-155 is induced during the macrophage inflammatory response. *Proc. Natl. Acad. Sci. U.S.A.* 104:1604. doi: 10.1073/pnas.0610731104

Ono, K., Kuwabara, Y., and Han, J. (2011). Micrornas and cardiovascular diseases. *FEBS J.* 278, 1619–1633.

Puri, R., Worthley, M. I., and Nicholls, S. J. (2011). Intravascular imaging of vulnerable coronary plaque: current and future concepts. *Nat. Rev. Cardiol.* 8, 131–139. doi: 10.1038/nrcardio.2010.210

Ross, R. (1999). Atherosclerosis — an inflammatory disease. *N. Engl. J. Med.* 340:115.

Shi, C., and Pamer, E. G. (2011). Monocyte recruitment during infection and inflammation. *Nat. Rev. Immunol.* 11:762. doi: 10.1038/nri3070

Suarez, Y., Wang, C., Manes, T. D., and Pober, J. S. (2010). Cutting edge: Tnf-induced micrornas regulate Tnf-induced expression of E-selectin and intercellular adhesion molecule-1 on human endothelial cells: feedback control of inflammation. *J. Immunol.* 184, 21–25. doi: 10.4049/jimmunol.0902369

Sun, X., Belkin, N., and Feinberg, M. W. (2013). Endothelial micrornas and atherosclerosis. *Curr. Atheroscler. Rep* 15:372. doi: 10.1007/s11883-013-0372-2

Tili, E., Michaille, J. J., Cimino, A., Costinean, S., Dumitru, C. D., Adair, B., et al. (2007). Modulation of miR-155 and miR-125b levels following lipopolysaccharide/Tnf-alpha stimulation and their possible roles in regulating the response to endotoxin shock. *J. Immunol.* 179:5082. doi: 10.4049/jimmunol.179.8.5082

Vanhoutte, P. M., Shimokawa, H., Tang, E. H. C., and Feletou, M. (2009). Endothelial dysfunction and vascular disease. *Acta Physiol.* 196, 193–222.

Wang, K. C., Yeh, Y. T., Nguyen, P., Limqueco, E., Lopez, J., Thorossian, S., et al. (2016). Flow-dependent Yap/Taz activities regulate endothelial phenotypes and atherosclerosis. *PNAS* 113, 11525–11530. doi: 10.1073/pnas.1613121113

Woollard, K. J., and Geissmann, F. (2010). Monocytes in atherosclerosis: subsets and functions. *Nat. Rev. Cardiol.* 7, 77–86. doi: 10.1038/nrcardio.2009.228

Wu, W., Xiao, H., Laguna-Fernandez, A., Villarreal, G., Wang, K.-C., Geary, G. G., et al. (2011). Flow-dependent regulation of kruppel-like factor 2 is mediated by microrna-92a. *Circulation* 124, 633–U231. doi: 10.1161/CIRCULATIONAHA.110.005108

Yamakuchi, M. (2012). Micrornas in vascular biology. *Int. J. Vasc. Med.* 2012:794898.

Zhang, L., Su, H. L., Cai, J., Cheng, D., Ma, Y., Zhang, J., et al. (2016). A multifunctional platform for tumor angiogenesis-targeted chemo-thermal therapy using polydopamine-coated gold nanorods. *ACS Nano* 10, 10404–10417. doi: 10.1021/acsnano.6b06267

Zhu, N., Zhang, D. Z., Chen, S. F., Liu, X., Lin, L., Huang, X., et al. (2011). Endothelial enriched micrornas regulate angiotensin Ii-induced endothelial inflammation and migration. *Atherosclerosis* 215, 286–293. doi: 10.1016/j.atherosclerosis.2010.12.024

10

An Aligned Patterned Biomimetic Elastic Membrane has a Potential as Vascular Tissue Engineering Material

Juanjuan Tan[1,2†], Jing Bai[1†] and Zhiqiang Yan[3]*

[1] School of Chemistry and Chemical Engineering, State Key Laboratory of Metal Matrix Composite Materials and Shanghai Key Lab of Electrical Insulation and Thermal Ageing, Shanghai Jiao Tong University, Shanghai, China, [2] Joint Research Center for Precision Medicine, Shanghai Jiao Tong University Affiliated Sixth People's Hospital South Campus, Shanghai, China, [3] Central Laboratory, Southern Medical University affiliated Fengxian Hospital, Shanghai, China

***Correspondence:**
Zhiqiang Yan
zqyan@sjtu.edu.cn

† These authors share first authorship

Cardiovascular disease is the leading cause of death worldwide, with an annual mortality incidence predicted to rise to 23.3 million worldwide by 2030. Synthetic vascular grafts as an alternative to autologous vessels have shown satisfactory long-term results for replacement of large- and medium-diameter arteries, but have poor patency rates when applied to small-diameter vessels. Nanoparticles with low toxicity, contrasting agent properties, tailorable characteristics, targeted/stimuli- response delivery potential, and precise control over behavior (via external stimuli such as magnetic fields) have made possible their use for improving engineered tissues. Poly (styrene-block-butadiene-block-styrene) (SBS) is a kind of widely used thermoplastic elastomer with good mechanical properties and biocompatibility. Here, we synthesized anthracene-grafted SBS (SBS-An) by the method for the fabrication of a biomimetic elastic membrane with a switchable Janus structure, and formed the patterns on the surface of SBS-An under ultraviolet (UV) light irradiation. By irradiating the SBS-An film at different times (0, 10, 20, 30, 60, and 120 s), we obtained six well-ordered surface-patterned biomimetic elastic film with SBS-An at different heights in the thickness direction and the same distances of intervals (named sample-0, 10, 20, 30, 60, and 120 s). The structural effects of the SBS-An films on the adhesion and proliferation of human umbilical vein endothelial cells (HUVECs) were studied, and the possible mechanism was explored. When the HUVECs were cultured on the SBS-An films at different heights in the thickness direction, the sample-30 s with approximately 4 μm height significantly promoted adhesion of the HUVECs at the early stage and proliferation during the culture period compared with the samples of the lower (0, 10, and 20 s) and higher (60 and 120 s) heights. Consistent with this, the sample 30 s showed a higher stimulatory effect on the proliferation- and angiogenesis-related genes. These results suggest that SBS-An with appropriate height could efficiently control bioactivities of the biomimetic elastic membrane and might have great potential in vascular tissue engineering application.

Keywords: vascular tissue engineering, nanoparticles, anthracene-grafted SBS, HUVECs, biocompatibility

INTRODUCTION

Cardiovascular diseases are a serious threat to human health. The number of deaths caused by cardiovascular disease is as high as 15 million worldwide every year, ranking first among various causes of death. Another statistic enumerates approximately 850,000 vascular reconstruction operations in the world each year, most of which use autologous blood vessels, though postoperative data show that the surgical effect is not ideal given the scarcity of autologous blood vessel sources (McBane et al., 2012; Schwann et al., 2012). Therefore, the research and development of artificial blood vessels have great application prospects and social significance.

An artificial blood vessel is a substitute that can be used to replace or repair a diseased blood vessel, and its source does not belong to the tissue or organ contributed by the host's own or a foreign body. Thus, the design of the artificial blood vessel should meet certain performance requirements, such as a suitable microporous structure on the surface and the long-term compliance of the blood vessel in the body (Chen et al., 2001; Nerem, 2004). Therefore, materials play a vital role in the successful application of tissue engineering, and choosing the right materials will have a profound impact on the regeneration of new tissues in the human body. The main challenge for tissue engineering is to develop materials that can promote the required cells and identify tissue behavior (O'Brien, 2011). The development of artificial blood vessels began in the early 20th century. Scholars from various countries first used tubular materials made of metal, glass, polyethylene, silicone rubber, and other materials for a large number of animal experiments (Nerem and Seliktar, 2001). However, they were not widely used in clinical practice because of their susceptibility to intraluminal thrombosis in the short term. In 1952, Voorhees et al. (1952) first studied the use of vinylon as a vascular prosthesis, which changed the impermeability of the previous vascular wall. In the next few years, Voorhees et al. did a large number of clinical trials to develop a meshed artificial blood vessel, which is a milestone in the history of the development of vascular substitutes. Subsequently, experts tested many materials such as PVC (polyvinyl chloride), polyacrylonitrile (acrylic), silk, nylon, and viscose (Guidoin, 1992). Artificial blood vessels made of polyacrylonitrile (acrylic) and nylon will degrade in the body; thus, these two materials were quickly eliminated. In addition, polyurethane (PU) has been used in tissue engineering as a vascular implant for 30 years due to its excellent blood compatibility, mechanical strength, and ideal long-term patency. It is considered by many researchers as an ideal artificial blood vessel material. However, some studies have pointed out that after long-term implantation, aging degradation and calcification can occur, which results in material cracking (Kannan et al., 2005). Although the clinical demand for bioengineered blood vessels continues to rise, currently there are still limited choices for blood vessels. Therefore, finding new materials remains the focus of research.

Natural blood vessels are mainly composed of three layers: intima, media, and adventitia (Li et al., 2014). The innermost layer is the endothelial cell layer. Intact endothelial cells adhere to the basement membrane containing collagen and laminin to prevent infection and thrombosis. Vascular endothelial cells are not only a physical barrier on the surface of blood vessels, but more importantly, they play an indispensable function and role in the regulation of vasoconstriction and the maintenance of the balance of the coagulation-fibrinolytic system. Constructing an endothelial cell layer with normal morphology and physiological functions is an important means to solve the thrombosis after the in vivo implantation of tissue-engineered blood vessels. The endothelialization of tissue-engineered blood vessels can effectively resist thrombosis and inhibit intimal hyperplasia (Ballyk et al., 1997; Chlupác et al., 2009). Therefore, a hot spot in the study of vascular stent biocompatibility is the rapid endothelialization of the stent surface and the maintenance of normal endothelial function after endothelialization.

In recent years, micrographics technology has received increasingly extensive attention, particularly in the fields of microelectronics, optics, tissue engineering, and biochip manufacturing due to its important research value. The topological surface structure of biological materials, such as their surface roughness, pore size, pore distribution, shape, size, and micro-pattern orientation greatly influence cell adhesion, proliferation, and differentiation (Lim and Donahue, 2007; Nel et al., 2009). Experiments have shown that a stripe structure with a large pitch (100 μm) can promote endothelial cell orientation, but does not form a capillary lumen structure. Among them, smaller-spaced stripe structures (10–50 μm) are more oriented to induce the growth of endothelial cells, and can promote the formation of a tubular structure of the lumen and a vascular network (Lei et al., 2013). Whited et al. studied the effect of PCL/gelatin electrospun materials with different fiber diameters and orientations on the angiogenic capacity of surface-grown ECs (Whited and Rylander, 2014). Their immunofluorescence staining image results showed that EC on the single-layer growth on the material surface, and the state of cell alignment and stretching increased with the degree of fiber orientation. Along the arrangement direction of the fibers, thicker actin bundles (F-actin bundles) were aligned, and strong expression of cadherin (VE-cadherin) was also observed at the junction between cells. The results indicated that the electrospun fiber materials with a directional arrangement structure helped enhance the adhesion ability of the ECs (Whited and Rylander, 2014). The aforementioned studies have demonstrated that the micro-pattern structure on the surface of the material effectively influenced and further regulated the cell-growth behavior on the material.

Interestingly, a series of studies have demonstrated that poly SBS is a widely used thermoplastic elastomer with good mechanical properties and biocompatibility, and more importantly, lower biotoxicity (Cho and Paul, 2001; Fu and Qutubuddin, 2001; Kim et al., 2001; Novak and Florián, 2004). However, in our previous study, a kind of biomimetic Janus membrane was fabricated with anthracene-grafted SBS and carbon nanotubes (CNTs), and the gradient Janus structure was obtained via the combination of UV light-induced dimerization of anthracene and control of the UV light penetration depth by the CNTs (Bai and Shi, 2017). These results demonstrated that this Janus membrane could be used as a shape actuator due to the Janus structure-induced impetus in its thickness direction. By designing different geometrical shapes and UV light irradiation conditions (time and location) or stimulated regions, the Janus membrane achieved more complex and diversified shape shifting or morphing triggered by the solvent effect or shape memory mechanism. In addition, we developed a new approach for making two-/three-dimensional (2D/3D) latent photopatterned morphologies on the modified SBS films. Therefore, we intend to investigate the potential of the SBS-An films as tissue-engineered vascular material. In this study, the branching ratio of anthracene was fixed at 10% of the double bonds on SBS chains, which can be crosslinked under UV light irradiation to easily form the pattern on the surface. Finally, the structure effects of the SBS-An films on the adhesion and proliferation of HUVECs were studied, and the possible mechanism was explored.

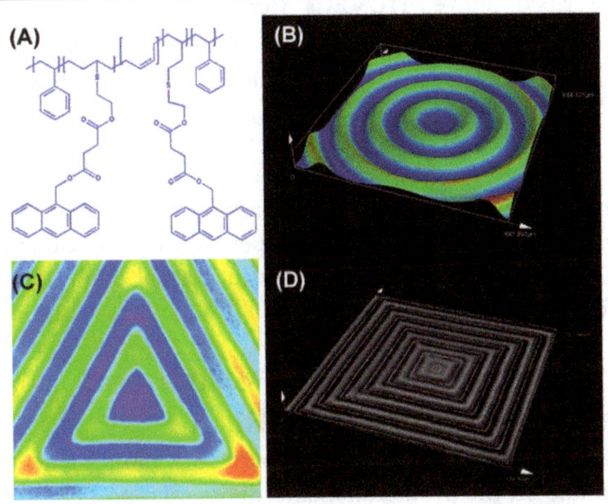

FIGURE 1 | (A) The chemical structure of the anthracene modified SBS. Laser scanning confocal microscopy (LSCM) images showing patterns written with different geometric configuration controlled with masks. **(B)** Positive and negative hybrid concentric rings (size width/space: 50/50 μm). **(C)** Positive and negative hybrid concentric triangles (size width/space: 100/100 μm). **(D)** Positive and negative hybrid concentric quadrangles (size width/space: 50/50 μm). The thickness of the polymer blend film was ≈200 μm. The intensity and exposure time of 365 nm UV light were ≈50 mW/cm^2 and 30 s, respectively.

MATERIALS AND METHODS

Materials

Toluene, 4-methylbenzenesulfonic acid, 4-dimethylaminopyridine, pyridine, and dichloromethane were purchased from Sinopharm Chemical Reagent Co., Ltd (Beijing, China). SBS (Mw∼153 000–185 000, 70 wt % PB block), 2-Mercaptoethanol, and succinic anhydride were purchased from Sigma-Aldrich. 9-anthracenemethanol was purchased from Alfa Aesar. All the reagents were used as received.

Preparation of the Anthracene-Grafted SBS

The UV light sensitive polymer (SBS-An) was prepared as our previous work (Bai and Shi, 2017). First, the hydroxyl-branched SBS was synthesized via the thiol-ene click reaction. The anthracene group was then grafted to the polymer chains via esterification. In the manuscript, the branching ratio of anthracene was fixed at 10% of the double bonds on the SBS chains. Due to the dimerization of anthracene, this kind of polymer can be crosslinked under UV light irradiation, while was utilized to form the pattern on the surface.

Preparation of the Surface Patterns

According to our previous study (Bai et al., 2019), the patterns can be written on the surface as shown in **Figure 1**. In detail, The SBS-An was dissolved in toluene, and the solution was cast on the glass plate. The films were then heated at approximately 80°C for 12 h to evaporate solvent. To write the patterns, the films were exposed to 365 nm UV light covered with a photomask at different times (0, 10, 20, 30, 60, and 120 s; marked as sample-0, 10, 20, 30, 60, and 120 s) to initiate the photo-dimerization of An to obtain a well-ordered surface pattern that transferred the pattern on the mask with different height in the thickness direction without cumbersome processing steps. The pattern on the surface of films can be obtained almost the same as the designed masks.

Cell Culture

According to a previous description with modification (Tan et al., 2017), the HUVECs were isolated from the human umbilical cord vein with 0.1% type I collagenase. The HUVECs were cultured in the endothelial cell medium (ECM) containing 5% FBS and 1% endothelial cell growth supplement kit (Sciencell, Carlsbad, CA, United States) at 37°C with 5% CO_2. The purity of the ECs was confirmed using the von Willebrand factor (vWF) antibody (Abcam, Cambridge, United Kingdom). Cells from passages 3–5 were employed for all experiments.

HUVEC Adhesion Assay

To evaluate the influence of the aligned patterned biomimetic elastic membrane on cell adhesion, samples were first sectioned into 10 × 10 mm^2 squares, and then soaked in ethanol for 0.5 h. The samples were then soaked in 75 vol% medical alcohol solution for another 2 h for sterilization and washed out with a large amount of sterile water prior to seeding cells on the samples.

The cell adhesion assay was performed as previously described (Winterbone et al., 2009). Briefly, the HUVECs were plated into the surfaces of those samples at a density of 2 × 10^4 cells per well in a 24-well culture plate. Following incubation for 6 h at 37°C in 5% CO_2, the wells were washed three times with 0.2 mL PBS, stained with 0.1% crystals, and the number of adherent cells in four high power fields of view were observed using a Leica BX-61 fluorescence microscope at ×100 magnification (Leica, Germany).

HUVEC Proliferation Assay

To investigate the influence of the aligned patterned biomimetic elastic membrane on cell proliferation, the samples were treated as described above. HUVECs were trypsinized and plated onto the surfaces of the samples at a density of 2×10^4 cells per well in a 24-well culture plate, and incubated in an atmosphere consisting of 5% CO_2 in air at 37°C for 72 h. The absorbance of HUVECs was determined with a CCK8 assay (Dojindo Molecular Technologies, Japan) according to the instructions of the manufacturer, and measured at 450 nm using an enzyme-linked immunosorbent assay plate reader (Bio-TEK, United States). Cells cultured in normal condition were regarded as controls.

Quantitative Real-Time Polymerase Chain Reaction (qRT-PCR)

To investigate the effect of aligned pattern of biomimetic elastic membrane on the proliferation and differentiation of HUVECs, the proliferation-related genes (p21, proliferating cell nuclear antigen (PCNA), cyclin-dependent kinase 2(CDK2), and Cyclin A2) and the angiogenesis-related genes [vascular endothelial growth factor receptor 2 (KDR), endothelial nitric oxide synthase (eNOS), and vascular endothelial cadherin (VE-cad)] from the cells cultured on different samples for 72 h were detected by qRT-PCR. TRIzol Reagent (Invitrogen, United States) was used to extract total RNAs according to the instructions of manufacturer. The concentration and purity of RNA were measured by a nanodrop 1000 reader (Thermo Scientific, United States). qRT-PCR was performed with the 2 × SYBR green master mix (Takara, Japan) with a 7500 Real-Time PCR System (Applied Biosystems, United States). After an initial incubation step of denaturation for 1 min at 95°C, 40 cycles (95°C for 15s, 60°C for 30s, 72°C for 20 s) of PCR were performed. Reactions were performed in triplicate. The PCR primer sequences of the above genes and glyceraldehyde 3-phosphate dehydrogenase (GAPDH) are summarized in **Table 1**. All fold changes were calculated by the method of $2^{-\Delta\Delta Ct}$. GAPDH was used as a housekeeping gene. Data were normalized to GAPDH mRNA expression of each condition and were quantified relative to the corresponding gene expression from the control samples (cells cultured on the surface of sample-0 s or in normal condition).

Statistical Analysis

Experimental data were expressed as a means ± standard deviation (SD). Three independent experiments were performed, and at least three samples per each test were taken for statistical analysis. The statistical significance was calculated by a Student's *t*-test or one-way ANOVA using GraphPad Prism 6.0 (GraphPad Software, San Diego, CA, United States). Differences were considered significant when $p < 0.05$ (*), $p < 0.01$ (**).

RESULTS

The Preparation of the Patterns on the Polymer Films

As shown in **Figure 1**, **Figure 1A** shows the chemical structure of the anthracene modified SBS. SBS-An films can be patterned with different geometric configuration controlled with masks, such as rings (**Figure 1B**), triangles (**Figure 1C**), and hexagons (**Figure 1D**). Due to the different irradiating time, the patterns exhibited different height which increased with the irradiation time as reported in our previous work. **Figure 2** shows the 3D/2D images and the height of SBS-An films exposed to 365 nm UV light covered with a quadrangular photomask for 0, 10, 20, 30, 60, and 120 s. With the same distance of interval(50 μm), the height of samples 0-, 10-, 20-, 30-, 60-, and 120-s were 0, 1.36 ± 0.12, 2.56 ± 0.09, 4.47 ± 0.08, 7.22 ± 0.05, and 22.86 ± 0.28 μm, respectively.

Effect of the Aligned Patterned Biomimetic Elastic Membrane on Cell Adhesion

The effect of the aligned patterned biomimetic elastic membranes on the adhesion of HUVECs were evaluated, as shown in **Figure 3**. On the whole, the adhesion of HUVECs cultured on the SBS-An films were lower than those in the normal condition. The number of adhesive HUVECs cultured on the sample-20 and 30 s biomimetic elastic membranes were higher than those on the sample-0 and 10 s biomimetic elastic membrane. Specifically, the number of adhesive HUVECs on sample-30 s biomimetic elastic membrane was a 2.28-fold increase compared with those on the sample-0 s. By contrast, the adhesion of HUVECs cultured on the sample-10 and 120 s biomimetic elastic membranes were no significant difference compared with those on the sample-0 s.

Effect of the Aligned Patterned Biomimetic Elastic Membrane on Cell Proliferation

To determine the HUVEC proliferation on the biomimetic elastic membrane, the viabilities of HUVECs were determined by CCK8 assay. **Figure 4** summarized the cell viability after incubation for 72 h. Overall, the proliferation of HUVECs cultured on the SBS-An films were lower than those in normal condition. However, after 72 h, the number of HUVECs cultured on sample-20, 30, and 60 s were significantly higher than those cultured on the sample-0 and 120 s, which indicates that those samples have stimulatory effects on HUVEC proliferation, while the number of HUVECs cultured on sample-10 and 120 s had no significantly difference compared with sample-0 s. Consistent with this, the proliferation-related genes showed the same trend. As shown in **Figures 4C–E**, the markers of proliferation (PCNA, CDK2, and cyclin A2) were lower expressed in SBS-An films than in normal condition. While p21, acting as an inhibitor of cell cycle progression, was significantly increased in SBS-An films compared with in normal condition(**Figure 4B**). Together, these results indicate that SBS-An films with different height in the thickness direction have effect on the proliferation of HUVECs.

Effect of the Aligned Patterned Biomimetic Elastic Membrane on Angiogenesis Related Gene Expression

To investigate the effect of the aligned patterned biomimetic elastic membrane on angiogenesis related genes, the expression

TABLE 1 | Primer sequences used in qRT-PCR.

Gene	Gene bank	Primer sequences	T_m (°C)
eNOS	NM_001160111	F: 5′-TGTCCAACATG CTGCTGGAAATTG-3′ R: 5′-AGGAGGTCTTCTTCCT GGTGATGCC-3′	55
KDR	NM_002253	F: 5′-GTGATCGGAAA TGACACTGGAG-3′ R: 5′-CATGTTGGTCACTA ACAGAAGCA-3′	60
VE-Cadherin	NM_001795	F: 5′-GGCTCAGAC ATCCACATAACC-3′ R: 5′-CTTACCAGGGCGT TCAGGGAC-3′	63
Cyclin A2	NM_001237	F: 5′-CGCTGGCG GTACTGAAGTC-3′ R: 5′-GAGGAACGGTGACA TGCTCAT-3′	60
P21	NM_000389	F: 5′-TGTCCGTCAGAACCC ATGC-3′ R: 5′-AAAGTCGAAGTTCC ATCGCTC-3′	63
PCNA	NM_002592	F: 5′-CCTGCTGGGA TATTAGCTCCA-3′ R: 5′-CAGCGGTAGGTG TCGAAGC-3′	60
CDK2	NM_001290230	F: 5′-CCAGGAGTTACT TCTATGCCTGA-3′ R: 5′-R TTCATCCAGGGGA GGTACAAC-3′	58
GAPDH	NM_002046	F: 5′-ACAAGATGGTGAA GGTCGGTGTGA-3′ R: 5′-AGCTTCCCATTCTC AGCCTTGACT-3′	60

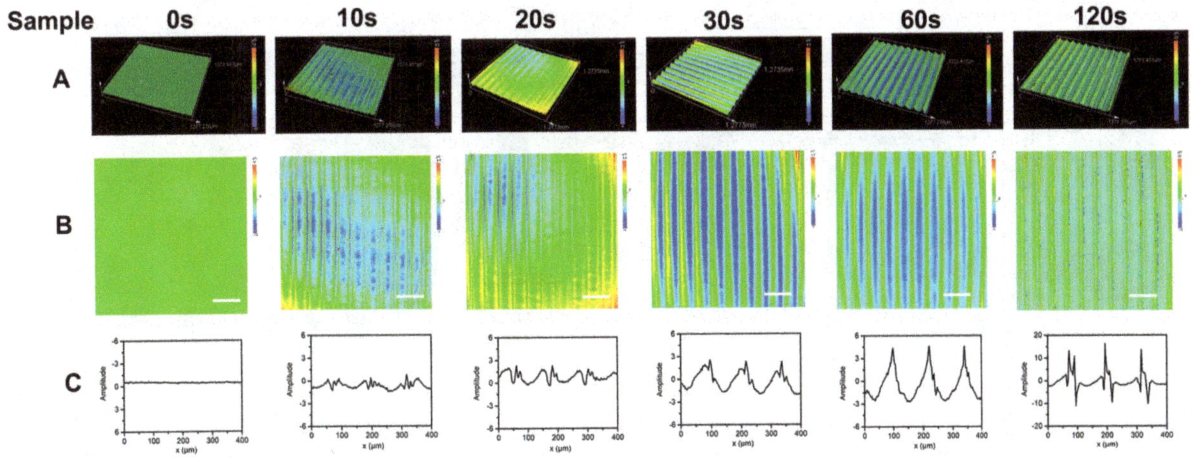

FIGURE 2 | (A) 3D images of sample-0, 10, 20 30, 60, and 120 s by LSCM, respectively. **(B)** 2D images of sample sample-0, 10, 20 30, 60, and 120 s by LSCM, respectively. **(C)** Height of the sample-0, 10, 20 30, 60, and 120 s, respectively. Scale bar: 100 μm.

of KDR, eNOS, and VE-Cadherin from HUVECs cultured on biomimetic elastic membrane with different aligned patterns has been investigated. **Figure 5** showed the mRNA expression of angiogenesis-related genes(KDR, eNOS and VE-Cad). The mRNA expression of KDR and VE-Cad were siginificantly higher in sample-30 s than in other samples and normal condition (**Figures 5A,C**). While, the mRNA expression of eNOS in sample-20, 30, and 60 s were significant differences compared with in sample-0, 10,120 s and normal condition. In a way, these results indicate that SBS-An films with different height in the thickness direction have effect on the differentiation of HUVECs.

DISCUSSION

With the development of micro/nano processing technology, many new methods such as soft lithography, laser particle beam engraving, electron beam etching, and hot stamping have been used to prepare morphologies on the surface of various substrates. There are three types of micro-nano pattern structures currently studied: micro-nano stripe/groove structure, micro-nano bump array, and micro-nano groove array. Among them, the micro-nano level stripe/groove structure has attracted much attention because it can make cells "contact guide" effect (Weiss and Hiscoe, 1948). Lei et al. used photolithography to prepare striped structures with different pitch sizes in polymer templates, and studied the effects of surfaces with striped structures on the adhesion, orientation, and morphological changes of endothelial cells (Lei et al., 2012). However, it is worth mentioning that the aforementioned micro-pattern preparation methods have their own limitations and disadvantages. For example, the requirements for the equipment are relatively high (electron beam etching), and they are limited by the limiting wavelength of the light source (lithography). It is difficult to control the elastic

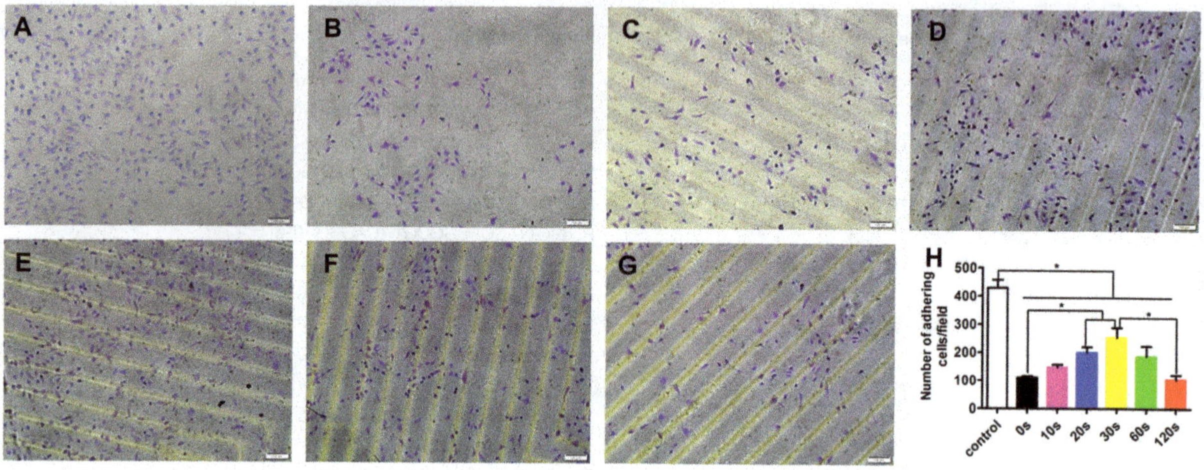

FIGURE 3 | Adhesion of HUVECs on the biomimetic elastic membrane with different height in the thickness direction (*$p < 0.05$). **(A–G)** HUVECs were stained with 0.1% crystals after cultured in normal condition and on the sample-0, 10, 20, 30, 60, and 120 s for 6 h. Scale bar: 100 μm. **(H)** Quantitation of adhesive cells. The data are shown as the mean ± SD of the number of adhesive cells from three independent experiments. *$p < 0.05$ represents statistical significance.

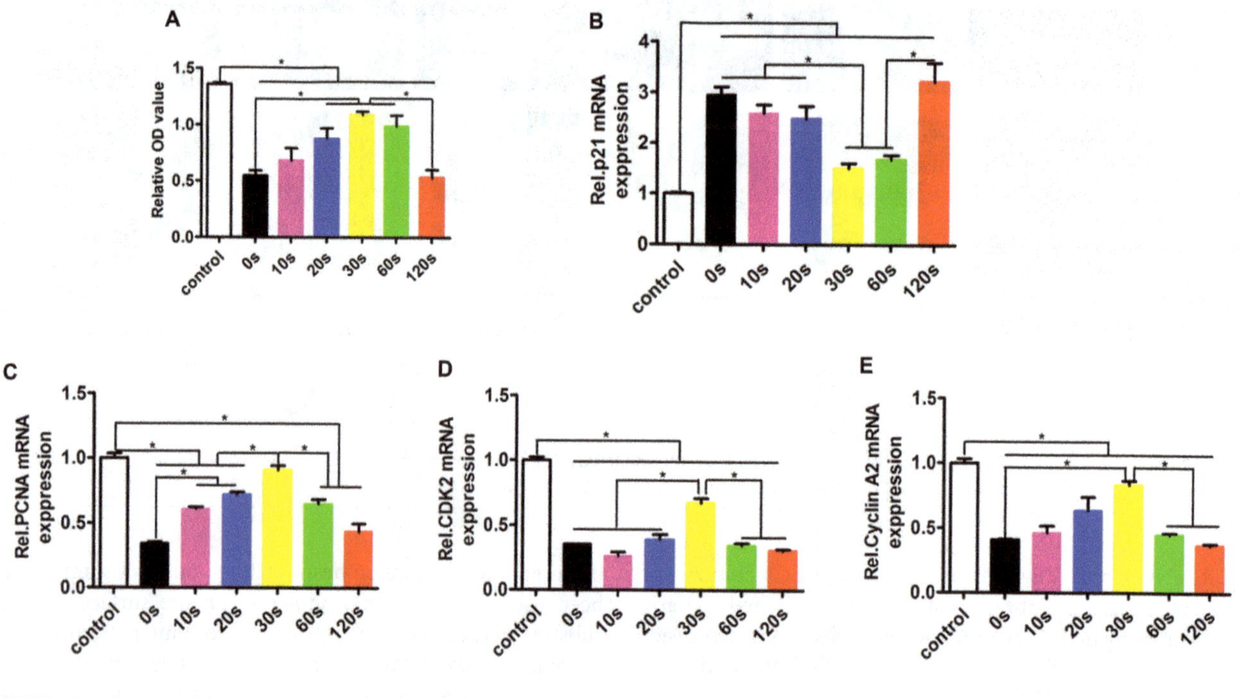

FIGURE 4 | Proliferation of HUVECs on the biomimetic elastic membrane with different height in the thickness direction. **(A)** The proliferation of HUVECs were assayed by CCK8 after cultured in normal condition and on the sample-0, 10, 20, 30, 60, and 120 s for 72 h. The mRNA expression of proliferation-related genes in HUVECs shown in each panel were **(B)** p21, **(C)** PCNA, **(D)** CDK2, and **(E)** cyclin A2, respectively (*$p < 0.05$).

deformation of the mold during operation to ensure the accuracy and repeatability of the pattern replication (soft lithography). In particular, due to the limited number of materials suitable for these technologies, it is not possible to directly achieve the controllable preparation of the micro-patterned structure on the surface of the required biodegradable material. In this work, the patterns were achieved via the UV light irradiation. This method is easy and convenient to operate, and can produce a variety of patterns. Meanwhile, the patterns can be design via the masks as needed.

Studies show that the choice of vascular endothelial cell carrier material and its traits have important effects on cell adhesion, growth, and expression of physiological functions (Jankowski and Wagner, 1999). In order to improve the adhesion and growth of endothelial cells on the surface of artificial blood vessels, people have tried to attach various cell adhesion factors such as collagen,

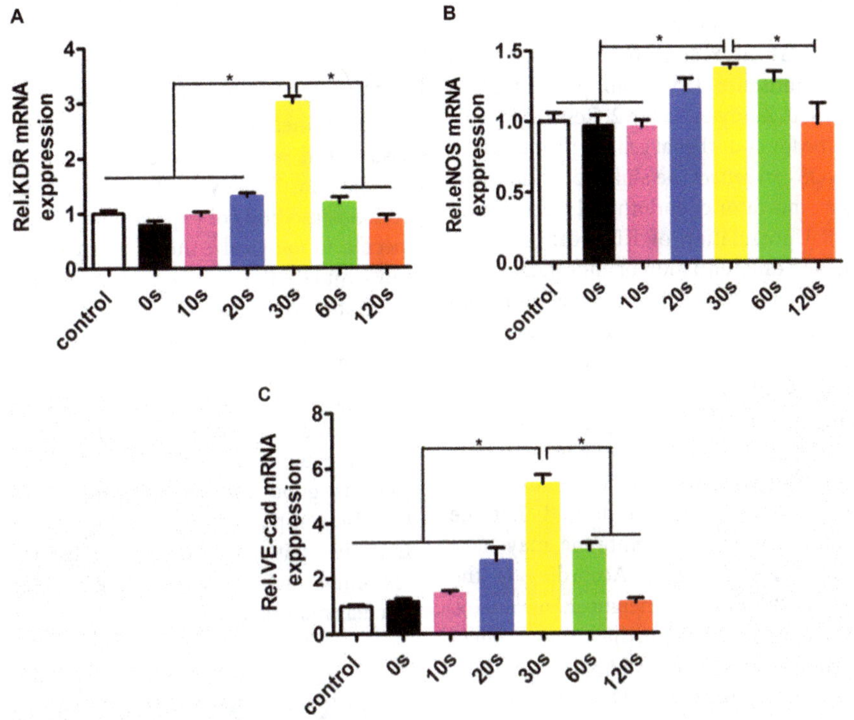

FIGURE 5 | The mRNA expressions of the angiogenesis-related genes in the HUVECs cultured in normal condition and on the sample-0, 10, 20, 30, 60, and 120 s for 72 h. The angiogenesis-related genes expression in HUVECs shown in each panel were **(A)** KDR, **(B)** eNOS, and **(C)** VE-Cad, respectively (*$p < 0.05$).

fibronectin, and laminin to the surface of vascular materials, and achieved relatively satisfactory results (Bellis, 2011). Later, it was discovered that the RGD (Arg-Gly-Asp) tripeptide is the smallest sequence for intercellular recognition shared by many cell membranes and multiple adhesion proteins in ECM, which plays a very important role in mediating cell adhesion and spreading (Pierschbacher and Ruoslahti, 1984; Ruoslahti, 1996; Arnaout et al., 2005). Currently, RGD has been widely used in the surface modification of biological materials to promote the adhesion and function of cells on the surface of biological materials (Barber et al., 2007). In addition to attaching various cell activation factors to the surface of the material, it has been found that the necessary 3D structure on the surface of the material is also one of the indispensable factors to promote cell adhesion and growth, especially to maintain cell functional differentiation. Numerous studies have well demonstrated that the appropriate surface topography of scaffolds could promote various cellular processes, including adhesion, proliferation, and migration (Dalby et al., 2007; Kirmizidis and Birch, 2009; Qi et al., 2010; Yang et al., 2010). Tunstall et al. (1994) compared the expression of tissue factor (TF) and prostacyclin (PG) during the growth of vascular endothelial cells on the surface of Dacron materials with different surface structures. During growth, the expression level of TF was significantly lower than that of endothelial cells grown on smooth surface Dacron membranes, while the expression level of PG was not significantly different between the two groups. Sun et al. have already demonstrated that the cell attachment would be greatly influenced by the diameter of electrospun fibers (Sun et al., 2007). Xu et al. (2015) investigated the effect of the fibrous patterns on cells, and found that the well-designed scaffolds with anisotropically and heterogeneously aligned patterns could significantly promote EC adhesion at the early stage and proliferation during the culture period.

Consistent with these studies, our results showed that biomimetic elastic membrane with different height in the thickness direction had an important influence on the adhesion and proliferation of HUVECs, which can significantly improve cell adhesion just inoculated cells, and cell proliferation during the cultivation process. However, the adhesion and proliferation of HUVECs cultured in SBS-An films were lower than these in normal condition. Therefore, future studies will try to attach some cell adhesion factors or the appropriate surface topography on the SBS-An films to improve the adhesion and growth of HUVECs on the biomimetic elastic membrane.

Moreover, we found that the biomimetic elastic membrane had a significant impact on the expression of the proliferation-related genes (such as p21, PCNA, CDK2, and cyclin A2) and angiogenic genes (such as eNOS, KDR, and VE-Cadherin). The tumor suppressor protein p21 Waf1/Cip1 acted as an inhibitor for cell cycle progression, and functioned in stoichiometric relationships to form heterotrimeric complexes with cyclins and cyclin-dependent kinases. In association with CDK2 complexes, it served to inhibit kinase activity and block progression through G1/S (Pestell et al., 1999). Proliferating cell nuclear antigen (PCNA) is a member of the DNA sliding clamp family of proteins that assist in DNA replication (Kelman and O'Donnell, 1995).

PCNA expression is a well-accepted marker of proliferation). A number of studies have described the ability of over-expressed cyclin A to accelerate the G1 to S transition causing DNA replication, and cyclin A antisense DNA can prevent DNA replication (D'Urso et al., 1990; Zindy et al., 1992; Resnitzky et al., 1995). eNOS is a key enzyme for endothelial cells to produce NO. The expression level of eNOS can reflect the ability of endothelial cells to secrete NO and is an indicator of endothelial cell integrity and vitality (Sessa, 2004). Upregulation of KDR can promote the survival, proliferation, and differentiation of endothelial cells, and is a better indicator of endothelial cell proliferation and differentiation (Santos et al., 2007). VE-cadherin is expressed at the cell adhesion junction, and its expression can specifically reflect the differentiation of endothelial cells (Schäfer et al., 2003). Examination of the abundance of the above gene expression can prove that biomimetic elastic membrane has an effect on the proliferation and differentiation of HUVECs. Different expression of these genes in SBS-An films indicated that the surface height of the biomimetic elastic membrane may have a significant influence on it (**Figures 4, 5**). According to the above results, the sample-20,30, and 60 s(height 2.56 ± 0.09, 4.47 ± 0.08, 7.22 ± 0.05 μm, respectively) had a stronger effect on the adhesion and proliferation of HUVECs, in contrast, sample-0,10, and 120 s (0, 1.36 ± 0.12, and 22.86 ± 0.28 μm, respectively.) had no siginificant difference. Therefore, this may be due to that too low or too high of the surface was not good for cell adhesion. However, the exact mechanism needs further study.

In conclusion, we easily achieved well-ordered surface patterned biomimetic elastic membrane with different height in the thickness direction through UV light-induced dimerization of anthracene grafted on SBS chains. All six membranes were found to be non-toxic against HUVECs. Among of them, sample-30 s had siginificantly effect on adhesion and proliferation of the HUVECs, and expression of the proliferation-related and angiogenic genes as compared with other samples, which makes it the best candidate for further improvement. Our results suggest that well-ordered surface-patterned biomimetic elastic membrane might have a potential in vascular tissue-engineering application.

The repair and reconstruction of tissues and organs make tissue engineering a hot research topic. However, the internal tissues and organs of organisms are complex structures with specific morphology and function composed of different cells. Previous methods of experiments are difficult to reconstruct the specific topological conformation of cells in tissues and organs and simulate the microenvironment in which cells are located. After the continuous development of chemical technology, it has gradually become an experimental tool for studying and controlling cell behavior, making it an asset in the fields of cell biology, tissue engineering, cell sensing, drug screening, and wound treatment. Although some defects are still present, such as its non-biodegradability, SBS-An films have many advantages, such as good mechanical properties, low cost, abundance, good biocompatibility, precise and controllable surface patterns, diversified patterns, fast and easy preparation method, and good flexibility, making them a great potential tissue engineering vascular material.

AUTHOR CONTRIBUTIONS

JT and JB carried out the experiments, analyzed the results, and wrote the manuscript, and were co-first authors. All authors contributed to conception and design of the study, and contributed to manuscript revision, read and approved the submitted version.

ACKNOWLEDGMENTS

We thank Central Laboratory and Southern Medical University affiliated Fengxian Hospital (Shanghai, China) for providing a research platform.

REFERENCES

Arnaout, M. A., Mahalingam, B., and Xiong, J. P. (2005). Integrin structure, allostery, and bidirectional signaling. *Annu. Rev. Cell Dev. Biol.* 21, 381–410. doi: 10.1146/annurev.cellbio.21.090704.151217

Bai, J., and Shi, Z. J. (2017). Shape memory: an efficient method to develop the latent photopatterned morphology for elastomer in two/three dimension. *Science* 6, 1025–1030. doi: 10.1021/acsmacrolett.7b00403

Bai, J., Zhang, L., Hou, H., Shi, Z., Yin, J., and Jiang, X. (2019). Light-written reversible 3D fluorescence and topography dual-pattern with memory and self-healing abilities. *Research* 2019:2389254. doi: 10.34133/2019/2389254

Ballyk, P. D., Walsh, C., Butany, J., and Ojha, M. J. (1997). Compliance mismatch may promote graft-artery intimal hyperplasia by altering suture-line stresses. *J. Biomech.* 31, 229–237. doi: 10.1016/S0197-3975(97)00111-115

Barber, T. A., Ho, J. E., De Ranieri, A., Virdi, A. S., Sumner, D. R., and Healy, K. E. (2007). Peri-implant bone formation and implant integration strength of peptide-modified p(AAM-co-EG/AAC) interpenetrating polymer network-coated titanium implants. *J. Biomed. Mater. Res. A* 80, 306–320. doi: 10.1002/jbm.a.30927

Bellis, S. L. (2011). Advantages of RGD peptides for directing cell association with biomaterials. *Biomaterials* 32, 4205–4210. doi: 10.1016/j.biomaterials.2011.02.029

Chen, G., Ushida, T., and Tateishi, T. (2001). Development of biodegradable porous scaffolds for tissue engineering. *Mater. Sci. Eng. C* 17, 63–69. doi: 10.1016/S0928-4931(01)00338-1

Chlupác, J., Filová, E., and Bacáková, L. (2009). Blood vessel replacement: 50 years of development and tissue engineering paradigms in vascular surgery. *Physiol. Res.* 58(Suppl. 2), S119–S139.

Cho, J., and Paul, D. R. (2001). Nylon 6 nanocomposites by melt compounding. *Polymer* 42, 1083–1094. doi: 10.1016/S0032-3861(00)00380-383

Dalby, M. J., Gadegaard, N., Tare, R., Andar, A., Riehle, M. O., Herzyk, P., et al. (2007). The control of human mesenchymal cell differentiation using nanoscale symmetry and disorder. *Nat. Mater.* 6, 997–1003. doi: 10.1038/nmat2013

D'Urso, G., Marraccino, R. L., Marshak, D. R., and Roberts, J. M. (1990). Cell cycle control of DNA replication by a homologue from human cells of the p34cdc2 protein kinase. *Science* 250, 786–791. doi: 10.1126/science.2173140

Fu, X., and Qutubuddin, S. J. P. (2001). Polymer-clay nanocomposites: exfoliation of organophilic montmorillonite nanolayers in polystyrene. *Polymer* 42, 807–813.

Guidoin, R. (1992). *Prostheses Arteriellesen: Principes Et Applications.* Paris: AERCV.

Jankowski, R. J., and Wagner, W. R. J. (1999). Directions in cardiovascular tissue engineering. *Clin. Plast. Surg.* 26, 605–616.

Kannan, R. Y., Salacinski, H. J., Butler, P. E., Hamilton, G., and Seifalian, A. M. (2005). Current status of prosthetic bypass grafts: a review. *J. Biomed. Mater. Res. B Appl. Biomater.* 74, 570–581. doi: 10.1002/jbm.b.30247

Kelman, Z., and O'Donnell, M. (1995). Structural and functional similarities of prokaryotic and eukaryotic DNA polymerase sliding clamps. *Nucleic Acids Res.* 23, 3613–3620.

Kim, G.-M., Lee, D.-H., Hoffmann, B., Kressler, J., and Stöppelmann, G. J. P. (2001). Influence of nanofillers on the deformation process in layered silicate/polyamide-12 nanocomposites. *Polymer* 42, 1095–1100. doi: 10.1016/S0032-3861(00)00468-467

Kirmizidis, G., and Birch, M. A. (2009). Microfabricated grooved substrates influence cell-cell communication and osteoblast differentiation in vitro. *Tissue Eng. Part. A* 15, 1427–1436. doi: 10.1089/ten.tea.2008.0137

Lei, Y., Zouani, O. F., Rami, L., Chanseau, C., and Durrieu, M. C. (2013). Modulation of lumen formation by microgeometrical bioactive cues and migration mode of actin machinery. *Small* 9, 1086–1095. doi: 10.1002/smll.201202410

Lei, Y., Zouani, O. F., Rémy, M., Ayela, C., and Durrieu, M. C. (2012). Geometrical microfeature cues for directing tubulogenesis of endothelial cells. *PLoS One* 7:e41163. doi: 10.1371/journal.pone.0041163

Li, S., Sengupta, D., and Chien, S. (2014). Vascular tissue engineering: from in vitro to in situ. *Wiley Interdiscip. Rev. Syst. Biol. Med.* 6, 61–76. doi: 10.1002/wsbm.1246

Lim, J. Y., and Donahue, H. J. (2007). Cell sensing and response to micro- and nanostructured surfaces produced by chemical and topographic patterning. *Tissue Eng.* 13, 1879–1891.

McBane, J. E., Sharifpoor, S., Labow, R. S., Ruel, M., Suuronen, E. J., and Paul Santerre, J. (2012). Tissue engineering a small diameter vessel substitute: engineering constructs with select biomaterials and cells. *Curr. Vasc. Pharmacol.* 10, 347–360.

Nel, A. E., Mädler, L., Velegol, D., Xia, T., Hoek, E. M., Somasundaran, P., et al. (2009). Understanding biophysicochemical interactions at the nano-bio interface. *Nat. Mater.* 8, 543–557. doi: 10.1038/nmat2442

Nerem, R. M. (2004). Tissue engineering of the vascular system. *Vox Sang.* 87(Suppl. 2), 158–160. doi: 10.1111/j.1741-6892.2004.00476.x

Nerem, R. M., and Seliktar, D. J. (2001). Vascular tissue engineering. *Annu. Rev. Biomed. Engin.* 3, 225–243. doi: 10.1146/annurev.bioeng.3.1.225

Novak, I., and Florián, ŠJ. (2004). Investigation of long-term hydrophobic recovery of plasma modified polypropylene. *J. Mater. Sci.* 39, 2033–2036.

O'Brien, F. J. (2011). Biomaterials & scaffolds for tissue engineering. *Mater. Today* 14, 88–95. doi: 10.1016/s1369-7021(11)70058-x

Pestell, R. G., Albanese, C., Reutens, A. T., Segall, J. E., Lee, R. J., and Arnold, A. (1999). The cyclins and cyclin-dependent kinase inhibitors in hormonal regulation of proliferation and differentiation. *Endocr. Rev.* 20, 501–534. doi: 10.1210/edrv.20.4.0373

Pierschbacher, M. D., and Ruoslahti, E. (1984). Cell attachment activity of fibronectin can be duplicated by small synthetic fragments of the molecule. *Nature* 309, 30–33. doi: 10.1038/309030a0

Qi, H., Du, Y., Wang, L., Kaji, H., Bae, H., and Khademhosseini, A. (2010). Patterned differentiation of individual embryoid bodies in spatially organized 3D hybrid microgels. *Adv. Mater.* 22, 5276–5281. doi: 10.1002/adma.201002873

Resnitzky, D., Hengst, L., and Reed, S. I. (1995). Cyclin A-associated kinase activity is rate limiting for entrance into S phase and is negatively regulated in G1 by p27Kip1. *Mol. Cell Biol.* 15, 4347–4352. doi: 10.1128/mcb.15.8.4347

Ruoslahti, E. (1996). RGD and other recognition sequences for integrins. *Annu. Rev. Cell Dev. Biol.* 12, 697–715. doi: 10.1146/annurev.cellbio.12.1.697

Santos, S. C., Miguel, C., Domingues, I., Calado, A., Zhu, Z., Wu, Y., et al. (2007). VEGF and VEGFR-2 (KDR) internalization is required for endothelial recovery during wound healing. *Exp. Cell Res.* 313, 1561–1574. doi: 10.1016/j.yexcr.2007.02.020

Schäfer, R., Abraham, D., Paulus, P., Blumer, R., Grimm, M., Wojta, J., et al. (2003). Impaired VE-cadherin/beta-catenin expression mediates endothelial cell degeneration in dilated cardiomyopathy. *Circulation* 108, 1585–1591.

Schwann, T. A., Engoren, M., Bonnell, M., Clancy, C., and Habib, R. H. (2012). Comparison of late coronary artery bypass graft survival effects of radial artery versus saphenous vein grafting in male and female patients. *Ann. Thorac. Surg.* 94, 1485–1491.

Sessa, W. C. (2004). eNOS at a glance. *J. Cell Sci.* 117, 2427–2429.

Sun, T., Norton, D., Mckean, R. J., Haycock, J. W., Ryan, A. J., and Macneil, S. (2007). Development of a 3D cell culture system for investigating cell interactions with electrospun fibers. *Biotechnol. Bioeng.* 97, 1318–1328. doi: 10.1002/bit.21309

Tan, J., Yang, L., Liu, C., and Yan, Z. (2017). MicroRNA-26a targets MAPK6 to inhibit smooth muscle cell proliferation and vein graft neointimal hyperplasia. *Sci. Rep.* 7:46602. doi: 10.1038/srep46602

Tunstall, A., Eberhart, R. C., and Prager, M. D. (1994). Comparison of tissue factor and prostacyclin production by human umbilical vein endothelial cells on dacron vascular prostheses and Dacron smooth films. *J. Biomed. Mater. Res.* 28, 1233–1238. doi: 10.1002/jbm.820281013

Voorhees, A. B. Jr., Jaretzki, A. III, and Blakemore, A. H. (1952). The use of tubes constructed from vinyon "N" cloth in bridging arterial defects. *Ann. Surg.* 135, 332–336.

Weiss, P., and Hiscoe, H. B. (1948). Experiments on the mechanism of nerve growth. *J. Exper. Zool.* 107, 315–395. doi: 10.1002/jez.1401070302

Whited, B. M., and Rylander, M. N. (2014). The influence of electrospun scaffold topography on endothelial cell morphology, alignment, and adhesion in response to fluid flow. *Biotechnol. Bioeng.* 111, 184–195. doi: 10.1002/bit.24995

Winterbone, M. S., Tribolo, S., Needs, P. W., Kroon, P. A., and Hughes, D. A. (2009). Physiologically relevant metabolites of quercetin have no effect on adhesion molecule or chemokine expression in human vascular smooth muscle cells. *Atherosclerosis* 202, 431–438.

Xu, H., Li, H., Ke, Q., and Chang, J. (2015). An anisotropically and heterogeneously aligned patterned electrospun scaffold with tailored mechanical property and improved bioactivity for vascular tissue engineering. *ACS Appl. Mater. Interf.* 7, 8706–8718. doi: 10.1021/acsami.5b00996

Yang, Y., Kusano, K., Frei, H., Rossi, F., Brunette, D. M., and Putnins, E. E. (2010). Microtopographical regulation of adult bone marrow progenitor cells chondrogenic and osteogenic gene and protein expressions. *J. Biomed. Mater. Res. A* 95, 294–304. doi: 10.1002/jbm.a.32838

Zindy, F., Lamas, E., Chenivesse, X., Sobczak, J., Wang, J., Fesquet, D., et al. (1992). Cyclin A is required in S phase in normal epithelial cells. *Biochem. Biophys. Res. Commun.* 182, 1144–1154. doi: 10.1016/0006-291x(92)91851-g

11

Nanoscale Technologies in Highly Sensitive Diagnosis of Cardiovascular Diseases

Chaohong Shi[1], Haotian Xie[2], Yifan Ma[3]*, Zhaogang Yang[4]* and Jingjing Zhang[3]*

[1] Department of Rehabilitation Medicine, The First People's Hospital of Wenling, Wenzhou Medical University, Wenling, China, [2] Department of Mathematics, The Ohio State University, Columbus, OH, United States, [3] Department of Chemical and Biomolecular Engineering, The Ohio State University, Columbus, OH, United States, [4] Department of Radiation Oncology, University of Texas Southwestern Medical Center, Dallas, TX, United States

***Correspondence:**
Yifan Ma
ma.1711@buckeyemail.osu.edu
Zhaogang Yang
Zhaogang.Yang@UTSouthwestern.edu
Jingjing Zhang
zhang.8211@osu.edu

Cardiovascular diseases (CVD) are the leading cause of death and morbidity in the world and are a major contributor to healthcare costs. Although enormous progress has been made in diagnosing CVD, there is an urgent need for more efficient early detection and the development of novel diagnostic tools. Currently, CVD diagnosis relies primarily on clinical symptoms based on molecular imaging (MOI) or biomarkers associated with CVDs. However, sensitivity, specificity, and accuracy of the assay are still challenging for early-stage CVDs. Nanomaterial platform has been identified as a promising candidate for improving the practical usage of diagnostic tools because of their unique physicochemical properties. In this review article, we introduced cardiac biomarkers and imaging techniques that are currently used for CVD diagnosis. We presented the applications of various nanotechnologies on diagnosis within cardiac immunoassays (CIAs) and molecular imaging. We also summarized and compared different cardiac immunoassays based on their sensitivities and working ranges of biomarkers.

Keywords: cardiovascular disease (CVD), biomarker, molecular imaging, diagnostic, nanotechnology

INTRODUCTION

Cardiovascular diseases (CVDs) are the most common causes of death in the world (Ho, 2018). CVDs can be medically defined as a group of disorders involving heart, brain, and blood vessels, including but not limited to coronary heart diseases, peripheral arterial diseases, rheumatic heart diseases, deep vein thrombosis, and cerebrovascular diseases – all of which result in ischemia and tissue death (Yang et al., 2009, 2012; Laflamme et al., 2012; Chakrabarti et al., 2013; Yu et al., 2015; Fan et al., 2020a,b). General CVDs can be characterized into five categories: atherosclerosis, acute myocardial infarction (AMI), heart failure (HF), stroke, and hypertension (Lichtenstein and Matthan, 2007; Govindappa et al., 2020; Joshi et al., 2020). Individuals who demonstrate tobacco smoking, high levels of low-density lipoproteins (LDL)-associated cholesterol, glucose, and diabetes as well as overweight and obesity, are especially susceptible to CVD morbidity and mortality (D'Agostino et al., 2008). Effectively diagnosing individuals who are most susceptible to CVDs opens the door to optimal treatment, thereby lowering the death rate. Given that early-stage CVDs demonstrate a high survival rate, predicting CVDs early on is essential.

Current common clinical CVD diagnosis methods include electrocardiography (ECG), plain X-ray, computed tomography (CT), and magnetic resonance imaging (MRI), and other MOI techniques (Anderson et al., 2013). ECG measures variations in the conduction system of the heart and monitors chest pain in AMI patients (Fesmire et al., 1998). CT scans X-ray images around the body and generates slices images of bones, blood vessels and tissues, which is appropriate for CVD diagnosis on grounds of its high signal contrast and accuracy (Kirkpatrick et al., 2003). MRI has been widely used in atherosclerosis and stroke detection given it scans three-dimensional images of bodies in a non-invasive manner (Pykett et al., 1983). However, these traditional methods were limited to low sensitivity and specificity.

To overcome these aforementioned difficulties, various new platforms such as cardiac immunoassays (CIAs) and advanced molecular imaging (MOI) were introduced, which significantly improved the efficiency of CVD diagnosis over the past decades (Qureshi et al., 2012; Osborn and Jaffer, 2013). Cardiac biomarkers are substances in the blood when the heart and brain are damaged or act abnormally. For example, cardiac troponin I (cTnI) has been demonstrated as a promising biomarker for AMI (Apple et al., 1997). MOI is capable of identifying cellular and molecular biology process, however, each technique has advantages and limitations. Therefore, advanced MOI combined different MOI techniques have been invented (e.g., dual-module, triple-module-CT) to obtain more detailed imaging information, which has increased the accuracy of diagnostic results (Hur et al., 2011, 2012).

Despite the great merits of previous methods, early-stage diagnosis is still challenging due to its complex pathophysiology, vague symptoms, and low expression levels of cardiac biomarkers. These difficulties increase the aggravation and mortality of CVDs. For instance, atherosclerosis shows no signs or symptoms and extremely low-level of related biomarkers in some patients even after a heart attack (Libby, 2002). Moreover, quick and convenient measurements are inadequate in addressing the expanded needs of CVD patients. Hence, rapid, accurate, and highly sensitive and specific platforms are needed for early-stage CVDs.

Nanotechnology involves nanoscale dimension systems (Johnson, 2012; Zhou et al., 2014), has specific physicochemical properties that make them appealing for improving current diagnosis (Kuriyama et al., 2011; Sun et al., 2016, 2019; Chen Z. et al., 2017; Liu et al., 2017; Yang et al., 2020a). Nanomaterials have been extensively applied to CIAs, including electrochemiluminescence (ECL), Electrochemical (EC), and photoelectrochemistry (PEC) due to their unique optical property, electrical property, and excellent biocompatibility (**Figure 1**) (Abdorahim et al., 2016). For example, Gold nanoparticles (AuNPs) can be incorporated with biotinylated antibodies to reduce non-specific binding, or conjugated with biomolecules with specific physical properties [e.g., hybridization chain reaction (HCR)] for signal amplification. Liu G. et al. (2016) detected cTnI via antigen-antibody affinity with a low limit of detection using AuNPs and graphene oxide. AuNPs and other metal nanoparticles can modify substrates (e.g., boron nitride nanosheets, titanium) in EC assays as well because of their attractive electrical properties (Golberg et al., 2010). Other nanomaterials, like silica/Pt NPs, are common signal enhancers in PEC and surface plasmon resonance (SPR) thanks to their efficient photocurrent quenching ability and unique plasmonic properties (Homola et al., 1999). Besides, upconversion nanoparticles (UCNPs) have been used in fluorescence assay because of their excellent photon conversion ability (Haase and Schäfer, 2011). Also, knotted and hollow nanomaterials (e.g., nanosheets, nanotubes, nanowires, and nanoclusters) with the large surface area that increases loading efficiency of biomolecules for signal enhancement (Kong et al., 2000). Nanomaterials also play important roles in MOI. Nanomaterials coupled with photoacoustic, fluorescent, radioactive, paramagnetic substances can work as contrast agents in MOI settings to enhance their detection signal (Van Schooneveld et al., 2010).

In this review, we will introduce the recent progress of nanotechnology for diagnosing CVDs. The nanotechnology facilitated CIA and MOI applications will be covered. Firstly, we summarized common clinical cardiac biomarkers and MOI settings. Then the applications on nanotechnology to identify cardiac biomarkers within different platforms based on unique properties of various nanomaterials will be introduced, including ECL, fluorescence, PEC, EC Surface-enhanced Raman scattering (SERS), SPR, Field effect transistor (FET), Enzyme-Linked Immunosorbent Assay (ELISA), and lateral flow assay (LFA). We compared different CIAs based on their sensitivities and working ranges of cardiac biomarkers as well. Besides, we concluded current diagnosis achievements on MOI with the help of functionalized nanoparticle.

CVD DIAGNOSTIC SETTINGS

Cardiac Immunoassay (CIA)

Cardiac biomarkers present in human bodyfluids are reliable and reproducible indicators of the risk and progression of CVDs. They can be detected and quantified through various CIAs based on antigen-antibody immunoaffinity. Measuring expression levels of cardiac biomarkers within CIAs shows advantages, including high sensitivity, rapid, cheap, and non-invasive for the prediction and diagnosis of disease. Cardiac biomarkers can be classified as circulating biomarkers and exosomal biomarkers. Circulating biomarkers present in bodyfluids freely, and exosomal biomarkers are bound into or on the surface of extracellular vesicles (EVs) that are mobile and secreted from cells.

Cardiac Circulating Biomarkers

Circulating biomarkers include miRNA, mRNA, long-non-coding RNA, proteins, and other substances that present in human blood, milk, saliva, urine, and cerebral spinal biofluids (Durrani-Kolarik et al., 2017; Wang et al., 2017a,b; Wang X. et al., 2018; Yang et al., 2020b). Currently, several cardiac biomarkers, such as cardiac troponin I (cTnI), troponin I (TnI), myoglobin (MB), C-reactive protein (CRP), and creatine kinase-MB (CK-MB), have attracted interests as potential biomarkers for AMI (Christenson and Christenson, 2013). Particularly, cTnI has high specificity and sensitivity toward AMI (Jo et al., 2015), and MB is a good candidate for early diagnosis of AMI (Korff et al., 2006).

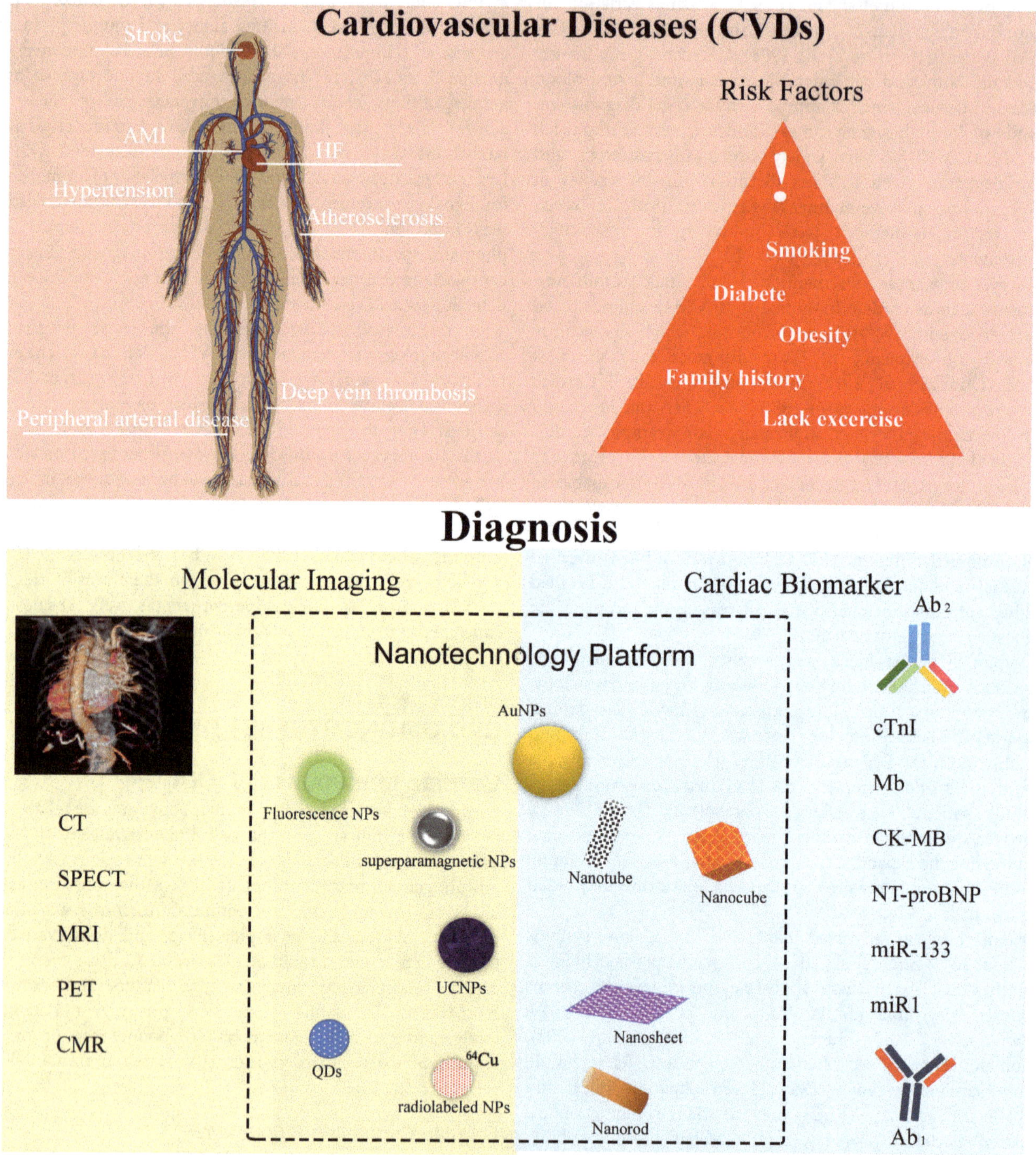

FIGURE 1 | Cardiovascular diseases (CVDs), their risk factors, and their diagnosis settings include molecular imaging and cardiac immunoassay within the nanotechnology platform. Ab_1, capture antibodies that immobilize the targets. Ab_2, detection or secondary antibodies that detect and quantify the targets.

Myeloperoxidase (MPO), glycogen phosphorylase isoenzyme BB (GPBB), B-type natriuretic peptide (BNP), N-terminal pro-B-type natriuretic peptide (NT-proBNP), C-type natriuretic peptide (c-TNP), Matrix metalloproteinase-8 (MMP-8), MMP-9 and tissue inhibitor of MMP-8 (TIMP-1), and leukotriene B4 are promising biomarkers as well (Anderon, 2005).

Recently, researchers discovered that some miRNAs circulating in serum or plasma were closely correlated with CVDs. For example, miR-208 was undetectable in healthy donors but was detected successfully in 90.9% of AMI patients (Ji et al., 2009). There are almost 50 circulating miRNAs proven to be relevant to CVDs. Specifically, miR-208a, miR-208b, and miR133 are up-regulated AMI biomarkers, while miR150, let-7b, and miR-126 are down-regulation AMI biomarkers (Corsten et al., 2010; Wang et al., 2010; Gidlöf et al., 2011; Long et al., 2012a,b; Devaux et al., 2013; Friese et al., 2013; Li et al., 2013). Furthermore, miR-423, miR-18b, miR-499, miR-142, miR-320a, miR-22, miR-20b, and miR-26b are positively associated with HF, but miR-103 is shown to be low in HF patients (Corsten et al., 2010; Tijsen et al., 2010; Goren et al., 2012; Ellis et al., 2013; Marfella et al., 2013). Additionally, let-7e, Hcmv-miR-UL112, miR-605, miR623, miR-516b, miR-132 are found to be relatively high in plasma in hypertension cases. In contrast, miR-296, miR-133b, miR-625, miR-1236 are down-regulation biomarkers (Li et al., 2011). Moreover, miR-145, miR21 are up-regulating biomarkers for strokes, and miR-221, miR-210, miR-30a, and miR-126 are shown to be low in human blood in stroke cases (Zeng et al., 2011; Gan et al., 2012; Long et al., 2012b; Tsai et al., 2013). In summary, circulating miRNAs are relatively stable and serve as sufficiently sensitive biomarkers for CVD diagnosis.

Cardiac Exosomal Biomarkers

EVs are submicron-sized vesicles ranging from 30 to 1000 nm secreted by cells. EVs play important roles in transferring proteins, mRNA, miRNA, and other molecules among cells (Yang et al., 2016; Ma et al., 2019; Walters et al., 2019; Liu et al., 2019). Increasing evidence showed that exosomal miRNAs are involved in the pathogenesis of CVDs (Zamani et al., 2019). It has been observed that exosomal miRNAs mediate intercellular communication in cardiovascular systems and play an indispensable role in the control of cellular functions (Bang et al., 2014). As such, exosomal miRNAs can be used as biomarkers for diagnosing subjects with CVDs (Rehman et al., 2017).

Recently, researchers found miR-1, miR-133a, miR-21, and miR-499 are AMI-related biomarkers (Cheng et al., 2012; Oerlemans et al., 2012). Also, miR-192, miR-194, miR-34a, miR-423-5p, miR320a, miR-22, and miR-92b are highly associated with HF (Goren et al., 2012; Matsumoto et al., 2013). Besides, miR-223 isolated from serum EVs is a potential biomarker for stroke (Chen Y. et al., 2017). Additionally, exosomal membrane proteins or internal proteins, such as TNF-α and fibronectin are also potential CVD biomarkers (de Jong et al., 2012; Yu et al., 2012). **Table 1** summarized the biomarkers mentioned above.

Molecular Imaging

Molecular imaging (MOI) is a common diagnostic tool for CVD in clinical practice. When paired with other approaches, MOI can reveal individual biology, including blood vessels, the brain, and the heart (Jaffer et al., 2007). Common MOI approaches include photoacoustic tomography (PAT), MRI, CT, positron emission tomography (PET), and single photon emission computed tomography (SPECT). PAT utilizes the photoacoustic effect that converts optical adsorption into acoustic energy and generates high-resolution imaged under optically ballistic and diffusive modules (Xia et al., 2014). Various materials such as dyes, nanoparticles, and probes can work as functional contrasts in PAT for vascular imaging (Li and Wang, 2009). CT takes X-ray images from different angles around the human body and produces cross-sectional images of the body to reveal blood vessels, tissues and organs (Article, 2018). MRI generates anatomical images based on the changes of protons in the body with a strong magnetic field (Hashemi et al., 2012). MRI sensors first turn on the radiofrequency current that spins the protons out of equilibrium and then detects the time and amount of released energy of realigning randomized protons within the magnetic field after turning off the radiofrequency current (McRobbie et al., 2017). Detected parameters are translated into images for diagnosis. PET uses injected radioactive tracers to review and evaluate tissues. The radiotracers used in PET produce positrons after decaying. Positrons react with electrons and produce photons that aggregate in specific, disease-related areas of the human body (Shan et al., 2013). The combination of PET with CT or MRI can create detailed, specific images. Similar to PET, SPECT provides tomographic images by recording and translating the activities of radioactive tracers that have gamma ray emissions (Hutton, 2014).

NANOTECHNOLOGY-BASED CARDIAC IMMUNOASSAY

Various advanced techniques like ECL, PEC, SERS, SPR, and ELISA have been utilized to detect cardiac biomarkers with precision. Despite satisfactory results from previous methods, pursuing high sensitivity and accuracy in testing results is still an ongoing endeavor. Combining nanotechnologies with cardiac immunoassays may serve as a solution for early-stage CVD diagnosis. Nanotechnologies may reduce non-specific binding sites, provide high binding efficiency of cardiac targets, offer excellent signal amplification, and possess multiple functions. **Table 2** summarized and compared performances of recent cardiac immunoassays based on various nanotechnology platforms.

Electrochemiluminescence (ECL) Immunoassay

Electrochemiluminescence (ECL) involves electron-transfer reactions that generate excited states and light emission, thus works as a common diagnostic assay to quantify expression levels of biomarkers because detected emission intensity in ECL is proportional to the concentration of the biomarkers (Richter, 2004). Luminol is one of the most important signal enhancers in ECL but has a weak signal and poor solubility. Fortunately, luminol-functionalized nanomaterials can overcome the limitations of traditional luminol and greatly enhance the intensity and sensitivity due to their large specific surface area (e.g., carbon nanotubes, nanosheets), the ability to functionalize signal amplification materials (e.g., nucleic acid isothermal amplification, HCR signal amplification), conductivity, and surface charge. All of these advantages have contributed to intense attention of ECL assay in biomolecule analysis (Hao et al., 2014; Feng et al., 2016).

Dong et al. (2019) detected NT-proBNP using ECL immunoassay based on ECL resonance energy transfer (RET). The ECL-RET transfer was between semicarbazide-modified

TABLE 1 | Summary of cardiac biomarkers.

Biomarker ID	Type	Pathology	Expression	References
cTnI, TnI, MB, C-CRP, CK-MB, MPO, GPBB, NT-proBNP, c-TNP, MMP-8, MMP-9, TIMP-1, leukotriene B4, TNF-α, and fibronectin	Protein	AMI, HF, Hypertension, Stroke	Upregulated	Anderon, 2005; Korff et al., 2006; de Jong et al., 2012; Yu et al., 2012; Christenson and Christenson, 2013; Jo et al., 2015
miR-208, miR-208a, miR-208b, miR133, miR-1, miR-133a, miR-21, and miR-499	RNA	AMI	Upregulated	Ji et al., 2009; Corsten et al., 2010; Wang et al., 2010; Gidlöf et al., 2011; Cheng et al., 2012; Long et al., 2012a,b; Oerlemans et al., 2012; Devaux et al., 2013; Friese et al., 2013; Li et al., 2013
miR150, let-7b, and miR-126	RNA	AMI	Downregulated	Devaux et al., 2013; Friese et al., 2013; Li et al., 2013
miR-423, miR-18b, miR-499, miR-142, miR-320a, miR-22, miR-20b, miR-26b, miR-192, miR-194, miR-34a, miR-423-5p, miR320a, miR-22, and miR-92b	RNA	HF	Upregulated	Corsten et al., 2010; Tijsen et al., 2010; Goren et al., 2012; Ellis et al., 2013; Marfella et al., 2013; Matsumoto et al., 2013
miR-103	RNA	HF	Downregulated	Ellis et al., 2013
let-7e, Hcmv-miR-UL112, miR-605, miR623, miR-516b, miR-132	RNA	Hypertension	Upregulated	Li et al., 2011
miR-296, miR-133b, miR-625, miR-1236	RNA	Hypertension	Downregulated	Li et al., 2011
miR-145, miR21, miR-223	RNA	Stroke	Upregulated	Zeng et al., 2011; Gan et al., 2012; Long et al., 2012b; Tsai et al., 2013; Chen Y. et al., 2017
miR-221, miR-210, miR-30a, and miR-126	RNA	Stroke	Downregulated	Zeng et al., 2011; Long et al., 2012b

gold nanoparticles (AgNC-sem@AuNPs) covered nanocubes (donor) and a Ti (IV)-based metal-organic framework of type MIL-125 (receptor). The partial overlap between the ECL emission of the AgNC-sem@AuNPs and the visible adsorption spectrum of MIL-135 created RET. The schematic was illustrated in **Figure 2A**. Firstly, 8 μL of AgNC-sem@AuNP solution was dropped on the pre-cleaned glassy carbon electrode (GCE) surface, then the primary antibody$_1$ (Ab_1) was immobilized on it via Au-NH_2 bond. Then, NT-proBNP analytes were added to the assay and captured by Ab_1. Finally, the MIL-125 labeled secondary antibody$_2$ (Ab_2) was incubated onto the electrode to form the sandwich format and quench the ECL strength of luminophore. The assay was able to recover 96.8%~100.2% of NT-proBNP and detect it as low as 0.11 pg/mL.

Zhu et al. (2019) detected cTnI using Au Nanocluster and HCR signal amplification. A sandwich immunocomplex composed of cTnI, Ab_1, and Ab_2-AuNP-T_1 was applied. Ab_2-AuNP-T_1 is a smart probe in which the DNA initiator strands (T_1) and Ab_2 are conjugated onto the AuNPs. The schematic was illustrated in **Figure 2B**. Once the cTnI was caught, the initiator strands T_1 of Ab_2-AuNP-T_1 opened the hairpin DNA structures (H1 and H2) that were dual-labeled on the Au nanoclusters (Au NCs). This process triggered hybridization events, thus modified a large number of Au NCs on the surface of the electrode. Finally, a strong ECL signal was emitted owing to the reaction of the modified Au NCs and the coreactant $K_2S_2O_2$. This ECL-HCR sensor was able to detect 1.01 fg/mL cTnI with high specificity stability and reproducibility.

Recently, various research groups have made great progress in CVD diagnosis using ECL assay. Wang et al. (2019) combined Co^{2+}-based metal organic frameworks (MOF), zeolitic imidazolate frameworks (ZIF-67), and luminol-capped Ag nanoparticles (luminol-AgNPs) for fast and ultrasensitive detection of cTnI, with a 0.58 fg/mL detection limit. Zou et al. (2019) developed an ECL immunosensor to detect MB in human serum. They fabricated a basal electrode using AuNPs and platinum nanowires that were deposited onto indium tin oxide-coated glass linked with 3-aminopropyl-trimethoxysilane. Besides, Adhikari et al. (2019) presented an ultrasensitive label-free ECL immunosensor for CK-MB detection using a novel nanocomposite-modified printed electrode. To fabricate this sensor, carbon nano-onions (CNOs)/Fe_3O_4/AuNP/chitosan (CS) nanocomposite was dropped in single-layered rolled-up carbon nanotubes (SWCNTs). Then Ab_1 against CK-MB was spiked onto the electrode and blocked by bovine serum albumin (BSA). Once CK-MB was captured on the electrode, the ECL signal was determined by Tris(2,2′-bipyridyl)-ruthenium(II) chloride ($[Ru(bpy)_3]^{2+}Cl$) and tri-*n*-propylamine (TPrA), in which $Ru(bpy)_3]^{2+}Cl$ was used as luminophore and TPrA was the co-reactant. Moreover, Lakshmanakumar et al. (2019) functionalized graphene quantum dots with acetic acid (fGQDs) on the Au electrode to detect cTnI. The cTnI was recognized via carbodiimide conjugation between the N-H group of cTnI and the COOH group on fGQDs instead of antibody-antigen interaction. The interaction of cTnI and fGQDs was examined by cyclic voltammetry (CV) and amperometry (Lakshmanakumar et al., 2019). They detected cTnI over a linear range of 0.17–3 ng/mL and offered a detection limit of 0.02 ng/mL with good stability and sensitivity. Based on the aforementioned discussion, ECL immunoassay is appealing for diagnosis since its high stability as well as sensitivity and specificity. Despite the considerable advantages for biomedical analysis, ECL often requires specialized and expensive equipment for generating excited states with light-emitting for detection, which to some extent impair its extensive application.

Fluorescence Immunoassay

Fluorescence immunoassay is by far the dominant analytical approach in biomedical engineering on account of its outstanding versatility and signal enhancement ability (Strianese et al., 2012).

TABLE 2 | Comparison of cardiac biomarker detection in developed immunoassays.

Target	Assay	Nanoplatform	Range	Detection limit	References
cTnI	ECL	Au nanocluster	5 fg/mL to 50 ng/mL	1.01 fg/mL	Zhu et al., 2019
	ECL	Ag Nanoparticles	NA	0.58 fg/mL	Wang et al., 2019
	ECL	QDs	0.17–3 ng/mL	0.02 ng/mL	Lakshmanakumar et al., 2019
	Fluorescence	QDs	1 pg/mL to 10 ng/mL	0.227 pg/mL	Miao et al., 2019
	Fluorescence	Pd-Ir nanocubes	1 pg/mL to 1 ng/mL	0.31 pg/mL	Tan et al., 2019
	Fluorescence	AuNP	NA	0.019 ng/mL	Han and Kim, 2019
	PEC	QDs	0.5 pg/mL to 10 ng/mL	0.5 pg/mL	Xue et al., 2019
	PEC	Nanospheres and QDs	0.08 ng/mL to 40 ng/mL	0.026 ng/mL	Dong et al., 2020
	PEC	Mesoporous silica nanoparticles	1.2 fg/mL to 20 ng/mL	0.47 fg/mL	Gao et al., 2019
	EC	AuNPs	1–1100 pM	0.18 pM	Lopa et al., 2019
	EC	Carbon nanotubes	NA	0.05 ng/mL	Vasantham et al., 2020
	EC	Nanospheres	0.005 ng/mL to 100 ng/mL	5 pg/mL	Singh et al., 2019
	EC	Carbon nanotubes	0.05 ng/mL to 30 ng/mL	0.03 ng/mL	Shen et al., 2019
	EC	Nanorods	0.01 ng/mL to 10 ng/mL	NA	Sandil et al., 2019
	EC	Nanocubes	NA	33.3 fg/mL	Zhang et al., 2019
	EC	Nanoparticles	1.0 pg/mL to 100 ng/mL	0.39 pg/mL	Ma et al., 2019
	EC	Nanocubes	100 fg/mL to 250 ng/mL	33 fg/mL	Lv et al., 2019
	SERS	AuNPs	0.01 ng/mL to 1000 ng/mL	5 pg/mL	Fu et al., 2019
	SPR	AuNPs	NA	3.75 ng/mL	Chen et al., 2019
	FET	Nanoribbon	NA	1 pg/mL	Liu Q. et al., 2016
	ELISA	Nanodendrites	0.1 pg/mL to 1000 ng/mL	0.056 pg/mL	Jiao et al., 2019
	LFA	AuNPs	NA	0.1 ng/mL	Lim et al., 2019
	LFA	Nanosphere	0.049 ng/mL to 50 ng/mL	0.049 ng/mL	Lou et al., 2019a
	LFA	Nanosphere		0.1 ng/mL	Lou et al., 2019b
NT-proBNP	ECL	Nanocube and AuNPs	0.25 pg/mL to 100 ng/mL	0.11 pg/mL	Dong et al., 2019
MB	ECL	AuNPs and platinum nanowires	3.0 ng/mL to 0.32 μg/mL	0.11 ng/mL	Zou et al., 2019
	Fluorescence	UCNPs	10 ng/mL to 400 ng/mL	0.21 ng/mL	Ji et al., 2019
	EC	AuNPs and nanosheets	0.1 μg/mL to 100 μg/mL	34.6 ng/mL	Adeel et al., 2019
cTnT	EC	Carbon nanotubes	0.1 pg/mL to 8.0 pg/mL	0.04 pg/mL	Phonklam et al., 2020
BNP	FET	Nanoribbon		10 pg/mL	Liu Q. et al., 2016
FABP	Fluorescence	Nanowires	2.5–60 ng/mL	1.36 ng/mL	Guo et al., 2019
CK-MB	ECL	AuNPs, Fe_3O_4, carbon nano-onions	10 ng/mL to 50 fg/mL	5 fg/mL	Adhikari et al., 2019
	SERS	AuNPs	NA	9.7 pg/mL	Cheng et al., 2019
	FET	Nanoribbon	NA	0.1 ng/mL	Liu Q. et al., 2016
	LFA	AuNPs	NA	5 ng/mL	Lim et al., 2019
Vaspin	Fluorescence	UCNPs	0.1 ng/mL to 55 ng/mL	39 pg/mL	Ali et al., 2020
GPBB	LFA	AuNPs	NA	10 ng/mL	Lim et al., 2019

Nanomaterials have promoted the efficiency of fluorescence assay because nanomaterials have good solubility, low toxicity, and high binding affinity of biomolecules, which can couple with various intensive fluorescence materials for amplification (e.g., Horseradish Peroxidase) (Yeh et al., 2010; Lu et al., 2017).

Miao et al. (2019) used a robust nanoceria-linked immunosorbent assay to detect cTnI based on colorimetric and ratiometric fluorescence. Ratiometric fluorescence overcomes some dependence defects, such as external environment luminophore, consequently, it can be used for trace detection. The schematic of the sensor was illustrated in **Figure 2C**. After the bonding of cTnI and Ab_1, *o*-phenylenediamine (OPD) as an organic substrate was oxidized and converted into 2,3-diaminophenazine (oxOPD) by the robust nanozyme of nanoceria with peroxidase-like properties and the addition of H_2O_2. OxOPD was immobilized on the surface of g-C_3N_4 QDs through hydrogen bonding and $\pi-\pi$ stacking interactions. The g-C_3N_4 QDs led to a ratiometric fluorescence response as a result of photoinduced electron transfer (PET). Besides, a visible color change was detected through the conversion of colorless OPD to an orange oxOPD, which acted as a colorimetric fluorescence. As a result, cTnI was quantified by combining the merits of the ratiometric assay and colorimetric assay. Similarly, Tan et al. (2019) oxidized the OPD to oxOPD through the Pd-Ir nanocubes catalysis, which possessed excellent peroxidase-like activity. The detection range of cTnI was between 1 pg/mL to 1 ng/mL, and the detection limit was 0.31 pg/mL.

Moreover, Guo et al. (2019) completed multiplexed detection of cTnI, human heart-type fatty acid binding protein (FABP), and MB using Zinc Oxide Nanowires to enhance fluorescence signal.

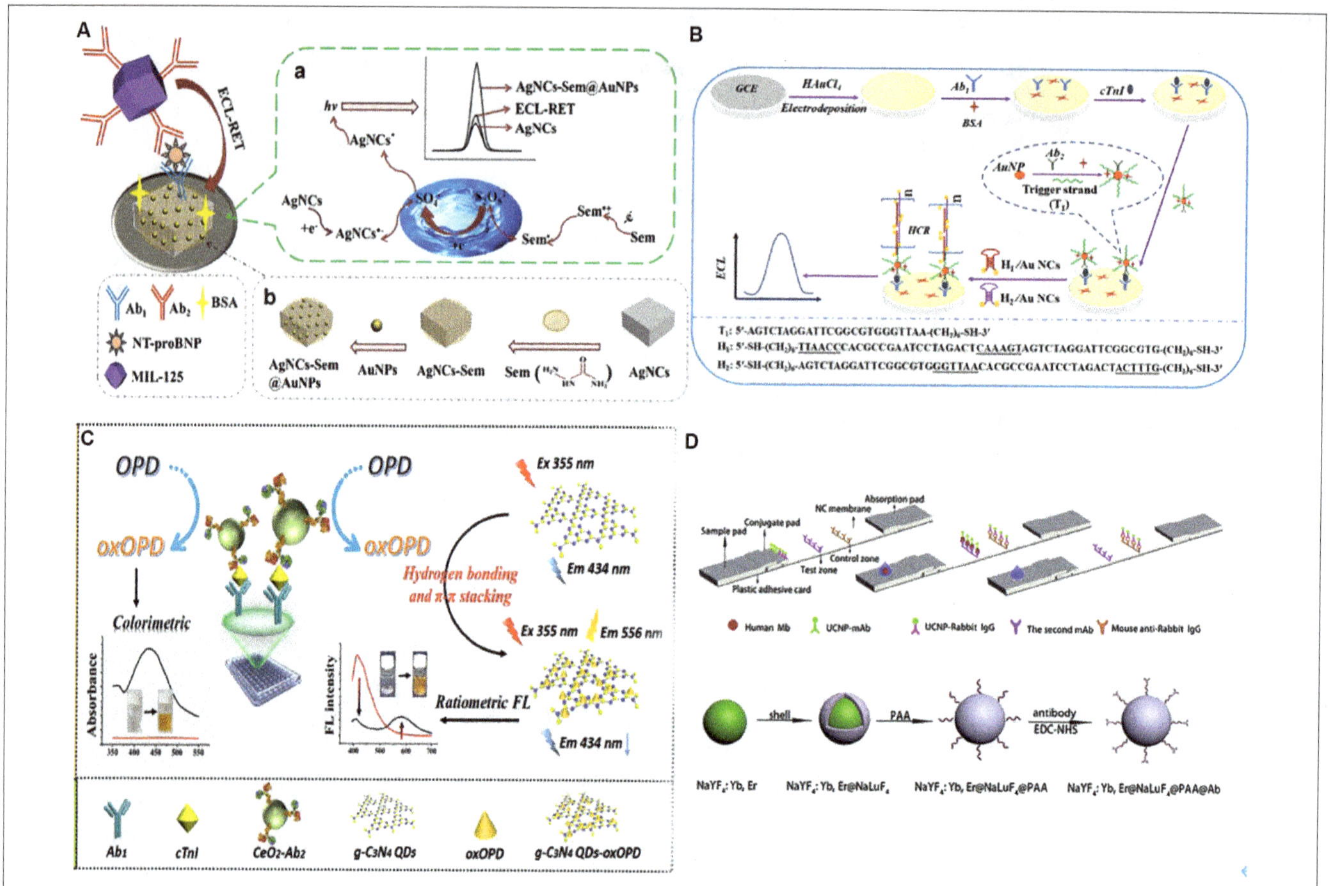

FIGURE 2 | (A) (a) The schematic of fabricating ECL immunoassay and its possible self-enhanced luminescence mechanism. A sandwich detection format was utilized to detect NT-proBNP. Ab_1 was immobilized via Au-NH_2 bond and dried on AgNC-sem@AuNP modified GCE surface, once the NT-proBNP was captured, the MIL-125 labeled Ab_2 was added to quench the ECL luminophore. The resonance energy transfer was due to the partial overlap between the ECL emission of the AgNC-sem@AuNPs (wavelength 470–900 nm) and the visible adsorption spectrum of MIL-135 (wavelength 406–900 nm). **(b)** The preparation of self-enhanced luminophore AgNC-Sem@AuNPs. AuNPs combined with Sem-AgNCs with Au-NH_2 bond. (Dong et al., 2019).
(B) Schematic Illustration of ECL-HCR Immunosensor. AuNPs modified GCE immobilized Ab_1 via Au-N and Au-S bonds, and then AuNPs/GCE was prepared by electrodepositing in $HAuCl_4$ solution. The Ab_2-AuNP-T_1 opened hairpin DNA structures (H1 and H2 after cTnI was caught), which triggered hybridization that modified Au NCs on the electrode. Au NCs reacted with $K_2S_2O_2$ thus emitted the ECL signal (Zhu et al., 2019). **(C).** The mechanism of nanozyme-linked immunosorbent assay for dual colorimetric and ratiometric fluorescent detection. OPD was oxidized and converted into oxOPD by the robust nanozyme of nanoceria with peroxidase-like properties, resulting an emission maximum of oxOPD at 578 nm. OxOPD was immobilized on the surface of g-C_3N_4 QDs, which led to a ratiometric fluorescence response as a result of photoinduced electron transfer (PET). The combination of ratiometric fluorescent assay with colorimetric assay could quantify cTnI (Miao et al., 2019).**(D)** Schematic of UCNPs based immunoassay and the synthesis, surface modification of core-shell UCNPs. UCNPs-Ab_1 and UCNPs-rabbit IgG were added on the conjugate pad, the second anti-(MB Ab_1) and anti- (rabbit IgG) antibodies were separately stripped onto the NC membrane. Samples will be captured on the sample pad. UCNPs on the test and control line was excited by a continuous wave laser diode at 908 nm for reading. The Poly (acrylic acid) PAA was added to the core-shell $NaYF_4$: Yb, Er@$NaLuF_4$ nanoparticles, and yield UCNPs@PAA particles. Then UCNPs@PAA were conjugated with Ab_1 using 1-Ethyl-3-(3-dimethyllaminopropyl) carbodiimide hydrochloride (EDC-HCl) and *N*-Hydroxysulfosuccinimide sodium salt (Sulfo-NHS) as cross-linking agents (Ji et al., 2019).

Han and Kim (2019) designed a AuNP-Antibody-HRP conjugate for cTnI detection. They bound aldehydeactivated(ald)HRP and the primary amine group based on adsorption or covalent coupling, to enhance the sensitivity of the AuNP-based conjugates.

Upconversion nanoparticles (UCNPs) are another type of fluorescent nanomaterials that have been used in luminescent and fluorescent detection (Tan et al., 2016). Ji et al. (2019) used core-shell upconversion nanoparticles (UCNP) to capture the MB in blood samples. MB was fixed between UCNPs-Ab_1 and second anti-(MB Ab_1) antibody to form a sandwich format. UCNPs were excited by a continuous wave laser diode at 908 nm for fluorescent reading by external equipment. The detailed procedure was illustrated in **Figure 2D**. Applied UCNPs increased the sensitivity of the assay, which reached a limit of detection as low as 0.21 ng/mL with a 90.6–110.5% MB recovery rate (Ji et al., 2019). Ali et al. (2020) also designed a biosensor assisted with UCNPs for ultrasensitive detection of Vaspin.

Photoelectrochemical (PEC)

The photoelectrochemical (PEC) process refers to the electricity conversion of photons resulting from photoactive materials absorbing photons upon illumination and forming electron-hole pairs. This, in turn, causes the oxidization-reduction reaction of the molecules and generates charge separation and subsequent charge transfer. PEC is a promising diagnostic tool since the detected photocurrent change is caused by the biological interactions between biomarkers and corresponding recognitions (Zhao et al., 2014). Nanomaterials have improved the sensitivity of PEC assay because they present a low background signal. For instance, AuNPs, QDs, TiO_2 nanotubes (NTs), Pt NPs, and Silica NPs are suitable candidates for PEC biosensors thanks to their efficient photocurrent quenching ability and unique plasmonic properties (Zhao et al., 2012).

Xue et al. (2019) reported a split-type liposomal PEC immunoassay composed of immunoaffinity, cadmium sulfide (CdS) quantum dots-loaded liposomes (QDLL), and TiO_2 nanotubes (NTs) that capture QDs for cTnI detection. The thioglycolic acid (TGA)-capped QDs and QDLL were linked with the Ab_2 as signaling probes. The schema was explained in **Figure 3A**. cTnI was captured by Ab_1 in the 96-well plates, and then QDLL-Ab_2 was introduced after the immunorecognition. Triton X-100 (10%) was introduced to damage the QDLL and release the QDs that were later captured by the TiO_2-NTs electrode. TGA-capped CdS QDs reacted with the Titania surface through the complexing between the carboxylic acid functionality on the CdS QDs and the hydroxyl groups of the TiO_2 NTs – via either chelating or bidentate binding modes (or both). Owing to the sensitization effect, the photocurrents were acquired for PEC immunoassay.

Similarly, Dong et al. (2020) modified the indium tin oxide-polyethylene terephthalate (ITO-PET) electrode with Bi_2Se_3 and the flower-like $ZnIn_2S_4$ nanospheres (ZIS). The latter was synthesized by a solvothermal method, which accelerated the electronic transition and improved the photocurrent conversion efficiency. Additionally, the cadmium selenide (CdSe) QDs, which modified Ab_2, were able to increase the photocurrent blocked by immunoaffinity binding. This resulted in a detection limit of 0.026 ng/mL of cTnI (Dong et al., 2020).

Gao et al. (2019) fabricated cellulose paper-based, single-crystalline, three-dimensional aloe like TiO_2 arrays (PSATs) as the electron transporting material. It was subsequently coupled with CdS to form PSATs/CdS to extend the solar spectrum response for cTnI detection (**Figure 3B**) (Gao et al., 2019). Single stranded DNAs (ssDNAs) that bound to cTnI specifically were coupled with positive-charged mesoporous silica nanoparticles (PMSNs). The complexes were prepared as the nanocarrier to entrap the Cu^{2+}, which was regarded as a signal quencher because of its reaction with CdS to form Cu_xS. After the formation of cTnI-ssDNAs complexes, Cu^{2+} formed Cu_xS, which decreased the photocurrent signal. This process was used to quantify the concentration of cTnI.

Despite the accomplishments of PEC assay in CVD diagnosis, PEC assay has some disadvantages, especially the inherent drawback of photoanodes. For example, the CdS photoanodes of PEC might have low charge separation and transfer efficiency. Notably, they are unstable in water upon illumination as well.

Electrical and Reduction

Electrochemical (EC) immunoassay has attracted considerable attention and is one of the most promising techniques for diagnosis owing to its high sensitivity and fast response time. Besides that, nanomaterials are highly appreciated for improving EC sensitivity and intensity because of their catalytic property, conductivity, binding affinity, and large surface area. Like, AuNPs can bind biomolecules and facilitate electron transfer for catalyzing electrochemical reactions (Zhang et al., 2014). Besides, nanosheets and other hollow-structured nanomaterials can increase the loading efficiency of agents on grounds of their large surface area that enhances signal (Zhu et al., 2017).

Lopa et al. (2019) developed a AuNP modified titanium (Ti) metal substrate to detect cTnI based on DNA aptamer. AuNPs were deposited on Ti sheets by the potential-step deposition method. They immobilized the DNA aptamer using a self-assembled monolayer mechanism. The sensor obtained high sensitivity and specificity with the assistance of the AuNP-Ti layer and detected cTnI with the minimum detection limit of ca. 0.18 pM (Lopa et al., 2019).

Moreover, Adeel et al. (2019) modified the boron nitride nanosheets (BNNS) with AuNPs to detect MB in a low-cost, label-free and simple way (**Figure 4A**). BNNSs were synthesized via the hydrothermal method and were deposited on the fluorine-doped tin oxide (FTO) electrode. Subsequently, AuNPs were chemically deposited on the BNNS/FTO electrode. The AuNPs/BNNSs/FTO electrode was then used as a transducer to fix a thiol-functionalized DNA aptamer (Apt) via the Au-S covalent. When the MB bound to the sensor, [Fe(CN)6]3-/4- was used as a redox probe to monitor the oxidation current variation. The Apt/AuNPs/BNNSs/FTO sensor showed a high signal response for MB, with a detection limit of 34.6 ng/mL.

Phonklam et al. (2020) presented a molecularly imprinted polymer-based (MIP) EC sensor using a screen-printed carbon electrode (SPCE) to detect cTnT. The MIP sensor possessed an electrodeposited polymethylene blue (PMB) redox probe on SPCE, which was functionalized with multi-walled carbon nanotubes (MWCNTs). Also, the electropolymerized polyaniline was around the cTnT immobilized platform. The sensor response was stimulated by pulse voltammetry, wherein the concentration of cTnT was negatively associated with the PMB current. The linearity range of the sensor was between 0.10–8.0 pg/mL, with a detection limit of 0.040 pg/mL. Similarly, Vasantham et al. (2020) integrated MWCNT with Ab_2 to detect cTnI via paper-based multi-frequency impedimetric transducers. The limit of detection was 0.05 ng/mL, and the response time was ~1 min.

Singh et al. (2019) developed a microfluidic biosensor-integrated mesoporous nickel vanadate hollow-nanosphere modified chitosan (Ch-$Ni_3V_2O_8$) to detect cTnI in patient samples. They synthesized chitosan-based (Ch) $Ni_3V_2O_8$ hollow-nanospheres that could load abundant antibodies made possible by their hydroxy and amino clusters in the nanocomposite, their good adhesion capability, and their larger surface. Moreover, they amplified the electrochemical readouts because

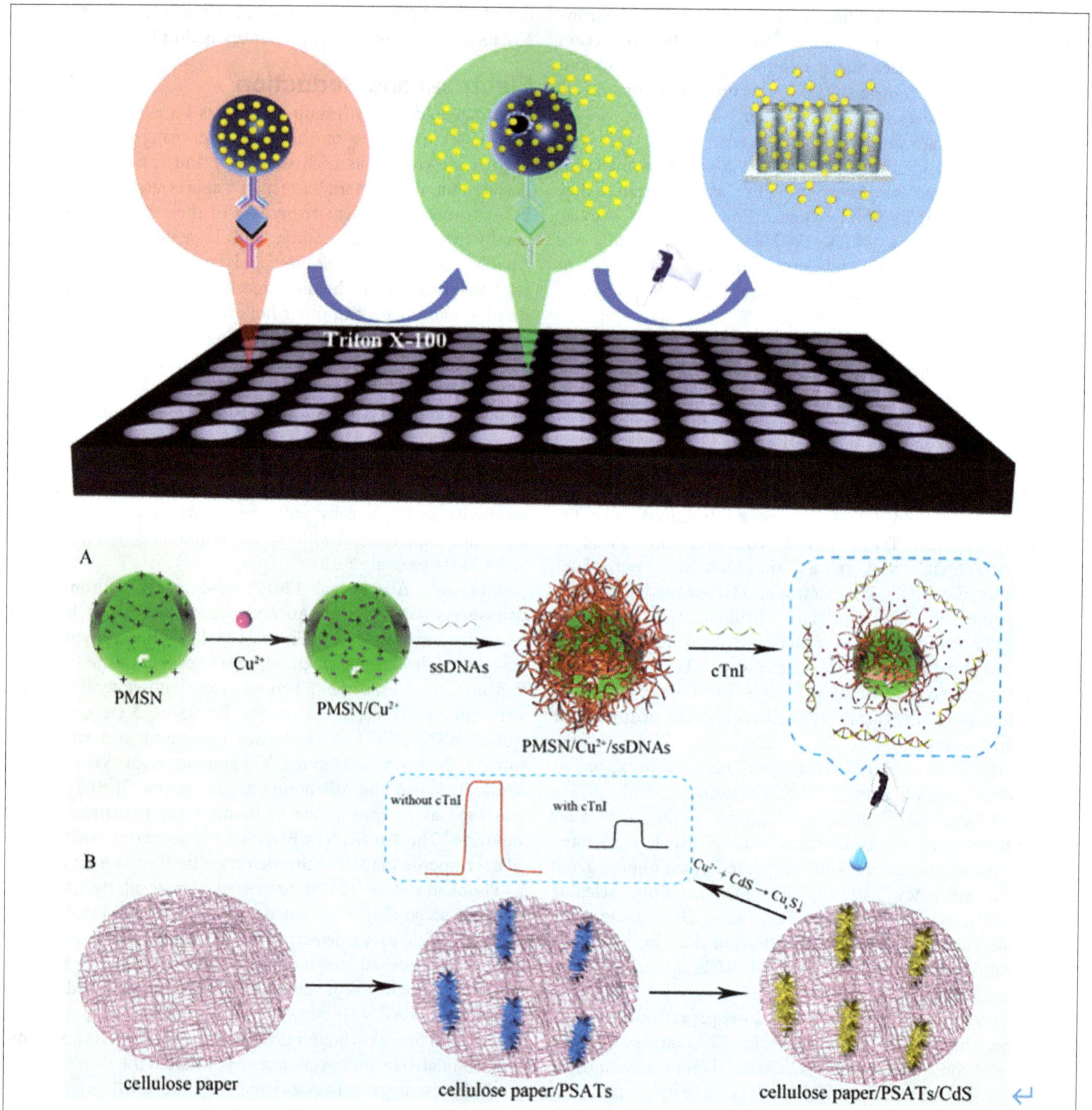

FIGURE 3 | (A) Scheme of the proposed liposomal PEC Immunoassay. Ab_1 were first loaded into 96-well plates, and then samples were incubated with Ab_1 for 1 h. The QDLL-Ab_2 was introduced after the immunorecognition of cTnI. Triton X-100 (10%) was introduced to release the QDs that were later captured by TiO_2-NTs electrode. The photocurrents were generated due to the sensitization effect (Xue et al., 2019). **(B)** Schematic principle of cTnI detection using PMSN/Cu2+/ssDNAs. Positive-charged PMSNs were added into Cu^{2+} solutions. Cu^{2+} entered the pores of PMSNs via diffusion. Later, ssDNAs bound cTnI specifically was added and attached on the surface of PMSNs. Once the cTnI was recognized by ssDNAs, the complexes reacted with CdS that was functionalized onto the PSATs, to form Cu_xS and diseased the photocurrent signal. The changes of photocurrent were correlated to the concentration of cTnI (Gao et al., 2019).

of tunable oxidation states of the Ch-$Ni_3V_2O_8$ matrix. The microfluidic biosensor was fabricated using a three-electrode system, including a patterned gold (Au), silver (Ag/AgCl), and Ch-$Ni_3V_2O_8$ electrodes on a glass substrate. A bare Au electrode represented as the counter electrode (CE). The Ch-$Ni_3V_2O_8$ composite was added on the Au-coated substrate to capture

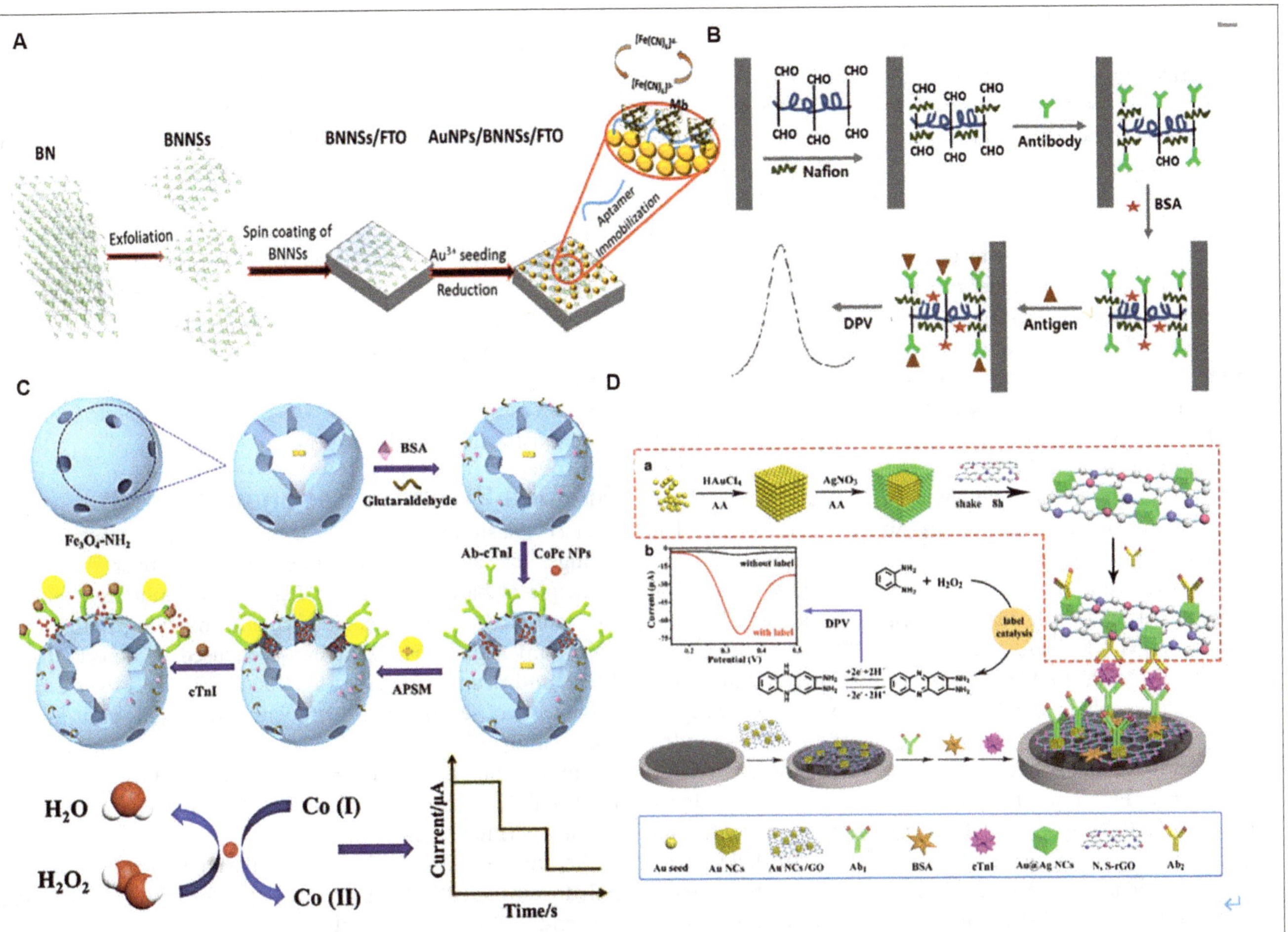

FIGURE 4 | (A) Schematic illustration for aptasensor fabrication and MB detection process. BNNSs were obtained from filtered BN powder dissolved solution via hydrothermal method. BNNSs were spinning deposited onto FTO electrode. AuNPs were then functionalized onto BNNS/FTO electrode to form AuNPs/BNNSs/FTO electrode acted a transducer to fix a thiol-functionalized DNA aptamer (Apt) via the Au-S covalent interaction. The [Fe(CN)6]3-/4- was used as a redox probe to monitor the oxidation current variation after MB binding to the Apt (Adeel et al., 2019). **(B)**. The illustration of electrochemical immunosensor. DIL was noncovalently non-covalently bonded with HCNTs to form the DIL-HCNTs composite, which provided sufficient binding sites for Ab1. After antigen was capture by Ab1, the sandwich immunocomplexes formed on the electrode hindered electron transfer thus decreased the peak current of DPV. The signals were corresponded to concentrations of cTnI (Shen et al., 2019). **(C)** The preparation procedure of the sandwich-type electrochemical immunosensor. Dispersed Fe_3O_4-NH_2 and glutaraldehyde was stirred to form Fe_3O_4-Ab_1, BSA was added to block remaining active sites on the surface of Fe_3O_4. CoPc NPs were first dispersed in the mesoporous of Fe_3O_4-Ab_1, then APSM was used to cap on the mesoporous of Fe_3O_4-Ab_1 by electrostatic interaction and formed APSM-capped CoPc NPs- Fe_3O_4-Ab_1. Once the target cTnI was captured, CoPC NPs were released after APSM was separated. The CoPC NPs oxidized the cobalt element from Co (I) to Co (II) with H_2O_2. The reduction current was corresponded to concentrations of cTnI (Ma et al., 2019). **(D)** The schematic diagrams of preparing Au@AgNC/N, S-rGO-Ab . Au solation was mixed with AA and AgNO3 in turn, then the Au@AgNC were collected using centrifugation. Later, Au@AgNC and S-rGO were reacted for 8 h for Au@AgNC and S-rGO composite. Ab_2 solution was added into Au@AgNC/N and S-rGO, and oscillated to form Au@AgNC/N, S-rGO-Ab_2. AuNC/GO immobilized Ab_1 via amino-Au affinity. Once cTnI was captured, the catalyzed-oxidation of o-phenylenediamine (o-PD) with H_2O_2 was accelerated. The oxidation generated 2,3-diaminophenazine that gained in electrons and hydrogen and generated a larger current signal of DPV at 0.34 V (Lv et al., 2019).

cTnI antibodies and connect the microchannels. Ag/AgCl was deposited on the substrate using e-beam evaporation for the reference electrode (RE). This device offered 5 pg/mL limit detection of cTnI with high stability, good selectivity, and high reproducibility, and detected BNP, MB, cardiac troponin C (cTnC), and cTnT with specific antigens (Singh et al., 2019).

Shen et al. (2019) presented a label-free electrochemical immunosensor using a helical carbon nanotube (HCNTs)-supported aldehyde-functionalized ionic liquid (DIL). The DIL-HCNTs provided binding sites for Ab_1, which simplified the sensor construction processes (**Figure 4B**) (Shen et al., 2019). The sandwich immunocomplexes influenced electron transfer on the electrode, thereby decreasing the peak current of differential pulse voltammetry (DPV). The signals corresponded to concentrations of cTnI.

Additionally, Sandil et al. (2019) immobilized cTnI (Ab_1) on tungsten trioxide nanorods (WO_3 NRs), which were deposited on indium tin oxide (ITO) using the electrophoretic deposition technique that worked as the electrode. The authors detected cTnI in a linear detection range of 0.01–10 ng/mL with high reproducibility (Sandil et al., 2019). Zhang et al. (2019) synthesized β-cyclodextrins-functionalized (CDs) 3D porous graphene-supported Pd@Au nanocubes (NCs) for cTnI detection. CDs were able to increase the dispersibility of the 3D-porous graphene and improve the capability of Ab_2 capture. Besides, the electrochemical signal was improving given the Pd@Au NCs. In addition, the amino-functionalized microporous carbon sphere was functionalized using AuNPs and Th (AuNPs-FMCS-Th) to immobilize Ab_1 effectively and accelerate the electron transfer process. The transfer was based on the reduction of H_2O_2 on the Th-modified electrode surface, which further amplified the signal response. The authors detected cTnI with a low detection limit of 33.3 fg/mL through the EC signal amplification labeling in the sandwich format (Zhang et al., 2019).

Similarly, Ma et al. (2019) utilized mesoporous Fe_3O_4-NH_2 for loading cobalt phthalocyanine NPs (CoPc NPs) and captured Ab_2 to form Fe_3O_4-Ab_1 to detect cTnI. The aminated polystyrene microsphere (APSM) was used to cap on the mesoporous of Fe_3O_4-Ab_1 by electrostatic interaction and presented as a molecular gate. Once the target cTnI was captured, CoPC NPs were released after APSM was separated. The CoPC NPs showed a superb catalytic performance that oxidized the cobalt element from Co (I) to Co (II) with the addition of H_2O_2. The reduction of current corresponded to concentrations of cTnI. This novel controlled release system-based EC immunoassay presented a broad linear range from 1.0 pg/mL to 100 ng/mL with a low detection limit of 0.39 pg/mL (**Figure 4C**) (Ma et al., 2019). Lv et al. (2019) functionalized the gold nanocube with graphene oxide (AuNC/GO) as the substrate to immobilize Ab_1 via amino-Au affinity. To detect cTnI, the authors utilized Au@Ag core–shell nanocubes and nitrogen/sulfur doped GO as signal amplification labels to conjugate with Ab_2 via Ag-N bonds. Once cTnI was captured, the catalyzed-oxidation of o-phenylenediamine (o-PD) with H_2O_2 was accelerated. The oxidation generated 2,3-diaminophenazine that gained in electrons and hydrogen and released an exaggerated current signal of DPV, which was used to electrochemical detect cTnI (**Figure 4D**) (Lv et al., 2019).

EC assay has shown advances in the sensitivity, but disadvantages remain. More specifically, the facility requires periodical calibration and care maintenance to guarantee accuracy, which is expensive and bothersome.

Surface-Enhanced Raman Scattering (SERS)

Surface-enhanced Raman scattering (SERS) immunoassay shows strong potential for CVD clinical diagnosis in view of their excellent multiplexing ability, high sensitivity, and large dynamic range (Huang et al., 2019). Typical SERS-based immunoassay uses substrates modified with Ab_1 to capture targets, and the concentration of the targets is quantified by the SERS immunoprobe (Wang et al., 2017c). Nanomaterials have simplified the preparation and attachment of Raman labels thus have improved the sensitivity. For example, Fu et al. (2019) developed a capture probe/target/SERS nanotags platform to detect cTnI. They functionalized graphene oxide (GO) with AuNPs, which acted as both SERS nanotags and signal amplification carriers. The GO/AuNP complexes provided strong SERS enhancement ability and detected cTnI with a 5 pg/mL detection limit (Fu et al., 2019). Similarly, Cheng et al. (2019) loaded targets and polyclonal-antibody-conjugated Au@Ag core–shell nanoparticles in a gold-patterned chip that ran as a SERS active template for the ultrasensitive detection of cTnI and CK-MB. The limits of detection were 8.9 pg/mL and 9.7 pg/mL for cTnI and CK-MB, respectively.

While large surface area and outstanding physical properties of nanomaterials have facilitated sensitive SERS immunoassays, additional work is required on stabilizing the tag functionalization in SERS assays.

Surface Plasmon Resonance (SPR)

Surface plasmon resonance (SPR) biosensor measures the changes of the refractive index at the sensor surface. Its principle is based on charge-density oscillation that exists at the interface of two media, normally involving a metal (i.e., gold) and a dielectric. SPR has been used to detect proteins, DNA, and drugs (Mullett et al., 2000). SPR sensors are mainly classified as sensors with angular wavelength and intensity modulation (Dudak and Boyaci, 2009). Nanomaterials with plasmonic and optical properties, good distributing ability, strong photostability have amplified signals, hence, improved SPR sensitivity (Liu et al., 2013).

Recently, Chen et al. (2019) modified Au film with AuNPs and polydopamine (PDA), which ran as platforms for immobilizing Ab_1 and SPR sensing. The films attracted the detection antibody on the PDA-coated Fe_3O_4 as the immune probe to detect cTnI (with a detection limit of 3.75 ng/mL) (Chen et al., 2019). The authors also introduced secondary antibody conjugated with multi-walled carbon nanotube (MWCNTs)-PDA-AgNPs to interact with cTnI exposed on the surface of probes, thus further amplifying the SPR response signal (**Figure 5A**).

Field Effect Transistor (FET)

Field effect transistor-based (FET) sensors have been applied in the biomedical analysis on grounds of their small size, high versatility, and low costs (Syedmoradi et al., 2019). FET-based sensors use an electric field to control the flow of current on platforms such as silicon nanowire and graphene (Kaisti, 2017).

Silicon nanoribbon fabricated biosensors are highly sensitive and uniform. However, they are expensive and complicated, requiring oxidation, photolithography, and wet etching. In contrast, semiconducting metal-oxide-based field-effect transistors (FET) biosensors show advantages, as simplicity and reliability. Photolithography-free shadow mask fabrication methods are also beneficial compared to silicon-based sensors. To give an example, Liu et al. developed a highly uniform, sensitive, and reusable In_2O_3 nanoribbon biosensor array using a lithography-free, scalable, and facile fabrication with high time efficiency (**Figure 5B**) (Liu Q. et al., 2016). The nanoribbons were formed through a first-layer shadow mask that was attached to a silicon substrate using In_2O_3 sputter-coating.

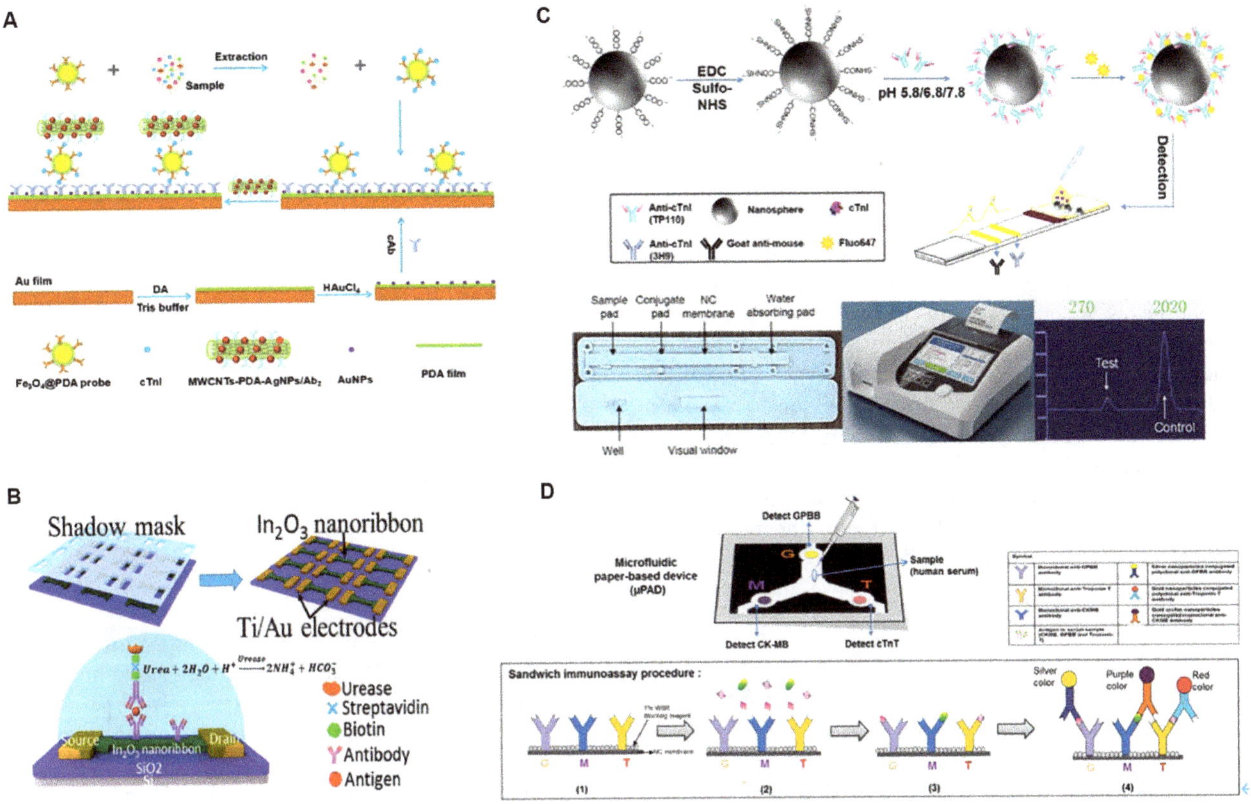

FIGURE 5 | (A) The schematic diagram of experimental procedure. A bare Au film with soaked into DA solution in Tris-buffer to form PDA-Au film. Afterward, AuNPs were deposited onto PDA-Au film with the help of $HAuCl_4$ to improve the sensitivity. After 30 min, Ab_1 was immobilized on the PDA-Au for further cTnI capture. As for detection probe, Fe_3O_4@PDA-detection antibody immune probe was collected with external magnet after Fe_3O_4@PDA and detection antibody were mixed and shake for 24 h. Then samples with different concentrations of cTnI were incubated with Fe_3O_4@PDA-detection antibody, and the nanoconjugates were collected by a magnet. Once the resonant wavelength of probes was stable, MWCNTS-PDA-AgNPs/secondary antibody was added to enhance SPR response signals (Chen et al., 2019). **(B)** Schematic of In O nanoribbon biosensor and electronic ELISA for cardiac biomarker detection. The first shadow mask was attached onto the SiO2/Si wafer, and then In_2O_3 ribbons were deposited using radio frequency (RF). Nanoribbons were obtained after removing first-layer shadow mask. A second shadow mask was attached to define the Ti/Au disposition, which used e-beam evaporation. Finally, a FET-based sensor was completed after removing shadow mask. Captured antibodies were fixed on the In_2O_3 surface and captured the biomarkers. Biomarkers were fixed between the capture antibody and a biotinylated secondary antibody that is specific to biomarkers. The biotin tales of the secondary antibody was to capture streptavidin, which bound to a biotinylated urease that led to deprotonation the hydroxyl groups on the nanoribbon and increased the negative surface charges. The change of surface charge was detected by FET sensor because negative charges decreased the conduction of nanoribbons (Liu Q. et al., 2016).
(C) Schematic representation of the preparation of antibody-modified nanoprobes involved in the lateral flow immunoassay. Carboxylated Nanospheres (CNs) were incubated with *N*-(3-dimethylaminopropyl)-*N'*-ethylcarbodiimide hydrochloride crystalline (EDC) and *N*-hydroxysulfosuccinimide sodium salt (sulfo-NHS), the mixtures were collected centrifugation. TP110 (detection antibody) was incubated with CNs at 5.8, 6.8, or 7.8 pH. Florescent molecules were conjugated with CNs-TP110 for later detection on LFA. Briefly, sample flowed through sample pad, and conjugated with fluorescent labeled CNs-TP110 on the conjugate pad. The complexes went through NC membrane that immobilized Ab1 (3H9) on the test line and Goat anti-mouse on the control line for further antigen capture. The strip was read by a fluorescent analyzer after 15 min (Lou et al., 2019b). **(D)** Scheme of fabrication of the microfluidic paper-based device (μPAD) for multiplex detection of cardiac markers. Capture antibodies were immobilized onto NC membrane at three positions (G for GPBB, M for CK-MB, and T for troponin T). Serum sample was added at central sample zone. After antibody-antigen capture, AuNPs conjugated anti-cTnT (red), silver-nanoparticles (AgNPs) conjugated anti-GPBB (yellow) and Gold urchin nanoparticles conjugated anti-CKMB (purple) were added for color detection (Lim et al., 2019).

The nanoribbons went through a metal electrode deposition process that was defined by a second-layer shadow mask. Two shadow masks were simply removed instead of being lifted off, as in the case in photolithography. Captured antibodies were fixed on the In_2O_3 surface using *N*-(3-dimethylaminopropyl)-*N'*-ethylcarbodiimide hydrochloride/*N*-hydroxysuccinimide (EDC/NHS) chemistry. A biotinylated secondary antibody was introduced to attach biomarkers, and its biotin tales were bounded to the streptavidin that attracted biotinylated urease later. Urea increased the pH of the solution, hence, causing the deprotonation of hydroxyl groups on the nanoribbon and lowering surface potential. Consequently, the conduction of the n-type nanoribbon FETs was decreased due to increased negative surface charges. They detected cTnI, CK-MB, and BNP down to 1 pg/mL, 0.1 ng/mL, and 10 pg/mL concentration range, respectively.

Enzyme-Linked Immunosorbent Assay (ELISA)

Enzyme-Linked Immunosorbent Assay (ELISA) is a commercialized method that identifies the concentration of targets through the color change of antigen-antibody reactions using an enzyme-linked conjugate and enzyme substrate. Even though ELISA shows advantages in reading results, it still requires more effort to improve sensitivity and accuracy (Aydin, 2015). Unique physical properties and biocompatibility of nanomaterials have greatly improved the performance of ELISA and below lateral flow assay (LFA). Nanofibers have the potential to reduce non-specific binding and improve binding efficiency due to their large surface area as an illustration. In addition, AuNPs conjugated with functional materials, such as HRP could amplify the detection signal in the assay (Wang W. et al., 2018).

Recently, Jiao et al. (2019) completed a multimodal ELISA diagnosis based on photothermal effect and the peroxidase-mimicking property in Au@Pt nanodendrites. The cTnI target was quantified using photothermal, colorimetric, and ratiometric fluorescent signals simultaneously.

Paper Based Lateral Flow Assay (LFA)

Lateral flow assay detects targets in a fast, simple, and cheap manner that has attracted much interests in recent years (Koczula and Gallotta, 2016). Lou et al. (2019a) functionalized the LFA with a multi-layer structure, including the BSA layer to increase biotinylation sites, a streptavidin layer loaded with a fluorescent dye, and an outermost layer on which the biotinylated antibody is bounded to the streptavidin. Due to the high loading efficiency of fluorescent molecules, the authors detected the cTnI within the range of 0.049–50 ng/mL (Lou et al., 2019a). Recently, Lou et al. (2019b) conjugated Ab_2 onto polystyrene nanospheres at pH 5.8 for fast and sensitive immunodetection. At pH 5.8, the tail-on orientated antibodies (TP110) were conjugated on the carboxylated nanospheres (CNs) because of the charge distribution and the hydrophobic area of antibodies. As a result, the loading capacity of TP110 was increased, thus the authors detected cTnI with high sensitivity. The detailed procedure was illustrated in **Figure 5C**. Lim et al. (2019) utilized AuNPs conjugated anti-cTnT, silver-nanoparticles (AgNPs) conjugated anti-GPBB, and Gold urchin nanoparticles conjugated anti-CKMB as probes to detect multiplexed biomarkers simultaneously. The serum sample was loaded on the central sample pad and flowed through the NC membrane where anti-GPBB, anti-CK-MB, and anti-cTnT were immobilized on at three positions. Nanoparticles-conjugated detection antibodies were added on the NC membrane for color detection in the end. The detailed illustration was in **Figure 5D** (Lim et al., 2019).

Despite the convenience of ELISA and LFA in analyzing biomolecules, they have some drawbacks. ELISA suffers from complicated procedures, long assay duration (at least 2–3 h), and large sample consumptions. LFA requires labor-intensive preparations and is highly susceptible to false positives/negatives due to improper operations.

NANOTECHNOLOGY-BASED MOI

Nanomaterials with good bioavailability and versatility have increased the accuracy and specificity of clinical MOI applications thanks to improved resolution, signal amplification, and simple manipulation. Among other nanomaterials, nanoparticles are suitable for MOI since their mobilities in both internal and external vascular systems, high surface area to volume ratio, and imaging functionality. These advantages allow them to circulate through human bodies with low restrictions and produce functional imaging vehicles as contrast agents when they are applied in MOI settings, which leads to significantly improved diagnosis efficiency.

Nanoparticles can be used for RNA detection in intravascular systems because of their mobility. Injected or swallowed nanoparticles that are functionalized with MOI detectable molecules can circulate through the human body and target specific RNA for diagnosis. However, the size, shape, morphology, and density of functionalized nanoparticles should be explored carefully since the RNA detection requires nanoparticles entering and interacting with cells.

In addition, nanoparticles can work as nanoscale contrast agents by incorporating materials such as photoacoustic, fluorescent, radioactive, paramagnetic, superparamagnetic, electron-dense, light-scattering particles, and multimodal functional groups that are detectable by MOI.

The fluorescent material is a popular choice to conjugate with nanoparticles. For example, fluorescence labeled quantum dots (QDs) exhibit good performance in atherosclerotic plagues imaging (Jaffer et al., 2007). Popular radionuclides, including ^{18}F, ^{64}Cu, ^{68}Ga, ^{124}I, ^{86}Y, have been conjugated with QDs, UCNPs, AuNPs, and NCs and have demonstrated good diagnostic functions (Saraste et al., 2009). For instance, radiolabeled nanoparticles play significant roles for atherosclerotic plagues under PET (Dobrucki and Sinusas, 2010). Radionuclides can be labeled either on the surface or encapsulated inside nanoparticles.

Additionally, superparamagnetic nanoparticles, like iron oxide (IO) nanoparticles and predominately magnetite (Fe_2O_3/Fe_3O_4), can improve the sensitivity of MRI by providing dark contrast to enhance the signal. For instance, MRI can detect thrombus (Chen and Wu, 2011), and the composition of plaques, including the fibrous cap and necrotic core, macrophage content, plaque neovascularization, intraplaque hemorrhage, and mural thrombus using superparamagnetic nanoparticles as contrasts (Avelar et al., 2017).

Also, AuNPs with good optical properties are good signal enhancers for photoacoustic tomography (PAT) (Taruttis et al., 2010). For example, Pan et al. (2014) successfully detected thrombus using gold nanobeacons under PAT. AuNPs can enhance the signal of coherence tomography (OCT) based on light-scattering as well.

Moreover, AuNPs were also widely used in CT as contrast agents. Hyafil et al. (2007) identified macrophages in atherosclerotic plagues using iodinated AuNPs facilitated CT. Kim et al. (2012) used polyethylene glycol (PEG)-coated AuNPs to improve the performance of CT scanning. They utilized PEG-coated GNPs as a contrast agent, in which the PEG-coating prevented antibiofouling and extended lifetime of AuNPs in the bloodstream. The PEG-coated GNPs obtained a better X-ray absorption coefficient and thus provided high-resolution images.

CONCLUSION AND FUTURE PERSPECTIVE

Current clinical challenges of CVDs include generating straightforward, accurate diagnostic clinical decisions, and monitoring drug responses frequently. To overcome these difficulties, various platforms have been proposed. Among these platforms, CIAs have gained attraction since they can measure and evaluate the expression of biomarkers for the prediction and diagnosis of disease in a sensitive, rapid, cheap, and non-invasive manner. Additionally, MOI settings have emerged as promising techniques for CVD diagnosis thanks to their excellent imaging capabilities that facilitate physicians to make decisions. Even though significant advances in CIAs and MOI have been made regarding CVD diagnosis, the early-stage diagnosis is still challenging since symptoms of early-stage CVDs are vague, and the expression level of cardiac biomarkers at early-stage is relatively low for detection.

Therefore, novel platforms with improved sensitivity and specificity are required. As summarized in this review, nanotechnology has greatly contributed to the developments of MOI and CIA on account of its specific physicochemical properties. By virtue of their excellent biocompatibility, nanomaterials can conjugate with various biomolecules because their excellent biocompatibility. These functional biomolecules were able to increase the sensitivity and specificity of diagnostic platforms. For example, AuNP-conjugated capture antibody can reduce non-specific bindings, thereby increasing the capture specificity and eliminating background noises in various CIAs. Besides, fluorescence lumiphore conjugated nanomaterials can work as enhancers to amplify the detective signals in ELISA, or as contrast agents in MOI. In addition, except for functionalized with other biomolecules, nanomaterial itself can serve as a signal enhancer. This is made possible by their unique optical, electrical and plasmonic properties, silica NPs can quench photocurrent effectively in PEC biosensors as an example. Moreover, nanomaterials with a large surface area (e.g., nanocubes) can improve the loading efficiency of biomolecules to increase the sensitivity of CIAs. To better elucidate CIAs in CVD diagnosis, the lasted outcomes of nanotechnology assisted CIAs (e.g., ECL) was introduced, with comparison to the sensitivity and detection range of cardiac targets among these assays. We also reviewed the clinical applications of nanoparticles in MOI settings. In this regard, we believe strongly bridging clinical platforms and nanotechnology is necessary for directing future research plans.

In this review, we have highlighted the advantages of CIAs. They are non-invasive, cheap, sensitivity, and convenient. Its repeat-sampling ability also makes it ideal for long-term diagnosis and prognosis. However, the CIA testing still faces challenges. An important concern is the sensitivity and specificity of the biomarker. Previous researchers have shown that a single marker may be insufficient, lack sensitivity and specificity for accurate CVD diagnosis. It is unrealistic to provide clear diagnosis results using only one biomarker owing to the complexity, heterogeneity and diversity of pathogenesis in different populations. Additionally, biomarkers may be regulated differently during the development of pathologies. Consequently, even though we can diagnosis some clinical subjects who have high risks for certain diseases using biomarkers (e.g., cTnI for AMI), we have insufficient information on the progression and states of the diseases (Madhurantakam et al., 2018). To solve this problem, multiplexed biomarker panels are critical. The multiplexed analysis of various biomarkers can establish correlations (or scores) with high specificities and predictive values, as a result, can improve the accuracy of diagnostic decisions. Hence, the fabrication of CIAs should focus on multiplexed analysis in the future. In addition, current findings on biomarkers are based on relatively small samples, which may possess large variations (Sayed et al., 2014). Most of the studies only focused on the correlation between biomarker expression level and single disease. The pathological significance behind the biomarker expression level changing is not addressed yet. As such, large-scale and systematic clinical studies are needed to recognize and better understand the mechanisms of biomarkers. Most importantly, combination with advanced analytic tools (e.g., machine learning) that is capable of developing objective and automatic algorithms to analyze large-scale and high-dimensional-multiplexed data should be highlighted in future studies, which are supposed to greatly improve the efficiency and accuracy of diagnosis.

AUTHOR CONTRIBUTIONS

ZY and JZ coordinated this project. CS and HX wrote this manuscript. CS and HX collected and summarized the literatures. YM edited the figures in this manuscript and revised this manuscript.

REFERENCES

Abdorahim, M., Rabiee, M., Alhosseini, S. N., Tahriri, M., Yazdanpanah, S., Alavi, S. H., et al. (2016). Nanomaterials-based electrochemical immunosensors for cardiac troponin recognition: an illustrated review. *TrAC Trends Anal. Chem.* 82, 337–347. doi: 10.1016/j.trac.2016.06.015

Adeel, M., Rahman, M. M., and Lee, J. J. (2019). Label-free aptasensor for the detection of cardiac biomarker myoglobin based on gold nanoparticles decorated boron nitride nanosheets. *Biosens. Bioelectron.* 126, 143–150. doi: 10.1016/j.bios.2018.10.060

Adhikari, J., Keasberry, N. A., Mahadi, A. H., Yoshikawa, H., Tamiya, E., and Ahmed, M. U. (2019). An ultra-sensitive label-free electrochemiluminescence CKMB immunosensor using a novel nanocomposite-modified printed electrode. *RSC Adv.* 9, 34283–34292. doi: 10.1039/c9ra05016g

Ali, M., Sajid, M., Khalid, M. A. U., Kim, S. W., Lim, J. H., Huh, D., et al. (2020). A fluorescent lateral flow biosensor for the quantitative detection of Vaspin using upconverting nanoparticles. *Spectrochim. Acta Part A Mol. Biomol. Spectrosc.* 226:117610. doi: 10.1016/j.saa.2019.117610

Anderon, L. (2005). Candidate-based proteomics in the search for biomarkers of cardiovascular disease. *J. Physiol.* 563(Pt 1), 23–60. doi: 10.1113/jphysiol.2004.080473

Anderson, T. J., Grégoire, J., Hegele, R. A., Couture, P., Mancini, G. B. J., McPherson, R., et al. (2013). 2012 update of the canadian cardiovascular society guidelines for the diagnosis and treatment of dyslipidemia for the prevention of cardiovascular disease in the adult. *Can. J. Cardiol.* 29, 151–167. doi: 10.1016/j.cjca.2012.11.032

Apple, F. S., Falahati, A., Paulsen, P. R., Miller, E. A., and Sharkey, S. W. (1997). Improved detection of minor ischemic myocardial injury with measurement of serum cardiac troponin I. *Clin. Chem.* 43, 2047–2051. doi: 10.1093/clinchem/43.11.2047

Article, E. (2018). CT SCAN. *Diagn. Radiol. Radiother.* 1, 162–169. doi: 10.22328/2079-5343-2018-9-1-162-169

Avelar, E., Strickland, C. R., and Rosito, G. (2017). Role of imaging in cardio-oncology. *Curr. Treat. Options Cardiovasc. Med.* 19:46. doi: 10.1007/s11936-017-0546-2

Aydin, S. (2015). A short history, principles, and types of ELISA, and our laboratory experience with peptide/protein analyses using ELISA. *Peptides* 72, 4–15. doi: 10.1016/j.peptides.2015.04.012

Bang, C., Batkai, S., Dangwal, S., Gupta, S. K., Foinquinos, A., Holzmann, A., et al. (2014). Cardiac fibroblast-derived microRNA passenger strand-enriched exosomes mediate cardiomyocyte hypertrophy. *J. Clin. Invest.* 124, 2136–2146. doi: 10.1172/JCI70577

Chakrabarti, S., Wu, X., Yang, Z., Wu, L., Yong, S. L., Zhang, C., et al. (2013). MOG1 rescues defective trafficking of nav1.5 mutations in brugada syndrome and sick sinus syndrome. *Circ. Arrhythmia Electrophysiol.* 6, 392–401. doi: 10.1161/CIRCEP.111.000206

Chen, F., Wu, Q., Song, D., Wang, X., Ma, P., and Sun, Y. (2019). Fe 3 O 4 @PDA immune probe-based signal amplification in surface plasmon resonance (SPR) biosensing of human cardiac troponin I. *Colloids Surf. B Biointerfaces.* 177, 105–111. doi: 10.1016/j.colsurfb.2019.01.053

Chen, I. Y., and Wu, J. C. (2011). Cardiovascular molecular imaging: focus on clinical translation. *Circulation* 123, 425–443. doi: 10.1161/CIRCULATIONAHA.109.916338

Chen, Y., Song, Y., Huang, J., Qu, M., Zhang, Y., Geng, J., et al. (2017). Increased circulating exosomal miRNA-223 is associated with acute ischemic stroke. *Front. Neurol.* 8:57. doi: 10.3389/fneur.2017.00057

Chen, Z., Zhang, A., Wang, X., Zhu, J., Fan, Y., Yu, H., et al. (2017). The advances of carbon nanotubes in cancer diagnostics and therapeutics. *J. Nanomater.* 2017:3418932. doi: 10.1155/2017/3418932

Cheng, Y., Wang, X., Yang, J., Duan, X., Yao, Y., Shi, X., et al. (2012). A translational study of urine miRNAs in acute myocardial infarction. *J. Mol. Cell. Cardiol.* 53, 668–676. doi: 10.1016/j.yjmcc.2012.08.010

Cheng, Z., Wang, R., Xing, Y., Zhao, L., Choo, J., and Yu, F. (2019). SERS-based immunoassay using gold-patterned array chips for rapid and sensitive detection of dual cardiac biomarkers. *Analyst* 144, 6533–6540. doi: 10.1039/c9an01260e

Christenson, E., and Christenson, R. H. (2013). The role of cardiac biomarkers in the diagnosis and management of patients presenting with suspected acute coronary syndrome. *Ann. Lab. Med.* 33, 309–318. doi: 10.3343/alm.2013.33.5.309

Corsten, M. F., Dennert, R., Jochems, S., Kuznetsova, T., Devaux, Y., Hofstra, L., et al. (2010). Circulating MicroRNA-208b and MicroRNA-499 reflect myocardial damage in cardiovascular disease. *Circ. Cardiovasc. Genet.* 3, 499–506. doi: 10.1161/CIRCGENETICS.110.957415

D'Agostino, R. B., Vasan, R. S., Pencina, M. J., Wolf, P. A., Cobain, M., Massaro, J. M., et al. (2008). General cardiovascular risk profile for use in primary care: the Framingham heart study. *Circulation.* 117, 743–753. doi: 10.1161/CIRCULATIONAHA.107.699579

de Jong, O. G., Verhaar, M. C., Chen, Y., Vader, P., Gremmels, H., Posthuma, G., et al. (2012). Cellular stress conditions are reflected in the protein and RNA content of endothelial cell-derived exosomes. *J. Extracell. Vesicles* 1:18396. doi: 10.3402/jev.v1i0.18396

Devaux, Y., Vausort, M., McCann, G. P., Kelly, D., Collignon, O., Ng, L. L., et al. (2013). A panel of 4 microRNAs Facilitates the prediction of left ventricular contractility after acute myocardial infarction. *PLoS One* 8:e70644. doi: 10.1371/journal.pone.0070644

Dobrucki, L. W., and Sinusas, A. J. (2010). PET and SPECT in cardiovascular molecular imaging. *Nat. Rev. Cardiol.* 7, 38–47. doi: 10.1038/nrcardio.2009.201

Dong, W., Mo, X., Wang, Y., Lei, Q., and Li, H. (2020). Photoelectrochemical immunosensor based on ZnIn2S4/Bi2Se3 nanocomposite for the determination of cardiac troponin I. *Anal. Lett.* doi: 10.1080/00032719.2020.1721003

Dong, X., Zhao, G., Li, X., Miao, J. C., Fang, J., Wei, Q., et al. (2019). Electrochemiluminescence immunoassay for the N-terminal pro-B-type natriuretic peptide based on resonance energy transfer between a self-enhanced luminophore composed of silver nanocubes on gold nanoparticles and a metal-organic framework of type MIL-125. *Microchim. Acta* 186:811. doi: 10.1007/s00604-019-3969-5

Dudak, F. C., and Boyaci, I. H. (2009). Rapid and label-free bacteria detection by surface plasmon resonance (SPR) biosensors. *Biotechnol. J.* 4, 1003–1011. doi: 10.1002/biot.200800316

Durrani-Kolarik, S., Pool, C. A., Gray, A., Heyob, K. M., Cismowski, M. J., Pryhuber, G., et al. (2017). miR-29b supplementation decreases expression of matrix proteins and improves alveolarization in mice exposed to maternal inflammation and neonatal hyperoxia. *Am. J. Physiol. Lung Cell. Mol. Physiol.* 313, L339–L349. doi: 10.1152/ajplung.00273.2016

Ellis, K. L., Cameron, V. A., Troughton, R. W., Frampton, C. M., Ellmers, L. J., and Richards, A. M. (2013). Circulating microRNAs as candidate markers to distinguish heart failure in breathless patients. *Eur. J. Heart Fail.* 15, 1138–1147. doi: 10.1093/eurjhf/hft078

Fan, C., Tang, Y., Zhao, M., Lou, X., Pretorius, D., Menasche, P., et al. (2020a). CHIR99021 and fibroblast growth factor 1 enhance the regenerative potency of human cardiac muscle patch after myocardial infarction in mice. *J. Mol. Cell. Cardiol.* 141, 1–10. doi: 10.1016/j.yjmcc.2020.03.003

Fan, C., Zhang, E., Joshi, J., Yang, J., Zhang, J., and Zhu, W. (2020b). Utilization of human induced pluripotent stem cells for cardiac repair. *Front. Cell Dev. Biol.* 8:36. doi: 10.3389/fcell.2020.00036

Feng, Q. M., Shen, Y. Z., Li, M. X., Zhang, Z. L., Zhao, W., Xu, J. J., et al. (2016). Dual-wavelength electrochemiluminescence ratiometry based on resonance energy transfer between au nanoparticles functionalized g-C3N4 Nanosheet and Ru(bpy)32+ for microRNA Detection. *Anal. Chem.* 88, 937–944. doi: 10.1021/acs.analchem.5b03670

Fesmire, F. M., Percy, R. F., Bardoner, J. B., Wharton, D. R., and Calhoun, F. B. (1998). Usefulness of automated serial 12-lead ECG monitoring during the initial emergency department evaluation of patients with chest pain. *Ann. Emerg. Med.* 31, 3–11. doi: 10.1016/S0196-0644(98)70274-4

Friese, R. S., Altshuler, A. E., Zhang, K., Miramontes-Gonzalez, J. P., Hightower, C. M., Jirout, M. L., et al. (2013). MicroRNA-22 and promoter motif polymorphisms at the Chga locus in genetic hypertension: functional andtherapeutic implications forgeneexpressionand the pathogenesis of hypertension. *Hum. Mol. Genet.* 22, 3624–3640. doi: 10.1093/hmg/ddt213

Fu, X., Wang, Y., Liu, Y., Liu, H., Fu, L., Wen, J., et al. (2019). A graphene oxide/gold nanoparticle-based amplification method for SERS immunoassay of cardiac troponin I. *Analyst* 144, 1582–1589. doi: 10.1039/c8an02022a

Gan, C. S., Wang, C. W., and Tan, K. S. (2012). Circulatory microRNA-145 expression is increased in cerebral ischemia. *Genet. Mol. Res.* 11, 147–152. doi: 10.4238/2012.January.27.1

Gao, C., Xue, J., Zhang, L., Zhao, P., Cui, K., Ge, S., et al. (2019). Paper based modification-free photoelectrochemical sensing platform with single-crystalline aloe like TiO 2 as electron transporting material for cTnI detection. *Biosens. Bioelectron.* 131, 17–23. doi: 10.1016/j.bios.2019.01.038

Gidlöf, O., Andersson, P., Van Der Pals, J., Götberg, M., and Erlinge, D. (2011). Cardiospecific microRNA plasma levels correlate with troponin and cardiac function in patients with ST elevation myocardial infarction, are selectively dependent on renal elimination, and can be detected in urine samples. *Cardiology.* 118, 217–226. doi: 10.1159/000328869

Golberg, D., Bando, Y., Huang, Y., Terao, T., Mitome, M., Tang, C., et al. (2010). Boron nitride nanotubes and nanosheets. *ACS Nano* 4, 2979–2993. doi: 10.1021/nn1006495

Goren, Y., Kushnir, M., Zafrir, B., Tabak, S., Lewis, B. S., and Amir, O. (2012). Serum levels of microRNAs in patients with heart failure. *Eur. J. Heart Fail.* 14, 147–154. doi: 10.1093/eurjhf/hfr155

Govindappa, P. K., Patil, M., Garikipati, V. N. S., Verma, S. K., Saheera, S., Narasimhan, G., et al. (2020). Targeting exosome-associated human antigen R attenuates fibrosis and inflammation in diabetic heart. *FASEB J.* 34, 2238–2251. doi: 10.1096/fj.201901995R

Guo, X., Zong, L., Jiao, Y., Han, Y., Zhang, X., Xu, J., et al. (2019). Signal-enhanced detection of multiplexed cardiac biomarkers by a paper-based fluorogenic immunodevice integrated with zinc oxide nanowires. *Anal. Chem.* 91, 9300–9307. doi: 10.1021/acs.analchem.9b02557

Haase, M., and Schäfer, H. (2011). Upconverting nanoparticles. *Angew. Chem. Int. Ed Engl.* 50, 5808–5829. doi: 10.1002/anie.201005159

Han, G. R., and Kim, M. G. (2019). Design, synthesis, and evaluation of gold nanoparticle-antibody-horseradish peroxidase conjugates for highly sensitive chemiluminescence immunoassay (hs-CLIA). *Biotechnol. Bioprocess. Eng.* 24, 206–214. doi: 10.1007/s12257-018-0369-3

Hao, N., Li, X. L., Zhang, H. R., Xu, J. J., and Chen, H. Y. (2014). A highly sensitive ratiometric electrochemiluminescent biosensor for microRNA detection based on cyclic enzyme amplification and resonance energy transfer. *Chem. Commun.* 50, 14828–14830. doi: 10.1039/c4cc06801g

Hashemi, R. H., Bradley, W. G., and Lisanti, C. J. (2012). *MRI: The Basics.* Philadelphia, PA: Lippincott Williams & Wilkins.

Ho, K. J. (2018). "Cardiovascular diseases," in *Nutritional Aspects of Aging*, Vol. 2, ed. L. H. Chen (Boca Raton, FL: CRC Press), doi: 10.1201/9781351075145

Homola, J., Yee, S. S., and Gauglitz, G. (1999). Surface plasmon resonance sensors: review. *Sens. Actuat. B Chem.* 54, 3–15. doi: 10.1016/S0925-4005(98)00321-9

Huang, Z., Zhang, A., Zhang, Q., and Cui, D. (2019). Nanomaterial-based SERS sensing technology for biomedical application. *J. Mater. Chem. B* 7, 3755–3774. doi: 10.1039/c9tb00666d

Hur, J., Kim, Y. J., Lee, H. J., Nam, J. E., Ha, J. W., Heo, J. H., et al. (2011). Dual-enhanced cardiac CT for detection of left atrial appendage thrombus in patients with stroke?: a prospective comparison study with transesophageal echocardiography. *Stroke* 42, 2471–2477. doi: 10.1161/STROKEAHA.110.611293

Hur, J., Kim, Y. J., Lee, H. J., Nam, J. E., Hong, J., Kim, H. Y., et al. (2012). Cardioembolic stroke: dual-energy cardiac CT for differentiation of left atrial appendage thrombus and circulatory stasis. *Radiology* 263, 688–695. doi: 10.1148/radiol.12111691

Hutton, B. F. (2014). The origins of SPECT and SPECT/CT. *Eur. J. Nucl. Med. Mol. Imaging.* 41(Suppl. 1), S3–S16. doi: 10.1007/s00259-013-2606-5

Hyafil, F., Cornily, J. C., Feig, J. E., Gordon, R., Vucic, E., Amirbekian, V., et al. (2007). Noninvasive detection of macrophages using a nanoparticulate contrast agent for computed tomography. *Nat. Med.* 13, 636–641. doi: 10.1038/nm1571

Jaffer, F. A., Libby, P., and Weissleder, R. (2007). Molecular imaging of cardiovascular disease. *Circulation* 116, 1052–1061. doi: 10.1161/CIRCULATIONAHA.106.647164

Ji, T., Xu, X., Wang, X., Zhou, Q., Ding, W., Chen, B., et al. (2019). Point of care upconversion nanoparticles-based lateral flow assay quantifying myoglobin in clinical human blood samples. *Sens. Actuat. B Chem.* 281, 309–316. doi: 10.1016/j.snb.2018.11.074

Ji, X., Takahashi, R., Hiura, Y., Hirokawa, G., Fukushima, Y., and Iwai, N. (2009). Plasma miR-208 as a biomarker of myocardial injury. *Clin. Chem.* 55, 1944–1949. doi: 10.1373/clinchem.2009.125310

Jiao, L., Zhang, L., Du, W., Li, H., Yang, D., and Zhu, C. (2019). Au@Pt nanodendrites enhanced multimodal enzyme-linked immunosorbent assay. *Nanoscale* 11, 8798–8802. doi: 10.1039/c8nr08741e

Jo, H., Gu, H., Jeon, W., Youn, H., Her, J., Kim, S. K., et al. (2015). Electrochemical aptasensor of cardiac Troponin I for the early diagnosis of acute myocardial infarction. *Anal. Chem.* 87, 9869–9875. doi: 10.1021/acs.analchem.5b02312

Johnson, S. (2012). "Nanotechnology," in *Encyclopedia of Applied Ethics*, ed. R. Chadwick (San Diego, CA: Academic Press).

Joshi, J., Rubart, M., and Zhu, W. (2020). Optogenetics: background, methodological advances and potential applications for cardiovascular research and medicine. *Front. Bioeng. Biotechnol.* 7:466. doi: 10.3389/fbioe.2019.00466

Kaisti, M. (2017). Detection principles of biological and chemical FET sensors. *Biosens. Bioelectron.* 98, 437–448. doi: 10.1016/j.bios.2017.07.010

Kim, S. H., Kim, E. M., Lee, C. M., Kim, D. W., Lim, S. T., Sohn, M. H., et al. (2012). Synthesis of PEG-iodine-capped gold nanoparticles and their contrast enhancement in in vitro and in vivo for X-ray/CT. *J. Nanomater.* 2012:504026. doi: 10.1155/2012/504026

Kirkpatrick, I. D. C., Kroeker, M. A., and Greenberg, H. M. (2003). Biphasic CT with mesenteric CT angiography in the evaluation of acute mesenteric ischemia: initial experience. *Radiology* 229, 91–98. doi: 10.1148/radiol.2291020991

Koczula, K. M., and Gallotta, A. (2016). Lateral flow assays. *Essays Biochem.* 60, 111–120. doi: 10.1042/EBC20150012

Kong, J., Franklin, N. R., Zhou, C., Chapline, M. G., Peng, S., Cho, K., et al. (2000). Nanotube molecular wires as chemical sensors. *Science* 287, 622–625. doi: 10.1126/science.287.5453.622

Korff, S., Katus, H. A., and Giannitsis, E. (2006). Differential diagnosis of elevated troponins. *Heart* 92, 987–993. doi: 10.1136/hrt.2005.071282

Kuriyama, R., Tanaka, Y., Akiyama, S., and Sato, Y. (2011). "Effect of electric double layer on near-wall ph in microfluidic device measured by nano-LIF," in *Proceedings of the 15th International Conference on Miniaturized Systems for Chemistry and Life Sciences 2011, MicroTAS 2011*, Seattle, WA.

Laflamme, M. A., Sebastian, M. M., and Buetow, B. S. (2012). 10 - Cardiovascular. *Comp. Anat. Histol.* 135–153. doi: 10.1016/B978-0-12-381361-9.00010-X

Lakshmanakumar, M., Nesakumar, N., Sethuraman, S., Rajan, K. S., Krishnan, U. M., and Rayappan, J. B. B. (2019). Functionalized graphene quantum dot interfaced electrochemical detection of cardiac Troponin I: an antibody free approach. *Sci. Rep.* 9:17348. doi: 10.1038/s41598-019-53979-5

Li, C., and Wang, L. V. (2009). Photoacoustic tomography and sensing in biomedicine. *Phys. Med. Biol.* 54, R59–R97. doi: 10.1088/0031-9155/54/19/R01

Li, S., Zhu, J., Zhang, W., Chen, Y., Zhang, K., Popescu, L. M., et al. (2011). Signature microRNA expression profile of essential hypertension and its novel link to human cytomegalovirus infection. *Circulation* 124, 175–184. doi: 10.1161/CIRCULATIONAHA.110.012237

Li, Y. Q., Zhang, M. F., Wen, H. Y., Hu, C. L., Liu, R., Wei, H. Y., et al. (2013). Comparing the diagnostic values of circulating microRNAs and cardiac troponin T in patients with acute myocardial infarction. *Clinics* 68, 75–80. doi: 10.6061/clinics/2013(01)OA12

Libby, P. (2002). Inflammation in atherosclerosis. *Nature* 1, 297–329. doi: 10.1038/nature01323

Lichtenstein, A. H., and Matthan, N. R. (2007). "Cardiovascular disease," in *Optimizing Women's Health through Nutrition*, eds L. U. Thompson and W. E. Ward (Boca Raton, FL: CRC Press).

Lim, W. Y., Thevarajah, T. M., Goh, B. T., and Khor, S. M. (2019). Paper microfluidic device for early diagnosis and prognosis of acute myocardial infarction via quantitative multiplex cardiac biomarker detection. *Biosens. Bioelectron.* 128, 176–185. doi: 10.1016/j.bios.2018.12.049

Liu, G., Qi, M., Zhang, Y., Cao, C., and Goldys, E. M. (2016). Nanocomposites of gold nanoparticles and graphene oxide towards an stable label-free electrochemical immunosensor for detection of cardiac marker troponin-I. *Anal. Chim. Acta* 909, 1–8. doi: 10.1016/j.aca.2015.12.023

Liu, P., Yang, X., Sun, S., Wang, Q., Wang, K., Huang, J., et al. (2013). Enzyme-free colorimetric detection of DNA by using gold nanoparticles and hybridization chain reaction amplification. *Anal. Chem.* 85, 7689–7695. doi: 10.1021/ac4001157

Liu, Q., Aroonyadet, N., Song, Y., Wang, X., Cao, X., Liu, Y., et al. (2016). Highly sensitive and quick detection of acute myocardial infarction biomarkers using In2O3 nanoribbon biosensors fabricated using shadow masks. *ACS Nano* 10, 10117–10125. doi: 10.1021/acsnano.6b05171

Liu, T., Yu, J., Deng, M., Yin, Y., Zhang, H., Luo, K., et al. (2017). CDK4/6-dependent activation of DUB3 regulates cancer metastasis through SNAIL1. *Nat. Commun.* 8:13923. doi: 10.1038/ncomms13923

Liu, Y., Ma, Y., Zhang, J., Yuan, Y., and Wang, J. (2019). Exosomes: a novel therapeutic agent for cartilage and bone tissue regeneration. *Dose Response* 17:1559325819892702. doi: 10.1177/1559325819892702

Long, G., Wang, F., Duan, Q., Chen, F., Yang, S., Gong, W., et al. (2012a). Human circulating microRNA-1 and microRNA-126 as potential novel indicators for acute myocardial infarction. *Int. J. Biol. Sci.* 8, 811–818. doi: 10.7150/ijbs.4439

Long, G., Wang, F., Duan, Q., Yang, S., Chen, F., Gong, W., et al. (2012b). Circulating miR-30a, miR-195 and let-7b associated with acute myocardial infarction. *PLoS One* 7:e50926. doi: 10.1371/journal.pone.0050926

Lopa, N. S., Rahman, M. M., Ahmed, F., Ryu, T., Sutradhar, S. C., Lei, J., et al. (2019). Simple, low-cost, sensitive and label-free aptasensor for the detection of cardiac troponin I based on a gold nanoparticles modified titanium foil. *Biosens. Bioelectron.* 136, 381–388. doi: 10.1016/j.bios.2018.11.012

Lou, D., Fan, L., Ji, Y., Gu, N., and Zhang, Y. (2019a). A signal amplifying fluorescent nanoprobe and lateral flow assay for ultrasensitive detection of cardiac biomarker Troponin I. *Anal. Methods* 11, 3506–3513. doi: 10.1039/c9ay01039d

Lou, D., Ji, L., Fan, L., Ji, Y., Gu, N., and Zhang, Y. (2019b). Antibody-oriented strategy and mechanism for the preparation of fluorescent nanoprobes for fast and sensitive immunodetection. *Langmuir* 35, 4860–4867. doi: 10.1021/acs.langmuir.9b00150

Lu, S., Wang, S., Zhao, J., Sun, J., and Yang, X. (2017). Fluorescence light-up biosensor for MicroRNA based on the distance-dependent photoinduced electron transfer. *Anal. Chem.* 89, 8429–8436. doi: 10.1021/acs.analchem.7b01900

Lv, H., Zhang, X., Li, Y., Ren, Y., Zhang, C., Wang, P., et al. (2019). An electrochemical sandwich immunosensor for cardiac troponin I by using nitrogen/sulfur co-doped graphene oxide modified with Au@Ag nanocubes as amplifiers. *Microchim. Acta* 186:416. doi: 10.1007/s00604-019-3526-2

Ma, N., Zhang, T., Yan, T., Kuang, X., Wang, H., Wu, D., et al. (2019). Novel electrochemical immunosensor for sensitive monitoring of cardiac troponin I using antigen–response cargo released from mesoporous Fe3O4. *Biosens. Bioelectron.* 143:111608. doi: 10.1016/j.bios.2019.111608

Madhurantakam, S., Babu, K. J., Rayappan, J. B. B., and Krishnan, U. M. (2018). Nanotechnology-based electrochemical detection strategies for hypertension markers. *Biosens. Bioelectron.* 116, 67–80. doi: 10.1016/j.bios.2018.05.034

Marfella, R., Di Filippo, C., Potenza, N., Sardu, C., Rizzo, M. R., Siniscalchi, M., et al. (2013). CirculatingmicroRNA changes in heart failure patients treated with cardiac resynchronization therapy: responders vs. non-responders. *Eur. J. Heart Fail.* 15, 1277–1288. doi: 10.1093/eurjhf/hft088

Matsumoto, S., Sakata, Y., Suna, S., Nakatani, D., Usami, M., Hara, M., et al. (2013). Circulating p53-responsive MicroRNAs are predictive indicators of heart failure after acute myocardial infarction. *Circ. Res.* 113, 322–326. doi: 10.1161/CIRCRESAHA.113.301209

McRobbie, D. W., Moore, E. A., and Graves, M. J. (2017). *MRI From Picture to Proton*. Cambridge: Cambridge University Press. doi: 10.2214/ajr.182.3.1820592

Miao, L., Jiao, L., Tang, Q., Li, H., Zhang, L., and Wei, Q. (2019). A nanozyme-linked immunosorbent assay for dual-modal colorimetric and ratiometric fluorescent detection of cardiac troponin I. *Sens. Actuat. B Chem.* 288, 60–64. doi: 10.1016/j.snb.2019.02.111

Mullett, W. M., Lai, E. P. C., and Yeung, J. M. (2000). Surface plasmon resonance-based immunoassays. *Methods* 22, 77–91. doi: 10.1006/meth.2000.1039

Oerlemans, M. I. F. J., Mosterd, A., Dekker, M. S., de Vrey, E. A., van Mil, A., Pasterkamp, G., et al. (2012). Early assessment of acute coronary syndromes in the emergency department: the potential diagnostic value of circulating microRNAs. *EMBO Mol. Med.* 4, 1176–1185. doi: 10.1002/emmm.201201749

Osborn, E. A., and Jaffer, F. A. (2013). The advancing clinical impact of molecular imaging in CVD. *JACC Cardiovasc. Imaging* 6, 1327–1341. doi: 10.1016/j.jcmg.2013.09.014

Pan, D., Schirra, C. O., Wickline, S. A., and Lanza, G. M. (2014). Multicolor computed tomographic molecular imaging with noncrystalline high-metal-density nanobeacons. *Contrast Media Mol. Imaging* 9, 13–25. doi: 10.1002/cmmi.1571

Phonklam, K., Wannapob, R., Sriwimol, W., Thavarungkul, P., and Phairatana, T. (2020). A novel molecularly imprinted polymer PMB/MWCNTs sensor for highly-sensitive cardiac troponin T detection. *Sens. Actuat. B Chem.* 308:127630. doi: 10.1016/j.snb.2019.127630

Pykett, I. L., Buonanno, F. S., Brady, T. J., and Kistler, J. P. (1983). True three-dimensional nuclear magnetic resonance neuro-imaging in ischemic stroke: correlation of nmr, x-ray ct and pathology. *Stroke* 14, 173–177. doi: 10.1161/01.STR.14.2.173

Qureshi, A., Gurbuz, Y., and Niazi, J. H. (2012). Biosensors for cardiac biomarkers detection: a review. *Sens. Actuat. B Chem.* 171–172, 62–76. doi: 10.1016/j.snb.2012.05.077

Rehman, S. A., Khurshid, Z., Niazi, F. H., Naseem, M., Waddani, H., Al Sahibzada, H. A., et al. (2017). Role of salivary biomarkers in detection of cardiovascular diseases (CVD). *Proteomes* 5, 4–9. doi: 10.3390/proteomes5030021

Richter, M. M. (2004). Electrochemiluminescence (ECL). *Chem. Rev.* 104, 3003–3036. doi: 10.1021/cr020373d

Sandil, D., Sharma, S. C., and Puri, N. K. (2019). Protein-functionalized WO3 nanorods-based impedimetric platform for sensitive and label-free detection of a cardiac biomarker. *J. Mater. Res.* 34, 1331–1340. doi: 10.1557/jmr.2018.481

Saraste, A., Nekolla, S. G., and Schwaiger, M. (2009). Cardiovascular molecular imaging: an overview. *Cardiovasc. Res.* 83, 643–652. doi: 10.1093/cvr/cvp209

Sayed, A. S. M., Xia, K., Salma, U., Yang, T., and Peng, J. (2014). Diagnosis, prognosis and therapeutic role of circulating miRNAs in cardiovascular diseases. *Heart Lung Circ.* 23, 503–510. doi: 10.1016/j.hlc.2014.01.001

Shan, B., Chai, P., and Zhang, Z. (2013). "Positron emission tomography," in *Advanced Topics in Science and Technology in China*, eds D. L. Bailey, D. W. Townsend, P. E. Valk, and M. N. Maisey (Berlin: Springer).

Shen, Q., Liu, M., Lü, Y., Zhang, D., Cheng, Z., Liu, Y., et al. (2019). Label-free electrochemical immunosensor based on a functionalized ionic liquid and helical carbon nanotubes for the determination of cardiac Troponin I. *ACS Omega* 4, 11888–11892. doi: 10.1021/acsomega.9b01152

Singh, N., Rai, P., Ali, M. A., Kumar, R., Sharma, A., Malhotra, B. D., et al. (2019). A hollow-nanosphere-based microfluidic biosensor for biomonitoring of cardiac troponin i. *J. Mater. Chem. B* 7, 3826–3839. doi: 10.1039/c9tb00126c

Strianese, M., Staiano, M., Ruggiero, G., Labella, T., Pellecchia, C., and D'Auria, S. (2012). Fluorescence-based biosensors. *Methods Mol. Biol.* 875, 193–216. doi: 10.1007/978-1-61779-806-1_9

Sun, J., Zhuang, J., Shi, J., Kormakov, S., Liu, Y., Yang, Z., et al. (2019). Highly elastic and ultrathin nanopaper-based nanocomposites with superior electric and thermal characteristics. *J. Mater. Sci.* 54, 8436–8449. doi: 10.1007/s10853-019-03472-1

Sun, Y., Kang, C., Zhang, A., Liu, F., Hu, J., Zhong, X., et al. (2016). Co-delivery of dual-drugs with nanoparticle to overcome multidrug resistance. *Eur. J. Biomed. Res.* 2, 12–18. doi: 10.18088/ejbmr.2.2.2016

Syedmoradi, L., Ahmadi, A., Norton, M. L., and Omidfar, K. (2019). A review on nanomaterial-based field effect transistor technology for biomarker detection. *Microchim. Acta* 186:739. doi: 10.1007/s00604-019-3850-6

Tan, G. R., Wang, M., Hsu, C. Y., Chen, N., and Zhang, Y. (2016). Small upconverting fluorescent nanoparticles for biosensing and bioimaging. *Adv. Opt. Mater.* 4, 984–997. doi: 10.1002/adom.201600141

Tan, X., Zhang, L., Tang, Q., Zheng, G., and Li, H. (2019). Ratiometric fluorescent immunoassay for the cardiac troponin-I using carbon dots and palladium-iridium nanocubes with peroxidase-mimicking activity. *Microchim. Acta.* 186:280. doi: 10.1007/s00604-019-3375-z

Taruttis, A., Herzog, E., Razansky, D., and Ntziachristos, V. (2010). Real-time imaging of cardiovascular dynamics and circulating gold nanorods with multispectral optoacoustic tomography. *Opt. Express.* 18, 19592–19602. doi: 10.1364/oe.18.019592

Tijsen, A. J., Creemers, E. E., Moerland, P. D., De Windt, L. J., Van Der Wal, A. C., Kok, W. E., et al. (2010). MiR423-5p as a circulating biomarker for heart failure. *Circ. Res.* 106, 1035–1039. doi: 10.1161/CIRCRESAHA.110.218297

Tsai, P. C., Liao, Y. C., Wang, Y. S., Lin, H. F., Lin, R. T., and Juo, S. H. H. (2013). Serum microrna-21 and microrna-221 as potential biomarkers for cerebrovascular disease. *J. Vasc. Res.* 50, 346–354. doi: 10.1159/000351767

Van Schooneveld, M. M., Cormode, D. P., Koole, R., Van Wijngaarden, J. T., Calcagno, C., Skajaa, T., et al. (2010). A fluorescent, paramagnetic and PEGylated gold/silica nanoparticle for MRI, CT and fluorescence imaging. *Contrast Media Mol. Imaging* 5, 231–236. doi: 10.1002/cmmi.376

Vasantham, S., Alhans, R., Singhal, C., Nagabooshanam, S., Nissar, S., Basu, T., et al. (2020). Paper based point of care immunosensor for the impedimetric detection of cardiac troponin I biomarker. *Biomed. Microdevices* 22:6. doi: 10.1007/s10544-019-0463-0

Walters, N., Nguyen, L. T. H., Zhang, J., Shankaran, A., and Reátegui, E. (2019). Extracellular vesicles as mediators of in vitro neutrophil swarming on a large-scale microparticle array. *Lab Chip* 19, 2874–2884. doi: 10.1039/c9lc00483a

Wang, G. K., Zhu, J. Q., Zhang, J. T., Li, Q., Li, Y., He, J., et al. (2010). Circulating microRNA: a novel potential biomarker for early diagnosis of acute myocardial infarction in humans. *Eur. Heart J.* 31, 659–666. doi: 10.1093/eurheartj/ehq013

Wang, S., Zhao, Y., Wang, M., Li, H., Saqib, M., Ge, C., et al. (2019). Enhancing luminol electrochemiluminescence by combined use of cobalt-based metal organic frameworks and silver nanoparticles and its application in ultrasensitive detection of cardiac Troponin I. *Anal. Chem.* 91, 3048–3054. doi: 10.1021/acs.analchem.8b05443

Wang, W., Zou, Y., Yan, J., Liu, J., Chen, H., Li, S., et al. (2018). Ultrasensitive colorimetric immunoassay for hCG detection based on dual catalysis of Au@Pt core–shell nanoparticle functionalized by horseradish peroxidase. *Spectrochim. Acta Part A Mol. Biomol. Spectrosc.* 193, 102–108. doi: 10.1016/j.saa.2017.12.014

Wang, X., Kwak, K. J., Yang, Z., Zhang, A., Zhang, X., Sullivan, R., et al. (2018). Extracellular mRNA detected by molecular beacons in tethered lipoplex nanoparticles for diagnosis of human hepatocellular carcinoma. *PLoS One* 13:e0198552. doi: 10.1371/journal.pone.0198552

Wang, X., Yang, Z., Tian, H., Li, Y., Li, M., Zhao, W., et al. (2017a). Circulating MIC-1/GDF15 is a complementary screening biomarker with CEA and correlates with liver metastasis and poor survival in colorectal cancer. *Oncotarget* 8, 24892–24901. doi: 10.18632/oncotarget.15279

Wang, X., Zhi, X., Yang, Z., Tian, H., Li, Y., Li, M., et al. (2017b). A novel serum based biomarker panel has complementary ability to preclude presence of early lung cancer for low dose CT (LDCT). *Oncotarget* 8, 45345–45355. doi: 10.18632/oncotarget.17477

Wang, Z., Zong, S., Wu, L., Zhu, D., and Cui, Y. (2017c). SERS-activated platforms for immunoassay: probes, encoding methods, and applications. *Chem. Rev.* 117, 7910–7963. doi: 10.1021/acs.chemrev.7b00027

Xia, J., Yao, J., and Wang, L. V. (2014). Photoacoustic tomography: principles and advances. *Prog. Electromagn. Res.* 147, 1–22. doi: 10.2528/PIER14032303

Xue, T. Y., Mei, L. P., Xu, Y. T., Liu, Y. L., Fan, G. C., Li, H. Y., et al. (2019). Nanoporous semiconductor electrode captures the quantum dots: toward ultrasensitive signal-on liposomal photoelectrochemical immunoassay. *Anal. Chem.* 91, 3795–3799. doi: 10.1021/acs.analchem.9b00170

Yang, Z., Ma, Y., Zhao, H., Yuan, Y., and Kim, B. Y. S. (2020a). Nanotechnology platforms for cancer immunotherapy. *Wiley Interdiscip. Rev. Nanomed. Nanobiotechnol.* 12, 1–28. doi: 10.1002/wnan.1590

Yang, Z., Shi, J., Xie, J., Wang, Y., Sun, J., Liu, T., et al. (2020b). Large-scale generation of functional mRNA-encapsulating exosomes via cellular nanoporation. *Nat. Biomed. Eng.* 4, 69–83. doi: 10.1038/s41551-019-0485-1

Yang, Z., Sun, W., and Hu, K. (2009). Adenosine A1 receptors selectively target protein kinase C isoforms to the caveolin-rich plasma membrane in cardiac myocytes. *Biochim. Biophys. Acta Mol. Cell Res.* 1793, 1868–1875. doi: 10.1016/j.bbamcr.2009.10.007

Yang, Z., Sun, W., and Hu, K. (2012). Molecular mechanism underlying adenosine receptor-mediated mitochondrial targeting of protein kinase C. *Biochim. Biophys. Acta Mol. Cell Res.* 1823, 950–958. doi: 10.1016/j.bbamcr.2011.12.012

Yang, Z., Xie, J., Zhu, J., Kang, C., Chiang, C., Wang, X., et al. (2016). Functional exosome-mimic for delivery of siRNA to cancer: in vitro and in vivo evaluation. *J. Control. Release* 243, 160–171. doi: 10.1016/j.jconrel.2016.10.008

Yeh, H. C., Sharma, J., Han, J. J., Martinez, J. S., and Werner, J. H. (2010). A DNA-silver nanocluster probe that fluoresces upon hybridization. *Nano Lett.* 10, 3106–3110. doi: 10.1021/nl101773c

Yu, H., Yang, Z., Pan, S., Yang, Y., Tian, J., Wang, L., et al. (2015). Hypoxic preconditioning promotes the translocation of protein kinase C ε binding with caveolin-3 at cell membrane not mitochondrial in rat heart. *Cell Cycle* 14, 3557–3565. doi: 10.1080/15384101.2015.1084446

Yu, X., Deng, L., Wang, D., Li, N., Chen, X., Cheng, X., et al. (2012). Mechanism of TNF-α autocrine effects in hypoxic cardiomyocytes: initiated by hypoxia inducible factor 1α, presented by exosomes. *J. Mol. Cell. Cardiol.* 53, 848–857. doi: 10.1016/j.yjmcc.2012.10.002

Zamani, P., Fereydouni, N., Butler, A. E., Navashenaq, J. G., and Sahebkar, A. (2019). The therapeutic and diagnostic role of exosomes in cardiovascular diseases. *Trends Cardiovasc. Med.* 29, 313–323. doi: 10.1016/j.tcm.2018.10.010

Zeng, L., Liu, J., Wang, Y., Wang, L., Weng, S., Tang, Y., et al. (2011). MicroRNA-210 as a novel blood biomarker in acute cerebral ischemia. *Front. Biosci.* 3:1265–1272. doi: 10.2741/e330

Zhang, J., Nie, H., Wu, Z., Yang, Z., Zhang, L., Xu, X., et al. (2014). Self-catalytic growth of unmodified gold nanoparticles as conductive bridges mediated gap-electrical signal transduction for DNA hybridization detection. *Anal. Chem.* 86, 1178–1185. doi: 10.1021/ac4032675

Zhang, X., Lv, H., Li, Y., Zhang, C., Wang, P., Liu, Q., et al. (2019). Ultrasensitive sandwich-type immunosensor for cardiac troponin i based on enhanced electrocatalytic reduction of H 2 O 2 using β-cyclodextrins functionalized 3D porous graphene-supported Pd@Au nanocubes. *J. Mater. Chem. B* 7, 1460–1468. doi: 10.1039/c8tb03362e

Zhao, W. W., Xu, J. J., and Chen, H. Y. (2014). Photoelectrochemical DNA biosensors. *Chem. Rev.* 114, 7421–7441. doi: 10.1021/cr500100j

Zhao, W. W., Yu, P. P., Shan, Y., Wang, J., Xu, J. J., and Chen, H. Y. (2012). Exciton-plasmon interactions between CdS quantum dots and Ag nanoparticles in photoelectrochemical system and its biosensing application. *Anal. Chem.* 84, 5892–5897. doi: 10.1021/ac300127s

Zhou, C., Yang, Z., and Teng, L. (2014). Nanomedicine based on nucleic acids: pharmacokinetic and pharmacodynamic perspectives. *Curr. Pharm. Biotechnol.* 15, 829–838. doi: 10.2174/1389201015666141020155620

Zhu, D., Liu, W., Zhao, D., Hao, Q., Li, J., Huang, J., et al. (2017). Label-free electrochemical sensing platform for MicroRNA-21 detection using thionine and gold nanoparticles co-functionalized MoS2 nanosheet. *ACS Appl. Mater. Interfaces* 9, 35597–35603. doi: 10.1021/acsami.7b11385

Zhu, L., Ye, J., Yan, M., Zhu, Q., Wang, S., Huang, J., et al. (2019). Electrochemiluminescence immunosensor based on Au nanocluster and hybridization chain reaction signal amplification for ultrasensitive detection of cardiac Troponin I. *ACS Sens.* 4, 2778–2785. doi: 10.1021/acssensors.9b01369

Zou, B., Cheng, H., and Tu, Y. (2019). An electrochemiluminescence immunosensor for myoglobin using an indium tin oxide glass electrode modified with gold nanoparticles and platinum nanowires. *Microchim. Acta* 186:598. doi: 10.1007/s00604-019-3703-3

12

Copper Sulfide Nanoparticles-Incorporated Hyaluronic Acid Injectable Hydrogel with Enhanced Angiogenesis to Promote Wound Healing

Wencheng Zhou[1,2†], Liu Zi[1,3†], Ying Cen[2], Chao You[1,4,5] and Meng Tian[1,2,4,5]*

[1] Neurosurgery Research Laboratory, National Clinical Research Center for Geriatrics, West China Hospital, Sichuan University, Chengdu, China, [2] Department of Burns and Plastic Surgery, West China Hospital, Sichuan University, Chengdu, China, [3] Department of Integrated Traditional and Western Medicine, West China Hospital, Sichuan University, Chengdu, China, [4] Department of Neurosurgery, West China Hospital, Sichuan University, Chengdu, China, [5] West China Brain Research Centre, West China Hospital, Sichuan University, Chengdu, China

***Correspondence:**
Meng Tian
tianmong007@gmail.com;
6744710@qq.com

† These authors have contributed equally to this work

Skin wound caused by trauma, inflammation, surgery, or burns remains a great challenge worldwide since there is no effective therapy available to improve its clinical outcomes. Herein, we report a copper sulfide nanoparticles-incorporated hyaluronic acid (CuS/HA) injectable hydrogel with enhanced angiogenesis to promote wound healing. The prepared hydrogel could not only be injected to the wound site but also exhibited good photothermal effect, with temperature increasing to 50°C from room temperature after 10 min of near-infrared light irradiation. The cell culture experiments also showed that the hydrogel has no cytotoxicity. In the rat skin wound model, the hydrogel treated wounds exhibited better healing performances. Masson's trichrome staining suggested that collagen deposition in wounds treated with the hydrogel was significantly higher than other groups. The immunohistochemical staining showed that the hydrogel can effectively upregulate the expression of vascular endothelial growth factor (VEGF) in the wound area at the incipient stage of healing, and the CD 31 immunofluorescence staining confirmed the enhanced angiogenesis of the hydrogel. Taken together, the prepared CuS/HA hydrogel can effectively increase the collagen deposition, upregulate the expression of VEGF, and enhance the angiogenesis, which may contribute to promote wound healing, making it a promising for application in treating skin wound.

Keywords: copper sulfide, nanoparticle, hydrogel, angiogenesis, wound healing

INTRODUCTION

Skin wound resulting from trauma, inflammation, surgery, or burns is a common issue that needs to be treated immediately (Browne and Pandit, 2015). However, up to now, an effective wound healing remains a significant challenge due to its complex biological process where various intracellular and intercellular pathways should be activated and coordinated to accelerate and enhance the healing

(Das and Baker, 2016). Among these biological processes, angiogenesis plays many important roles during the healing since the newly formed vessels are of great significance to nutrients and growth factors transport and granular tissue growth, and thus encouraging angiogenesis is regarded as one of the most essential steps for promotion of wound healing. In this regard, earlier studies mainly focused on the introduction of angiogenic growth factors such as vascular endothelial growth factor (VEGF), and basic fibroblast growth factor (bFGF). Nevertheless, the use of growth factors was limited by their high cost and side effects.

Recently, some metal ions have attracted more and more research interest due to their vascularization effect (Yu et al., 2019). For example, copper ions have been reported that could stimulate angiogenesis by secretion of VEGF and thus promote wound healing. Moreover, nano-formed copper such as copper sulfide nanoparticles (CuS NPs) is capable of photothermal therapy induced by near-infrared (NIR) light irradiation which would be effective in killing bacteria as a non-resistant and minimally invasive process (Zhou et al., 2015; Feng et al., 2019). As a result, CuS NPs may offer both angiogenesis and antibacterial ability, both of which are beneficial to accelerate wound healing (Li Z. et al., 2018; Shanmugapriya and Kang, 2019). However, the use of copper ions or CuS NPs alone is not suitable for wound healing since direct contact may produce inflammation in skin tissues and the administration will easily detach from the wound as well. Considering these shortages, it is potential to incorporate copper ions or CuS NPs into carriers for wound healing.

Hydrogel composed of cross-linked hydrophilic polymer chains has its innate merits as wound dressing or drug carrier for wound healing, resulting not only from its good water-reserving ability that is suitable for absorption of wound exudates and skin cell survival and metabolism but also from its interconnected pores that provide three-dimensional networks with large volume and surface area for the incorporation of a drug (Li S. et al., 2018). The hydrogel can be prepared by natural polymers or synthesized ones. Compared to synthesized polymers, natural ones are more biocompatible, and more importantly, they are usually derived from the extracellular matrix (ECM). For instance, hyaluronic acid (HA) is one of the major components of the ECM consisting of disaccharide units of D-glucuronic acid-N-acetylglucosamine which contains many carboxyl and hydroxyl groups that is beneficial to water conservation for the skin. Furthermore, it was found that HA also plays an important role in the process of angiogenesis, suggesting that HA is a promising candidate to prepared hydrogel for wound healing.

In this work, we hypothesize to prepare a CuS NPs-incorporated HA injectable hydrogel, which can not only be injected to the wound site but can also be capable of photothermal therapy induced by NIR light irradiation (as shown in **Figure 1**). Moreover, both the use of CuS NPs and HA may benefit to enhance angiogenesis and thus promote wound healing. To address this hypothesis, CuS NPs and thiolated HA were first synthesized, and then CuS/HA hydrogel was prepared and characterized in terms of gelation time, morphology, photothermal effect, and cytotoxicity, before the *in vivo* angiogenesis and wound healing ability was evaluated in a rat skin wound model.

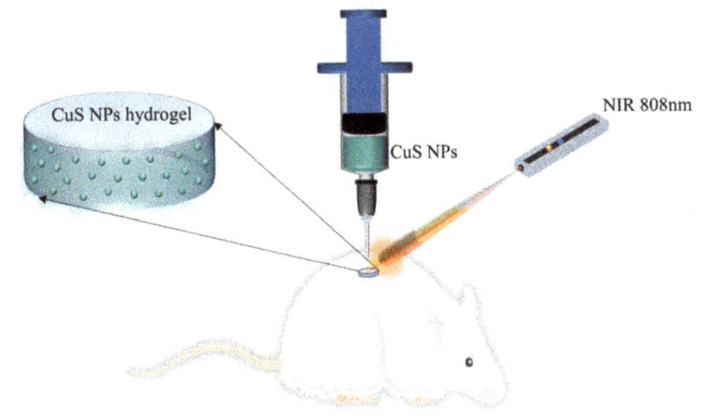

FIGURE 1 | Schematic presentation of CuS NPs-incorporated HA injectable hydrogel for wound healing.

MATERIALS AND METHODS

Materials

Copper chloride ($CuCl_2$), sodium sulfide (Na_2S $9H_2O$), and sodium citrate were purchased from Kelong Co., Ltd. (Chengdu, China). Methoxy-PEG-thiol (SH-PEG, molecular weight 5000 Da) was purchased from ToYongBio Co., Ltd. (Shanghai, China). HA sodium salt from Streptococcus Equi was supplied by Aladdin Co., Ltd. (Shanghai, China) 0.5, 5′-Dithiobis (2-nitrobenzoic acid; DTNB), N-(3-Dimethylaminopropyl)-N'-ethyl carbodiimide hydrochloride (EDAC), cysteamine, and dithiothreitol (DTT) were purchased from Sigma (St. Louis, MO, United States). N-hydroxysuccinimide (NHS) was obtained from Pierce. Isoflurane was obtained from RWD Life Science Co., Ltd. (Shenzhen, China). Cell counting kit-8 (CCK-8) was obtained from Dongren Chemical Technology Co., Ltd. (Shanghai, China). Hematoxylin and eosin (H&E) stains and Masson's Trichrome Stain Kit were purchased from Beijing Solarbio Science & Technology Co., Ltd. (Beijing, China). The antibody of endothelial growth factor anti-VEGF was bought from Proteintech (Chicago, United States). The anti-CD31 antibody was from Affinity Biosciences, Inc. (Cincinnati, OH, United States). Deionized water (18 MΩ) was obtained from a Milli-Qsynthesis system (Millipore, Billerica, MA, United States). All the above reagents are used directly without further purification.

Synthesis and Characterization of CuS Nanoparticles (NPs)

The synthesis of CuS NPs was carried out as a facile hydrothermal route as follows (Zhou et al., 2010). Briefly, 10 mL of sodium citrate (1.0 mg mL^{-1}), and 10 mL of $CuCl_2{\cdot}2H_2O$ (0.85 mg mL^{-1}) aqueous solutions were added into 30 mL of ultrapure water in sequence. The whole solution was protected by argon and stirred for 30 min at room temperature. After that, dropwise added 50 μL of $Na_2S{\cdot}9H_2O$ (78 mg mL^{-1}) aqueous solution into the reaction and kept on stirring another 5 min. In this process, the color of the reaction solution gradually changed from light blue to light yellow, orange, and finally to dark brown. Next, the reaction was transferred to a 90°C oil bath to react for 15 min to form green-colored CuS-citrate NPs. The whole mixture was moved to ice-cold water. To obtain PEG-coated NPs, 1 mg of SH-PEG was added to the 1 mL CuS-citrate NPs solution (200 μgmL^{-1}) to introduce the PEG coating. The reaction was performed overnight at room temperature to obtain PEG-coated CuS NPs.

The morphology of the CuS NPs was observed by transmission electron microscopy (TEM) performed on a Hitachi HT7700 (Japan). Specimens were prepared by adding 50 μL micellar solutions onto a copper grid followed by staining with phosphotungstic acid (1 wt%) for 1 min and then dried with filter paper. The size, zeta potential, and polymer dispersity index (PDI) of the CuS NPs were determined by dynamic light scattering (DLS) on a NanoBrook Series Particle/Protein Size and Zeta Potential Analyzer.

Synthesis and Characterization of Thiolated HA

The synthesis of thiolated HA is illustrated in **Supplementary Figure S1A**. The thiolated HA was synthesized by the coupling of cysteamine onto the HA molecular chains through EDC chemistry. Briefly, 1 g of HA sodium salt was dissolved in 200 ml distilled water, and then cysteamine and EDAC were added as solids to the reaction with a molar ratio of -COOH/cysteamine/EDAC 1:2:2. The pH of the reaction solution was maintained at 4.75 by the addition of 1 M HCl. After 4 h the reaction was stopped by neutralizing the solution by addition of 4 M NaOH. The solution was dialyzed (3500 cutoffs) against distilled water for 3 days at room temperature. 5 g DTT was then added to the resulting solution and the pH of the solution adjusted to 8.5. After stirring for 8 h under N_2, the pH of the solution was adjusted to 4.0 by the addition of 1 M HCl. The resulting solution was first dialyzed (3500 cutoffs) against HCl solution (pH 4.0) containing 100 mM NaCl under N_2, followed by dialysis (8000 cutoffs) against HCl solution (pH 4.0) under N_2. The solution was clarified by centrifugation, and the supernatant was sterilized with a 0.2 μm Millipore filter and then lyophilized. The product was stored at −20°C and protected under N_2. The degree of substitution (DS) of free thiols was determined using the Ellman method (Shu et al., 2002). The structure of thiolated hyaluronan was characterized by 1H NMR spectrum in D_2O.

Preparation of the Injectable CuS/HA Hydrogel

The CuS/HA hydrogel was prepared by simply mixing with thiolated HA solution and CuS NPs solution to obtain the precursor gelation solution, and then the gelation was initiated with the hydrogen peroxide solution. Gelation time was determined by a test tube inverting method. The final concentration of thiolated HA, CuS NPs, and hydrogen peroxide was 2% w/v, 200 μg/ml, and 0.03% v/v, respectively. This injectable CuS/HA hydrogel was named G II. The blank hydrogel without CuS NPs was used as a control (named G I). Scanning electron microscopy (SEM) was used to observe the morphology of the freeze-dried hydrogel. After coating with gold, the cross-sectional morphology was viewed with a ZEISS EVO 10 microscope. The storage and loss modulus were measured with a plate-to-plate rheometer (MCR 302, Anton Paar, Ashland, VA, United States) using a 25 mm plate under a constant strain of 1% and frequency of 10 rad/s.

In vitro Photothermal Effect

The photothermal effect of CuS NPs was carried out in two parts, nanoparticles solution, and hydrogels. For the solution, different concentrations (200, 100, 50, 20, and 10 μg/mL) were exposed to 808 nm laser at 1 W/cm^2 for 10 min and the temperatures were recorded every other min interval by an infrared imaging camera (FLIR ONE PRO, United States). To further test the stability of the photothermal effect, 200 μg/mL CuS NPs were determined to heat by the laser in the same condition and then cool down naturally for several cycles. On the other hand, the photothermal effect of CuS/HA hydrogels was evaluated in the same approach as above.

Cell Experiments

Mouse embryonic fibroblast (NIH/3T3) cell lines were chosen to perform the cell experiments. The cells were purchased from the ATCC and cultured in Dulbecco's modified Eagle's medium (DMEM) supplemented with 10% fetal bovine serum (FBS; Gibco, United States), 100 mg/ml penicillin, and 100 mg/ml streptomycin. The cells were grown at 37°C in an atmosphere of 95% humidified air containing 5% CO_2. Experiments were carried out when cells were in the logarithmic phase of growth. Cytotoxicity is a classic problem for biomaterials. According to ISO10993 part 5 guidelines 3, CCK-8 was used to examine the cytotoxic effects of the hydrogel, and solution of CuS NPs. For the test of CuS NPs solution, samples of three concentrations were used for testing (200, 100, and 50 μg/ml). For the injectable hydrogel test, both GI and GII were included. The extracts of these samples were prepared by the incubation of each sample with 1 ml of DMEM supplemented with 10% FBS for 48 h at 37°C.3T3 cells were cultured with common conditions [DMEM supplemented with penicillin (100 mg/ml), streptomycin (100 mg/ml), and 10% FBS, 37°C, 5% CO_2] until they reached approximately 80% confluency before cytotoxicity assay. After that, the cells were seeded into 96-well plates at a density of 3000 cells/well. After another 24 h incubation, the cells cultured in medium without test samples were used as a control group and the culture media of other wells were discarded and replaced with the medium containing the three concentration solutions of samples or two extracts (12.5%, v/v). After further cultured for designed time (0, 24, 48, and 72 h), the cells were subjected to cell toxicity assays by CCK-8. Briefly, the cells washed by phosphate buffer saline (PBS) and were incubated in a fresh culture medium containing 10% CCK-8 to incubate for 3 haway from light. Finally, the supernatant was transferred and the absorbance of the solution was determined at a test wavelength of 450 nm. The ratio of the optical density (OD) of the test samples to that of the control group presented the cell proliferation rate.

Cutaneous Wound Healing Experiments

The wound healing experiment *in vivo* for samples was conducted on Sprague–Dawley male rats (SD rats). All the animal experiments and procedures were approved by the Animal Ethical Committee of the West China Hospital of Sichuan University in compliance with Chinese national guidelines for the care and use of laboratory animals. Eight weeks old SD male rats ($200 \sim 220\ g$) were purchased from Da-Shuo Laboratory Animal Co., Ltd. (Chengdu, China). The rats were kept under controlled temperature and humidity with food and water *ad libitum*. After standard anesthetization with anesthetic ventilator using isoflurane (4%for induction in an induction chamber, and 2% for maintenance), the back of each animal was shaved to expose the injection site. A skin biopsy apparatus (6 mm) was used to make the round section of the full-thickness skin injury on the back of the rat skin. All procedures were performed under aseptic conditions during the surgery process. There were six round wounds (6 mm in diameter) created on the back of each rat and 7 rats were included, so there were 30 wounds served as experimental subjects, and 12 wounds as back-ups in case of experimental animal death. After the removal of wound skin, 100 μL of different injectable hydrogels were synthesized *in situ* (methods as mentioned before) 0.30 wounds were randomly divided into 6 groups (I-VI). Group I was the blank control group with nothing dressed after a skin injury, group II wounds received NIR radiation after the operation, group III wounds were dressed with the hydrogel G II, wounds in group IV were dressed with the hydrogel G II and treated with NIR, group V wounds were dressed with the hydrogel G I, and group VI wounds were dressed with the hydrogel G I and treated with NIR. For NIR treated groups, the wound area was irradiated with an 808 nm NIR laser (1 W/cm^2) for 10 min after the operation 10 min, 2 days, and 3 days and infrared photos were taken at the same time. The gross image of the wounds was taken after the operation on days 0, 3, 7, 10, and 14. To monitor the wound healing process, ImageJ software was employed to process the images to obtain the wound area. The healing rate (HR) was calculated, according to the formula as below:

$$HR = \frac{(S_0 - S_x)}{S_0} \times 100\%$$

where S_0 was the initial area on day 0 and S_x represented the wound areas on days 3, 7, 10, and 14, respectively.

Hematoxylin-Eosin and Masson's Trichrome Staining

Rats were sacrificed on the 3rd, 7th, and 14th days after the operation, respectively, and the skin tissue (1×1 cm^2) containing the wound was taken for dermatological examination. The samples were fixed in 4% paraformaldehyde, dehydrated in graded alcohol, and embedded in paraffin. The tissue blocks were sectioned into 5 μm thick slices. The sections were stained via H&E and Masson's trichrome to carry on histological analysis and collagen formation assessment. 8 All photos were captured by a microscope (BX43, Olympus, Japan). Histopathological scores of HE slices were employed to a semiquantitative evaluation of wound healing according to the criterion of Eldad et al. (1998). Collagen volume fraction (CVF) was utilized to assess collagen formation (Singh et al., 2019). Specifically, 6 regions of interest (ROIs) per HPF were recorded under a microscope. Then, the CVF of each ROI was assessed using the ImageJ software to semiquantitative analysis collagen content.

Immunohistochemical and Immunofluorescence Staining

Angiogenic vessel markers CD31 and VEGF were chosen in our experiment because they play an important role in angiogenesis (Nowak-Sliwinska et al., 2018). Immunofluorescence and immunohistochemical staining of CD31 and VEGF were carried out as previous literature. The rehydrated skin tissue sections were boiled in sodium citrate buffer for about 20 min before anti-CD31 and anti-VEGF (vascular endothelial growth factor) antibody incubated the sections overnight at 4°C, respectively. For CD31, DAPI stained the nuclei. The distribution of CD31 was observed by a fluorescence microscope and vascular density (VD) was expressed as the percentage of positive CD31 staining per ROI which were calculated using ImageJ software (Du et al., 2017). For VEGF, hematoxylin counterstained the nuclei and the integral optical density (IOD) of each view was assessed using the ImageJ software to determine its content (Zhou et al., 2020).

Statistical Analysis

The experimental data are expressed as mean ± standard deviation. Multiple comparisons among groups were determined using two-way ANOVA followed by Tukey's multiple comparisons test with adjusted P value. Significance was presented as: ****for $P < 0.0001$, ***for $P < 0.001$, **for $P < 0.01$, and *for $P < 0.05$.

RESULTS AND DISCUSSION

Synthesis and Characterization of CuS NPs

The CuS NPs were synthesized by a simple one-pot approach where CuS-citrate NPs were first prepared by reacting $CuCl_2$ and Na_2S in the presence of sodium citrate, and then PEG coating was introduced by incubation of CuS-citrate NPs with thiolated-PEG to disperse the NPs in the solution and incorporate into the hydrogel uniformly. The morphology of the synthesized CuS NPs was confirmed by TEM showing in **Figure 2A** where the NPs were in good dispersion and uniform size, with an average diameter of 12 nm. This diameter is of great significance for drug delivery through the blood vessels (Ding et al., 2019). The hydrodynamic average diameter of the CuS NPs

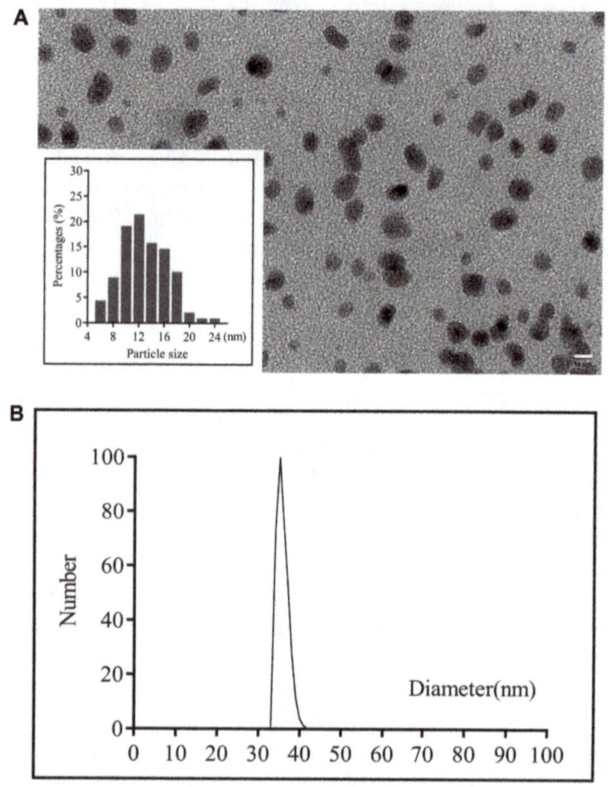

FIGURE 2 | **(A)** TEM images of the CuS NPs (scale bar 50 nm) and **(B)** Particle sizes of the CuS NPs detected by DLS.

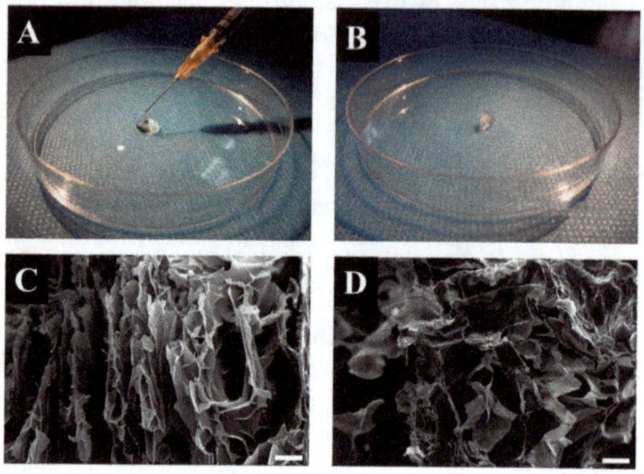

FIGURE 3 | **(A)** Injection operation of the CuS/HA hydrogel before gelation. **(B)** The gelated CuS/HA hydrogel. **(C)** SEM image of a cross-section of CuS/HA hydrogel, scale bar 100 μm. **(D)** SEM image of a cross-section of HA hydrogel, scale bar 100 μm.

was 35 nm as shown in **Figure 2B** determined by DLS. The Zeta-potential and PDI of the NPs was -6.07 mV, and 0.219, respectively. The negative charge of the NPs was probably due to the PEG layer, which is consistent with a previous report (Lin et al., 2019).

Synthesis and Characterization of Thiolated HA

Thiolated HA was synthesized using an amide condensation reaction between HA and cysteamine in the presence of EDC and followed by reduced using DTT. As shown in Supporting Information **Supplementary Figure S1**, the chemical structure of the final product was confirmed by 1H NMR spectrum in D_2O where two new peaks have appeared, one is at 2.8 ppm corresponding to the hydrogen of methylene close to thiol, and the other is at 2.6 ppm that assigned to the hydrogen of methylene adjacent to amide, suggesting that the Thiolated HA was successfully synthesized. The content of thiol was 0.49 mmol/g corresponding to 40% of the substitution degree as determined by the Ellman method.

Preparation of the Injectable CuS/HA Hydrogel

Both the CuS/HA hydrogel and blank hydrogel were formed by crosslinking with the disulfide bonds that initiate by oxidization of the thiolated groups along the HA chains with hydrogen peroxide. The gelation time of the CuS/HA and blank hydrogel was similar, approximately 6 min. Within this gelation time, the hydrogel could be injected into the skin wounds. **Figures 3A,B** show the injection operation of the CuS/HA hydrogel before gelation and the gelated CuS/HA hydrogel, respectively. The SEM images of a cross-section of CuS/HA hydrogel and blank hydrogel were shown in **Figures 3C,D**, both of which exhibited interconnected pores that provide three-dimensional networks with large volume and surface area. The storage (G') and loss modulus (G") were measured with a plate-to-plate rheometer. As shown in **Supplementary Figure S2**, the G' for HA hydrogel was 1820 Pa, while the one for CuS/HA hydrogel was 1930 Pa, and indicating that the hydrogel containing CuS NPs exhibited a higher modulus.

In vitro Photothermal Effect

The *in vitro* photothermal effect of the CuS NPs and CuS/HA hydrogel was studied to confirm their photothermal conversion. As shown in **Figures 4A,B**, the CuS NPs with different concentration (10, 20, 50, 100, and 200 μg/ml) was irradiated with NIR light at 808 nm and the results showed that the CuS NPs exhibited a significant increase in temperature upon 808 nm irradiation at all concentrations. In particular, the increase in temperature was dependent on the concentration of the CuS NPs, with the final temperature of the five concentrations reaching 34.4, 38.2, 46.7, 50.9, and 53.1°C after 10 min exposure, respectively, indicating that the synthesized CuS NPs has a good photothermal effect. The photothermal stability of the synthesized CuS NPs was also studied. As shown in **Figure 4C**, the heating curve of the CuS NPs of each cycle was identical upon repeated irradiation, with temperature from 27 to 53°C, and there was no significant change after repeated laser exposure. These results suggested that the synthesized CuS NPs displayed good photothermal stability. The photothermal

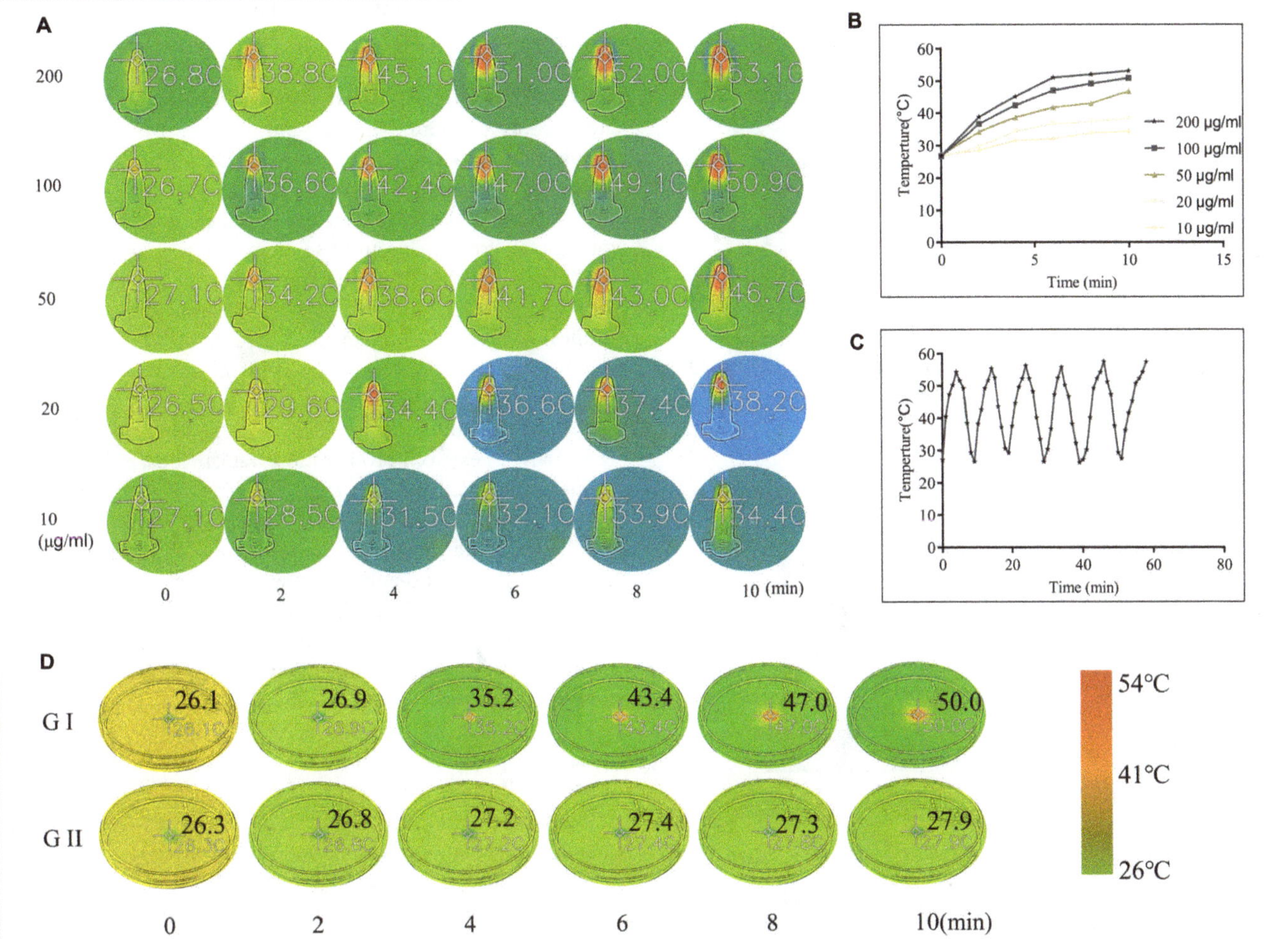

FIGURE 4 | (A,B) Photothermal images and corresponding heating curves of CuS NPs with different concentrations upon 808 nm laser exposure. **(C)** The heating curve of the CuS NPs upon repeated 808 nm irradiation and followed natural cooling. **(D)** Photothermal images of CuS/HA (GI) and blank hydrogels (GII) upon 808 nm laser exposure. (**A** and **D** share the same color scale).

images of CuS/HA and blank hydrogels upon 808 nm laser exposure were shown in **Figure 4D**. Like NPs, the CuS/HA hydrogel also exhibited good photothermal effect, with increasing temperature of 50°C after 10 min exposure. In contrast, there was no increase in temperature for blank hydrogel due to without CuS NPs.

Cytotoxicity

The evaluation of biocompatibility such as cytotoxicity is the primary problem in the application of biomaterials before further experiments that can only be carried out when the material is proved to be non-toxic (Savoji et al., 2018). Herein, we first tested the cytotoxicity of the CuS NPs and CuS/HA hydrogel. As shown in **Figure 5A**, the CuS NPs with different concentrations show not only hardly any toxicity to the cells, but also promoting the proliferation of cells with the culture time prolonged. Cell viability shows significantly CuS NPs concentration dependency, e.g., the higher the NPs concentration, the better the cell growth. In particular, the NPs with a concentration of 200 μg/ml can significantly promote cell proliferation during the whole test. The mechanism underlying the promotion of the proliferation of the cells has been suggested to relate with them directly or indirectly stimulation effects of the copper ions (Li M. et al., 2018). For example, the copper ions stimulated the cells to secrete growth factors such as bFGF, which is known to promote the proliferation of the cells (Gopal et al., 2014). **Figure 5B** demonstrates that both hydrogels do not have toxicity to cells too. The above results indicated that the CuS NPs could be biosafe for the following experiment and application.

Animal Experiments

To evaluate the effects of CuS/HA injectable hydrogel on the wound healing process, a full-thickness skin wound model was used. As shown in **Figures 6A,B**, in general, the wound area of all groups decreased with the prolongation of the healing time. On day 0, immediately after injection the hydrogel onto the wounds, the hydrogel can effectively stop bleeding. On day 3, compared with the blank control group I, the wounds were going to form a scar in all the other groups, and while

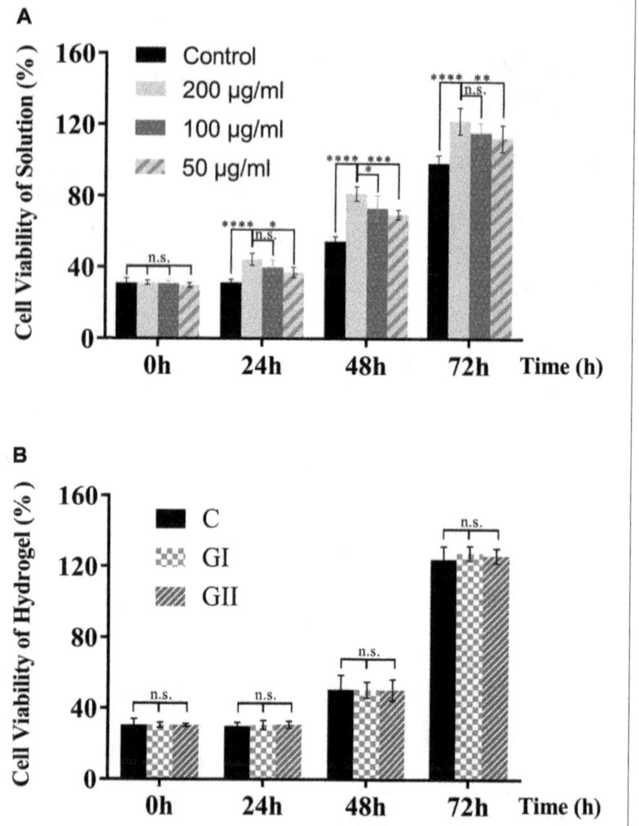

FIGURE 5 | Cytotoxicity of the CuS NPs and CuS/HA hydrogel. **(A)** The cytotoxicity of the CuS NPs solutions with different concentrations. **(B)** The cytotoxicity of the hydrogels (G I and G II) compared with the blank control. Error bars represent means ± SD for $n = 5$, ****for $P < 0.0001$, ***for $P < 0.001$, ** for$P < 0.01$, and *for $P < 0.05$.

the edema and exudation in group I were observed. By the 7th day, the difference in the healing area in each group was gradually obvious. On the 10th day, to observe and measure the area of wound healing, the hair around the rat's wound was shaved off and we could perceive that the scars in the groups without NIR irradiated were smaller than those in the corresponding control groups. At the end of the experiment (Day 14), it is easy to notice that the groups with NIR treated present better recovery outcomes than their counterparts, not only from the smaller areas of the scars but also the lighter degree of pigmentation. Consistently, the HR for each group was shown in **Figure 6C**. To evaluate the safety of the photothermal effect *in vivo*, the temperature change on the wound site was also recorded. As shown in **Supplementary Figure S3** the temperature of CuS/HA injectable hydrogel in the wound site changed from 32.4 to 50.3°C. On the other hand, the temperature of HA injectable hydrogel changed from 34.2 to 37.7°C. The time-temperature relationship determines the burn injury. It has been reported that burn injury occurs when the temperature reaches 50°C and the time need at least 60 min. The treated time of the highest temperature is shorter than 10 min in our experiment. Thus, the treatment is safe for animals (Martin and Falder, 2017).

Pathomorphological Evaluation

The process of wound healing was further evaluated on the pathological level through HE staining. **Figure 7A** demonstrated pathological changes of skin in each group on day 14 post-operation. The skin structure was formed without a residual wound in all groups. For groups I, III, and V without NIR treated, the thickness of epidermal was thin and there were few layers of epidermal cells. They all shared these commonalities: edematous bundles of collagen, no obvious proliferation, more lasting inflammatory cells infiltration in the wound, slow formation of granulation tissue, and less neovascularization. On the contrary, the groupII, IV, and Vexposed to NIR exhibited better healing performances, e.g., cell proliferation was obvious; epidermis and dermis were thickened to a certain extent; clear epidermis cell structure was seen; inflammatory cells were reduced; necrotic tissue fell off, and cells were found to crawl. Especially in group VI, most of the wound epithelium was completely covered; there was more neovascularization; granulation tissue was thicker and collagen was more and arranged in order. To semiquantitative evaluation of wound healing, histopathological scores of HE slices were calculated based on the research of Eldad et al. As shown in **Figure 7B**, the scores of all groups were calculated on days 3,7, and 14, respectively. The results were following the wound healing tendency that all groups were going to heal with different degrees. It is intriguing to notice that there are differences between groups V and VI, but there is no statistical significance discrepancy between groups III and IV. Therefore, it indicates that NIR promotes wound healing on account of CuS/HA hydrogel. Furthermore, it is uncalled for to discuss the groups without NIR treated in the following tests.

Collagen deposition played an important role in the course of repair (Yen et al., 2018). It can be a temporary scaffold and a bed enabling migration of epithelium, keratinocytes, and microvasculature. Thus, collagen deposition was chosen as an indirect indicator to reflect the wound healing. More collagen deposition would promote wound repair in a better way and CVF would be on behalf of the collagen deposition. To determine the formation of collagen, Masson's trichrome staining was used in this study. As depicted in **Figure 8A**, collagen was dyed blue in all groups. CVF was calculated using ImageJ to the semiquantitative analysis of collagen content. As shown in **Figure 8B**, collagen deposition in group VI had been significantly higher than other groups, even though all groups were growing. This trend consistent with HE results further clued that CuS/HA hydrogel might accelerate wound healing through increasing collagen deposition.

Angiogenic Evaluation

Vascular endothelial growth factor, a specific growth factor, can bind to specific receptors on the surface of endothelial cells, which effectively stimulates the mitosis of cells and make them proliferate. Additionally, VEGF acts a pivotal part in stimulating the formation of granulation tissue and epithelium,

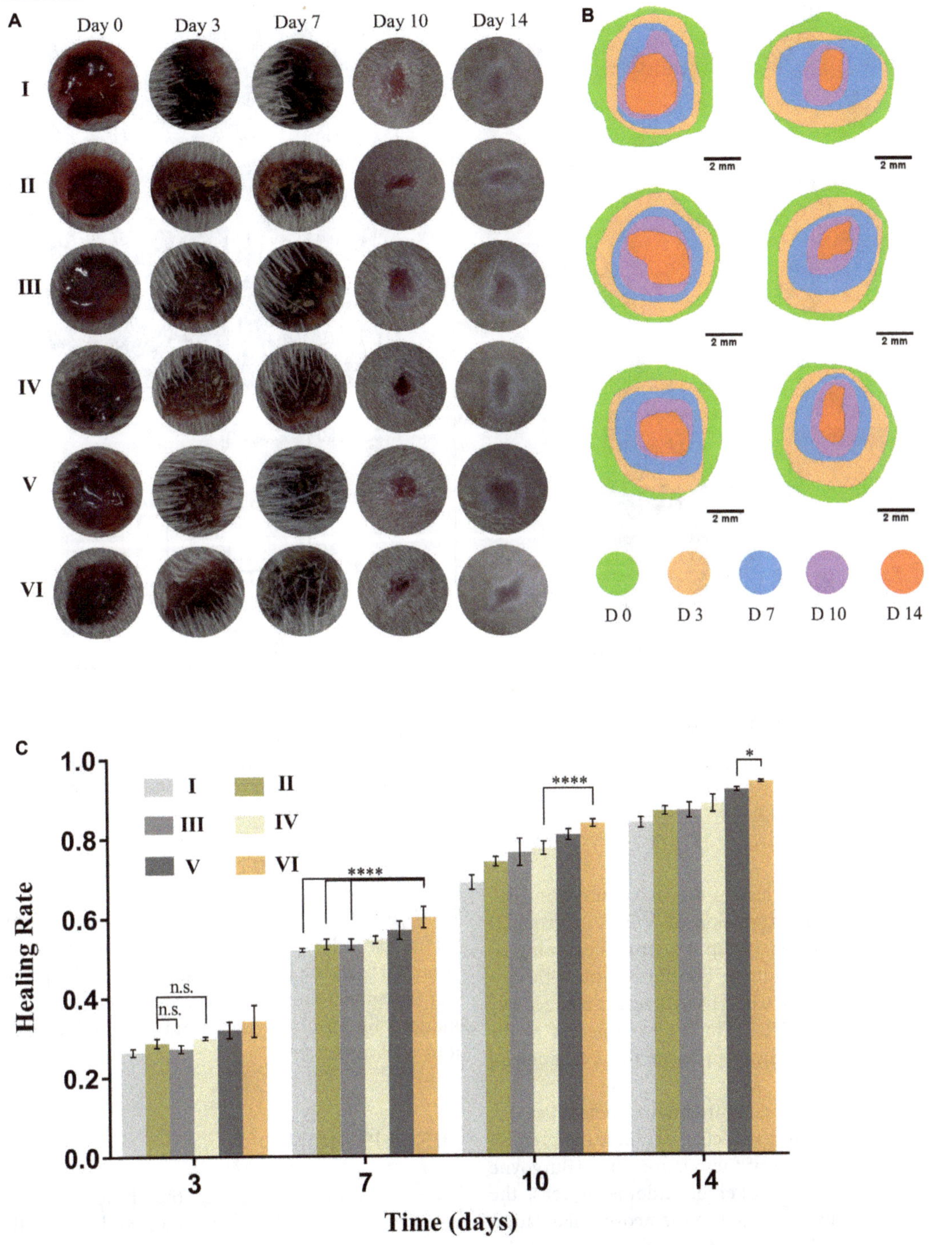

FIGURE 6 | Performance of hydrogels on wound healing. **(A)** Representative gross views of wounds at predetermined time points. **(B)** Traces of wound closure area for 14 days. **(C)** Healing rate for each group, $n = 5$, data = mean ± SD. (I: blank control; II: NIR; III: HA hydrogel; IV: HA hydrogel + NIR; V: CuS/HA hydrogel; and VI: CuS/HA hydrogel + NIR).

keratinocytes, and fibroblasts, and promotes the healing of the wound. Therefore, VEGF was employed to unveil the truth of wound healing at a molecular level. As shown in **Figure 9A**, the skin samples of the groups treated NIR were dyed by immunohistochemical staining at predesigned day (3, 7, and 14). Further statistical analysis results in **Figure 9B** revealed that the tendencies among the three groups were different. Specifically, the expression of VEGF in group VI reached the peak value at the beginning (the 3rd day), then it weakened gradually over time. However, for groups II and IV, they

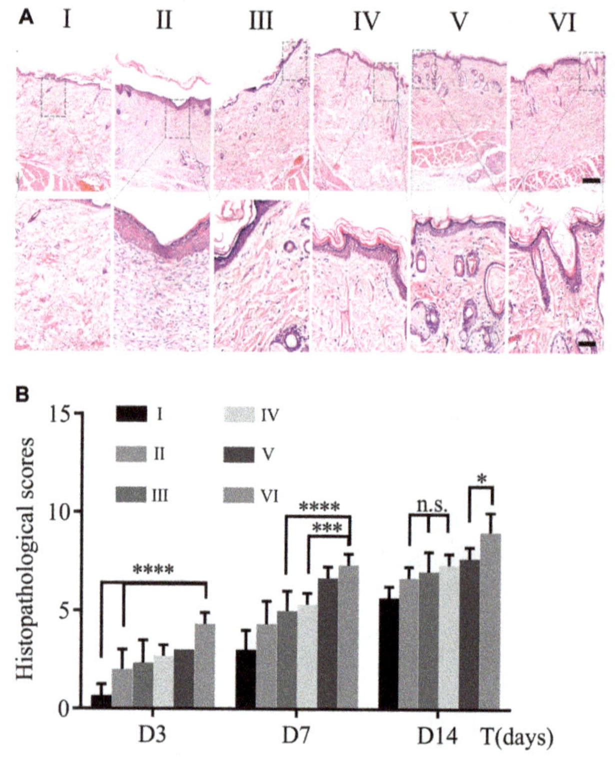

FIGURE 7 | (A) HE staining of wound section on day 14. The scale bar of the upper panel is 200 μm; nether, 50 μm. **(B)** Histopathological scores were calculated by HE staining on day 3, 7, and 14. (*n* = 3, data = mean ± SD.) (I: blank control; II: NIR; III: HA hydrogel; IV: HA hydrogel + NIR; V: CuS/HA hydrogel; and VI: CuS/HA hydrogel + NIR).

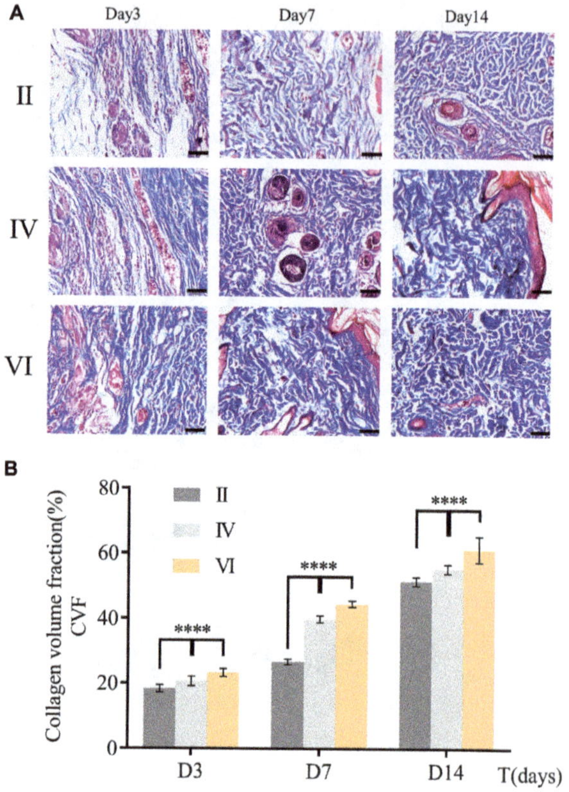

FIGURE 8 | (A) Masson's trichrome staining of skin sample in group B, D, and F during wound healing at different days (3, 7, and 14). Scale bar = 200 μm. **(B)** Collagen volume fraction was calculated by ImageJ. (*n* = 3, data = mean ± SD.) (II: NIR; IV: HA hydrogel + NIR; and VI: CuS/HA hydrogel + NIR).

both gradually increased from less to the maximum and then decreased. In particular, the expression of VEGF in group II and IV had never outstripped group VI from beginning to end, even though all of them hitting bottom on the 14th day. These observations indicate that CuS/HA hydrogel can effectively upregulate the expression of VEGF in the wound area at the incipient stage of wound healing to promote the formation of new blood vessels.

Wound healing requires enough nutrients and metabolism for repair and reconstruction, and neovascularization is the premise and basis for the transportation of these ingredients (Burgoyne and Morgan, 2003). As a biomarker of endothelial cells, the expression of CD31 was used to evaluate the neovascularization of the wounds. As shown in **Figure 10A**, immunofluorescence staining of CD31 confirmed the number of newly formed blood vessels in the wounds of different groups. The expression of CD31 in group VI was always higher than the other groups and reached a peak on the 7th day (**Figure 10B**). However, for groups II and IV, CD31 gradually increased and finally hit the maximum on the 14th day. These observations indicated that the CuS/HA hydrogel enhanced the angiogenesis of the wound at the early stage of wound healing.

To figure out whether the VEGF expression was induced by PTT or not, we compared the VEGF expression in groups I, II, V, and VI. As shown in **Supplementary Figure S4**, there was a relatively low expression of VEGF in groups I and II. In contrast, both the PTT and copper ions released from CuS NPs can upregulate the VEGF expression, and the VEGF expression induced by PTT was significantly higher than that of copper ions release alone.

DISCUSSION

Wound healing refers to the process of healing after disconnection or defect of skin and other tissues caused by external forces on the body, including regeneration of various tissues, hyperplasia of granulation tissues and complex combination of scar formation, and showing the synergistic effect of various processes. Among them, granulation tissue has an important function of anti-infection to protect the wound and filling the gap of tissue defects (Suarato et al., 2018). Especially, angiogenesis is the critical process to form granulation tissue, because newly formed blood vessels, like a farm irrigation system, and can provide nutrients and oxygen to cells in the wound site. Therefore, promoting angiogenesis can be used as a strategy to promote wound healing.

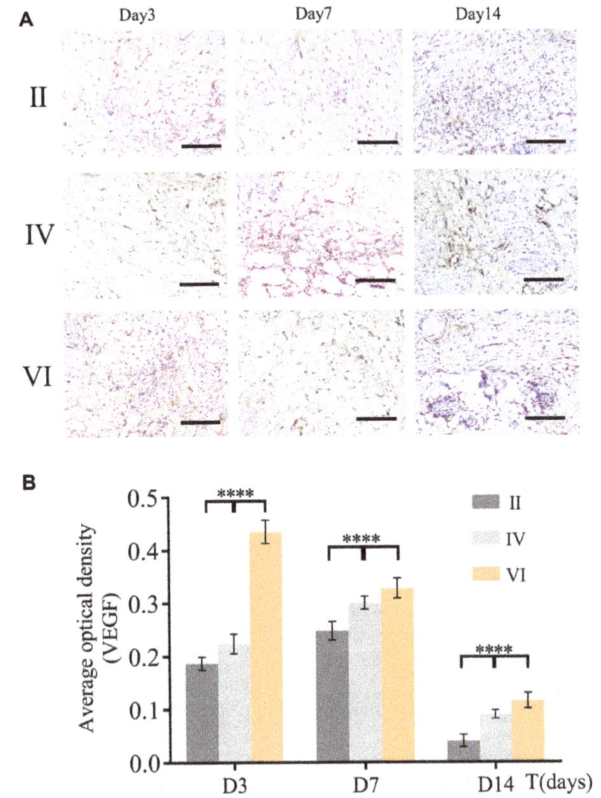

FIGURE 9 | (A) Immunohistochemical staining for angiogenic factor VEGF of the wound tissues during the healing at different days (3, 7, and 14). Scale bar, 200 μm. **(B)** The average optional density was calculated by ImageJ. (*n* = 6, data = mean ± SD.) (II: NIR; IV: HA hydrogel + NIR; and VI: CuS/HA hydrogel + NIR).

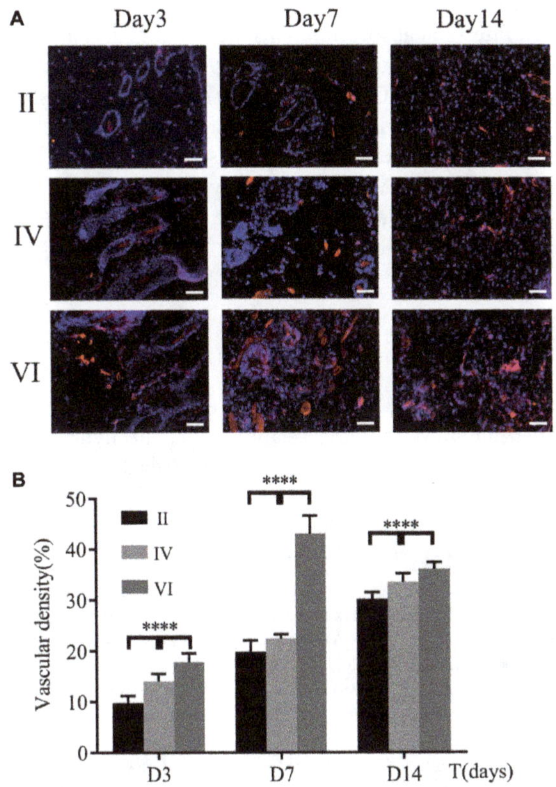

FIGURE 10 | (A) Immunofluorescence staining for CD31 of the wound tissues during the healing on days 3, 7, and 14, respectively. Scale bar, 200 μm. **(B)** Vascular density was calculated by ImageJ. (*n* = 6, data = mean ± SD.) (II: NIR; IV: HA hydrogel + NIR; and VI: CuS/HA hydrogel + NIR).

In our study, we have found that the CuS/HA hydrogel can promote the secretion of VEGF at the beginning of the healing process. This time is pivotal for the angiogenesis, while VEGF in the other groups does not increase rapidly and sensitively. As time went on, the VEGF in the other groups then increased gradually, but they might miss the golden window phase. In the initial stage of healing, the more angiogenesis appears, the faster wound healing will be. However, the increased expression of angiogenesis in the middle and later stages is not beneficial to epidermal remodeling for the healing. The wound healing process generally consists of several intersecting and fused parts, including thrombosis, inflammation, hyperplasia, and remodeling (Wang et al., 2019). Each part is not independent, but a complex whole of intersecting and interacting with each other. The cellular proliferation status, granulation tissue formation, collagen matrix deposition, and remodeling processes are all making great contributions to efficient wound healing. Our CuS/HA hydrogels accelerate the wound healing not only by angiogenesis but also through boosting collagen matrix deposition which was proved by the observation of Masson's trichrome staining. Why could our CuS/HA hydrogels have this talent to kill two birds with one stone? These good characteristics should attribute the success to the biological effect of copper. Copper ion is involved in the activity of many transcription factors and combines with the release complex of the cell membrane to promote the release of growth factors and cytokines. Moreover, copper can stimulate angiogenesis and collagen deposition at the same time, which has been proved by Gérard et al. (2010).

As a wound dressing, the long-term stability of CuS NPs *in vivo* should be considered. When ingested by the organism, what is the fate of NPs? All forms [zero-valent state (Cu0), ionic copper (Cu1 + orCu2 +), copper NPs] of copper may cause varying degrees of biotoxicity at high exposure concentrations (Ameh and Sayes, 2019). Some studies have shown that copper NPs have cytotoxic and genotoxic effects on human skin epidermal cells (HaCaT), which is mediated by mitochondrial pathways triggered by reactive oxygen species (ROS; Alarifi et al., 2016). Because the size of copper NPs is very small, a single copper nanoparticle can be transferred through intercellular or permeated through the cell membrane. Eventually, the particles enter the bloodstream. Most copper nanoparticles were mainly found in feces. This suggests that the colon removes most of the unabsorbed particles (Lee et al., 2016).

To make sure the needs of copper can meet while minimizing adverse effects associated with defects or overages, organisms have developed a series of strategies to maintain homeostasis. As for mammalians, they can make the Cu change not significantly through intestinal absorption, biliary excretion, and intrahepatic storage, when the organisms expose in mild to moderate concentration of Cu (Gaetke et al., 2014). These mechanisms have significant meanings in exploring the appropriate concentration of copper nanoparticles in the process of fabricating Cu NPs contained biomaterials. In our study, there was no obvious toxicity appearance, indicating that the concentration of Cu NPs used might be safe in our condition.

CONCLUSION

In conclusion, we successfully prepared CuS/HA hydrogel for wound healing. Within the gelation time, the hydrogel could be injected into the skin wounds. The hydrogel exhibited good photothermal effect, with increasing temperature of 50°C after 10 min irradiation with NIR light at 808 nm, as well as no toxicity to the cells *in vitro*. In the rat skin wound model, the CuS/HA hydrogel can effectively increase the collagen deposition, upregulate the expression of VEGF, and enhance angiogenesis, which might contribute to promote wound healing.

AUTHOR CONTRIBUTIONS

WZ performed the experiments, writing the manuscript, and the discussion of the results. LZ performed the experiments. YC and CY were involved in the discussion of the results. MT was responsible for conceptualizing, performed the experiments, the discussion of the results, and revising the manuscript.

REFERENCES

Alarifi, S., Ali, D., Verma, A., Alakhtani, S., and Ali, B. A. (2016). Cytotoxicity and genotoxicity of copper oxide nanoparticles in human skin keratinocytes cells. *Int. J. Toxicol.* 32, 296–307. doi: 10.1177/1091581813487563

Ameh, T., and Sayes, C. M. (2019). The potential exposure and hazards of copper nanoparticles: a review. *Environ. Toxicol. Pharmacol.* 71:103220. doi: 10.1016/j.etap.2019.103220

Browne, S., and Pandit, A. (2015). Biomaterial-Mediated modification of the local inflammatory environment. *Front. Bioeng. Biotechnol.* 3:67. doi: 10.3389/fbioe.2015.00067

Burgoyne, R. D., and Morgan, A. (2003). Secretory granule exocytosis. *Physiol. Rev.* 83, 581–632. doi: 10.1152/physrev.00031.2002

Das, S., and Baker, A. B. (2016). Biomaterials and nanotherapeutics for enhancing skin wound healing. *Front. Bioeng. Biotechnol.* 4:82. doi: 10.3389/fbioe.2016.00082

Ding, J., Chen, J., Gao, L., Jiang, Z., Zhang, Y., Li, M., et al. (2019). Engineered nanomedicines with enhanced tumor penetration. *Nano Today* 29:100800. doi: 10.1016/j.nantod.2019.100800

Du, P., Suhaeri, M., Ha, S. S., Oh, S. J., Kim, S. H., and Park, K. (2017). Human lung fibroblast-derived matrix facilitates vascular morphogenesis in 3D environment and enhances skin wound healing. *Acta Biomater.* 54, 333–344. doi: 10.1016/j.actbio.2017.03.035

Eldad, A., Weinberg, A., Breiterman, S., Chaouat, M., Palanker, D., and Ben-Bassat, H. (1998). Early nonsurgical removal of chemically injured tissue enhances wound healing in partial thickness burns. *Burns* 24, 166–172. doi: 10.1016/S0305-4179(97)00086-7

Feng, X., Xu, W., Li, Z., Song, W., Ding, J., and Chen, X. (2019). Immunomodulatory nanosystems. *Adv. Sci.* 6:1900101. doi: 10.1002/advs.201900101

Gaetke, L. M., Chow-Johnson, H. S., and Chow, C. K. (2014). Copper: toxicological relevance and mechanisms. *Arch. Toxicol.* 88, 1929–1938. doi: 10.1007/s00204-014-1355-y

Gérard, C., Bordeleau, L., Barralet, J., and Doillon, C. J. (2010). The stimulation of angiogenesis and collagen deposition by copper. *Biomaterials* 31, 824–831. doi: 10.1016/j.biomaterials.2009.10.009

Gopal, A., Kant, V., Gopalakrishnan, A., Tandan, S. K., and Kumar, D. (2014). Chitosan-based copper nanocomposite accelerates healing in excision wound model in rats. *Eur. J. Pharmacol.* 731, 8–19. doi: 10.1016/j.ejphar.2014.02.033

Lee, I. C., Ko, J. W., Park, S. H., Lim, J. O., Shin, I. S., Moon, C., et al. (2016). Comparative toxicity and biodistribution of copper nanoparticles and cupric ions in rats. *Int. J. Nanomedicine* 11, 2883–2900. doi: 10.2147/IJN.S106346

Li, M., Liu, X., Tan, L., Cui, Z., and Yang, X. (2018). Noninvasive rapid bacteria-killing and acceleration of wound healing through photothermal/photodynamic/copper ion synergistic action of a hybrid hydrogel. *Biomater. Sci.* 6, 2110–2121. doi: 10.1039/C8BM00499D

Li, S., Dong, S., Xu, W., Tu, S., and Yan, L. (2018). Antibacterial hydrogels. *Adv. Sci.* 5:1700527. doi: 10.1002/advs.201700527

Li, Z., Zhou, F., Li, Z., Lin, S., and Chen, L. (2018). Hydrogel cross-linked with dynamic covalent bonding and micellization for promoting burn wound healing. *ACS Appl. Mater. Interfaces* 10, 25194–25202. doi: 10.1021/acsami.8b08165

Lin, H., Wang, Q., Zhong, R., Li, Z., Zhao, W., Chen, Y., et al. (2019). Biomimetic phosphorylcholine strategy to improve the hemocompatibility of pH-responsive micelles containing tertiary amino groups. *Coll. Surf. B Biointerfaces* 184:110545. doi: 10.1016/j.colsurfb.2019.110545

Martin, N. A., and Falder, S. (2017). A review of the evidence for threshold of burn injury. *Burns* 43, 1624–1639. doi: 10.1016/j.burns.2017.04.003

Nowak-Sliwinska, P., Alitalo, K., Allen, E., Anisimov, A., Aplin, A. C., Auerbach, R., et al. (2018). Consensus guidelines for the use and interpretation of angiogenesis assays. *Angiogenesis* 21, 425–532. doi: 10.1007/s10456-018-9613-x

Savoji, H., Godau, B., Hassani, M. S., and Akbari, M. (2018). Skin tissue substitutes and biomaterial risk assessment and testing. *Front. Bioeng. Biotechnol.* 6:86. doi: 10.3389/fbioe.2018.00086

Shanmugapriya, K., and Kang, H. W. (2019). Engineering pharmaceutical nanocarriers for photodynamic therapy on wound healing: review. *Mater. Sci. Eng. C* 105:110110. doi: 10.1016/j.msec.2019.110110

Shu, X. Z., Liu, Y., Luo, Y., Roberts, M. C., and Prestwich, G. D. (2002). Disulfide cross-linked hyaluronan hydrogels. *Biomacromolecules* 3, 1304–1311. doi: 10.1021/bm025603c

Singh, W. R., Devi, H. S., Kumawat, S., Sadam, A., Appukuttan, A. V., Patel, M. R., et al. (2019). Angiogenic and MMPs modulatory effects of icariin improved cutaneous wound healing in rats. *Eur. J. Pharmacol.* 858:172466. doi: 10.1016/j.ejphar.2019.172466

Suarato, G., Bertorelli, R., and Athanassiou, A. (2018). Borrowing from nature: biopolymers and biocomposites as smart wound care materials. *Front. Bioeng. Biotechnol.* 6:137. doi: 10.3389/fbioe.2018.00137

Villegas, M. R., Baeza, A., and Vallet-Regí, M. (2019). Engineered nanomedicines with enhanced tumor penetration. *Nano Today* 29:100800. doi: 10.1016/j.nantod.2019.100800

Wang, Y., Jiang, Z., Xu, W., Yang, Y., Zhuang, X., Ding, J., et al. (2019). Chiral polypeptide thermogels induce controlled inflammatory response as potential immunoadjuvants. *ACS Appl. Mater. Interfaces* 11, 8725–8730. doi: 10.1021/acsami.9b01872

Yen, Y. H., Pu, C. M., Liu, C. W., Chen, Y. C., Chen, Y. C., Liang, C. J., et al. (2018). Curcumin accelerates cutaneous wound healing via multiple biological actions: the involvement of TNF-??, MMP-9, ??-SMA, and collagen. *Int. Wound J.* 15, 605–617. doi: 10.1111/iwj.12904

Yu, Y., Xu, Q., He, S., Xiong, H., Zhang, Q., Xu, W., et al. (2019). Recent advances in delivery of photosensitive metal-based drugs. *Coord. Chem. Rev.* 387, 154–179. doi: 10.1016/j.ccr.2019.01.020

Zhou, M., Li, J., Liang, S., Sood, A. K., Liang, D., and Li, C. (2015). CuS nanodots with ultrahigh efficient renal clearance for positron emission tomography imaging and Image-Guided photothermal therapy. *ACS Nano* 9, 7085–7096. doi: 10.1021/acsnano.5b02635

Zhou, M., Zhang, R., Huang, M., Lu, W., Song, S., Melancon, M. P., et al. (2010). A Chelator-Free multifunctional [64 cu]CuS nanoparticle platform for simultaneous Micro-PET/CT imaging and photothermal ablation therapy. *J. Am. Chem. Soc.* 132, 15351–15358. doi: 10.1021/ja106855m

Zhou, W. C., Tan, P. F., Chen, X. H., Cen, Y., You, C., Tan, L., et al. (2020). Berberine-Incorporated shape memory fiber applied as a novel surgical suture. *Front. Pharmacol.* 10:1506. doi: 10.3389/fphar.2019.01506

13

Scalable Biomimetic Coaxial Aligned Nanofiber Cardiac Patch: A Potential Model for "Clinical Trials in a Dish"

*Naresh Kumar[1,2†], Divya Sridharan[1,2†], Arunkumar Palaniappan[1,2,3], Julie A. Dougherty[1,2], Andras Czirok[4], Dona Greta Isai[5], Muhamad Mergaye[1,2], Mark G. Angelos[1,2], Heather M. Powell[5,6,7] and Mahmood Khan[1,2,8]**

[1] Department of Emergency Medicine, The Ohio State University Wexner Medical Center, Columbus, OH, United States, [2] Dorothy M. Davis Heart & Lung Research Institute, The Ohio State University Wexner Medical Center, Columbus, OH, United States, [3] Centre for Biomaterials, Cellular and Molecular Theranostics, Vellore Institute of Technology, Vellore, India, [4] Department of Anatomy and Cell Biology, University of Kansas Medical Center, Kansas City, KS, United States, [5] Department of Biomedical Engineering, The Ohio State University, Columbus, OH, United States, [6] Department of Materials Science and Engineering, The Ohio State University, Columbus, OH, United States, [7] Research Department, Shriners Hospitals for Children, Cincinnati, OH, United States, [8] Department of Physiology and Cell Biology, The Ohio State University Wexner Medical Center, Columbus, OH, United States

Correspondence:
Mahmood Khan
mahmood.khan@osumc.edu

† These authors have contributed equally to this work

Recent advances in cardiac tissue engineering have shown that human induced-pluripotent stem cell-derived cardiomyocytes (hiPSC-CMs) cultured in a three-dimensional (3D) micro-environment exhibit superior physiological characteristics compared with their two-dimensional (2D) counterparts. These 3D cultured hiPSC-CMs have been used for drug testing as well as cardiac repair applications. However, the fabrication of a cardiac scaffold with optimal biomechanical properties and high biocompatibility remains a challenge. In our study, we fabricated an aligned polycaprolactone (PCL)-Gelatin coaxial nanofiber patch using electrospinning. The structural, chemical, and mechanical properties of the patch were assessed by scanning electron microscopy (SEM), immunocytochemistry (ICC), Fourier-transform infrared spectroscopy (FTIR)-spectroscopy, and tensile testing. hiPSC-CMs were cultured on the aligned coaxial patch for 2 weeks and their viability [lactate dehydrogenase (LDH assay)], morphology (SEM, ICC), and functionality [calcium cycling, multielectrode array (MEA)] were assessed. Furthermore, particle image velocimetry (PIV) and MEA were used to evaluate the cardiotoxicity and physiological functionality of the cells in response to cardiac drugs. Nanofibers patches were comprised of highly aligned core-shell fibers with an average diameter of 578 ± 184 nm. Acellular coaxial patches were significantly stiffer than gelatin alone with an ultimate tensile strength of 0.780 ± 0.098 MPa, but exhibited gelatin-like biocompatibility. Furthermore, hiPSC-CMs cultured on the surface of these aligned coaxial patches (3D cultures) were elongated and rod-shaped with well-organized sarcomeres, as observed by the expression of cardiac troponin-T and α-sarcomeric actinin. Additionally, hiPSC-CMs cultured on these coaxial patches formed a functional syncytium evidenced by the expression of connexin-43 (Cx-43) and synchronous calcium transients. Moreover, MEA analysis showed that the hiPSC-CMs cultured on aligned patches showed an improved response to cardiac drugs like Isoproterenol (ISO), Verapamil (VER), and E4031, compared to the corresponding 2D cultures. Overall, our results demonstrated that an aligned, coaxial 3D cardiac patch can be used for culturing of hiPSC-CMs. These biomimetic cardiac patches could further be used as a potential 3D *in vitro* model for "clinical trials in a dish" and for *in vivo* cardiac repair applications for treating myocardial infarction.

Keywords: nanofibers, cardiac patch, myocardial infarction, cardiovascular disease, multielectrode array (MEA), 3D model, induced pluripotent stem cell-derived cardiomyocytes

INTRODUCTION

Cardiovascular diseases (CVDs) are the number one cause of morbidity in North America. However, the development of therapeutics for CVDs has been limited by the paucity of efficient model systems for drug screening and toxicology studies (Schroer et al., 2019). Most pharmacological studies make use of primary cell lines or model organisms like rodents, rabbits, pigs, and non-human primates for assessing the effect of putative drug molecules (Savoji et al., 2019). Small animal models like rodents, which have been extensively used for pre-clinical cardiovascular drug testing, are not ideal models, since their cardiomyocytes differ significantly from humans in their structure and function (Milani-Nejad and Janssen, 2014). On the other hand, large animal models (pigs and non-human primates) are good systems as their cardiovascular system and the associated hemodynamics are similar to humans. However, the costs associated with their housing, maintenance, and ethical concerns make them less favorable for pre-clinical drug testing applications (Milani-Nejad and Janssen, 2014). While primary cultures of adult cardiomyocytes are a good, cost-effective system to study drug effects *in vitro*, their use is restrained by their limited availability and lack of efficient culture protocols (Ribeiro et al., 2019).

In this context, human induced-pluripotent stem cell-derived cardiomyocytes (hiPSC-CMs) have become increasingly popular for use as an *in vitro* model system (Karakikes et al., 2015). These cells have shown great potential in developing strategies for cardiac repair (Park and Yoon, 2018). Additionally, the advances in techniques for hiPSC generation, ease of scalability of hiPSC-CMs, and development of next-generation genetic manipulation techniques make hiPSC-CMs an attractive model for the development of patient-specific personalized precision medicine (Park and Yoon, 2018; Gintant et al., 2019; Ribeiro et al., 2019). Hence, hiPSC-CMs have become increasingly popular as an *in vitro* model for cardioprotective and cardiotoxic drug screening (Lynch et al., 2019; Ribeiro et al., 2019). However, in most of these studies, hiPSC-CMs used were cultured in two-dimensional (2D) culture dishes (Antoni et al., 2015; Savoji et al., 2019). The 2D culture system has multiple drawbacks: (a) immature phenotype of hiPSC-CMs, (b) heterogeneity of the cells in culture, (c) lack of alignment of hiPSC-CMs, and (d) inconsistent response to drug treatment (Karakikes et al., 2015; da Rocha et al., 2017). However, recent studies have shown improved function and maturation of hiPSC-CMs in 2D cultures with increased culture time (Kumar et al., 2019) or electrical and mechanical stimulation (Machiraju and Greenway, 2019).

Overall, three-dimensional (3D) culture systems have been shown to improve the maturation as well as functionality of hiPSC-CMs (Savoji et al., 2019). Cells cultured in a 3D environment are shown to have better physiological characteristics and more closely resemble native tissue than the same cells grown in classical 2D culture flasks (Savoji et al., 2019). Hence, 3D cultures provide a better and more relevant model for cardiotoxicity and drug screening studies (Zuppinger, 2016, 2019; Archer et al., 2018; Savoji et al., 2019). The 3D models currently explored as CVD models include: (a) hydrogel-based engineered heart tissue (Weinberger et al., 2017), (b) self-assembling spheroids formed *via* hanging drop method (Figtree et al., 2017), (c) cardiac cell-sheets (Shimizu et al., 2003), and (d) bioengineered scaffolds (Khan et al., 2015, 2018; Kc et al., 2019). Of these, the scaffold-based models have been extensively studied for the development of engineered heart tissues (Gao et al., 2018; Dattola et al., 2019; Jabbour et al., 2019).

Three-dimensional scaffolds have been fabricated using different bioengineering techniques, like microfluidics (Wang et al., 2010), 3D bioprinting (Zhu et al., 2016), gas foaming (Costantini and Barbetta, 2018), and electrospinning (Jun et al., 2018). Of these, electrospinning provides for reduced batch-to-batch variation, better uniformity within scaffolds, nano-dimensional architecture similar to cardiac tissue, and controlled alignment of nanofibers (Kai et al., 2011; Khan et al., 2015; Kitsara et al., 2017). Further, nanofiber-based scaffolds have been fabricated using a wide variety of natural and synthetic biocompatible materials. It has been reported that scaffolds made using natural polymers like gelatin and collagen (Aldana and Abraham, 2017) exhibit efficient cell adhesion but poor mechanical properties. Alternatively, the scaffolds made using synthetic polymers like poly(lactic-co-glycolic) acid (PLGA; Khan et al., 2015), polylactic acid (PLA; Wang et al., 2017), and polycaprolactone (PCL; Chen et al., 2015) have poor biomimetic and cell adhesion properties but improved mechanical support (Bhattarai et al., 2018). In our study, we fabricated an aligned coaxial nanofibrous scaffold, with nanofibers having a PCL core with a gelatin shell. The PCL imparts mechanical strength while gelatin provides the required biomimetic properties, thereby improving cell attachment. The hiPSC-CMs were seeded and cultured on the surface of a 3D aligned coaxial nanofibrous scaffold to obtain a functional 3D 'cardiac patch,' which was then used for drug screening and toxicity studies.

MATERIALS AND METHODS

Fabrication of PCL-Gelatin Aligned Coaxial Nanofibrous Patch

Gelatin (12% w/v) [gelatin from bovine skin, Sigma-Aldrich, St. Louis, MO] and PCL (8% w/v) [Sigma-Aldrich, St. Louis, MO; Mn = 42,500] solutions were prepared in 1,1,1,3,3,3-hexafluoro-2-propanol. The gelatin and PCL solutions were fed to the outer (at a flow rate of 4 ml/h) and inner tube (at a flow rate of 1 ml/h), respectively, of the coaxial spinneret as shown in **Figure 1A**. The distance between the spinneret tip and the grounded rotating collector was maintained at 20 cm and a 20 kV voltage was applied at the spinneret tip. The aligned coaxial nanofibers collected were dried inside a chemical fume hood overnight, to remove remnant solvent.

The morphology of the nanofibrous patch was assessed by scanning electron microscopy (SEM). To confirm the coaxial morphology of the nanofibrous patch, gelatin and PCL solutions were mixed with 1% w/v fluorescein (Sigma-Aldrich, St. Louis, MO) and rhodamine (Sigma-Aldrich, St. Louis, MO), respectively, and nanofibrous patches were fabricated as mentioned above and imaged using a confocal microscope (Olympus FV3000 Confocal microscope).

Patches were first cross-linked, sterilized, and hydrated using the protocol described previously (Drexler and Powell, 2011). Briefly, patches were cut into the desired diameter using biopsy punches (8 mm) and treated with 7 mM 1-ethyl-3-(3Dimethylamino propyl)carbodiimide hydrochloride (EDC) solution in ethanol for 24 h, followed by incubation in 70% ethanol for hydration and sterilization. The patches were then washed in phospahate-buffered saline (PBS), two times for 24 h each. Patches were then used for confocal imaging, mechanical testing, and cell seeding.

Fourier-Transform Infrared Spectroscopy (FTIR) Studies

Surface chemical analysis of the gelatin-only, PCL-only, and coaxial patches was performed using attenuated total reflection Fourier transform infrared spectroscopy (ATR-FTIR) between the range of 400–4000 cm^{-1} (Thermo Nicolet Nexus 670 FTIR spectrometer, MN). Approximately 25–40 scans were performed on the three types of patches.

Mechanical Testing of Nanofiber Scaffolds

The mechanical properties of acellular aligned PCL, gelatin, and PCL-gelatin coaxial nanofibrous patches were tested using a TestResources 100R (Shakopee, MN) as per the American Society for Testing and Materials (ASTM) D638 Type V standard, using the protocol described previously (Johnson et al., 2007; Blackstone et al., 2018). For aligned gelatin and coaxial patches, tests were performed after crosslinking in EDC solution and further hydration in PBS (described above). For aligned PCL patches, incubation was carried out in ethanol (to mimic the crosslinking process) before hydration in PBS. The thickness of each sample was measured using digital calipers. Samples were strained (along the axis of alignment) at a grip speed of 2 mm/s until failure. Samples were made using a dog-bone shaped punch, 3 mm gauge width, and 10 mm gauge length. The thickness of each sample was quantified using digital calipers. Stress-strain curves were generated for each sample and the ultimate tensile strength and Young's modulus were determined and reported as mean $\pm$ SD. Ultimate tensile strength was determined at the point of greatest stress, before failure. Young's modulus was calculated from the stress-strain curve using linear regression analysis for the first linear region of the curve (where $R^2 \sim 0.98$) past the toe-in region, if present.

Degradation Studies

The scaffold was cut into small 8 mm diameter circular patches and incubated in medium at 37°C for 2 weeks. After 1 and 2 weeks, the patches were rinsed in water, air-dried and weighed to determine their weight loss by degradation. The weights of four independent samples were measured for each time point. Additionally, the patches were imaged using SEM to assess any morphological changes in the fibers during the 2-week culture duration.

Culturing and Maintenance of hiPSC-CMs on Aligned Coaxial Nanofibrous Patches

The hiPSC-CMs were obtained from Fujifilm Cellular Dynamics International (CDI, Madison, WI, United States, Cat# R 1007). The cells were plated in sterile six-well plates according to the manufacturer's protocol and after 48 h, cells were cultured in CDI hiPSC-CMs maintenance medium in a humidified atmosphere at 37°C at 5% CO_2, as previously described (Citro et al., 2014; Khan et al., 2015).

Once the hiPSC-CMs showed contractions, the cells were seeded onto aligned coaxial nanofibrous patches. For this, sterile cross-linked 8 mm aligned coaxial patches were transferred onto N-terface (Winfield Labs, Richardson, TX, United States) and coated with 30 µl of fibronectin (50 µg/ml) for 1 h in a humidified atmosphere at 37°C. The patches on N-terface were then transferred onto sterile sponges soaked in the hiPSC-CMs' culture medium placed in a 100 mm culture dish. The hiPSC-CMs were harvested using 0.25% trypsin-EDTA and seeded onto the coaxial patches at a final density of 1×10^6 cells/cm^2 (50 µl of cell suspension/patch) and incubated at 5% CO_2 at 37°C for 1 h. After 4–6 h, the aligned coaxial cardiac patches (aligned coaxial nanofibrous patches seeded with hiPSC-CMs) were transferred to six-well plates (one patch/well) containing 2 ml CDI hiPSC-CMs maintenance medium. The medium was replaced every alternate day for 2 weeks.

Scanning Electron Microscopy (SEM)

Scanning electron microscopy was used to observe the morphology of the aligned PCL, gelatin, and PCL-gelatin

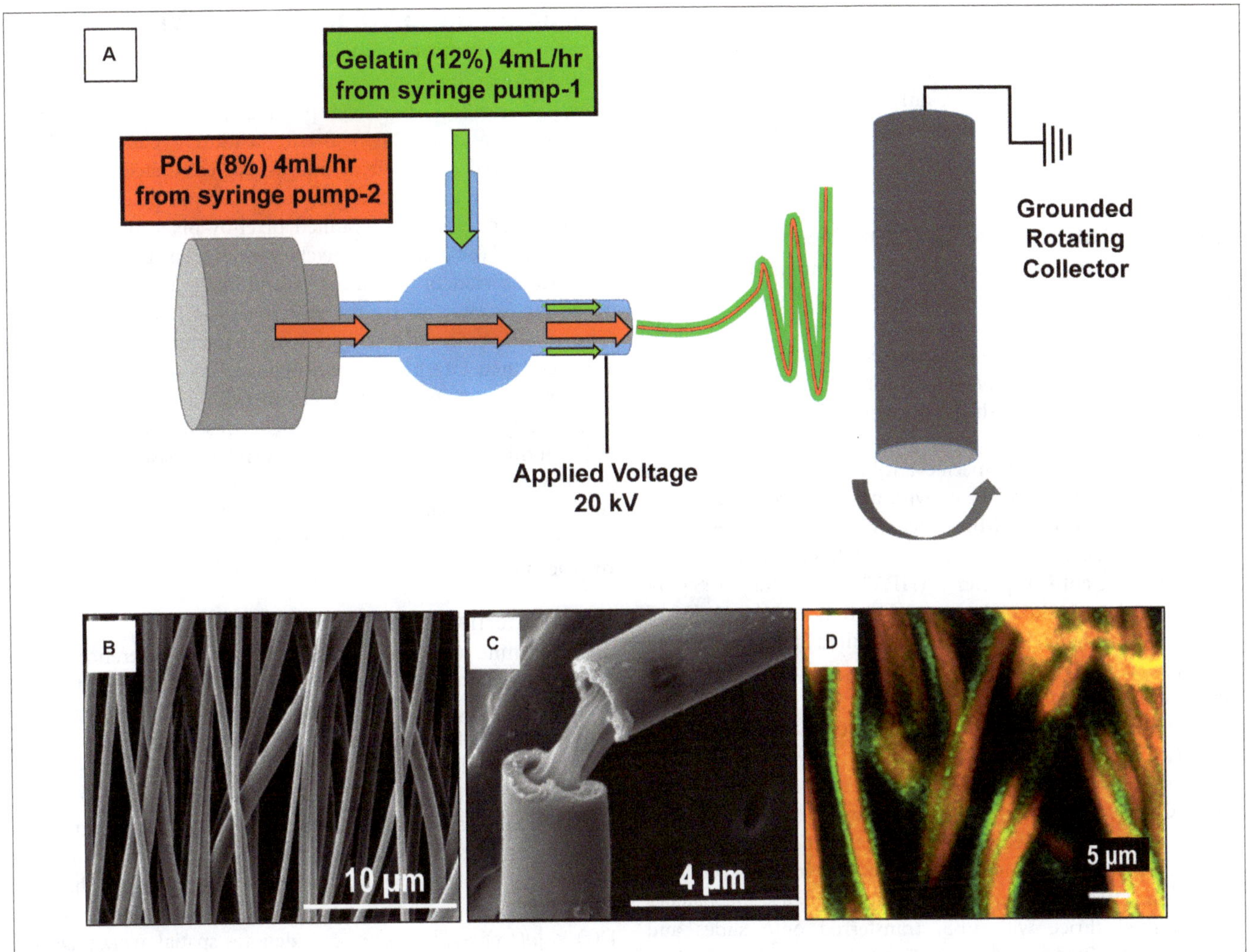

FIGURE 1 | Schematic of the aligned coaxial nanofibrous cardiac patch fabrication process. **(A)** Polycaprolactone (PCL; 8% w/v) and Gelatin (12% w/v) were employed for the fabrication of aligned coaxial (CoA) nanofibrous patches by an electrospinning method. **(B)** SEM image of the aligned CoA nanofibrous patch. **(C)** SEM image of a single CoA nanofiber showing a core-shell structure. **(D)** Confocal image of aligned CoA nanofibers showing the presence of PCL (red) in the core and gelatin (green) in the shell.

coaxial nanofibrous patches. SEM was also performed on aligned coaxial cardiac patches to determine the distribution and alignment of the seeded hiPSC-CMs. For these studies, the samples were prepared as described previously (Huang et al., 2013; McBane et al., 2013; Khan et al., 2015). In brief, the cardiac patches were fixed in 4% paraformaldehyde (PFA, MilliporeSigma, Milwaukee, WI, United States) for 1 h. Patches were then washed with de-ionized water and further dehydrated by gradually increasing ethanol concentration (50, 70, 80, 95, and 100%). The patches were then dried chemically using an increasing gradient of hexamethyldisilazane. Finally, patches were sputter-coated with gold-palladium (Pelco Model 3) and imaged on FEI NOVA nanoSEM.

Cellular Viability Staining of hiPSC-CMs

LIVE/DEAD™ Cell Imaging Kit (Cat # R37601) was procured from Invitrogen (Life Technologies Corporation, Carlsbad, CA, United States) and used to stain the live and dead cells in culture per the manufacturer's instructions. After staining, the hiPSC-CMs were washed with maintenance medium three times and imaging was performed on an EVOS™ FL Auto 2 Fluorescent microscope (Thermo Fisher Scientific, Waltham, MA, United States).

Lactate Dehydrogenase (LDH) Assay

To measure the cytotoxicity of the aligned coaxial patch on hiPSC-CMs, LDH assay was performed using the *in vitro* toxicology assay kit, lactic dehydrogenase based (Cat# TOX7-1KT, MilliporeSigma, Milwaukee, WI, United States). The culture medium was collected from hiPSC-CMs cultured in tissue culture plates or on aligned coaxial patches after 48 h of culture and LDH release assay was performed according to the manufacturer's protocols. Background and primary absorbance of the plate were measured on a spectrophotometer (2030 Multilabel Reader, Victor™

×3, PerkinElmer, Inc., Waltham, MA, United States) at 690 and 490 nm, respectively. The assay was performed in quadruplicate ($n = 4$) and data obtained was analyzed on WorkOut 2.5 (build 0428, PerkinElmer, Inc., Waltham, MA, United States), by subtracting background absorbance from primary absorbance.

Immunostaining for Cardiac Markers

As described previously (Khan et al., 2015), immunofluorescence staining was performed to analyze the expression of cardiac markers in aligned coaxial cardiac patches. Briefly, aligned coaxial cardiac patches, after 2 weeks in culture, were washed twice with PBS and fixed with 4% PFA for 10 min at room temperature. The patches were then washed twice with PBS and incubated in blocking buffer (PBS, 5% normal goat serum, and 0.3% Triton X) for 1 h to block non-specific antibody binding. Following this, the patches were incubated with anti-α-sarcomeric actinin (A7811, MilliporeSigma, Milwaukee, WI, United States), anti-GATA4 (PA1-102, Thermo Fisher Scientific, Waltham, MA, United States), anti-Troponin-T (HPA017888, MilliporeSigma, Milwaukee, WI, United States), and anti-Connexin-43 (MAB 3067, MilliporeSigma, Milwaukee, WI, United States) antibodies, overnight at 4°C and after which the patches were washed thrice in PBS, 5 min. each. Cells were then incubated with the corresponding secondary antibodies conjugated either with Texas Red or FITC against rabbit (1:5000, 8889S, Cell Signaling Technology, Danvers, MA, United States) or mouse (1:5000, 4408S, Cell Signaling Technology, Danvers, MA, United States) for 1 h at room temperature in the dark and washed thrice in PBS. Nuclei were counterstained with NucBlue (R37605, Invitrogen, Carlsbad, CA, United States). Finally, the patches were washed thrice with PBS, transferred onto slides and mounted with ProLong™ Glass Antifade mounting medium (Cat# P36984, Invitrogen, Carlsbad, CA, United States). Imaging was performed on a confocal microscope (Olympus FV 1000 spectral, Olympus Corporation, Center Valley, PA, United States) and images were processed using the Olympus FLUOVIEW Ver. 4.2a Viewer.

Assessment of Calcium Cycling in hiPSC-CMs

Calcium transients were imaged in hiPSC-CMs cultured on fibronectin-coated glass coverslips and aligned coaxial cardiac patches using the calcium-binding dye Fluo-3, AM (F1242, Invitrogen, Carlsbad, CA, United States). For staining, the hiPSC-CMs cultured on coverslips or patches were washed three times with Dulbecco's Modified Eagle's Medium (DMEM) and incubated in 5 μM Fluo 3-AM in DMEM for 1 h in dark at 37°C, 5% CO_2 in a humidified atmosphere. The cells were then washed three times in DMEM and incubated for an additional 30 min in serum-containing medium at 37°C, 5% CO_2 in a humidified atmosphere. The cell culture plate was then placed on the microscope (Leica Microsystems, Wetzlar, Germany) stage to record a movie using Leica Application Suite X 3.0.6.17580 software.

Particle Image Velocimetry (PIV)

Cross-Correlation ("PIV") Analysis of Images

Cell contractility kinetics were assessed using the optical flow/PIV method described previously (Zamir et al., 2005; Aleksandrova et al., 2012). Briefly, a motion pattern (velocity field) captured on a pair of images was calculated by dividing the first image into overlapping tiles, each 64 pixels wide. The second image was then scanned pixel-by-pixel, by shifting an equally sized (64 pixels × 64 pixels) window. The most similar (by Euclidean distance) tile on the second image was then assumed to be the location where the pattern in the first image moved. The resulting displacement vectors characterizing each image tile were then interpolated and denoised by a thin-plate spline fit, yielding our coarse displacement field. The coarse estimate was used to construct a second, higher resolution displacement field. In this second step, the cross-correlation search for pattern similarity was repeated with tiles that were only 32 pixels wide but in a much smaller search area allowing only for four-pixel displacements around the location predicted by the coarse displacement field.

Beat Patterns

To determine the beat patterns, a suitable reference image taken at time t^*, which is a frame between two contraction cycles, where movement is minimal: $V(t) \geq V(t^*)$, in a motion-free state, was first identified. This reference image was then compared to all other images of the recordings with cross-correlation ("PIV") analysis. The result is a series of displacement vector fields $d(t,x)$, which estimate for each time point t and location x the total movement (magnitude and directionality) relative to a resting state. For each time point t the beat pattern $D(t)$ is the spatial average of the magnitude of $d(t,x)$ as $D(t) \leq |d(t,x)| >_x$, where $<\ldots>_x$ denotes spatial averaging over all possible locations x.

Frequency Analysis

Fourier spectra were calculated from $D(t)$ beat patterns using the discrete Fourier transform algorithm as described previously (Rajasingh et al., 2018). Power densities were calculated as the magnitudes of the squared Fourier spectra, and indicate periodicity within the signal in the form of peaks at the corresponding frequencies. When the analyzed signal is not a pure sine wave, harmonics are expected to appear at integer multiples of the fundamental frequency f ($2f$, $3f$, etc.). The magnitude of a peak in the power spectrum indicates the amplitude of the signal oscillating with the corresponding frequency.

Convergence Analysis

Cell layers often move passively without actively contracting. The optical flow-based method does not distinguish between active and passive (elastic response of the adjacent cell layer) contractility. To identify contractile centers, we estimated the convergence maps of the displacement field as its negative divergence from optical flow data $d(t,x)$ as previously described (Czirok et al., 2017).

Functional Characterization Using a Multi-Electrode Array (MEA) System

The field potentials of hiPSC-CMs cultured in 2D or on aligned coaxial patches (3D) were measured using an MEA system. For this, hiPSC-CMs were either cultured directly on 24-well MEA plates (M384-tMEA-24W, Axion Biosystems, Atlanta, GA, United States) having 16 PEDOT microelectrodes per well (as described previously; Kumar et al., 2019) or on 8 mm aligned coaxial patches; both were cultured for 2 weeks. The aligned coaxial cardiac patches were transferred into a sterile six-well MEA plate (M384-tMEA-6W, Axion Biosystems, Atlanta, GA, United States) having 64 PEDOT microelectrodes per well. The plate was equilibrated in the MEA system (Maestro Edge, Axion Biosystems, Atlanta, GA, United States) for 30 min in 5% CO_2 with a humidified atmosphere at 37°C. For the patches, the excess culture medium was removed to facilitate better contact with the electrodes. The baseline was recorded for each well for 5 min. After which the hiPSC-CMs in 2D, as well as the cardiac patches, were treated with different cardiac drugs: (a) Isoproterenol (ISO, 10 and 100 nM), (b) Verapamil (VER, 0.1 and 0.3 μM), and (c) E4031 hydrochloride (E4031, 50 and 100 nM). The stock solutions of all drugs were prepared in dimethylsulphoxide (DMSO). The plates were equilibrated for 5 min after the addition of drugs and the field potentials were recorded for 5 min for each drug treatment. AxIS Navigator version™ 1.4.1.9 was used for data recording while CiPA™ analysis tool version 2.1.10 (Axion Biosystems, Atlanta, GA, United States) was used for data analysis. The beat period, field potential duration (FPD), spike amplitude, and the incidences of arrhythmias were calculated. Further, the Fredericia's correction was applied to the FPD, to interpret the effect of drugs on the QT interval. Data are expressed as mean ± SD ($n = 3$).

Statistical Analysis

Data acquired is expressed as mean ± SD. Statistical significance was determined using one-way ANOVA. All pairwise multiple comparison procedures were performed by the Holm–Sidak method. p-value < 0.05 was considered statistically significant.

RESULTS

Fabrication of Aligned Nanofibrous Coaxial, PCL, and Gelatin Patches

Aligned nanofibrous PCL-gelatin coaxial patches were successfully fabricated via electrospinning (**Figure 1A**). Coaxial nanofibers were highly aligned with a mean diameter of 578 ± 184 nm (**Figure 1B**). The overall mean thickness of the aligned coaxial nanofibrous patches was 115 ± 11 μm. SEM imaging of a single nanofiber showed a core-shell structure indicating successful coaxial morphology (**Figure 1C**). Further, confocal microscope images of the coaxial patches after mixing of rhodamine and fluorescein with PCL and gelatin, respectively, validated the coaxial morphology. These images clearly showed the presence of PCL (red) in the core and gelatin (green) in the shell (**Figure 1D**). Following hydration, confocal image analysis showed that the nanofibers had a diameter of 2.21 ± 0.50 μm. Additionally, a comparison of the SEM images of pure PCL and pure gelatin nanofibrous patches versus coaxial patches clearly showed that the coaxial nanofibers were more uniform and cylindrical in morphology (**Figure 2A**). AFTIR analysis of the PCL and gelatin patches showed peaks corresponding to C = O ester of PCL at 1722 cm^{-1} (green) and peaks corresponding to the amide groups of gelatin at 1544 and 1657 cm^{-1} (brown; **Figure 2B**). Coaxial patches exhibited all three peaks (**Figure 2B**), further reiterating the presence of both polymers in the nanofibers.

Mechanical Testing of Aligned Coaxial Patches

The mechanical strength of PCL, gelatin, and the PCL-gelatin coaxial patches was determined by tensile testing. The stress-strain curves obtained showed that the aligned PCL-only patch had the highest values for both tensile strength (1.490 ± 0.290 MPa) as well as Young's modulus (0.093 ± 0.017 MPa; **Figures 2C,D**). This was followed by the aligned coaxial patch, which had a tensile strength and Young's modulus of 0.780 ± 0.098 and 0.039 ± 0.007 MPa, respectively (**Figures 2C,D**). The aligned gelatin patches had the least mechanical strength with tensile strength and Young's modulus of 0.308 ± 0.032 and 0.009 ± 0.001 MPa (**Figures 2C,D**), respectively. However, in terms of percent elongation, gelatin showed the highest elongation, while no significant difference was observed between the PCL and coaxial patches (**Figure 2E**). Therefore, the aligned coaxial patches had strength and stiffness intermediate to PCL and gelatin, a percent elongation at failure similar to PCL alone, and their elongation at failure matched the PCL patches.

Degradation of Aligned Coaxial Nanofiber Scaffolds

The degradation of the coaxial scaffolds at 1 and 2 weeks was determined by measuring their weight loss and studying their morphology. SEM images of the scaffolds after 7 and 14 days (**Figures 3A,B**) in culture did not show any striking differences when compared to the crosslinked patches at the beginning of the experiment (**Figure 1B**). Furthermore, no significant difference was observed in the weight of the scaffold after 7 and 14 days in the culture (**Figure 3C**). Taken together, this data suggests that the scaffolds did not undergo rapid degradation under the culture conditions used in our study.

Morphology and Viability of hiPSC-CMs on Aligned Coaxial Nanofibrous Patches

The hiPSC-CMs cultured on aligned coaxial patches and their morphology was assessed at 2 weeks by SEM. The SEM images showed a uniform distribution and attachment of the hiPSC-CMs on the coaxial patches (**Figure 3D**). The hiPSC-CMs also showed a parallel alignment with the nanofibers (**Figure 3E**). The viability of the hiPSC-CMs cultured on the coaxial patches was assessed by staining the cardiomyocytes with Calcein-AM (for live cells), BOBO-3 iodide (for dead

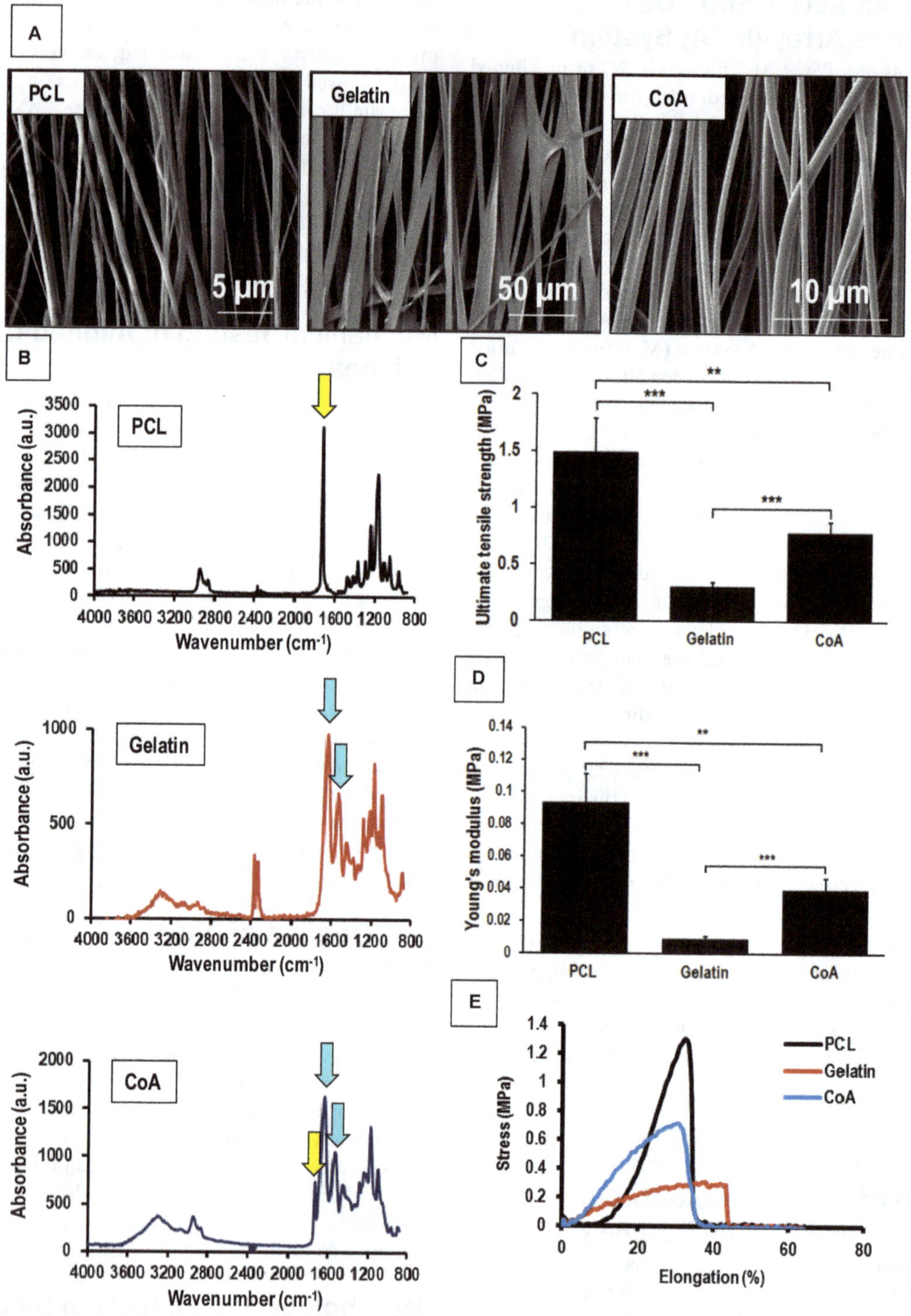

FIGURE 2 | Mechanical testing of aligned nanofibrous patches and comparison with aligned coaxial patch. **(A)** SEM images of aligned PCL, aligned gelatin, and aligned coaxial (CoA) PCL/Gel nanofibrous patches. **(B)** FTIR spectra of aligned PCL, aligned gelatin, and aligned CoA PCL/Gel nanofibrous patches. **(C)** Tensile strength, yellow and blue arrows indicate functional groups corresponding to PCL and gelatin, respectively, **(D)** Young's modulus, and **(E)** Stress vs. elongation% for aligned PCL, aligned gelatin, and aligned CoA PCL/Gel nanofibrous patches. n = 4; $^{**}p < 0.01$; $^{***}p < 0.001$.

cells), and LDH assay (**Figure 3F**). Fluorescence images showed that a majority of cardiomyocytes stained positive for calcein-AM, indicating that they are viable and metabolically active (**Figures 3G,I**). Additionally, some cardiomyocytes stained positive for BOBO-3 iodide (**Figures 3H,I**), indicating that the patch was biocompatible. Furthermore, no significant differences

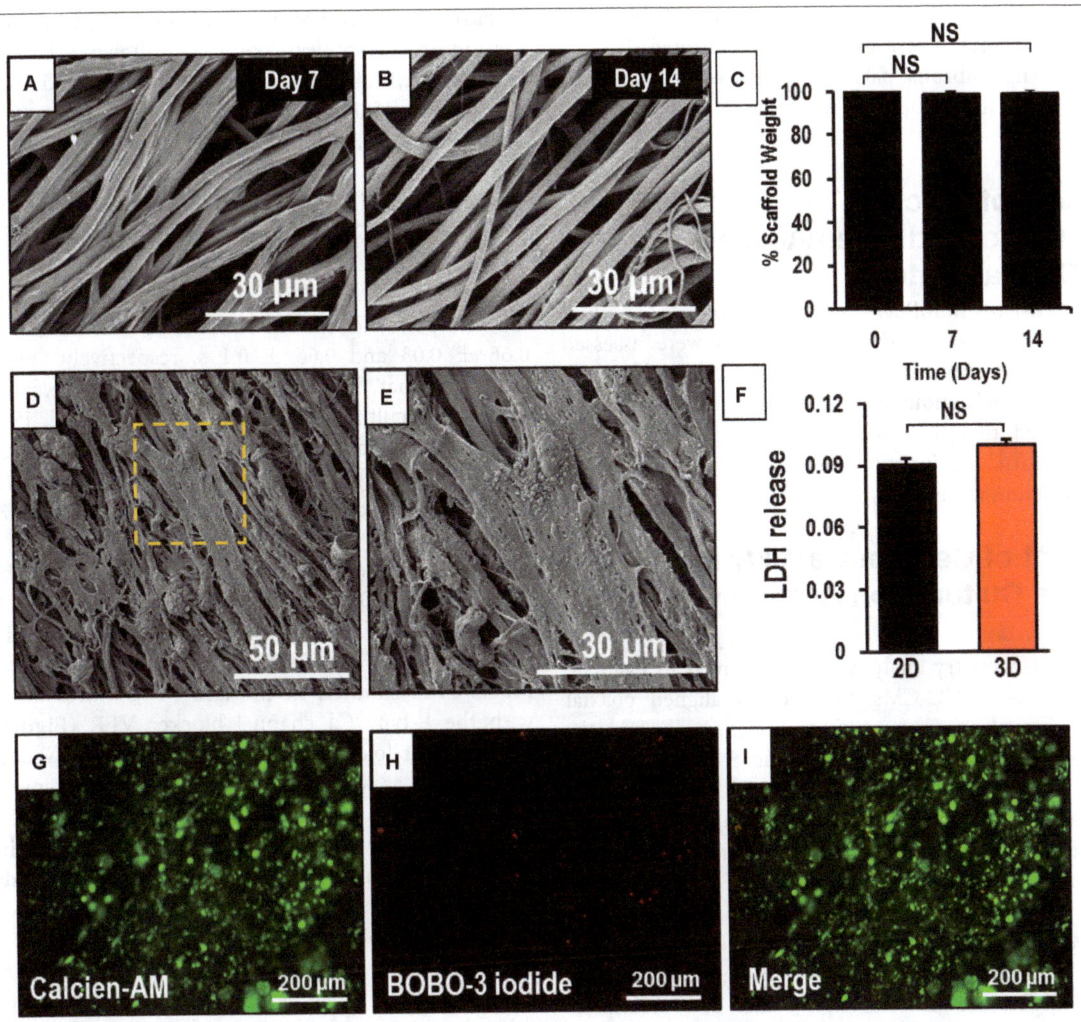

FIGURE 3 | Assessment of degradability and biocompatibility of human induced-pluripotent stem cell-derived cardiomyocytes (hiPSC-CMs) seeded on an aligned coaxial patch. **(A,B)** SEM images of the aligned coaxial patches after 1 and 2 weeks in culture. **(C)** Weight of the coaxial scaffolds after 1 and 2 weeks in culture. NS, not significant. **(D,E)** SEM images of hiPSC-CMs cultured on aligned coaxial (CoA) PCL/Gel nanofibrous patches. **(F)** Fold change in LDH released by hiPSC-CMs cultured in tissue culture plates (2D) and CoA patches (3D) as compared control. Data expressed as mean ± SD, *n* = 3. NS, not significant. **(G–I)** Live-dead cell staining of hiPSC-CMs cultured on coaxial aligned scaffolds showing live cells stained with Calcein-AM (green) and dead cells stained with BOBO-3 iodide (red) after 2 weeks in culture.

were observed in LDH released from hiPSC-CMs cultured on the aligned coaxial nanofibrous patches (3D) versus on a flat-plate (2D) (**Figure 3F**). Taken together, these results showed that aligned coaxial PCL/Gel patches are biocompatible and support the 3D culture of hiPSC-CMs.

Confocal Imaging to Assess the Expression of Cardiac Markers in hiPSC-CMs Cultured on an Aligned Coaxial Patch

The expression of cardiac makers in hiPSC-CMs was assessed by confocal imaging to understand the intracellular sarcomere arrangement in the cells following culture on the aligned coaxial patches. At 2 weeks, the hiPSC-CMs cultured on aligned coaxial patches stained positive for the cardiac lineage markers; GATA 4, Nkx2.5, α-sarcomeric actinin (α-SA), cardiac Troponin T (TnT), and connexin-43 (Cx-43) (**Figure 4**). Expression of the cardiac transcription factors GATA4 (**Figures 4A–F**) and Nkx2.5 (**Figures 4J,K**) was detected in the nucleus of the hiPSC-CMs. Additionally, these hiPSC-CMs showed parallelly arranged sarcomeres, as observed by α-SA (**Figures 4A–F,I**) and TnT staining (**Figures 4G,H,J,K**). Also, the hiPSC-CMs showed the expression of Cx-43, indicating good intercellular contact between neighboring cardiomyocytes (**Figures 4G,H**). The distribution of the hiPSC-CMs was also assessed across the depth of the patch. The cross-sections and Z-stack confocal images of aligned coaxial cardiac patches showed migration of the hiPSC-CMs up to 40–50 microns below the surface of the scaffold (**Figures 4C,D,F,J**), evidenced by the expression of α-SA, TnT, GATA4, and Nkx2.5. Additionally, increased magnification of a single hiPSC-CM imaged on the patch showed a multi-nucleated rod-shaped morphology with well-organized sarcomeres (**Figure 4I**). These observations indicated that the aligned coaxial nanofibrous patch can be used as a model for understanding the structural maturation of hiPSC-CMs on 3D scaffolds.

Assessment of Calcium Transients in hiPSC-CMs Seeded on an Aligned Coaxial Cardiac Patch

The calcium transients in hiPSC-CMs cultured on tissue culture plates (2D) and aligned coaxial patches (3D) were assessed after 2 weeks in culture. The hiPSC-CMs cultured in 2D and 3D showed synchronous calcium transients (**Figure 5A**). This data showed that the hiPSC-CMs cultured on aligned coaxial patches formed a functional syncytium as indicated by synchronous calcium waves.

Assessment of Cell Contractility in hiPSC-CMs Cultured on Aligned Coaxial Patches

Particle image velocimetry analysis was performed to evaluate the contractility of hiPSC-CMs cultured on aligned coaxial patches. For this, the response of the patches, at 2 weeks of culture, to 100 nM ISO, a non-specific β-adrenoreceptor agonist, was analyzed by an optical measure of contractility (**Figures 5B–G**). For both treated and control cultures, six videomicroscopic recordings were obtained from two parallel cultures. Beat patterns (**Figures 5B,E**) indicated an ISO-induced increase in spontaneous beat frequency and amplitude. Also, Fourier power spectra of the beat patterns indicated an increase in frequency by shifting the dominant peak toward higher frequencies (right) after ISO treatment (**Figures 5C,F**). A significant increase ($p < 0.0004$) in the average frequency of spontaneous beating from 0.136 ± 0.0069 to 1.497 ± 0.0394 SEM Hz was observed following ISO treatment (**Figures 5C,F**). Additionally, ISO treatment also promoted better-defined beating activity that is indicated by the tall narrow peaks. The contractility maps showed a stronger, spatially extended beating activity in ISO-treated patches (**Figures 5D,G**). These results demonstrate the ability of the aligned coaxial patches to respond to cardiac drugs in a reproducible manner.

Electrophysiological Assessment of hiPSC-CMs Cultured on Aligned Coaxial Patches

The hiPSC-CMs cultured in 2D and 3D (aligned coaxial patch) was assessed on the MEA system for field potentials, which result from spontaneous cardiac action potentials propagating across cells on neighboring electrodes. The hiPSC-CMs were treated with different concentrations of ISO, VER, and E4031, and the changes in their field potential was measured. An increase in the beating frequency (beats per minute) was observed in both the 2D as well as 3D cultures following treatment with ISO (**Figures 6A,B**) and VER (**Figures 6A,C**), while a decrease in beating frequency was observed following E4031 treatment (**Figures 7A,B**). These changes were as expected for these drugs' mechanisms of action.

A significant, dose-dependent decrease in the beat period was observed in hiPSC-CMs in both 2D and 3D cultures after treatment with ISO. After treatment with 10 nM ISO, the beat period in the 2D and 3D cultures decreased from 1.04 ± 0.04 and 1.22 ± 0.16 s to 0.67 ± 0.04 and 0.8 ± 0.15 s, respectively (**Figures 6D,E**). Similarly, after treatment with 100 nM ISO, the beat period of the hiPSC-CMs in 2D and 3D cultures was 0.66 ± 0.03 and 0.66 ± 0.1 s, respectively (**Figures 6D,E**), indicating that the dose-dependent response was improved in case of 3D cultures. Furthermore, as expected, ISO treatment resulted in a dose-dependent shortening of the QT interval, as evidenced by the decrease in Friedrica's corrected field potential duration (FPDc) in both the 2D and 3D cultures (**Figures 6D–F**). Also, between the 2D and 3D cultures, a significant difference in the FPDc was observed after treatment with 10 and 100 nM ISO, indicating that the 3D cultures responded more robustly to the treatment (**Figure 6F**). A similar decrease in the beat period and FPDc was observed in the hiPSC-CMs cultured in 2D and 3D cultures after treatment with the L-type Ca channel blocker VER (**Figures 6C,G–I**). A significant fold decrease in the beat period was observed in both the 2D as well as 3D cultures after treatment with 0.1 and 0.3 μM VER, as compared to their respective baseline controls (**Figure 6I**). However, a dose-dependent decrease in the FPDc was observed only in the case of the 3D culture indicating that the 3D culture system was a more responsive model for drug testing (**Figure 6I**).

We also assessed the effect of the hERG-type K^+ channel blocker E4031, which is an anti-arrhythmic drug. However, this drug is pro-arrhythmic *in vitro* especially at higher doses (Goto et al., 2018). As expected, following treatment with the E4031, a significant increase in the beat period and FPDc was observed in the 2D cultures following treatment with 50 and 100 nM of E4031, while a significant increase was observed in 3D cultures only after treatment with 100 nM E4031 (**Figures 7C–E**). Furthermore, we also observed higher variability in the FPDc in 3D cultures as compared to the 2D cultures (**Figure 7C**). This was reiterated by a Comprehensive *in vitro* Pro-arrhythmia Assay (CiPA), which showed that 16.67% (4/24) and 33% (8/24) of the samples in 2D cultures showed beat period irregularity after treatment with 50 and 100 nM E4031, respectively, while patches showed beat period irregularity of 60% following treatment with E4031(6/10). This data indicated the increased occurrence of arrhythmias in these cardiac patches (**Figure 7G**) making them a more powerful system for arrhythmia detection. Additionally, a significant decrease in the spike amplitude was observed in both the 2D and 3D cultures, following treatment with 100 nM E4031 (**Figure 7F**). Taken together, these results showed that while hiPSC-CMs cultured in 2D and 3D cultures responded to drug treatments, the 3D cultured hiPSC-CMs had more efficacious responses and would be a better model for *in vitro* drug testing.

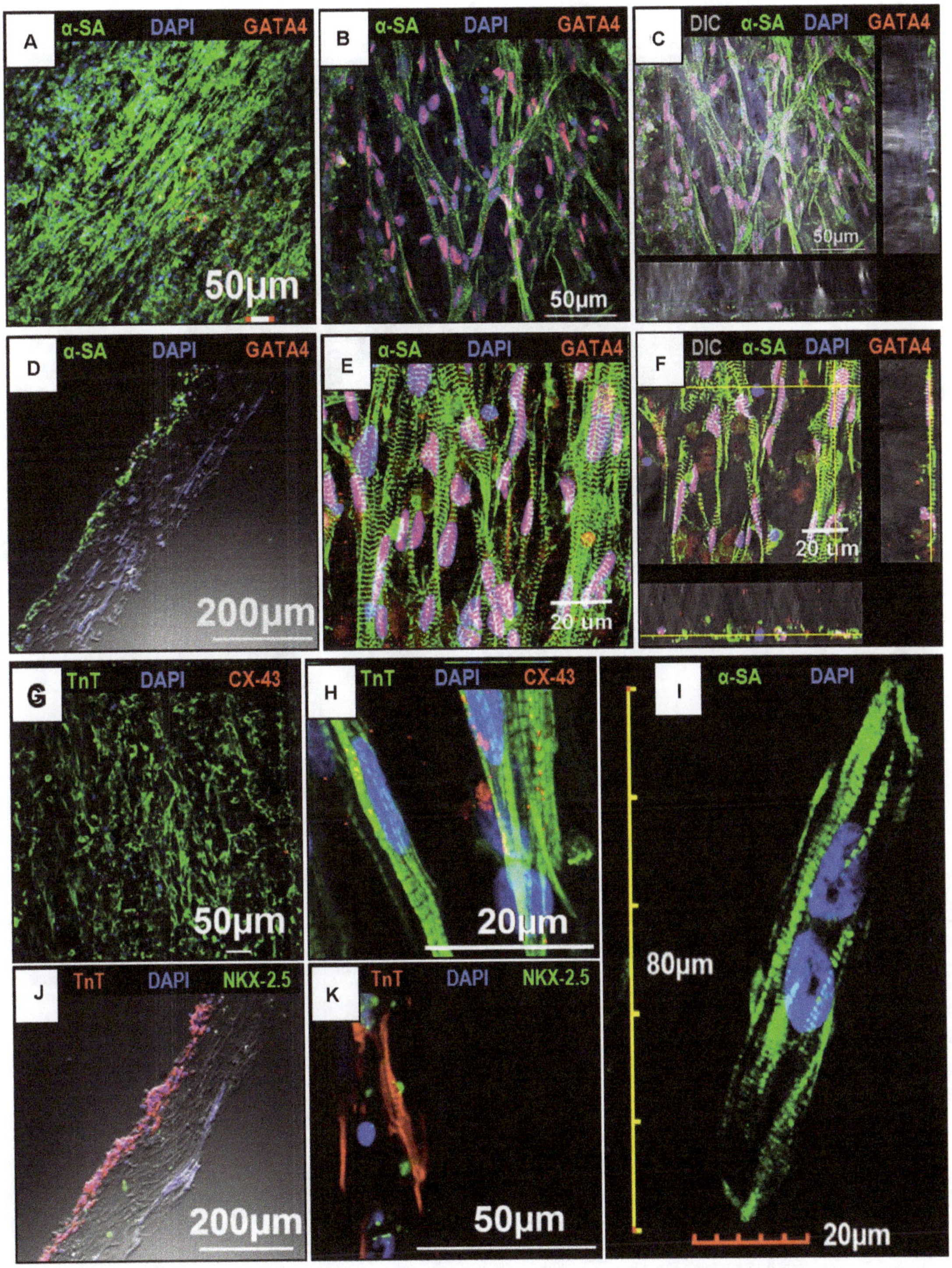

FIGURE 4 | Confocal imaging to assess the expression of cardiac markers in human induced-pluripotent stem cell-derived cardiomyocytes (hiPSC-CMs) cultured on the aligned coaxial nanofiber patch. **(A–F)** Confocal images showing the expression of α-SA and GATA4 in hiPSC-CMs cultured on aligned coaxial patches. **(G,H)** Confocal images showing the expression of TnT and Cx-43 in hiPSC-CMs cultured on aligned coaxial patches. **(J,K)** Confocal images showing the expression of TnT and Nkx2.5 in hiPSC-CMs cultured on aligned coaxial patches. **(C,F)** Z-stack images showing the distribution of the hiPSC-CMs through the depth of the coaxial patches. **(D,J)** Cross-section images of the coaxial patches showing the distribution of hiPSC-CMs in the patch. **(I)** Confocal image of a single hiPSC-CM cultured on an aligned coaxial patch.

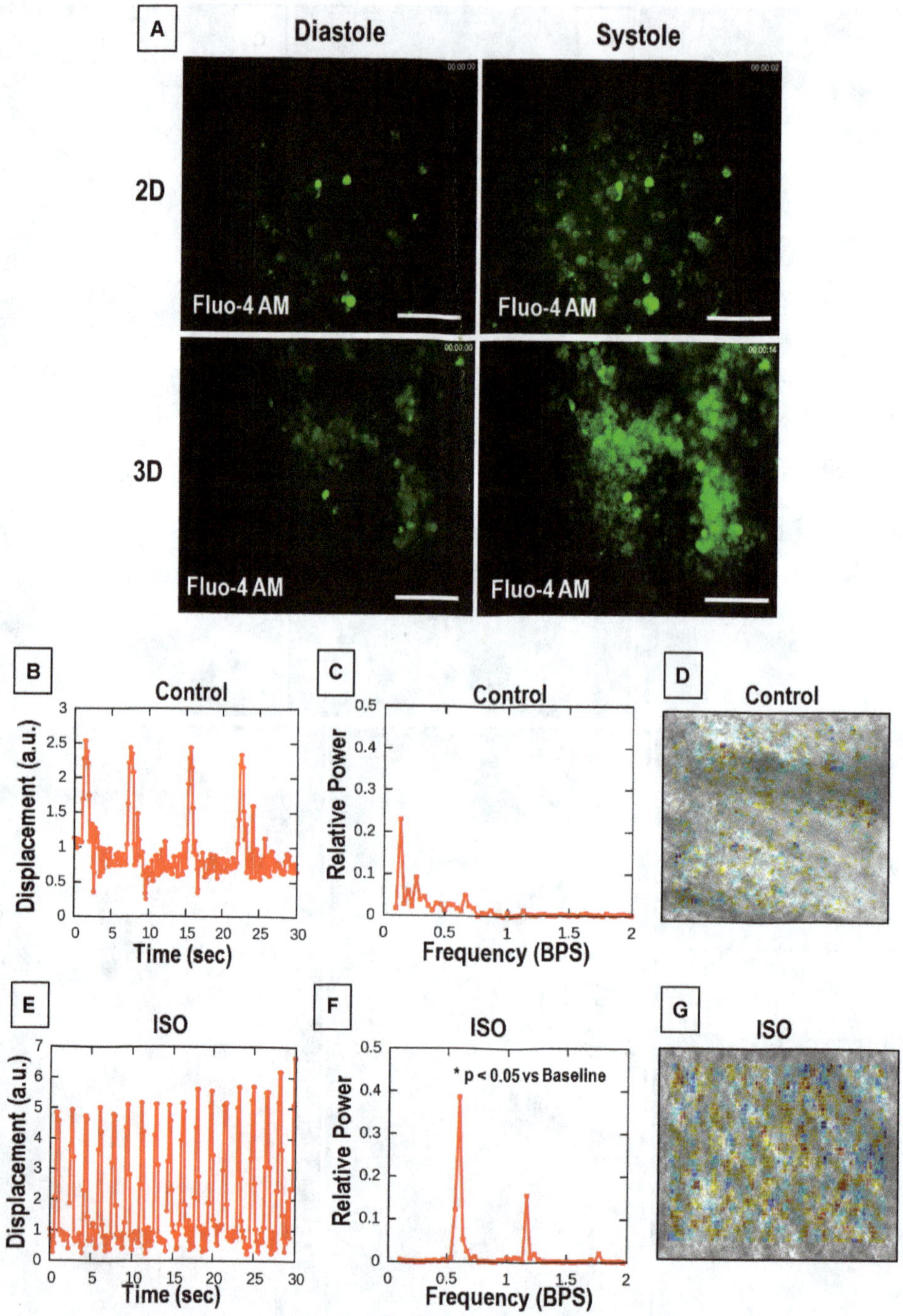

FIGURE 5 | Calcium cycling and optical contractility analysis of the aligned coaxial cardiac patch. **(A)** Representative images of calcium transients in 2D and 3D cultures. **(B–D)** Representative data of untreated control aligned coaxial (CoA) cardiac patches **(B–D)**, and **(E–G)** aligned CoA cardiac patches treated with 100 nM Isoproterenol (ISO). **(B,E)** Spontaneous beat patterns expressed as displacement relative to a resting reference state vs. time. **(C,F)** Fourier power spectra of beat patterns show the dominant beat frequency as a peak and spatially resolved contractility analysis. **(D,G)** Representation of particle image velocimetry (PIV) with warmer colors corresponding to higher divergence, a numerical estimate of contractile strength.

DISCUSSION

The main focus of the present study was to develop a potent and efficient 3D culture system for cardiac drug testing. Our findings demonstrate that aligned PCL-Gel coaxial nanofibrous scaffolds successfully culture hiPSC-CMs in a 3D microenvironment. The comparative assessment of hiPSC-CMs cultured in 2D and 3D culture systems carried out in the present study showed improved functional characteristics and increased responsiveness to cardiac drugs in the latter.

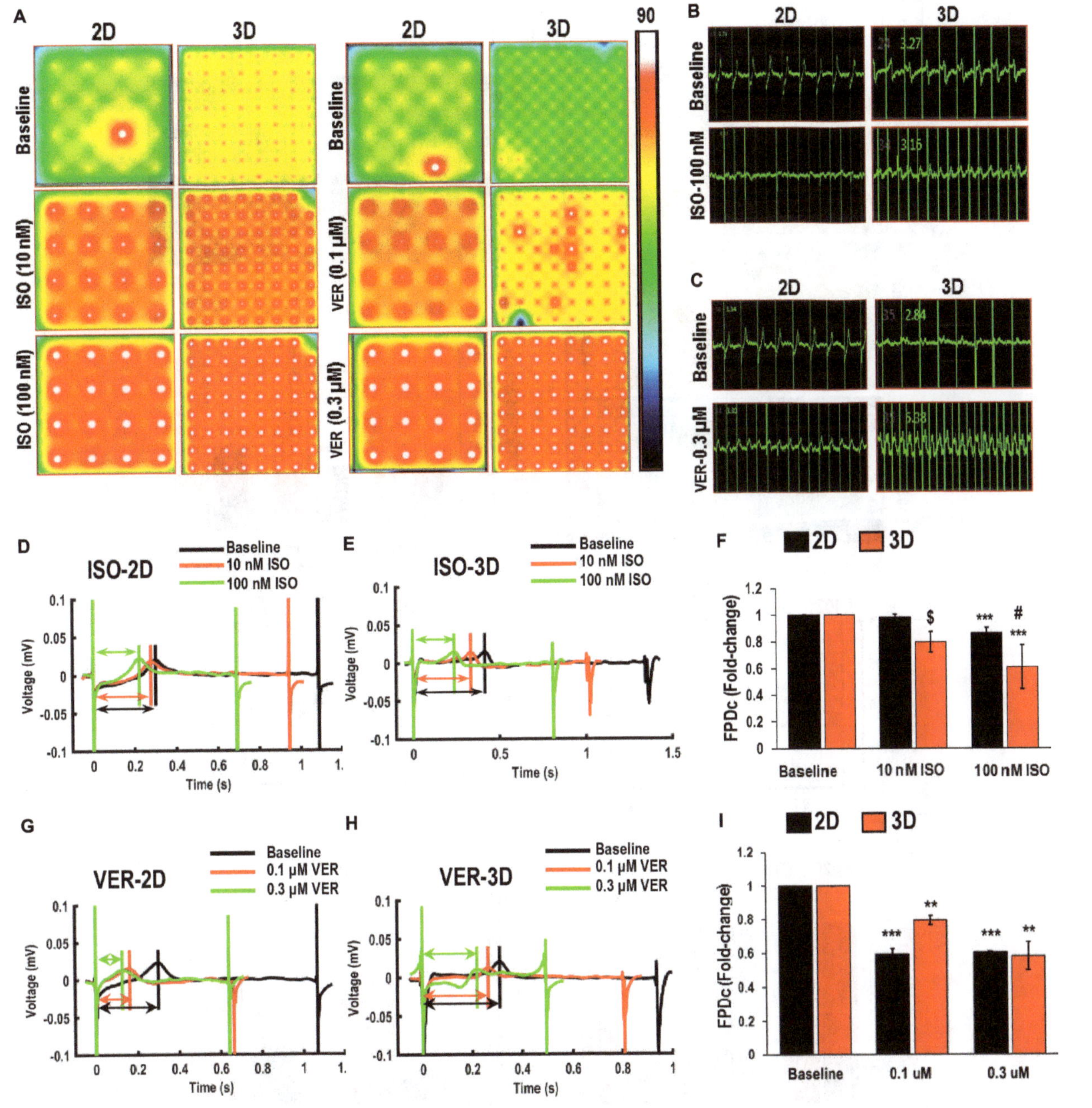

FIGURE 6 | Functional assessment of human induced-pluripotent stem cell-derived cardiomyocytes (hiPSC-CMs) cultured in 2D and 3D cultures in response to Isoproterenol (ISO) and Verapamil (VER). **(A)** Heat maps showing the beat rate in representative wells of 2D and 3D cultures before treatment (baseline) and after treatment with ISO or VER at different concentrations. Representative images showing changes in beat detection before (baseline) and after treatment with **(B)** 100 nM ISO and **(C)** 0.3 μM VER. Representative images showing changes in beat period in **(D,G)** 2D and **(E,H)** 3D cultures after treatment with **(D,E)** ISO and **(G,H)** VER. Quantitative assessment of change in corrected field potential duration (FPDc) after treatment with **(F)** ISO and **(I)** VER, respectively, in 2D and 3D cultures. Dotted arrows in **(D,E,G,H)** show field potential duration (FPD). Scale in A represents the beats per minute. Data shown in **(F,I)** is mean ± SD, $n = 8$, from three independent cultures. $^{**}p < 0.01$, $^{***}p < 0.001$ vs. corresponding baseline; $^{\$}p < 0.001$, $^{\#}p < 0.01$ vs. corresponding 2D cultures.

Coaxial PCL-gelatin scaffolds demonstrated excellent biological properties including cell attachment, organization, and expression of cardiac lineage markers along with high mechanical strength and Young's modulus allowing for the scaffold to be handled easily. Our observations are consistent with previous reports, which have shown coaxial electrospinning is an efficient strategy for surface modification of nanofibrous scaffolds made from synthetic polymers like PCL, PLGA, and polyvinyl alcohol (PVA) (Kim and Cho, 2016). While coaxial electrospinning has been more commonly used for controlled drug/biomolecule release (Zhang et al., 2006; Ji et al., 2010; Sun et al., 2019), it has also been used to coat

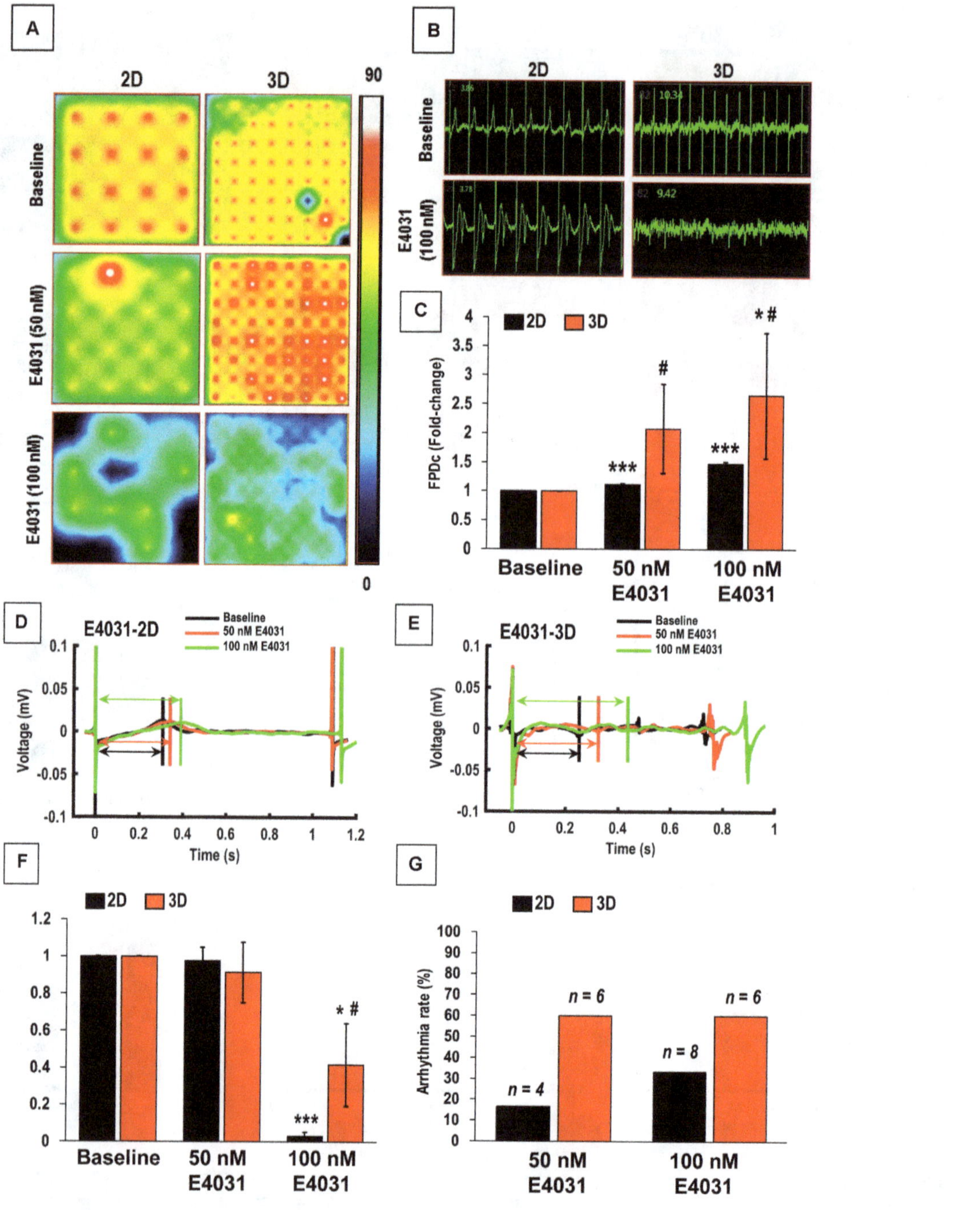

FIGURE 7 | Functional assessment of human induced-pluripotent stem cell-derived cardiomyocytes (hiPSC-CMs) cultured in 2D and 3D cultures after treatment with E4031. **(A)** Heat maps showing the beat rate in representative wells of 2D and 3D cultures before treatment (baseline) and after treatment with E4031. **(B)** Representative images showing changes in beat detection before (baseline) and after treatment with E4031. **(C)** Quantitative assessment of fold change in corrected field potential duration (FPDc) following E4031 treatment in 2D and 3D cultures. Representative images showing changes in beat period in **(D)** 2D and **(E)** 3D cultures after treatment with E4031. Quantitative assessment of change in **(F)** spike amplitude and **(G)** arrhythmicity after E4031 treatment in 2D and 3D cultures. Arrows in **(D,E)** show field potential duration (FPD). Scale in A represents the beats per minute. Data shown in **(C,F,G)** is mean ± SD, $n = 8$, from three independent cultures. $^{*}p < 0.05$, $^{***}p < 0.001$ vs. corresponding baseline; $^{\#}p < 0.01$ vs. corresponding 2D cultures.

synthetic polymer-based nanofibers with a natural polymer (like gelatin, alginate, and collagen) to make them more biomimetic (Zhang et al., 2007; Hu et al., 2020). The use of coaxial nanofibers with a PCL inner core and gelatin outer shell has previously been used for wound healing (Blackstone et al., 2014) and vascular (Coimbra et al., 2017) and bone (Alissa Alam et al., 2020) tissue engineering applications. This coaxial structure has been shown to improve the biocompatibility of the scaffolds as well as provide structural support to the cells for *in vivo* applications.

Another striking observation made in our study was the alignment of hiPSC-CMs with the nanofibers in the scaffold. As a result, the hiPSC-CMs cultured on the aligned scaffolds showed an elongated rod-shaped morphology. Additionally, the sarcomeres in these hiPSC-CMs showed parallel organization inside the cell, with some cells being binucleated. These observations indicate the maturation of the cells cultured on the coaxial scaffolds. Our observations are consistent with previous reports demonstrating a similar alignment of hiPCMs when cultured on aligned scaffolds (Khan et al., 2015; Han et al., 2016; Wanjare et al., 2017). These studies have clearly shown enhanced maturation of hiPSC-CMs cultured on aligned 3D scaffolds based on increased expression of cardiac genes, re-organization of sarcomeres, and an adult cardiomyocyte-like rod-shaped morphology of the cells. Additionally, it has been observed that scaffolds with fibrous, aligned structures mimic the structure of heart tissue, thereby providing a 3D microenvironment for anisotropic arrangement of hiPSC-CMs similar to cardiomyocytes in the heart (Kitsara et al., 2017). Of relevance is another observation made in a previous study by our group (Kumar et al., 2019), wherein hiPSC-CMs cultured in 2D showed similar morphological maturation, but only after 4 weeks in culture. This further reiterates that 3D cultures would be more relevant for structural and functional maturation of hiPSC-CMs, when compared to 2D cultures.

Another important aspect of an *in vitro* model system for cardiac tissue, is the development of a functional syncytium of beating cardiomyocytes. It is a well-established fact that the electrical interconnectivity of cardiomyocytes is an essential pre-requisite for developing *in vitro* cardiac tissues for drug testing applications. This is especially important to determine the effect of a drug molecule on the heart function (e.g., heart rate, arrhythmia-inducing potential; Stoppel et al., 2016; Ugolini et al., 2017). Hence, cell-cell interaction between cardiomyocytes is extremely critical. Previous studies have shown the formation of a functional syncytium in 2D cultures mainly due to hypertrophic growth of hiPSC-CMs (Kumar et al., 2019). On the contrary, functional coupling between cardiomyocytes cultured on 3D constructs has been reported only after mechanical or electrical stimulation (Valls-Margarit et al., 2019). Interestingly, in our study, we observed the formation of a functional syncytium of hiPSC-CMs cultured on the coaxial patches, evidenced by the expression of the gap junction protein, Cx-43, and synchronous calcium transients across the patch. These observations are similar to the behavior of hiPSC-CMs cultured in 2D (Kumar et al., 2019), further indicating that the aligned coaxial scaffolds can be used as an *in vitro* culture system.

It has been shown that 3D culture systems making use of hiPSC-CMs are better suited for cardiac drug testing and toxicity studies because they mimic the *in vivo* response (Kussauer et al., 2019). However, the use of 3D cultures has been restrained due to lack of (a) extensive literature, (b) reproducible culture protocols, and (c) precise analysis tools (Zuppinger, 2019). In recent years, several different techniques have been developed and optimized for analyzing the effect of different cardiac drugs on hiPSC-CMs in 3D cultures, such as calcium imaging using fluorescent dyes, PIV, and measurement of field potentials by MEA (Zuppinger, 2019). In our study, these analysis tools were used to monitor the effectiveness of a few commonly used cardiac drugs on hiPSC-CMs cultured in 2D *vis-à-vis* 3D cultures. As expected, an increase in the beat rate along with a decrease in beat period and FPDc was observed in both the 2D as well as the 3D cultures after ISO treatment. Our observations are consistent with previous studies, where a dose-dependent increase in contractility was observed in 2D cultured hiPSC-CMs following treatment with ISO (Mehta et al., 2011; Blazeski et al., 2012; Kitaguchi et al., 2017), as a result of β1 and β2 receptor stimulation. Additionally, although VER has been known to inhibit voltage-dependent calcium channels (Harris et al., 2013), an increase in contractility was observed in both 2D and 3D cultures. However, consistent with our observation. a recent study identified that this discrepancy in the effect of VER *in vitro* and *in vivo*, resulted from the low potassium concentration in cell culture medium (Zeng et al., 2019). On the other hand, E4031, an hERG channel blocker, resulted in prolonged QT interval (FPDc) in addition to decreased spike amplitude in a dose-dependent manner for 3D cultured cells. The incidence of arrhythmicity increased following the addition of E4031 in both the 2D as well as 3D cultures. However, 3D cultures showed a four-times greater response to drugs than 2D cultures. Our observations are in agreement with earlier reports (Harris et al., 2013) using hiPSC-CMs. Overall, these results strongly indicated an elevated sensitivity of hiPSC-CMs in 3D cultures to various drugs used in this study. Similar observations were reported in the case of 3D culture of primary hepatocytes (Bell et al., 2018; Zhou et al., 2019) and cancer cells (Chaicharoenaudomrung et al., 2019). Likewise, a recent study demonstrated that 3D cardiac spheroids mimics an *in vivo* environment for drug testing and cardiotoxicity studies (Polonchuk et al., 2017).

CONCLUSION

Overall, our study demonstrated the fabrication and testing of an aligned coaxial PCL-gelatin nanofiber patch with mechanical and biomimetic properties desired for cardiac applications. hiPSC-CMs cultured on these patches showed a rod-shaped morphology and were aligned in parallel with the nanofibers. These cells on the cardiac patch showed synchronous contractions and exhibited quick response to cardiac drugs. Finally, these cardiac patches can be scaled and used as an *in vitro* drug screening platform for cardiotoxicity studies, as well as to developed into future strategies of cardiac patch transplantation for ischemic heart disease.

AUTHOR CONTRIBUTIONS

MK, NK, DS, and AP conceived and designed the experiments. MK, NK, DS, AP, JD, DI, AC, HP, and MM performed the experiments and data analysis. NK, DS, AP, JD, and MM analyzed the data. MK, HP, MA, and AC contributed reagents, materials, and analysis tools. DS, NK, AP, JD, HP, DS, and MK wrote and reviewed the manuscript. The input from all the authors was incorporated in finalizing the manuscript draft.

REFERENCES

Aldana, A. A., and Abraham, G. A. (2017). Current advances in electrospun gelatin-based scaffolds for tissue engineering applications. *Int. J. Pharm.* 523, 441–453. doi: 10.1016/j.ijpharm.2016.09.044

Aleksandrova, A., Czirok, A., Szabo, A., Filla, M. B., Hossain, M. J., Whelan, P. F., et al. (2012). Convective tissue movements play a major role in avian endocardial morphogenesis. *Dev. Biol.* 363, 348–361. doi: 10.1016/j.ydbio.2011.12.036

Alissa Alam, H., Dalgic, A. D., Tezcaner, A., Ozen, C., and Keskin, D. (2020). A comparative study of monoaxial and coaxial PCL/gelatin/Poloxamer 188 scaffolds for bone tissue engineering. *Int. J. Polym. Mater. Polym. Biomater.* 69, 339–350. doi: 10.1080/00914037.2019.1581198

Antoni, D., Burckel, H., Josset, E., and Noel, G. (2015). Three-dimensional cell culture: a breakthrough *in vivo*. *Int. J. Mol. Sci.* 16, 5517–5527. doi: 10.3390/ijms16035517

Archer, C. R., Sargeant, R., Basak, J., Pilling, J., Barnes, J. R., and Pointon, A. (2018). Characterization and validation of a human 3D cardiac microtissue for the assessment of changes in cardiac pathology. *Sci. Rep.* 8:10160.

Bell, C. C., Dankers, A. C. A., Lauschke, V. M., Sison-Young, R., Jenkins, R., Rowe, C., et al. (2018). Comparison of hepatic 2D sandwich cultures and 3D spheroids for long-term toxicity applications: a multicenter Study. *Toxicol. Sci.* 162, 655–666. doi: 10.1093/toxsci/kfx289

Bhattarai, D. P., Aguilar, L. E., Park, C. H., and Kim, C. S. (2018). A review on properties of natural and synthetic based electrospun fibrous materials for bone tissue engineering. *Membranes* 8:62. doi: 10.3390/membranes8030062

Blackstone, B. N., Drexler, J. W., and Powell, H. M. (2014). Tunable engineered skin mechanics via coaxial electrospun fiber core diameter. *Tissue Eng. Part A* 20, 2746–2755. doi: 10.1089/ten.tea.2013.0687

Blackstone, B. N., Hahn, J. M., McFarland, K. L., DeBruler, D. M., Supp, D. M., and Powell, H. M. (2018). Inflammatory response and biomechanical properties of coaxial scaffolds for engineered skin in vitro and post-grafting. *Acta Biomater.* 80, 247–257. doi: 10.1016/j.actbio.2018.09.014

Blazeski, A., Zhu, R., Hunter, D. W., Weinberg, S. H., Zambidis, E. T., and Tung, L. (2012). Cardiomyocytes derived from human induced pluripotent stem cells as models for normal and diseased cardiac electrophysiology and contractility. *Prog. Biophys. Mol. Biol.* 110, 166–177. doi: 10.1016/j.pbiomolbio.2012.07.013

Chaicharoenaudomrung, N., Kunhorm, P., and Noisa, P. (2019). Three-dimensional cell culture systems as an in vitro platform for cancer and stem cell modeling. *World J. Stem Cells* 11, 1065–1083. doi: 10.4252/wjsc.v11.i12.1065

Chen, Y., Zeng, D., Ding, L., Li, X. L., Liu, X. T., Li, W. J., et al. (2015). Three-dimensional poly-(epsilon-caprolactone) nanofibrous scaffolds directly promote the cardiomyocyte differentiation of murine-induced pluripotent stem cells through Wnt/beta-catenin signaling. *BMC Cell Biol.* 16:22. doi: 10.1186/s12860-015-0067-3

Citro, L., Naidu, S., Hassan, F., Kuppusamy, M. L., Kuppusamy, P., Angelos, M. G., et al. (2014). Comparison of human induced pluripotent stem-cell derived cardiomyocytes with human mesenchymal stem cells following acute myocardial infarction. *PLoS One* 9:e116281. doi: 10.1371/journal.pone.0116281

Coimbra, P., Santos, P., Alves, P., Miguel, S. P., Carvalho, M. P., Correia, I. J., et al. (2017). Coaxial electrospun PCL/Gelatin-MA fibers as scaffolds for vascular tissue engineering. *Colloids Surf. B Biointerfaces* 159, 7–15. doi: 10.1016/j.colsurfb.2017.07.065

Costantini, M., and Barbetta, A. (2018). "6 - Gas foaming technologies for 3D scaffold engineering," in *Functional 3D Tissue Engineering Scaffolds*, eds Y. Deng and J. Kuiper (Sawston: Woodhead Publishing), 127–149. doi: 10.1016/b978-0-08-100979-6.00006-9

Czirok, A., Isai, D. G., Kosa, E., Rajasingh, S., Kinsey, W., Neufeld, Z., et al. (2017). Optical-flow based non-invasive analysis of cardiomyocyte contractility. *Sci. Rep.* 7:10404.

da Rocha, A. M., Campbell, K., Mironov, S., Jiang, J., Mundada, L., Guerrero-Serna, G., et al. (2017). hiCM monolayer maturation state determines drug responsiveness in high throughput pro-arrhythmia screen. *Sci. Rep.* 7:13834.

Dattola, E., Parrotta, E. I., Scalise, S., Perozziello, G., Limongi, T., Candeloro, P., et al. (2019). Development of 3D PVA scaffolds for cardiac tissue engineering and cell screening applications. *RSC Adv.* 9, 4246–4257. doi: 10.1039/c8ra08187e

Drexler, J. W., and Powell, H. M. (2011). Regulation of electrospun scaffold stiffness via coaxial core diameter. *Acta Biomater.* 7, 1133–1139. doi: 10.1016/j.actbio.2010.10.025

Figtree, G. A., Bubb, K. J., Tang, O., Kizana, E., and Gentile, C. (2017). Vascularized cardiac spheroids as novel 3D in vitro models to study cardiac fibrosis. *Cells Tissues Organs* 204, 191–198. doi: 10.1159/000477436

Gao, L., Gregorich, Z. R., Zhu, W., Mattapally, S., Oduk, Y., Lou, X., et al. (2018). Large cardiac muscle patches engineered from human induced-pluripotent stem cell-derived cardiac cells improve recovery from myocardial infarction in swine. *Circulation* 137, 1712–1730. doi: 10.1161/circulationaha.117.030785

Gintant, G., Burridge, P., Gepstein, L., Harding, S., Herron, T., Hong, C., et al. (2019). Use of human induced pluripotent stem cell-derived cardiomyocytes in preclinical cancer drug cardiotoxicity testing: a scientific statement from the american heart association. *Circ. Res.* 125, e75–e92.

Goto, A., Izumi-Nakaseko, H., Hagiwara-Nagasawa, M., Chiba, K., Ando, K., Naito, A. T., et al. (2018). Analysis of torsadogenic and pharmacokinetic profile of E-4031 in dogs bridging the gap of information between in vitro proarrhythmia assay and clinical observation in human subjects. *J. Pharmacol. Sci.* 137, 237–240. doi: 10.1016/j.jphs.2018.06.005

Han, J., Wu, Q., Xia, Y., Wagner, M. B., and Xu, C. (2016). Cell alignment induced by anisotropic electrospun fibrous scaffolds alone has limited effect on cardiomyocyte maturation. *Stem Cell Res.* 16, 740–750. doi: 10.1016/j.scr.2016.04.014

Harris, K., Aylott, M., Cui, Y., Louttit, J. B., McMahon, N. C., and Sridhar, A. (2013). Comparison of electrophysiological data from human-induced pluripotent stem cell-derived cardiomyocytes to functional preclinical safety assays. *Toxicol. Sci.* 134, 412–426. doi: 10.1093/toxsci/kft113

Hu, Q., Wu, C., and Zhang, H. (2020). Preparation and optimization of a biomimetic triple-layered vascular scaffold based on coaxial electrospinning. *Appl. Biochem. Biotechnol.* 190, 1106–1123. doi: 10.1007/s12010-019-03147-2

Huang, H., Ding, Y., Sun, X. S., and Nguyen, T. A. (2013). Peptide hydrogelation and cell encapsulation for 3D culture of MCF-7 breast cancer cells. *PLoS One* 8:e59482. doi: 10.1371/journal.pone.0059482

Jabbour, R., Owen, T., Reinsch, M., Pandey, P., Terracciano, C., Weinberger, F., et al. (2019). BS27 Development and preclinical testing of a large heart muscle patch. *Heart* 105:A157.

Ji, W., Yang, F., van den Beucken, J. J., Bian, Z., Fan, M., Chen, Z., et al. (2010). Fibrous scaffolds loaded with protein prepared by blend or coaxial electrospinning. *Acta Biomater.* 6, 4199–4207. doi: 10.1016/j.actbio.2010.05.025

Johnson, J., Ghosh, A., and Lannutti, J. (2007). Microstructure-property relationships in a tissue-engineering scaffold. *J. Appl. Polym. Sci.* 104, 2919–2927. doi: 10.1002/app.25965

Jun, I., Han, H. S., Edwards, J. R., and Jeon, H. (2018). Electrospun fibrous scaffolds for tissue engineering: viewpoints on architecture and fabrication. *Int. J. Mol. Sci.* 19:745. doi: 10.3390/ijms19030745

Kai, D., Prabhakaran, M. P., Jin, G., and Ramakrishna, S. (2011). Polypyrrole-contained electrospun conductive nanofibrous membranes for cardiac tissue engineering. *J. Biomed. Mater. Res. A* 99, 376–385. doi: 10.1002/jbm.a.33200

Karakikes, I., Ameen, M., Termglinchan, V., and Wu, J. C. (2015). Human induced pluripotent stem cell-derived cardiomyocytes: insights into molecular, cellular, and functional phenotypes. *Circ. Res.* 117, 80–88. doi: 10.1161/circresaha.117.305365

Kc, P., Hong, Y., and Zhang, G. (2019). Cardiac tissue-derived extracellular matrix scaffolds for myocardial repair: advantages and challenges. *Regen. Biomater.* 6, 185–199. doi: 10.1093/rb/rbz017

Khan, K., Gasbarrino, K., Mahmoud, I., Makhoul, G., Yu, B., Dufresne, L., et al. (2018). Bioactive scaffolds in stem-cell-based therapies for cardiac repair: protocol for a meta-analysis of randomized controlled preclinical trials in animal myocardial infarction models. *Syst. Rev.* 7:225.

Khan, M., Xu, Y., Hua, S., Johnson, J., Belevych, A., Janssen, P. M., et al. (2015). Evaluation of changes in morphology and function of human induced pluripotent stem cell derived cardiomyocytes (HiCMs) cultured on an aligned-nanofiber cardiac patch. *PLoS One* 10:e0126338. doi: 10.1371/journal.pone.0126338

Kim, P. H., and Cho, J. Y. (2016). Myocardial tissue engineering using electrospun nanofiber composites. *BMB Rep.* 49, 26–36. doi: 10.5483/bmbrep.2016.49.1.165

Kitaguchi, T., Moriyama, Y., Taniguchi, T., Maeda, S., Ando, H., Uda, T., et al. (2017). CSAHi study: detection of drug-induced ion channel/receptor responses, QT prolongation, and arrhythmia using multi-electrode arrays in combination with human induced pluripotent stem cell-derived cardiomyocytes. *J. Pharmacol. Toxicol. Methods* 85, 73–81. doi: 10.1016/j.vascn.2017.02.001

Kitsara, M., Agbulut, O., Kontziampasis, D., Chen, Y., and Menasche, P. (2017). Fibers for hearts: a critical review on electrospinning for cardiac tissue engineering. *Acta Biomater.* 48, 20–40. doi: 10.1016/j.actbio.2016.11.014

Kumar, N., Dougherty, J. A., Manring, H. R., Elmadbouh, I., Mergaye, M., Czirok, A., et al. (2019). Assessment of temporal functional changes and miRNA profiling of human iPSC-derived cardiomyocytes. *Sci. Rep.* 9:13188.

Kussauer, S., David, R., and Lemcke, H. (2019). hiPSCs derived cardiac cells for drug and toxicity screening and disease modeling: what micro- electrode-array analyses can tell us. *Cells* 8:1331. doi: 10.3390/cells8111331

Lynch, S., Pridgeon, C. S., Duckworth, C. A., Sharma, P., Park, B. K., and Goldring, C. E. P. (2019). Stem cell models as an in vitro model for predictive toxicology. *Biochem. J.* 476, 1149–1158. doi: 10.1042/bcj20170780

Machiraju, P., and Greenway, S. C. (2019). Current methods for the maturation of induced pluripotent stem cell-derived cardiomyocytes. *World J. Stem Cells* 11, 33–43. doi: 10.4252/wjsc.v11.i1.33

McBane, J. E., Vulesevic, B., Padavan, D. T., McEwan, K. A., Korbutt, G. S., and Suuronen, E. J. (2013). Evaluation of a collagen-chitosan hydrogel for potential use as a pro-angiogenic site for islet transplantation. *PLoS One* 8:e77538. doi: 10.1371/journal.pone.0077538

Mehta, A., Chung, Y. Y., Ng, A., Iskandar, F., Atan, S., Wei, H., et al. (2011). Pharmacological response of human cardiomyocytes derived from virus-free induced pluripotent stem cells. *Cardiovasc. Res.* 91, 577–586. doi: 10.1093/cvr/cvr132

Milani-Nejad, N., and Janssen, P. M. (2014). Small and large animal models in cardiac contraction research: advantages and disadvantages. *Pharmacol. Ther.* 141, 235–249. doi: 10.1016/j.pharmthera.2013.10.007

Park, M., and Yoon, Y. S. (2018). Cardiac regeneration with human pluripotent stem cell-derived cardiomyocytes. *Korean Circ. J.* 48, 974–988. doi: 10.4070/kcj.2018.0312

Polonchuk, L., Chabria, M., Badi, L., Hoflack, J. C., Figtree, G., Davies, M. J., et al. (2017). Cardiac spheroids as promising in vitro models to study the human heart microenvironment. *Sci. Rep.* 7:7005.

Rajasingh, S., Isai, D. G., Samanta, S., Zhou, Z. G., Dawn, B., Kinsey, W. H., et al. (2018). Manipulation-free cultures of human iPSC-derived cardiomyocytes offer a novel screening method for cardiotoxicity. *Acta Pharmacol. Sin.* 39, 1590–1603. doi: 10.1038/aps.2017.183

Ribeiro, A. J. S., Guth, B. D., Engwall, M., Eldridge, S., Foley, C. M., Guo, L., et al. (2019). Considerations for an in vitro, cell-based testing platform for detection of drug-induced inotropic effects in early drug development. part 2: designing and fabricating microsystems for assaying cardiac contractility with physiological relevance using human iPSC-cardiomyocytes. *Front. Pharmacol.* 10:934. doi: 10.3389/fphar.2019.00934

Savoji, H., Mohammadi, M. H., Rafatian, N., Toroghi, M. K., Wang, E. Y., Zhao, Y., et al. (2019). Cardiovascular disease models: a game changing paradigm in drug discovery and screening. *Biomaterials* 198, 3–26. doi: 10.1016/j.biomaterials.2018.09.036

Schroer, A., Pardon, G., Castillo, E., Blair, C., and Pruitt, B. (2019). Engineering hiPSC cardiomyocyte in vitro model systems for functional and structural assessment. *Prog. Biophys. Mol. Biol.* 144, 3–15. doi: 10.1016/j.pbiomolbio.2018.12.001

Shimizu, T., Yamato, M., Kikuchi, A., and Okano, T. (2003). Cell sheet engineering for myocardial tissue reconstruction. *Biomaterials* 24, 2309–2316. doi: 10.1016/s0142-9612(03)00110-8

Stoppel, W. L., Kaplan, D. L., and Black, L. D. III (2016). Electrical and mechanical stimulation of cardiac cells and tissue constructs. *Adv. Drug Deliv. Rev.* 96, 135–155. doi: 10.1016/j.addr.2015.07.009

Sun, Y., Cheng, S., Lu, W., Wang, Y., Zhang, P., and Yao, Q. (2019). Electrospun fibers and their application in drug controlled release, biological dressings, tissue repair, and enzyme immobilization. *RSC Adv.* 9, 25712–25729. doi: 10.1039/c9ra05012d

Ugolini, G. S., Visone, R., Cruz-Moreira, D., Redaelli, A., and Rasponi, M. (2017). Tailoring cardiac environment in microphysiological systems: an outlook on current and perspective heart-on-chip platforms. *Future Sci. OA* 3:FSO191.

Valls-Margarit, M., Iglesias-Garcia, O., Di Guglielmo, C., Sarlabous, L., Tadevosyan, K., Paoli, R., et al. (2019). Engineered macroscale cardiac constructs elicit human myocardial tissue-like functionality. *Stem Cell Rep.* 13, 207–220. doi: 10.1016/j.stemcr.2019.05.024

Wang, J., Bettinger, C. J., Langer, R. S., and Borenstein, J. T. (2010). Biodegradable microfluidic scaffolds for tissue engineering from amino alcohol-based poly(ester amide) elastomers. *Organogenesis* 6, 212–216. doi: 10.4161/org.6.4.12909

Wang, L., Wu, Y., Hu, T., Guo, B., and Ma, P. X. (2017). Electrospun conductive nanofibrous scaffolds for engineering cardiac tissue and 3D bioactuators. *Acta Biomater.* 59, 68–81. doi: 10.1016/j.actbio.2017.06.036

Wanjare, M., Hou, L., Nakayama, K. H., Kim, J. J., Mezak, N. P., Abilez, O. J., et al. (2017). Anisotropic microfibrous scaffolds enhance the organization and function of cardiomyocytes derived from induced pluripotent stem cells. *Biomater. Sci.* 5, 1567–1578. doi: 10.1039/c7bm00323d

Weinberger, F., Mannhardt, I., and Eschenhagen, T. (2017). Engineering cardiac muscle tissue: a maturating field of research. *Circ. Res.* 120, 1487–1500. doi: 10.1161/circresaha.117.310738

Zamir, E. A., Czirok, A., Rongish, B. J., Little, C. D., and digital, A. (2005). image-based method for computational tissue fate mapping during early avian morphogenesis. *Ann. Biomed. Eng.* 33, 854–865. doi: 10.1007/s10439-005-3037-7

Zeng, H., Wang, J., Clouse, H., Lagrutta, A., and Sannajust, F. (2019). Resolving the reversed rate effect of calcium channel blockers on human-induced pluripotent stem cell-derived cardiomyocytes and the impact on in vitro cardiac safety evaluation. *Toxicol. Sci.* 167, 573–580. doi: 10.1093/toxsci/kfy264

Zhang, Y. Z., Su, B., Venugopal, J., Ramakrishna, S., and Lim, C. T. (2007). Biomimetic and bioactive nanofibrous scaffolds from electrospun composite nanofibers. *Int. J. Nanomedicine* 2, 623–638.

Zhang, Y. Z., Wang, X., Feng, Y., Li, J., Lim, C. T., and Ramakrishna, S. (2006). Coaxial electrospinning of (fluorescein isothiocyanate-conjugated bovine serum albumin)-encapsulated poly(epsilon-caprolactone) nanofibers for sustained release. *Biomacromolecules* 7, 1049–1057. doi: 10.1021/bm050743i

Zhou, Y., Shen, J. X., and Lauschke, V. M. (2019). Comprehensive evaluation of organotypic and microphysiological liver models for prediction of drug-induced liver injury. *Front. Pharmacol.* 10:1093. doi: 10.3389/fphar.2019.01093

Zhu, W., Ma, X., Gou, M., Mei, D., Zhang, K., and Chen, S. (2016). 3D printing of functional biomaterials for tissue engineering. *Curr. Opin. Biotechnol.* 40, 103–112. doi: 10.1016/j.copbio.2016.03.014

Zuppinger, C. (2016). 3D culture for cardiac cells. *Biochim. Biophys. Acta* 1863, 1873–1881. doi: 10.1016/j.bbamcr.2015.11.036

Zuppinger, C. (2019). 3D cardiac cell culture: a critical review of current technologies and applications. *Front. Cardiovasc. Med.* 6:87. doi: 10.3389/fcvm.2019.00087

14

Extracellular Matrix Mimicking Nanofibrous Scaffolds Modified with Mesenchymal Stem Cell-Derived Extracellular Vesicles for Improved Vascularization

Dake Hao[1,2], *Hila Shimshi Swindell*[1,2], *Lalithasri Ramasubramanian*[1,2], *Ruiwu Liu*[3], *Kit S. Lam*[3], *Diana L. Farmer*[1,2] and *Aijun Wang*[1,2,4*]

[1] *Department of Surgery, School of Medicine, University of California, Davis, Sacramento, CA, United States,* [2] *Institute for Pediatric Regenerative Medicine, Shriners Hospitals for Children, Sacramento, CA, United States,* [3] *Department of Biochemistry and Molecular Medicine, School of Medicine, University of California, Davis, Sacramento, CA, United States,* [4] *Department of Biomedical Engineering, University of California, Davis, Davis, CA, United States*

Correspondence:
Aijun Wang
aawang@ucdavis.edu

The network structure and biological components of natural extracellular matrix (ECM) are indispensable for promoting tissue regeneration. Electrospun nanofibrous scaffolds have been widely used in regenerative medicine to provide structural support for cell growth and tissue regeneration due to their natural ECM mimicking architecture, however, they lack biological functions. Extracellular vesicles (EVs) are potent vehicles of intercellular communication due to their ability to transfer RNAs, proteins, and lipids, thereby mediating significant biological functions in different biological systems. Matrix-bound nanovesicles (MBVs) are identified as an integral and functional component of ECM bioscaffolds mediating significant regenerative functions. Therefore, to engineer EVs modified electrospun scaffolds, mimicking the structure of the natural EV-ECM complex and the physiological interactions between the ECM and EVs, will be attractive and promising in tissue regeneration. Previously, using one-bead one-compound (OBOC) combinatorial technology, we identified LLP2A, an integrin α4β1 ligand, which had a strong binding to human placenta-derived mesenchymal stem cells (PMSCs). In this study, we isolated PMSCs derived EVs (PMSC-EVs) and demonstrated they expressed integrin α4β1 and could improve endothelial cell (EC) migration and vascular sprouting in an *ex vivo* rat aortic ring assay. LLP2A treated culture surface significantly improved PMSC-EV attachment, and the PMSC-EV treated culture surface significantly enhanced the expression of angiogenic genes and suppressed apoptotic activity. We then developed an approach to enable "Click chemistry" to immobilize LLP2A onto the surface of electrospun scaffolds as a linker to immobilize PMSC-EVs onto the scaffold. The PMSC-EV modified electrospun scaffolds significantly promoted EC survival and angiogenic gene expression, such as KDR and TIE2, and suppressed the expression of apoptotic markers, such as caspase 9 and caspase 3. Thus, PMSC-EVs hold promising potential to functionalize biomaterial constructs and improve the vascularization and regenerative potential. The EVs modified biomaterial scaffolds can be widely used for different tissue engineering applications.

Keywords: electrospun nanofibrous scaffold, mesenchymal stem cell, extracellular vesicle, integrin-based ligand, vascularization, tissue regeneration

INTRODUCTION

Natural extracellular space is a dynamic and responsive environment consisting of non-cellular components such as soluble factors, non-soluble extracellular matrix (ECM), and extracellular vesicles (EVs) (Mathivanan, 2017). The ECM regulates many important processes including cellular proliferation, adhesion, migration, differentiation, tissue homeostasis and remodeling. These functions do not only depend on ECM's three-dimensional network, but also on its biological components (Huleihel et al., 2016). Electrospinning is a powerful technology to manufacture nano/microfibrous scaffolds that imitate the natural ECM architecture for allowing the integration of the scaffolds with surrounding cells and promoting tissue regeneration (Sarkar et al., 2006; Gao et al., 2018). We have successfully constructed electrospun scaffolds for various tissue regeneration applications, such as vascular tissue regeneration (Yu et al., 2012; Hao et al., 2020a), wound healing (Lee et al., 2012), peripheral nerve regeneration (Wang et al., 2011; Zhu et al., 2011), spinal cord regeneration (Zhu et al., 2010; Saadai et al., 2011; Downing et al., 2012) and drug delivery (Qi et al., 2006). However, the electrospun scaffolds lack biological motifs that are also included in the natural ECM and can mediate biological signaling and intercellular communication (Lu et al., 2011; Demircan et al., 2014). Surface modification plays a key role in regulating the biological interactions between cell/tissue and biomaterials (Wang et al., 2003). The functionalities of biomaterials, such as biocompatibility, adhesion and biological signaling, can be further improved by surface modification with bioactive motifs (Jiao and Cui, 2007; de Mel et al., 2012). Our previous studies have successfully improved the biological functions of electrospun scaffolds for different types of stem cells by surface modification (Hao et al., 2017, 2020b). Thus, surface modification is essential for the new functional biomaterial development and innovative medical devices design, which are contributive for advancing biomaterials in tissue regeneration and clinical applications (Wu et al., 2012; Bose et al., 2018). Vascularization is crucial for tissue development, maintenance and regeneration by to supplying nutrients and oxygen for cells and tissue (Santos and Reis, 2010; Muangsanit et al., 2018). Thus, many different approaches have been used to functionalize the electrospun scaffolds for enhancing vascularization, such as growth factors (Zhao et al., 2016; Janse van Rensburg et al., 2017), functional molecules (Lee et al., 2015; Garcia and Garcia, 2016), DNA (Scharnweber et al., 2018) and so on. In our previous studies, we demonstrated that an integrin-based ligand modified electrospun scaffold improved EC functions *in vitro* and vascularization *in vivo* (Hao et al., 2017, 2020a). However, these approaches only improve the cell and tissue functions by promoting cell/tissue-biomaterial interaction, but do not promote the biological information and substance transfer simulating the dynamic native ECM (Teodori et al., 2014; Sood et al., 2019). Therefore, to construct biofunctional scaffolds with biological information exchange and transmission will further promote the applications of biological materials in tissue regeneration.

EVs are produced in the endosomal compartment of most eukaryotic cells (Yanez-Mo et al., 2015; van Niel et al., 2018), enriched with various molecular constituents of their original cell, including lipids, proteins and RNAs, and are capable of transferring cell-to-cell signaling (van der Pol et al., 2012; Dhondt et al., 2016). Therefore, EVs have been widely used in tissue engineering area due to their multiple functions, such as pro-angiogenesis, cancer dormancy, anti-inflammation, mineralization (Azoidis et al., 2018; Casson et al., 2018; Baruah and Wary, 2019; Zhang H. et al., 2019). It is also known that physiologically native EVs actively interact with the ECM (Buzas et al., 2018) and the EV-ECM complexes are mediating significant biological functions of both ECMs and EVs (Sung et al., 2015). Recently, matrix-bound vesicles (MBVs) are identified to play a significant role in mediating the regenerative functions of ECM scaffolds (Huleihel et al., 2016, 2017; van der Merwe et al., 2017; Rilla et al., 2019), which highlights the biological functions of the EV-ECM structural complexes. Therefore, designing and constructing biomaterial scaffolds to mimic the structure of the EV-ECM complex and the physiological interactions between the ECM and EVs, represents an attractive and promising novel approach for tissue engineering applications. Mesenchymal stem cells (MSCs) isolated from various tissues are multipotent stem cells (Fridenshtein et al., 1968; Jo et al., 2007; Oh et al., 2008; Zannettino et al., 2008; Xue et al., 2018), represent a promising regenerative treatment for a variety of diseases (Bouffi et al., 2010; Lankford et al., 2015, 2017; Wang et al., 2015; Brown et al., 2016; Hofer and Tuan, 2016; Kabagambe et al., 2017; Galganski et al., 2019; Vanover et al., 2019; Zhang Z. et al., 2019), especially vascular diseases (Pankajakshan and Agrawal, 2014; Premer et al., 2019), due to the biofunctional paracrine secretion, including EVs. However, in many of the cases where therapeutic effects were observed using MSCs, the transplanted stem cells did not persist following injection and thus did not contribute to tissue regeneration by integration. Therefore, MSC derived EVs represent a promising alternative with sustained paracrine functions of live MSCs and have great potential for cell-free therapy. Although the functions of the EVs are not as comprehensive as the MSCs, EVs derived from different types of MSCs also have been demonstrated for improving tissue regeneration (Zhang et al., 2015; Liang et al., 2016; Merino-Gonzalez et al., 2016). Among other molecules, integrins on the surface of EVs are of critical functional significance as they regulate the interactions between EVs and the surrounding micro milieu, especially ECM molecules (Clayton et al., 2004; de Jong et al., 2016; Buzas et al., 2018). Therefore, developing integrin-based conjugation approaches to immobilize MSC-derived EVs onto biomaterial scaffolds will mimic the EV-ECM complexes and hold promise for tissue engineering applications.

One-bead one-compound (OBOC) combinatorial technology is an ultra-high throughput chemical library synthesis and screening method, which is suitable for integrin-based ligand discovery (Lam et al., 1991). Previously, we have identified various potent ligands, such as LXY30, LXW7, and LLP2A targeting integrins α3β1, αvβ3, and α4β1, respectively, by employing the OBOC combinatorial technology (Peng et al., 2006; Xiao et al., 2010, 2016). We also have identified LLP2A had strong binding to human placental chorionic villus MSCs (PMSCs) (Hao et al., 2019) via integrin α4β1 and established an approach to immobilize LLP2A onto electrospun scaffold (Hao et al., 2020b). It has been shown that EVs derived from MSCs, especially from PMSCs, could stimulate angiogenesis (Komaki et al., 2017). Thus, in this study, we propose to immobilize PMSC-derived EVs (PMSC-EVs) onto native ECM mimicking electrospun nanofibrous scaffold by using LLP2A as the conjugation linker to construct the functional biomaterial scaffold to mimic the natural EV-ECM structural complexes and promote the vascularization and regeneration potential for tissue regeneration applications.

MATERIALS AND METHODS

Cell Culture

We used PMSCs isolated from early gestation placental chorionic villus tissue as described in our previous studies (Lankford et al., 2017; Hao et al., 2019; Kumar et al., 2019). PMSCs were expanded in D5 medium containing high-glucose DMEM (HyClone), 5% fetal bovine serum (FBS, HyClone), 20 ng/mL recombinant human basic fibroblast growth factor (bFGF, R&D systems), 20 ng/mL recombinant human epidermal growth factor (EGF, R&D systems), 100 UI/mL of penicillin and 100 μg/mL of streptomycin and incubated at 37°C, 5% CO_2. PMSCs were used between P3 and P5 for all experiments. Human umbilical vein endothelial cells (HUVECs) were purchased from Lonza and expanded in EGM-2 media (Lonza). HUVECs were used between P3 and P6 for all experiments.

EV Isolation and Characterization

EV isolation and characterization were performed using an established protocol described in our previous study (Kumar et al., 2019). Briefly, PMSCs were seeded at a density of 20,000 cells/cm^2 in tissue culture–treated T175 flasks in 20 mL of EV-depleted FBS containing D5 medium for 48 h at 37°C, 5% CO_2. Conditioned medium was collected and sequentially centrifuged at 300 g for 10 min, 2,000 g for 20 min, and passed through a 0.2 mm filter. Then, the medium was concentrated using Amicon Ultra 15 Centrifugal Filter Units with a 100 kDa MW cutoff (MilliporeSigma), transferred to thickwall polypropylene tubes (Beckman Coulter), and centrifuged at 8,836 g using the SW28 rotor and L7 Ultracentrifuge (Beckman Coulter). The supernatant was transferred to fresh tubes, centrifuged at 112,700 g for 90 min, and the pellet was resuspended in PBS (HyClone) and spun again at the same speed and time. The final pellet was resuspended in 10 mL of PBS per T175 flask and stored in aliquots at −80°C. The number and size distribution of isolated EVs were characterized by nanoparticle tracking analysis (NTA) using the NanoSight LM10 (Malvern Panalytical, Malvern, United Kingdom) equipped with a 404-nm laser and sCMOScamera. The morphology of isolated EVs was characterized by Transmission electron microscopy (TEM) using a CM120 transmission electron microscope (Philips/FEI BioTwin, Amsterdam, Netherlands) at 80 kV. For Western blot analysis, 10 mL of EVs were treated with either NuPAGE LDS Sample Buffer (Thermo Fisher Scientific) containing reducing agent DTT, for detecting ALIX, tumor susceptibility gene 101 (TSG101), calnexin, integrin α4 and integrin β1 proteins, or without DTT, for detecting CD9 and CD63 proteins), and heated to 90°C. The samples were run, transferred, probed with primary antibodies ALIX, TSG101, CD9 (MilliporeSigma), calnexin (Cell Signaling Technology), CD63 (Thermo Fisher Scientific), Integrin α4 (MilliporeSigma) and Integrin β1 (MilliporeSigma) at 4°C overnight. Subsequently, membranes were incubated for 1 h with conjugated secondary antibodies (Cell Signaling Technology) at room temperature and blots were imaged using a ChemiDoc MP$^+$ imaging system (Bio-Rad).

Cell Migration Assay

HUVECs were seeded in Culture-Insert 2 Well in μ-Dish (ibidi) and cultured in EBM-2 with 1% BSA (Thermo Fisher Scientific) with EVs or without EVs and incubated at 37°C, 5% CO_2 for 12 h. Images were taken using a Carl Zeiss Axio Observer D1 inverted microscope. The cell migration area was quantified using ImageJ software (NIH).

Rat Aortic Ring Assay

All procedures were approved by the Institutional Animal Care and Use Committee at the University of California, Davis. Ten-week-old male Sprague Dawley rats were purchased from the Charles River animal facility. Rat abdominal aortas were dissected and sliced into 1 mm sections. Aortic rings were embedded in Matrigel® Growth Factor Reduced (GFR) Basement Membrane Matrix (Corning) and cultured in EBM-2 medium with 1% BSA with or without EVs and incubated at 37°C, 5% CO_2. Angiogenic sprouts were counted after 7 days of culture. The number of sprouts was quantified using Wimasis Image Analysis.

Exo-Glow Labeling of EVs

EVs were labeled using Exo-Glow (Green) (System Biosciences) according to manufacturer's instructions. Briefly, Exo-Glow (Green) was diluted 1:500 in PBS and added to EVs. The sample was mixed gently by flicking the tube and incubated at

37°C for 10 min. Twenty microliters of ExoQuick-TC (System Biosciences) were added to stop the labeling reaction and the sample was incubated on ice for 30 min. Excess dye was removed by centrifuging at 16,000 g for 3 min at 4°C. The EV pellet was resuspended in 500 μL of cold PBS, placed on ice for 5 min, and centrifuged again at 16,000 g for 3 min at 4°C. Washes were repeated for a total of 3 times. After the final wash, labeled EVs were resuspended in 500 μL of PBS. As a control, the same process was repeated using with same volume of PBS that the EVs were re-suspended in.

EV Attachment on LLP2A Treated Surface

To modify the culture surface with ligands, cell culture wells in a 48-well plates were coated with 150 μL of 20 μg/mL Avidin (Thermo Fisher Scientific) and incubated for 1 h at 37°C. Avidin coated wells were rinsed three times with PBS and were treated with 150 μL molar equivalents (2 μM) of D-biotin (Thermo Fisher Scientific) or LLP2A-bio. After 1 h, the wells were washed three times with PBS and blocked with 1% BSA for 1 h. After the wells were rinsed three times with PBS, for the EV attachment assay, 5×10^6 EVs suspended in PBS was added into each well and incubated for 10 min at 37°C and 5% CO_2. Then the wells were washed three times with PBS, and the adhered EVs were imaged using a Carl Zeiss Axio Observer D1 inverted microscope. Quantification of images was performed using the ImageJ software.

Quantitative Reverse Transcription Polymerase Chain Reaction (qRT-PCR) Assay and Caspase 3 Assay

For the treated culture surface assay, three different groups, untreated, LLP2A treated and EV treated were set up in 24-well plates. As described above, the untreated wells were coated with D-bio, the LLP2A treated wells were coated with LLP2A and the EV treated wells were seeded with EVs on the LLP2A treated surface. HUVECs were seeded in wells with different treatments and cultured in EBM-2 media with 1% BSA at 37°C and 5% CO_2 for 48 h. RNA extraction from cells was performed using RNeasy Mini Kit (Qiagen) according to the manufacturer's instructions, and cDNA was synthesized using Superscript II Reverse transcriptase (ThermoFisher Scientific). PCR was performed using the Biorad CFX96 Real-Time PCR Detection System (BioRad Laboratories) machinewith the SsoAdvanced SYBR Green Supermix (Bio-Rad). Amplification conditions after an initial denaturation step for 90 s at 95°C were 40 cycles of 95°C, 10 s, for denaturation, 55°C, 10 s, for annealing and 72°C, 30 s, for elongation. GAPDH was used as the reference gene for calculations. Data were analyzed by the 2DDCT threshold cycle method. Primer sequences are listed in **Table 1**. For caspase 3 assay, to mimic the ischemic environment when ECs often experience after implantation *in vivo* into the wounded or defect area, EC survival was characterized in a hypoxic chamber as described previously (Hao et al., 2019). HUVECs were seeded on different treated surfaces and cultured in hypoxia chamber in EBM-2 media at 37°C, 1% O_2 and 5% CO_2 for 6 h, and then lysed and analyzed by using a caspase 3 Assay Kit (Cell Signaling Technology) according to the manufacturer's instruction. Fluorescence (ex 380 nm/em 450 nm) was measured using a SpectraMax i3x Multi-Mode Detection Platform (Molecular Devices).

TABLE 1 | Primers used for qRT-PCR.

Gene	Forward primer	Reverse primer
KDR	CCAAGAACTCCATGCCCCTTA	ATCCCTGGGATCTGAAACG
TIE2	TAGAGCCTGAAACAGCATACCAGG	CTATTGGAATGGCAAATGCTGGG
GAPDH	ACCACAGTCCATGCCATCAC	TCCACCACCCTGTTGCTGTA

Preparation of EV-Modified Electrospun Scaffolds

Preparation of EV-modified electrospun scaffolds included three steps as shown in **Figure 5**: (1) construction of electrospun scaffolds using the established electrospinning technology, (2) LLP2A immobilization on the electrospun scaffolds via "Click chemistry," and (3) EV immobilization on the LLP2A modified electrospun scaffolds via integrin-based conjugation. Construction of electrospun scaffolds was performed as previously reported (Hao et al., 2020b). Briefly, The polymer blends (e.g., 19% PLLA and 5% PCL; w/v) were completely dissolved in 1,1,1,3,3,3-hexafluoro-2-propanol (HFIP, Aladdin). Electrospun scaffolds were prepared by electrospinning polymer fibers onto the rotating drum collector. A negative voltage of 4.5 kV was applied to the mandrel, and a positive voltage of 4 kV was applied to the spinneret, by using a high voltage generator (Gamma High Voltage). LLP2A was grafted onto the PLLA/PCL membrane surface as our previously reported in three steps (Hao et al., 2020b). First, scaffolds were incubated in 0.01 M sodium hydroxide for 10 min to expose the carboxyl groups on the surface. Second, the scaffolds were further incubated in a solution of 1-ethyl-3-(3-(dimethylamino)propyl)-carbodiimide hydrochloride (EDC, Thermo Fisher Scientific) and N-hydroxysulfosuccinimide (sulfo-NHS, Thermo Fisher Scientific) in 0.5 M morpholino ethanesulfonic acid (MES) buffer (Thermo Fisher Scientific) for 30 min. After washing with PBS, the scaffolds were incubated in a solution of azido-PEG11-amine (N_3-PEG11-NH_2, BroadPharm) in alkalescent PBS (pH = 7.8) for 2 h on a shaker. Third, 20 mM LLP2A-DBCO was conjugated to azido-decorated scaffolds via "Click chemistry" in water for 16 h.

To evaluate the EV immobilization on the LLP2A modified electrospun scaffolds, EVs were seeded on electrospun scaffolds modified with different density of LLP2A (0, 50% or 100%). Briefly, we used another peptide ligand LXW7, specifically binds to $\alpha v\beta 3$ integrin, but not integrin $\alpha 4\beta 1$, described in our previous studies (Hao et al., 2017, 2020a) as the competitor ligand to LLP2A to modify the electrospun scaffolds. We used three conditions with different molar ratios of LLP2A-DBCO/LXW7-DBCO to modify the scaffolds: (1) PBS, (2) solution with equal molar ratio of LLP2A-DBCO/LXW7-DBCO (0.5:0.5), and (3) solution with LLP2A only (LLP2A-DBCO/LXW7-DBCO=1:0) to represent 0, 50% density of LLP2A, and 100% density of

LLP2A. The scaffolds were washed with PBS for three times. The EV immobilization was characterized by using Scanning Electron Microscope (SEM, Hitachi TM-1000). Quantification of images was performed using the ImageJ software.

Evaluation of Angiogenic Gene Expression, Apoptosis and Survival of HUVECs

For angiogenic gene expression, HUVECs were seeded on electrospun scaffolds modified with or without EVs and cultured in EGM-2 medium at 37°C, 20% O_2 and 5% CO_2 for 48 h, and the gene expression was evaluated by qRT-PCR as described above. For apoptosis and survival assay, the ischemic environment was set up as described above. HUVECs were seeded on electrospun scaffolds modified with or without EVs and cultured in hypoxia chamber in EBM-2 medium at 37°C, 1% O_2 and 5% CO_2. For Annexin V staining, the cells were cultured for 6 h, the staining was performed by using the Annexin V-FITC antibody (Abcam) according to the manufacturer's instructions. The images were collected using a Carl Zeiss Axio Observer D1 inverted microscope. Quantification of images was performed using the ImageJ software. For caspase 9 assay and caspase 3 assay, the cells were cultured for 6 h, and then lysed and analyzed by using a caspase-9 Activity Assay Kit (Abcam) or the caspase 3 Assay Kit, respectively, according to the manufacturer's instructions. Fluorescence (ex 380 nm/em 450 nm) was measured using a SpectraMax i3x Multi-Mode Detection Platform. For cell survival assay, the cells were cultured for 4 days and then determined using the MTS assay according to the manufacturer's instruction. The amount of soluble formazan product produced by the reduction of MTS by metabolically active cells was measured at the 490 nm absorbance using the SpectraMax i3x Multi-Mode Detection Platform.

Statistical Analysis

For two-sample comparison, a student's t-test was used. For multiple-sample comparison, analysis of variance (ANOVA) was performed to detect whether a significant difference existed between groups with different treatments. A p-value of 0.05 or less indicates a significant difference between samples in comparison.

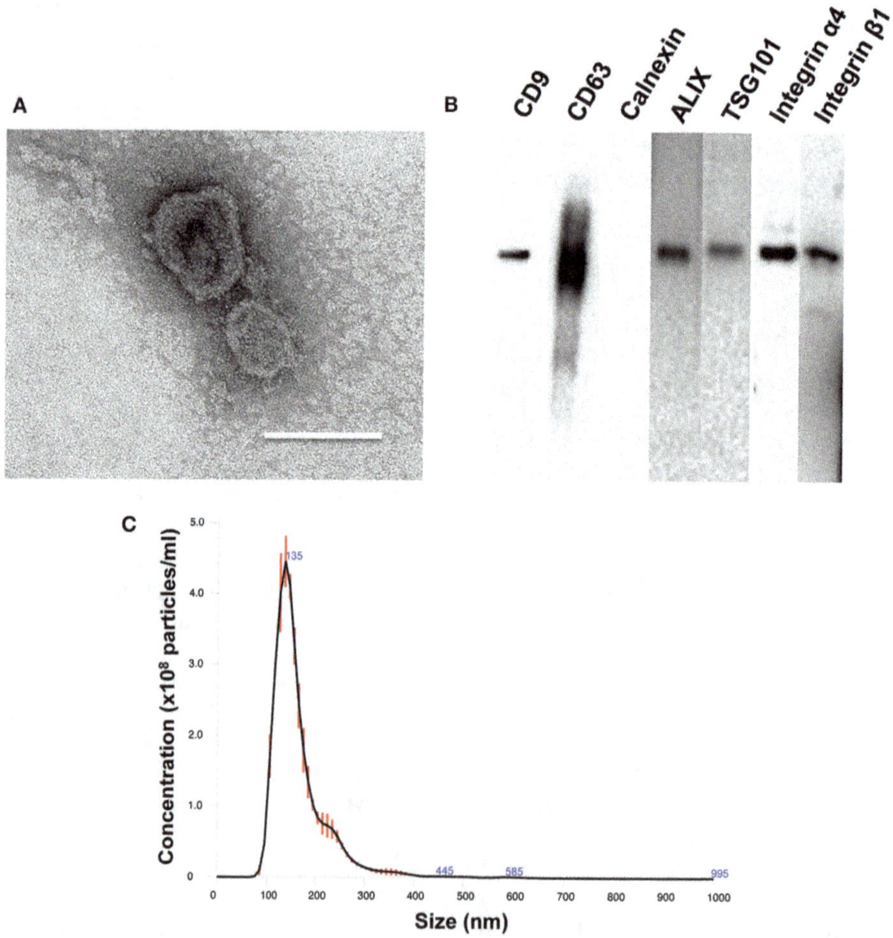

FIGURE 1 | Characterization of PMSC-EVs. **(A)** TEM image of PMSC-EVs. Scale bar = 150 nm. **(B)** Western blot analysis of CD9, CD63, calnexin, ALIX, TSG101, integrin α4 and integrin β1 of PMSC-EVs. **(C)** NTA analysis of PMSC-EVs.

RESULTS AND DISCUSSION

Characterization of PMSC-EVs

TEM analysis showed the characteristic cup shape and size of PMSC-EVs (**Figure 1A**). NTA showed that PMSC-EVs have a size range of 137.4 ± 3.6 nm, which is within the expected size range of EVs (**Figure 1C**). Western blot analysis confirmed the presence of characteristic EV markers CD9, CD63, ALIX and TSG101, and the absence of endoplasmic reticulum marker calnexin (**Figure 1B**). The mechanism of EV binding to natural ECM is important to explore the applications of EVs in tissue regeneration, especially to achieve the conjugation of EVs to biomaterials for modification (Huang et al., 2016). EVs adhere to ECM constituents in the integrin dependent manner (Clayton et al., 2004). Thus, the integrin expression on PMSC-EVs was also determined. Our previous study showed that PMSCs highly expressed integrin α4 and integrin β1 (Hao et al., 2020b). Also, EVs carry markers of their original cells (van der Pol et al., 2012). Thus, in addition to the characteristic EV markers, the Western blot results also confirmed that PMSC-EVs expressed integrin α4 and integrin β1 that could be used as the junction to conjugate PMSC-EVs to biomaterial for simulating the natural ECM. The integrin α4 and integrin β1 expression results were also consistent with the report related to protein identification of EVs in our previous study (Kumar et al., 2019).

PMSC-EVs Promoted EC Migration and Sprouting

Angiogenesis is the crucial need for tissue regeneration (Bi et al., 2012). MSC derived EVs have already developed for the

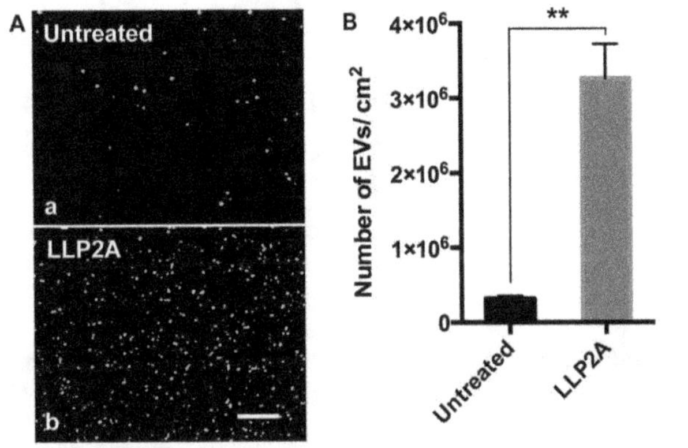

FIGURE 3 | Attachment of PMSC-EVs on different treated surfaces. **(A)** Images of attached PMSC-EVs on untreated surface (a) and LLP2A treated surface (b). Scale bar = 5 μm. **(B)** Quantification of the numbers of PMSC-EVs attached on different surfaces. Data were expressed as mean ± standard deviation: $^{**}p < 0.01$ ($n = 5$).

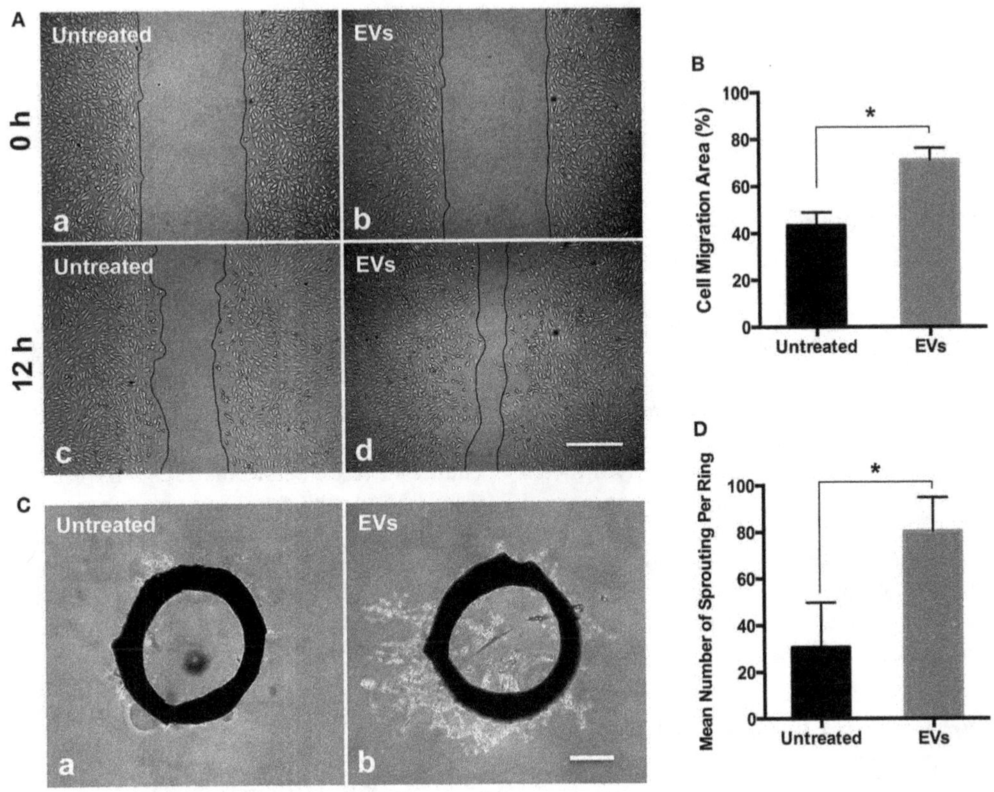

FIGURE 2 | Proangiogenic capacities of PMSC-EVs. **(A)** HUVEC migration treated with PMSC-EVs (b, d) or without PMSC-EVs (a, c). Scale bar = 100 μm. **(B)** Quantification of HUVEC migration area. Data were expressed as mean ± standard deviation: $^{*}p < 0.05$ ($n = 3$). **(C)** Rat aortic ring assay treated with PMSC-EVs (b) or without PMSC-EVs (a). Scale bar = 500 μm. **(D)** Quantification of the number of sprouting per ring. Data were expressed as mean ± standard deviation: $^{*}p < 0.05$ ($n = 3$).

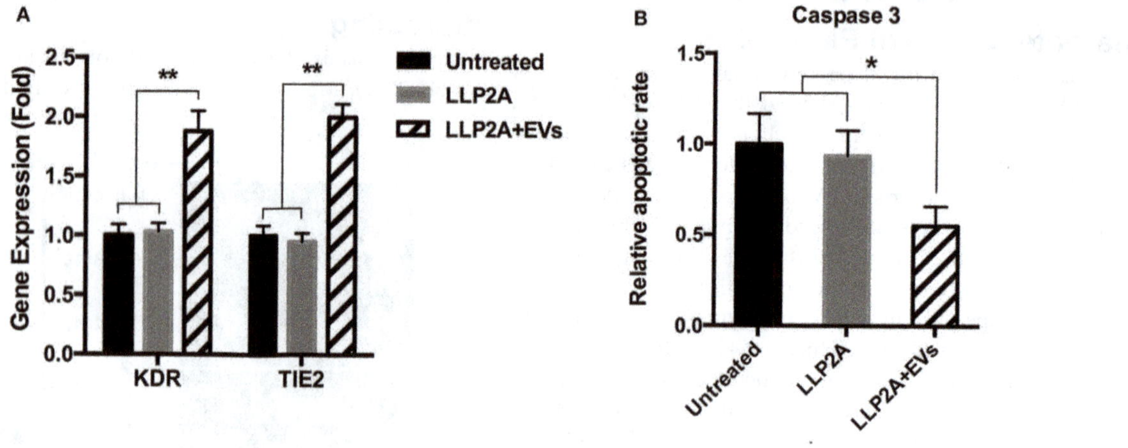

FIGURE 4 | Effects of PMSC-EV treated surface on angiogenic and apoptotic activity of HUVECs. **(A)** KDR and TIE2 expression of HUVECs cultured on untreated surface, LLP2A treated surface or PMSC-EV treated surface. **(B)** Caspase 3 activity of HUVECs cultured on untreated surface, LLP2A treated surface or PMSC-EV treated surface. Data are expressed as mean ± standard deviation: $^*p < 0.05$, $^{**}p < 0.01$ ($n = 4$).

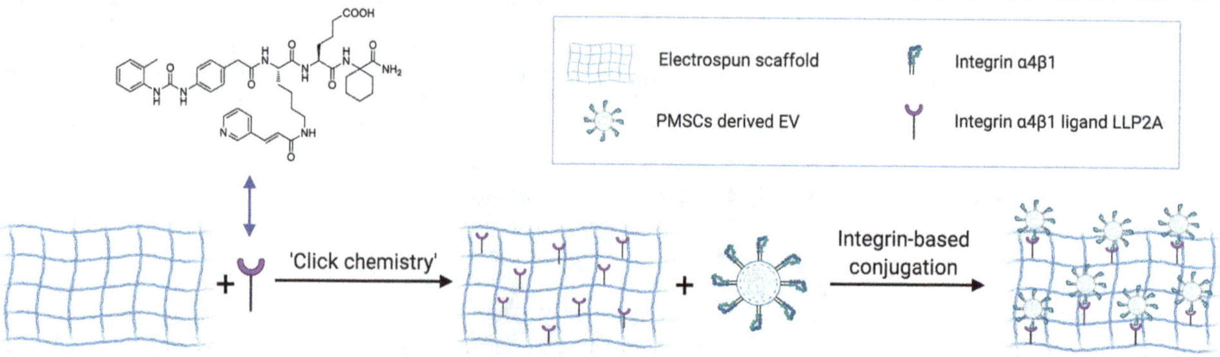

FIGURE 5 | Schematic diagram showing the use of "Click chemistry" to introduce LLP2A to the electrospun scaffold, and the use of immobilized LLP2A to capture PMSC-EVs onto the scaffold surface.

new impetus for improving angiogenesis in tissue regeneration, and EVs derived from different types of MSCs have been demonstrated promoted angiogenesis (Shi et al., 2019). The EC migration results showed that PMSC-EVs significantly enhanced the migration of HUVECs compared to the control group (**Figures 2A,B**). The rat aortic ring assay is an *ex vivo* model of angiogenesis that studies the effects of mediators on normal vessel sprouting, which showed that PMSC-EVs significantly promoted vessel sprouting compared to the control group (**Figures 2C,D**). These results indicate that PMSC-EVs prossess strong proangiogenic capacitiy that will extend the PMSC-EV applications in tissue regeneration.

LLP2A Treated Surface Improved the Attachment of PMSC-EVs

The addition of tool molecules, such as biotin, to ligands can be advantageous when used in combination with other components and when used to expand the bioengineering applications of the ligands (Hao et al., 2020b). Our previous work has shown that biotinylation of the ligand did not decrease its binding affinity and showed nearly identical binding strength to the targeted integrin (Hao et al., 2017). Therefore, we conjugated LLP2A to biotin (LLP2A-bio), as described in our previous study (Peng et al., 2006). We used LLP2A-bio or D-biotin (untreated, as control) to treat the culture surfaces and investigated the attachment of PMSC-EVs on different culture surfaces. Before the PMSC-EV seeding, the PMSC-EVs were labeled with Exo-Glow (green) to facilitate the imaging. The results showed that only a few PMSC-EVs attached on the untreated surface (**Figure 3A**, a) and a number of PMSC-EVs attached on the LLP2A untreated surface (**Figure 3A**, b). The numbers of attached PMSC-EVs on different treated surfaces were quantified, which showed the LLP2A-treated surface significantly improved PMSC-EV attachment compared to the untreated surface (**Figure 3B**).

PMSC-EV Treated Surface Improved Angiogenic Activity and Suppressed Apoptotic Activity of ECs

Angiogenic gene expression, such as KDR and TIE2, is the result of new vessel formation and the improvement of the process of tissue regeneration (Malecki et al., 2005). Upon ligand

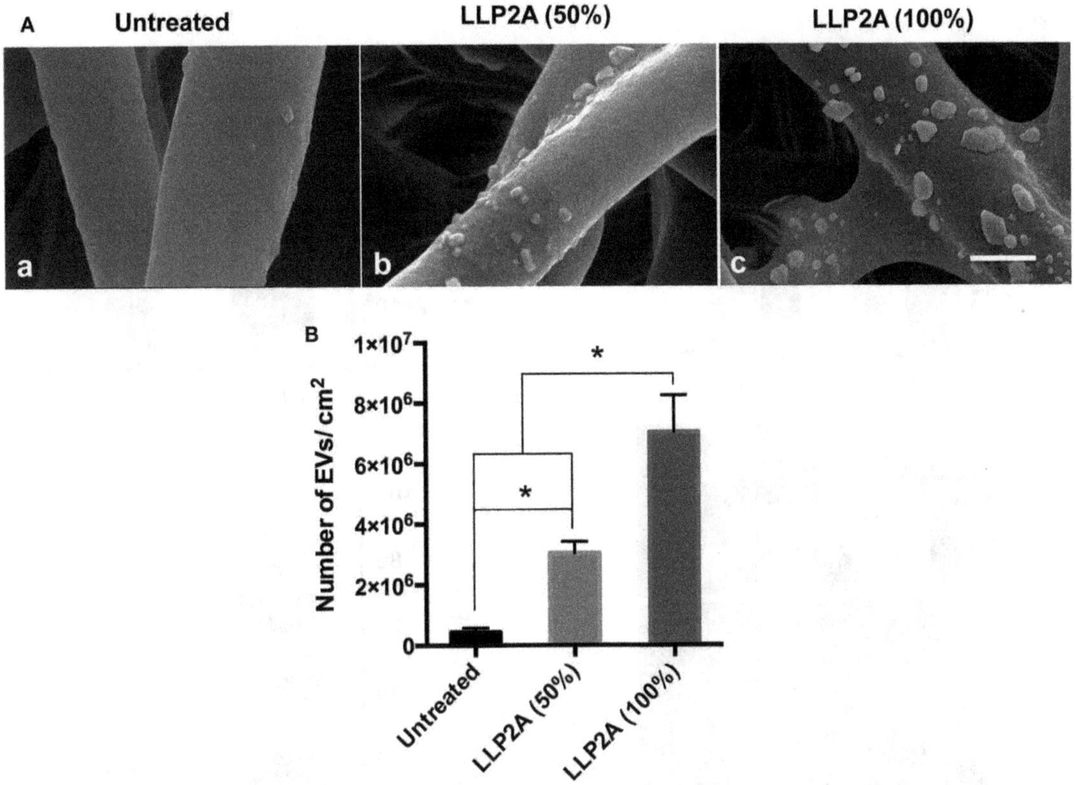

FIGURE 6 | Effect of LLP2A modification on PMSC-EV attachment on electrospun scaffolds. **(A)** SEM images of PMSC-EV attachment on untreated electrospun scaffold (a), 50% LLP2A modified electrospun scaffold (b) and 100% LLP2A modified electrospun scaffold (c). Scale bar = 500 μm. **(B)** Quantification of the numbers of PMSC-EVs on the different modified electrospun scaffolds. Data were expressed as mean ± standard deviation: $^*p < 0.05$ ($n = 5$).

binding, integrins activate signal transduction pathways that mediate cellular signals (Giancotti and Ruoslahti, 1999). Our previous study has demonstrated that LLP2A was an integrin α4β1 ligand (Hao et al., 2020b). To avoid the effect of LLP2A on the gene and protein expression of cells, we set up LLP2A treated surface as another control group. The results showed that PMSC-EV treated surface significantly increased the expression of the angiogenic genes, KDR and TIE2, compared to untreated surface and LLP2A untreated surface, and no significant difference was shown between untreated surface and LLP2A untreated surface (**Figure 4A**). Caspase-3 has been found to be necessary in apoptosis due to it is responsible for chromatin condensation and DNA fragmentation (Porter and Janicke, 1999). The results showed that PMSC-EV treated surface significantly decreased the expression of caspase 3 compared to untreated surface and LLP2A untreated surface, and no significant difference was shown between untreated surface and LLP2A untreated surface (**Figure 4B**). These results indicate that PMSC-EV treated surface is able to improve angiogenic activity and suppressed apoptotic activity of ECs, but LLP2A treated surface does not have impact on angiogenic and apoptotic activity of ECs.

Preparation and Characterization of PMSC-EV Modified Electrospun Scaffold

ECM is a three-dimensional (3D) network of extracellular macromolecules and the crucial need to provide structural and biochemical support to surrounding cells (Bonnans et al., 2014; Rabelink et al., 2017). To mimic the natural ECM structure, we employed electrospinning technology to construct network electrospun scaffolds as the description in our previous study (Hao et al., 2020b). To increase the integrin binding sites on the electrospun scaffolds, we developed a protocol to immobilize LLP2A, an integrin α4β1 ligand, onto the electrospun scaffolds via "Click chemistry" as the description in our previous study (Hao et al., 2020b). To mimic the biological EV-ECM complexes of natural ECM, we conjugated the integrin α4β1 expressing PMSC-EVs onto the electrospun scaffolds via integrin-based binding approach (**Figure 5**). The PMSC-EV modified electrospun scaffold was evaluated using SEM. The results showed the 50% LLP2A modified electrospun scaffolds showed significantly increased immobilization of PMSC-EVs compared to the control untreated electrospun scaffolds, and the 100% LLP2A modified electrospun scaffolds further significantly increased the PMSC-EV immoblization compared to the 50% LLP2A modified electrospun scaffolds (**Figure 6A**), and the quantification of the numbers of immobilized PMSC-EVs on the electrospun scaffolds showed linear correlation with the densities of LLP2A used indicates that the PMSC-EV immobilization system we developed in this study is mechanistically mediated by the densities of LLP2A molecules (**Figure 6B**) and the PMSC-EVs have been successfully immobilized on the electrospun scaffold via LLP2A binding approach. The SEM results showed that some

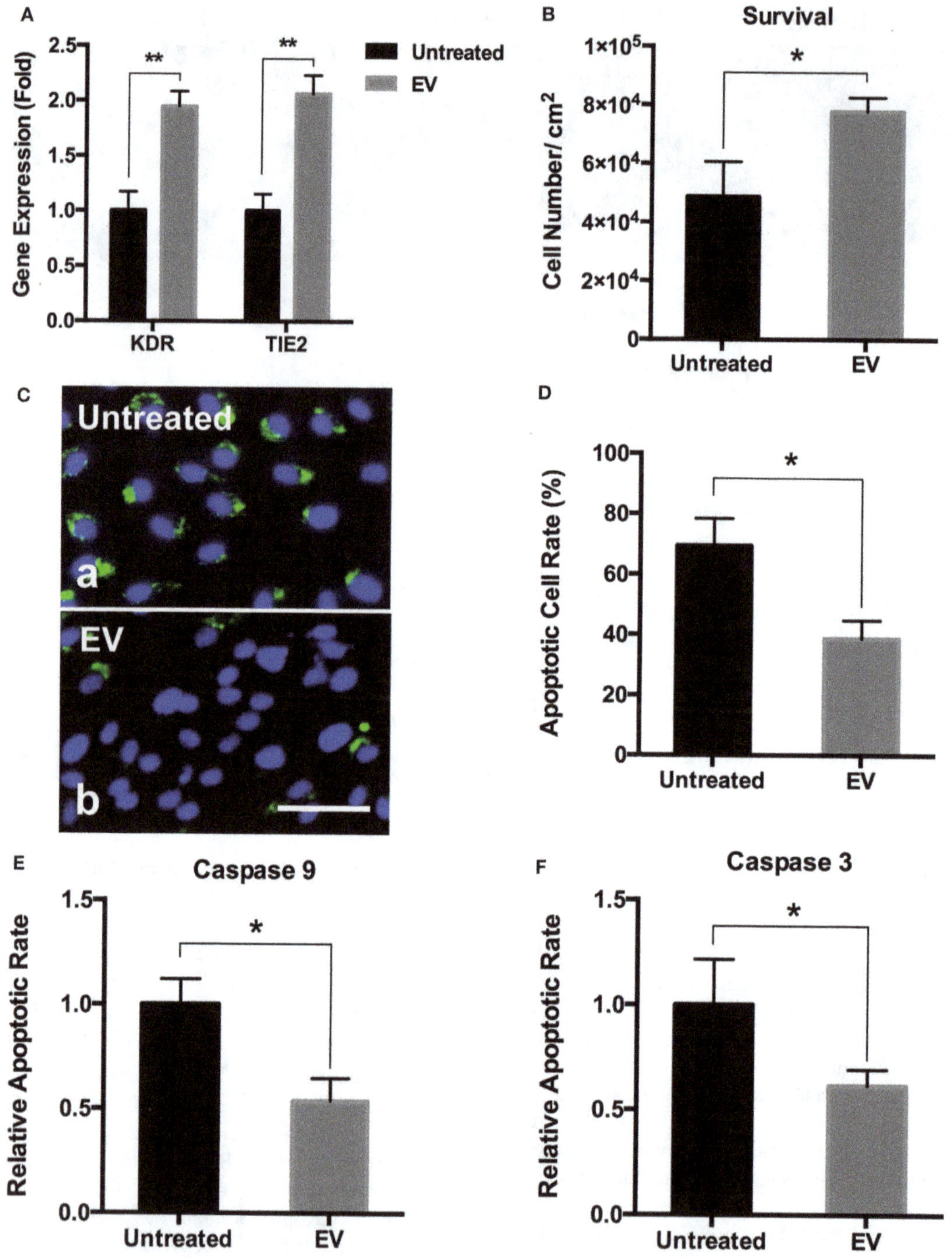

FIGURE 7 | Effects of PMSC-EV modified electrospun scaffolds on angiogenic gene expression and apoptotic rate and protein expression of HUVECs. **(A)** Quantification of KDR and TIE2 expression of HUVECs cultured on untreated electrospun scaffolds and PMSC-EV modified electrospun scaffolds. **(B)** Quantification of HUVEC survival on untreated electrospun scaffolds and PMSC-EV modified electrospun scaffolds. **(C)** Annexin V staining of HUVECs cultured on untreated electrospun scaffolds (a) and PMSC-EV modified electrospun scaffolds (b). **(D)** Quantification of apoptotic rate of HUVECs cultured on untreated electrospun scaffolds and PMSC-EV modified electrospun scaffolds. **(E)** Quantification of caspase 9 expression of HUVECs cultured on untreated electrospun scaffolds and PMSC-EV modified electrospun scaffolds. **(F)** Quantification of caspase 3 expression of HUVECs cultured on untreated electrospun scaffolds and PMSC-EV modified electrospun scaffolds. Data were expressed as mean standard deviation: $^{*}p < 0.05$, $^{**}p < 0.01$ ($n = 4$).

EVs seemed aggregated on the ligand modified scaffolds. It is known that EV aggregation could occur during isolation, storage or upon freeze and thaw (Bosch et al., 2016) and the EVs we used in this study were frozen stored before the immobilization process. Therefore, we believe that the aggregation of EVs seen on the scaffolds happened due to the storage of the EVs. To minimize EV aggregation, avoiding the freeze-thaw cycles of EVs and adding Trehalose into the frozen stock solution could prevent aggregation and cryodamage of EVs according to the previous study (Bosch et al., 2016). We do not anticipate that the EV immobilization strategy we developed in this study will facilitate EV aggregation, because in our design, we conjugated EVs onto electrospun scaffolds by using LLP2A as a linker, and LLP2A was first conjugated onto the electrospun scaffold, then the EVs were immobilized onto the LLP2A modified electrospun scaffold. EVs were never in direct contact with free LLP2A molecules, therefore EV aggregation, if any, should not be caused due to their interactions with free LLP2A molecules. In addition, LLP2A is a small peptide molecule that can bind to integrin molecules on the surface of EVs, and one LLP2A molecule that is immobilized to the scaffold surface can only bind to one integrin molecule. Therefore, we do not anticipate the immobilized LLP2A molecules would affect the aggregation of EVs directly.

PMSC-EV Modified Electrospun Scaffolds Improved the Angiogenic Activity and Survival of ECs

Angiogenic gene expression is essential for the regulation of new vessel formation that is fundamental to the development and maintenance of regenerative tissues (Holden and Nair, 2019). The results showed that compared to the untreated electrospun scaffolds, PMSC-EV modified electrospun scaffolds significantly improved the expression of angiogenic genes, KDR and TIE2, of HUVECs (**Figure 7A**). EC transplantation is an effective approach to improve vascularization and integration of the transplanted biomaterial-based scaffolds, however, EC survival is a significant challenge for the success of cell-based functional biomaterial implants for tissue regeneration (Foster et al., 2018). Apoptosis is a form of programmed cell death that is regulated by the caspase family of proteins, such as caspase 9 and caspase 3, activation of which is the result of intrinsic apoptosis (Hassan and Amer, 2011; Brentnall et al., 2013). Many previous studies have demonstrated that MSC derived EVs prevent cell apoptosis by regulating the activation of caspase 9 and caspase 3 (Li et al., 2019; Liu et al., 2019). In addition, Annexin V is commonly used to detect apoptotic cells by its ability to bind to phosphatidylserine, a marker of apoptosis expressed on the outer leaflet of the plasma membrane. The results showed PMSC-EV modified electrospun scaffolds significantly improved HUVEC survival (**Figure 7B**), decreased the apoptotic rate (**Figures 7C,D**) and the expression of caspase 9 and caspase 3 of HUVECs (**Figures 7E,F**). These results indicate PMSC-EV modified electrospun scaffolds will be worth expecting in vascular tissue regeneration. The main innovation of this study is that it established a novel approach to immobilize the PMSC-EVs onto the electrospun scaffolds by using an integrin-based method that mimics the MBVs in native ECM. This EV delivery system was to modify the polymeric scaffold with EVs to confer the biological functions of EVs to the scaffold. The EVs possess multiple functions, therefore, the EV-modified scaffolds could be widely applied in different areas. Further detailed evaluation of the functions of EV-modified scaffolds in different *in vivo* models is warranted in future studies.

The release of the EVs from the scaffold is crucial for the regenerative capacity of this EVs modified scaffold. We anticipate that when used *in vivo*, the PMSC-EVs modified scaffold could transfer the biological information inside the EVs to the cells that are in direct contact with the scaffolds via EV-cell fusion without the need of releasing the EVs to the body system. Meanwhile, immobilized PMSC-EVs on the scaffold could also be released from the scaffold to the body system. The EV delivery system we designed in this study is based on chemical modification of the scaffolds with the N_3-PEG11-NH_2 linker and DBCO-LLP2A via "Click chemistry" and then the molecular interaction mediated by LLP2A and integrin $\alpha4\beta1$ on the surface of EVs. Since the LLP2A-integrin binding is an "on-and-off" non-covalent interaction, therefore, we anticipate PMSC-EVs will be released first off from the scaffold by the dissociation of the LLP2A from the binding pocket of integrin $\alpha4\beta1$. In the long-term, PMSC-EVs will be released from the scaffold because of the break of the covalent bonds between LLP2A and electrospun scaffold as well as the biodegradation of the electrospun scaffold.

CONCLUSION

In this study, we isolated EVs from PMSCs and demonstrated the PMSC-EVs possessed pro-angiogenic capacity and anti-apoptotic capacity. We successfully established an integrin-based binding technology to immobilize the PMSC-EVs onto the electrospun ECM-mimicking scaffolds to mimic the EV-ECM complexes. The PMSC-EV modified electrospun scaffolds promoted EC angiogenesis and prevented EC apoptosis in ischemic environment. This study demonstrates that EV modified biomaterials represent a new functional biomaterial and hold promise for tissue engineering and regenerative medicine applications.

AUTHOR CONTRIBUTIONS

DH performed the evaluation of PMSC-EVs, performed the construction and evaluation of the PMSC-EVs modified electrospun ECM-mimicking scaffolds, wrote the manuscript, and discussed the results. DH and HS performed the isolation and characterization of the PMSC-EVs. LR performed the labeling of PMSC-EVs. KL and RL performed the chemical synthesis and discussed the results. DF discussed the results. AW was responsible for conceptualization, results discussion revising the manuscript. All authors contributed to the article and approved the submitted version.

ACKNOWLEDGMENTS

The authors would also like to thank the Combinatorial Chemistry and Chemical Biology Shared Resource at University of California Davis for design and synthesis of LLP2A-Bio and LLP2A-DBCO. Utilization of this Shared Resource was supported by the UC Davis Comprehensive Cancer Center Support Grant awarded by the National Cancer Institute (P30CA093373). We acknowledge Jordan Elizabeth Jackson and Mounika LS Bhaskara for their help with the rat aortic ring collection. We acknowledge Alexandra Maria Iavorovschi and Olivia K Vukcevich for their help with manuscript editing and submission.

REFERENCES

Azoidis, I., Cox, S. C., and Davies, O. G. (2018). The role of extracellular vesicles in biomineralisation: current perspective and application in regenerative medicine. *J. Tissue Eng.* 9:2041731418810130. doi: 10.1177/2041731418810130

Baruah, J., and Wary, K. K. (2019). Exosomes in the regulation of vascular endothelial cell regeneration. *Front. Cell Dev. Biol.* 7:353. doi: 10.3389/fcell.2019.00353

Bi, L., Jung, S., Day, D., Neidig, K., Dusevich, V., Eick, D., et al. (2012). Evaluation of bone regeneration, angiogenesis, and hydroxyapatite conversion in critical-sized rat calvarial defects implanted with bioactive glass scaffolds. *J. Biomed. Mater. Res. Part A* 100, 3267–3275. doi: 10.1002/jbm.a.34272

Bonnans, C., Chou, J., and Werb, Z. (2014). Remodelling the extracellular matrix in development and disease. *Nat. Rev. Mol. Cell Biol.* 15, 786–801. doi: 10.1038/nrm3904

Bosch, S., de Beaurepaire, L., Allard, M., Mosser, M., Heichette, C., Chretien, D., et al. (2016). Trehalose prevents aggregation of exosomes and cryodamage. *Sci. Rep.* 6:36162. doi: 10.1038/srep36162

Bose, S., Robertson, S. F., and Bandyopadhyay, A. (2018). Surface modification of biomaterials and biomedical devices using additive manufacturing. *Acta Biomater.* 66, 6–22. doi: 10.1016/j.actbio.2017.11.003

Bouffi, C., Bony, C., Courties, G., Jorgensen, C., and Noel, D. (2010). IL-6-dependent PGE2 secretion by mesenchymal stem cells inhibits local inflammation in experimental arthritis. *PLoS ONE* 5:e14247. doi: 10.1371/journal.pone.0014247

Brentnall, M., Rodriguez-Menocal, L., De Guevara, R. L., Cepero, E., and Boise, L. H. (2013). Caspase-9, caspase-3 and caspase-7 have distinct roles during intrinsic apoptosis. *BMC Cell Biol.* 14:32. doi: 10.1186/1471-2121-14-32

Brown, E. G., Keller, B. A., Lankford, L., Pivetti, C. D., Hirose, S., Farmer, D. L., et al. (2016). Age does matter: a pilot comparison of placenta-derived stromal cells for in utero repair of myelomeningocele using a lamb model. *Fetal Diagn. Ther.* 39, 179–185. doi: 10.1159/000433427

Buzas, E. I., Toth, E. A., Sodar, B. W., and Szabo-Taylor, K. E. (2018). Molecular interactions at the surface of extracellular vesicles. *Semin. Immunopathol.* 40, 453–464. doi: 10.1007/s00281-018-0682-0

Casson, J., Davies, O. G., Smith, C. A., Dalby, M. J., and Berry, C. C. (2018). Mesenchymal stem cell-derived extracellular vesicles may promote breast cancer cell dormancy. *J. Tissue Eng.* 9:2041731418810093. doi: 10.1177/2041731418810093

Clayton, A., Turkes, A., Dewitt, S., Steadman, R., Mason, M. D., and Hallett, M. B. (2004). Adhesion and signaling by B cell-derived exosomes: the role of integrins. *FASEB J.* 18, 977–979. doi: 10.1096/fj.03-1094fje

de Jong, O. G., van Balkom, B. W., Gremmels, H., and Verhaar, M. C. (2016). Exosomes from hypoxic endothelial cells have increased collagen crosslinking activity through up-regulation of lysyl oxidase-like 2. *J. Cell. Mol. Med.* 20, 342–350. doi: 10.1111/jcmm.12730

de Mel, A., Cousins, B. G., and Seifalian, A. M. (2012). Surface modification of biomaterials: a quest for blood compatibility. *Int. J. Biomater.* 2012:707863. doi: 10.1155/2012/707863

Demircan, K., Comertoglu, I., Akyol, S., Yigitoglu, B. N., and Sarikaya, E. (2014). A new biological marker candidate in female reproductive system diseases: matrix metalloproteinase with thrombospondin motifs (ADAMTS). *J. Turk. Ger. Gynecol. Assoc.* 15, 250–255. doi: 10.5152/jtgga.2014.14206

Dhondt, B., Rousseau, Q., De Wever, O., and Hendrix, A. (2016). Function of extracellular vesicle-associated miRNAs in metastasis. *Cell Tissue Res.* 365, 621–641. doi: 10.1007/s00441-016-2430-x

Downing, T. L., Wang, A., Yan, Z. Q., Nout, Y., Lee, A. L., Beattie, M. S., et al. (2012). Drug-eluting microfibrous patches for the local delivery of rolipram in spinal cord repair. *J. Control. Release* 161, 910–917. doi: 10.1016/j.jconrel.2012.05.034

Foster, A. A., Dewi, R. E., Cai, L., Hou, L., Strassberg, Z., Alcazar, C. A., et al. (2018). Protein-engineered hydrogels enhance the survival of induced pluripotent stem cell-derived endothelial cells for treatment of peripheral arterial disease. *Biomater. Sci.* 6, 614–622. doi: 10.1039/C7BM00883J

Fridenshtein, A., Petrakova, K. V., Kuralesova, A. I., and Frolova, G. I. (1968). [Precursor cells for osteogenic and hemopoietic tissues. Analysis of heterotopic transplants of bone marrow]. *Tsitologiia* 10, 557–567.

Galganski, L. A., Kumar, P., Vanover, M. A., Pivetti, C. D., Anderson, J. E., Lankford, L., et al. (2019). *In utero* treatment of myelomeningocele with placental mesenchymal stromal cells - selection of an optimal cell line in preparation for clinical trials. *J. Pediatr. Surg.* doi: 10.1016/j.jpedsurg.2019.09.029. [Epub ahead of print].

Gao, J., Jiang, L., Liang, Q., Shi, J., Hou, D., Tang, D., et al. (2018). The grafts modified by heparinization and catalytic nitric oxide generation used for vascular implantation in rats. *Regen. Biomater.* 5, 105–114. doi: 10.1093/rb/rby003

Garcia, J. R., and Garcia, A. J. (2016). Biomaterial-mediated strategies targeting vascularization for bone repair. *Drug Deliv. Transl. Res.* 6, 77–95. doi: 10.1007/s13346-015-0236-0

Giancotti, F. G., and Ruoslahti, E. (1999). Integrin signaling. *Science* 285, 1028–1032. doi: 10.1126/science.285.5430.1028

Hao, D., Fan, Y., Xiao, W., Liu, R., Pivetti, C., Walimbe, T., et al. (2020a). Rapid endothelialization of small diameter vascular grafts by a bioactive integrin-binding ligand specifically targeting endothelial progenitor cells and endothelial cells. *Acta Biomater.* 108, 178–193. doi: 10.1016/j.actbio.2020.03.005

Hao, D., He, C., Ma, B., Lankford, L., Reynaga, L., Farmer, D. L., et al. (2019). Hypoxic preconditioning enhances survival and proangiogenic capacity of human first trimester chorionic villus-derived mesenchymal stem cells for fetal tissue engineering. *Stem Cells Int.* 2019:9695239. doi: 10.1155/2019/9695239

Hao, D., Ma, B., He, C., Liu, R., Farmer, D. L., Lam, K. S., et al. (2020b). Surface modification of polymeric electrospun scaffolds via a potent and high-affinity integrin alpha4beta1 ligand improved the adhesion, spreading and survival of human chorionic villus-derived mesenchymal stem cells: a new insight for fetal tissue engineering. *J. Mater. Chem. B* 8, 1649–1659. doi: 10.1039/C9TB02309G

Hao, D., Xiao, W., Liu, R., Kumar, P., Li, Y., Zhou, P., et al. (2017). Discovery and characterization of a potent and specific peptide ligand targeting endothelial progenitor cells and endothelial cells for tissue regeneration. *ACS Chem. Biol.* 12, 1075–1086. doi: 10.1021/acschembio.7b00118

Hassan, H., and Amer, A. O. (2011). Cell intrinsic roles of apoptosis-associated speck-like protein in regulating innate and adaptive immune responses. *ScientificWorldJournal* 11, 2418–2423. doi: 10.1100/2011/429192

Hofer, H. R., and Tuan, R. S. (2016). Secreted trophic factors of mesenchymal stem cells support neurovascular and musculoskeletal therapies. *Stem Cell Res. Ther.* 7:131. doi: 10.1186/s13287-016-0394-0

Holden, P., and Nair, L. S. (2019). Deferoxamine: an angiogenic and antioxidant molecule for tissue regeneration. *Tissue Eng. Part B Rev.* 25, 461–470. doi: 10.1089/ten.teb.2019.0111

Huang, C. C., Narayanan, R., Alapati, S., and Ravindran, S. (2016). Exosomes as biomimetic tools for stem cell differentiation: applications in dental pulp tissue regeneration. *Biomaterials* 111, 103–115. doi: 10.1016/j.biomaterials.2016.09.029

Huleihel, L., Bartolacci, J. G., Dziki, J. L., Vorobyov, T., Arnold, B., Scarritt, M. E., et al. (2017). Matrix-bound nanovesicles recapitulate extracellular matrix effects on macrophage phenotype. *Tissue Eng. Part A* 23, 1283–1294. doi: 10.1089/ten.tea.2017.0102

Huleihel, L., Hussey, G. S., Naranjo, J. D., Zhang, L., Dziki, J. L., Turner, N. J., et al. (2016). Matrix-bound nanovesicles within ECM bioscaffolds. *Sci. Adv.* 2:e1600502. doi: 10.1126/sciadv.1600502

Janse van Rensburg, A. J., Davies, N. H., Oosthuysen, A., Chokoza, C., Zilla, P., and Bezuidenhout, D. (2017). Improved vascularization of porous scaffolds through growth factor delivery from heparinized polyethylene glycol hydrogels. *Acta Biomater.* 49, 89–100. doi: 10.1016/j.actbio.2016.11.036

Jiao, Y. P., and Cui, F. Z. (2007). Surface modification of polyester biomaterials for tissue engineering. *Biomed. Mater.* 2, R24–R37. doi: 10.1088/1748-6041/2/4/R02

Jo, Y. Y., Lee, H. J., Kook, S. Y., Choung, H. W., Park, J. Y., Chung, J. H., et al. (2007). Isolation and characterization of postnatal stem cells from human dental tissues. *Tissue Eng.* 13, 767–773. doi: 10.1089/ten.2006.0192

Kabagambe, S., Keller, B., Becker, J., Goodman, L., Pivetti, C., Lankford, L., et al. (2017). Placental mesenchymal stromal cells seeded on clinical grade extracellular matrix improve ambulation in ovine myelomeningocele. *J. Pediatr. Surg.* 53, 178–182. doi: 10.1016/j.jpedsurg.2017.10.032

Komaki, M., Numata, Y., Morioka, C., Honda, I., Tooi, M., Yokoyama, N., et al. (2017). Exosomes of human placenta-derived mesenchymal stem cells stimulate angiogenesis. *Stem Cell Res. Ther.* 8:219. doi: 10.1186/s13287-017-0660-9

Kumar, P., Becker, J. C., Gao, K., Carney, R. P., Lankford, L., Keller, B. A., et al. (2019). Neuroprotective effect of placenta-derived mesenchymal stromal cells: role of exosomes. *FASEB J.* 33, 5836–5849. doi: 10.1096/fj.201800972R

Lam, K. S., Salmon, S. E., Hersh, E. M., Hruby, V. J., Kazmierski, W. M., and Knapp, R. J. (1991). A new type of synthetic peptide library for identifying ligand-binding activity. *Nature* 354, 82–84. doi: 10.1038/354082a0

Lankford, L., Chen, Y. J., Saenz, Z., Kumar, P., Long, C., Farmer, D., et al. (2017). Manufacture and preparation of human placenta-derived mesenchymal stromal cells for local tissue delivery. *Cytotherapy* 19, 680–688. doi: 10.1016/j.jcyt.2017.03.003

Lankford, L., Selby, T., Becker, J., Ryzhuk, V., Long, C., Farmer, D., et al. (2015). Early gestation chorionic villi-derived stromal cells for fetal tissue engineering. *World J. Stem Cells* 7, 195–207. doi: 10.4252/wjsc.v7.i1.195

Lee, B. L., Jeon, H., Wang, A., Yan, Z., Yu, J., Grigoropoulos, C., et al. (2012). Femtosecond laser ablation enhances cell infiltration into three-dimensional electrospun scaffolds. *Acta Biomater.* 8, 2648–2658. doi: 10.1016/j.actbio.2012.04.023

Lee, T. T., Garcia, J. R., Paez, J. I., Singh, A., Phelps, E. A., Weis, S., et al. (2015). Light-triggered *in vivo* activation of adhesive peptides regulates cell adhesion, inflammation and vascularization of biomaterials. *Nat. Mater.* 14, 352–360. doi: 10.1038/nmat4157

Li, L., Wang, R., Jia, Y., Rong, R., Xu, M., and Zhu, T. (2019). Exosomes derived from mesenchymal stem cells ameliorate renal ischemic-reperfusion injury through inhibiting inflammation and cell apoptosis. *Front. Med.* 6:269. doi: 10.3389/fmed.2019.00269

Liang, X., Zhang, L., Wang, S., Han, Q., and Zhao, R. C. (2016). Exosomes secreted by mesenchymal stem cells promote endothelial cell angiogenesis by transferring miR-125a. *J. Cell Sci.* 129, 2182–2189. doi: 10.1242/jcs.170373

Liu, Z., Xu, Y., Wan, Y., Gao, J., Chu, Y., and Li, J. (2019). Exosomes from adipose-derived mesenchymal stem cells prevent cardiomyocyte apoptosis induced by oxidative stress. *Cell Death Discov.* 5, 1–7. doi: 10.1038/s41420-019-0159-5

Lu, P., Takai, K., Weaver, V. M., and Werb, Z. (2011). Extracellular matrix degradation and remodeling in development and disease. *Cold Spring Harb. Perspect. Biol.* 3:a005058. doi: 10.1101/cshperspect.a005058

Malecki, M., Kolsut, P., and Proczka, R. (2005). Angiogenic and antiangiogenic gene therapy. *Gene Ther.* 12 (Suppl. 1), S159–S169. doi: 10.1038/sj.gt.3302621

Mathivanan, S. (2017). Extracellular matrix and the extracellular environment. *Proteomics* 17:7700185. doi: 10.1002/pmic.2017700185

Merino-Gonzalez, C., Zuniga, F. A., Escudero, C., Ormazabal, V., Reyes, C., Nova-Lamperti, E., et al. (2016). Mesenchymal stem cell-derived extracellular vesicles promote angiogenesis: potencial clinical application. *Front. Physiol.* 7:24. doi: 10.3389/fphys.2016.00024

Muangsanit, P., Shipley, R. J., and Phillips, J. B. (2018). Vascularization strategies for peripheral nerve tissue engineering. *Anat. Rec.* 301, 1657–1667. doi: 10.1002/ar.23919

Oh, W., Kim, D. S., Yang, Y. S., and Lee, J. K. (2008). Immunological properties of umbilical cord blood-derived mesenchymal stromal cells. *Cell. Immunol.* 251, 116–123. doi: 10.1016/j.cellimm.2008.04.003

Pankajakshan, D., and Agrawal, D. K. (2014). Mesenchymal stem cell paracrine factors in vascular repair and regeneration. *J. Biomed. Technol. Res.* 1:09. doi: 10.19104/jbtr.2014.107

Peng, L., Liu, R., Marik, J., Wang, X., Takada, Y., and Lam, K. S. (2006). Combinatorial chemistry identifies high-affinity peptidomimetics against alpha4beta1 integrin for *in vivo* tumor imaging. *Nat. Chem. Biol.* 2, 381–389. doi: 10.1038/nchembio798

Porter, A. G., and Janicke, R. U. (1999). Emerging roles of caspase-3 in apoptosis. *Cell Death Differ.* 6, 99–104. doi: 10.1038/sj.cdd.4400476

Premer, C., Wanschel, A., Porras, V., Balkan, W., Legendre-Hyldig, T., Saltzman, R. G., et al. (2019). Mesenchymal stem cell secretion of SDF-1α modulates endothelial function in dilated cardiomyopathy. *Front. Physiol.* 10:1182. doi: 10.3389/fphys.2019.01182

Qi, H., Hu, P., Xu, J., and Wang, A. (2006). Encapsulation of drug reservoirs in fibers by emulsion electrospinning: morphology characterization and preliminary release assessment. *Biomacromolecules* 7, 2327–2330. doi: 10.1021/bm060264z

Rabelink, T. J., van den Berg, B. M., Garsen, M., Wang, G., Elkin, M., and van der Vlag, J. (2017). Heparanase: roles in cell survival, extracellular matrix remodelling and the development of kidney disease. *Nat. Rev. Nephrol.* 13, 201–212. doi: 10.1038/nrneph.2017.6

Rilla, K., Mustonen, A. M., Arasu, U. T., Harkonen, K., Matilainen, J., and Nieminen, P. (2019). Extracellular vesicles are integral and functional components of the extracellular matrix. *Matrix Biol.* 75–76, 201–219. doi: 10.1016/j.matbio.2017.10.003

Saadai, P., Nout, Y. S., Encinas, J., Wang, A., Downing, T. L., Beattie, M. S., et al. (2011). Prenatal repair of myelomeningocele with aligned nanofibrous scaffolds-a pilot study in sheep. *J. Pediatr. Surg.* 46, 2279–2283. doi: 10.1016/j.jpedsurg.2011.09.014

Santos, M. I., and Reis, R. L. (2010). Vascularization in bone tissue engineering: physiology, current strategies, major hurdles and future challenges. *Macromol. Biosci.* 10, 12–27. doi: 10.1002/mabi.200900107

Sarkar, S., Lee, G. Y., Wong, J. Y., and Desai, T. A. (2006). Development and characterization of a porous micro-patterned scaffold for vascular tissue engineering applications. *Biomaterials* 27, 4775–4782. doi: 10.1016/j.biomaterials.2006.04.038

Scharnweber, D., Bierbaum, S., and Wolf-Brandstetter, C. (2018). Utilizing DNA for functionalization of biomaterial surfaces. *FEBS Lett.* 592, 2181–2196. doi: 10.1002/1873-3468.13065

Shi, Y., Shi, H., Nomi, A., Lei-Lei, Z., Zhang, B., and Qian, H. (2019). Mesenchymal stem cell-derived extracellular vesicles: a new impetus of promoting angiogenesis in tissue regeneration. *Cytotherapy* 21, 497–508. doi: 10.1016/j.jcyt.2018.11.012

Sood, D., Tang-Schomer, M., Pouli, D., Mizzoni, C., Raia, N., Tai, A., et al. (2019). 3D extracellular matrix microenvironment in bioengineered tissue models of primary pediatric and adult brain tumors. *Nat. Commun.* 10:4529. doi: 10.1038/s41467-019-12420-1

Sung, B. H., Ketova, T., Hoshino, D., Zijlstra, A., and Weaver, A. M. (2015). Directional cell movement through tissues is controlled by exosome secretion. *Nat. Commun.* 6:7164. doi: 10.1038/ncomms8164

Teodori, L., Costa, A., Marzio, R., Perniconi, B., Coletti, D., Adamo, S., et al. (2014). Native extracellular matrix: a new scaffolding platform for repair of damaged muscle. *Front. Physiol.* 5:218. doi: 10.3389/fphys.2014.00218

van der Merwe, Y., Faust, A. E., and Steketee, M. B. (2017). Matrix bound vesicles and miRNA cargoes are bioactive factors within extracellular matrix bioscaffolds. *Neural Regen Res.* 12, 1597–1599. doi: 10.4103/1673-5374.217324

van der Pol, E., Boing, A. N., Harrison, P., Sturk, A., and Nieuwland, R. (2012). Classification, functions, and clinical relevance of extracellular vesicles. *Pharmacol. Rev.* 64, 676–705. doi: 10.1124/pr.112.005983

van Niel, G., D'Angelo, G., and Raposo, G. (2018). Shedding light on the cell biology of extracellular vesicles. *Nat. Rev. Mol. Cell Biol.* 19, 213–228. doi: 10.1038/nrm.2017.125

Vanover, M., Pivetti, C., Lankford, L., Kumar, P., Galganski, L., Kabagambe, S., et al. (2019). High density placental mesenchymal stromal cells provide neuronal preservation and improve motor function following in utero treatment of ovine myelomeningocele. *J. Pediatr. Surg.* 54, 75–79. doi: 10.1016/j.jpedsurg.2018.10.032

Wang, A., Brown, E. G., Lankford, L., Keller, B. A., Pivetti, C. D., Sitkin, N. A., et al. (2015). Placental mesenchymal stromal cells rescue ambulation in ovine myelomeningocele. *Stem Cells Transl. Med.* 4, 659–669. doi: 10.5966/sctm.2014-0296

Wang, A., Tang, Z., Park, I. H., Zhu, Y., Patel, S., Daley, G. Q., et al. (2011). Induced pluripotent stem cells for neural tissue engineering. *Biomaterials* 32, 5023–5032. doi: 10.1016/j.biomaterials.2011.03.070

Wang, Y. C., Kao, S. H., and Hsieh, H. J. (2003). A chemical surface modification of chitosan by glycoconjugates to enhance the cell-biomaterial interaction. *Biomacromolecules* 4, 224–231. doi: 10.1021/bm0256294

Wu, Z. J., Garimella, N., Larsson, R., and Brynda, E. (2012). Advanced surface modifications for blood-contacting surfaces of medical devices. *Int. J. Biomater.* 2012:291735. doi: 10.1155/2012/291735

Xiao, W., Li, T., Bononi, F. C., Lac, D., Kekessie, I. A., Liu, Y. et al. (2016) Discovery and characterization of a high-affinity and high-specificity peptide ligand LXY30 for in vivo targeting of α3 integrin-expressing human tumors. *EJNMMI Res.* 6, 1–18. doi: 10.1186/s13550-016-0165-z

Xiao, W., Wang, Y., Lau, E. Y., Luo, J., Yao, N., Shi, C., et al. (2010). The use of one-bead one-compound combinatorial library technology to discover high-affinity αvβ3 integrin and cancer targeting arginine-glycine-aspartic acid ligands with a built-in handle. *Mol. Cancer Ther.* 9, 2714–2723. doi: 10.1158/1535-7163.MCT-10-0308

Xue, Q., Yin, Z., Varshithreddy, N., Liang, H. S., Wang, M. Y., Dong, W. L., et al. (2018). The immunomodulatory function of human amniotic fluid stromal cells on B lymphocytes. *J. Neurorestoratol.* 6, 122–133. doi: 10.26599/JNR.2018.9040010

Yanez-Mo, M., Siljander, P. R., Andreu, Z., Zavec, A. B., Borras, F. E., Buzas, E. I., et al. (2015). Biological properties of extracellular vesicles and their physiological functions. *J. Extracell. Vesicles* 4:27066. doi: 10.3402/jev.v4.27066

Yu, J., Wang, A., Tang, Z., Henry, J., Li-Ping Lee, B., Zhu, Y., et al. (2012). The effect of stromal cell-derived factor-1α/heparin coating of biodegradable vascular grafts on the recruitment of both endothelial and smooth muscle progenitor cells for accelerated regeneration. *Biomaterials* 33, 8062–8074. doi: 10.1016/j.biomaterials.2012.07.042

Zannettino, A. C., Paton, S., Arthur, A., Khor, F., Itescu, S., Gimble, J. M., et al. (2008). Multipotential human adipose-derived stromal stem cells exhibit a perivascular phenotype *in vitro* and *in vivo*. *J. Cell. Physiol.* 214, 413–421. doi: 10.1002/jcp.21210

Zhang, B., Wu, X., Zhang, X., Sun, Y., Yan, Y., Shi, H., et al. (2015). Human umbilical cord mesenchymal stem cell exosomes enhance angiogenesis through the Wnt4/β-catenin pathway. *Stem Cells Transl. Med.* 4, 513–522. doi: 10.5966/sctm.2014-0267

Zhang, H., Wang, L., Li, C., Yu, Y., Yi, Y., Wang, J., et al. (2019). Exosome-induced regulation in inflammatory bowel disease. *Front. Immunol.* 10:1464. doi: 10.3389/fimmu.2019.01464

Zhang, Z., Wang, F., and Song, M. (2019). The cell repair research of spinal cord injury: a review of cell transplantation to treat spinal cord injury. *J. Neurorestoratol.* 7, 55–62. doi: 10.26599/JNR.2019.9040011

Zhao, L., Ma, S., Pan, Y., Zhang, Q., Wang, K., Song, D., et al. (2016). Functional modification of fibrous PCL scaffolds with fusion protein VEGF-HGFI enhanced cellularization and vascularization. *Adv. Healthc. Mater.* 5, 2376–2385. doi: 10.1002/adhm.201600226

Zhu, Y., Wang, A., Patel, S., Kurpinski, K., Diao, E., Bao, X., et al. (2011). Engineering bi-layer nanofibrous conduits for peripheral nerve regeneration. *Tissue Eng. Part C Methods* 17, 705–715. doi: 10.1089/ten.tec.2010.0565

Zhu, Y., Wang, A., Shen, W., Patel, S., Zhang, R., Young, W., et al. (2010). Nanofibrous patches for spinal cord regeneration. *Adv. Funct. Mater.* 20, 1433–1440. doi: 10.1002/adfm.200901889

15

Nanomedicine in Oncocardiology: Contribution and Perspectives of Preclinical Studies

Gabriel Silva Marques Borges[1,2†], *Eduardo Burgarelli Lages*[1,2†], *Pierre Sicard*[2,3], *Lucas Antônio Miranda Ferreira*[1] *and Sylvain Richard*[2,3*]

[1] *Departamento de Produtos Farmacêuticos, Faculdade de Farmácia, Universidade Federal de Minas Gerais, Belo Horizonte, Brazil,* [2] *PhyMedExp, Université de Montpellier, INSERM, CNRS, Montpellier, France,* [3] *IPAM, BioCampus, CNRS, INSERM, Université de Montpellier, Montpellier, France*

Correspondence:
Sylvain Richard
sylvain.richard@inserm.fr

† These authors have contributed equally to this work and share first authorship

Cancer and cardiovascular diseases are the leading causes of death and morbidity worldwide. Strikingly, cardiovascular disorders are more common and more severe in cancer patients than in the general population, increasing incidence rates. In this context, it is vital to consider the anticancer efficacy of a treatment and the devastating heart complications it could potentially cause. Oncocardiology has emerged as a promising medical and scientific field addressing these aspects from different angles. Interestingly, nanomedicine appears to have great promise in reducing the cardiotoxicity of anticancer drugs, maintaining or even enhancing their efficacy. Several studies have shown the benefits of nanocarriers, although with some flaws when considering the concept of oncocardiology. Herein, we discuss how preclinical studies should be designed as closely as possible to clinical protocols, considering various parameters intrinsic to the animal models used and the experimental protocols. The sex and age of the animals, the size and location of the tumors, the doses of the nanoformulations administered, and the acute vs. the long-term effects of treatments are essential aspects. We also discuss the perspectives offered by non-invasive imaging techniques to simultaneously assess both the anticancer effects of treatment and its potential impact on the heart. The overall objective is to accelerate the development and validation of nanoformulations through high-quality preclinical studies reproducing the clinical conditions.

Keywords: anticancer drugs, cardiotoxicity, nanoformulations, non-invasive imaging, echography, photoacoustic, small animals

INTRODUCTION

Recent advances in the treatment of cancers have improved patient care and cure rates. Cancer, once fatal, is now emerging as a chronic disease, often at the cost of cardiovascular complications. Moreover, cardiovascular diseases (CVD) are more common and more severe in cancer patients (1–5). In this context, the development of novel treatments with antineoplastic agents still raises concerns about undesirable effects at the acute phase of the treatment and potentially during long-term therapy (6). Therefore, the management of cancer patients has moved from general cardiology to a specialized discipline, oncocardiology, with in-depth cardiovascular monitoring at each stage of cancer therapy (1, 7). Among various areas that can help solve these problems, nanotechnology is being increasingly investigated in preclinical studies to improve anticancer treatments and reduce their cardiotoxicity. This review will discuss the potential of nanocarriers to optimize the use of anticancer drugs through tailored preclinical approaches that can help understand/control their adverse effects and how preclinical models can be better designed to represent an oncocardiology approach truly.

REDUCING CARDIOTOXICITY OF ANTICANCER DRUGS THROUGH NANOTECHNOLOGY

Cardiotoxicity is a broad term that embraces toxic effects on cardiac structure, morphology, rest parameters, and the dynamic function of the heart. Cytotoxic drugs and targeted therapies used to treat cancer, including classic chemotherapeutic agents, tyrosine kinase inhibitors, antiangiogenic drugs, and immunotherapy, often impair the cardiovascular system (8). Of note, cancer itself may promote CVD (6).

The cardiotoxicity evoked by conventional chemotherapy is widely known and occur through multiple mechanisms, including overproduction of free radical species, inhibition of topoisomerase 2β causing DNA double-strand breaks and activation of apoptosis, profound changes in the transcriptome leading to the generation of reactive oxygen species, and inhibition of VEGF receptors causing endothelial dysfunction and vascular injury. In turn, the novel immunotherapeutic agents can lead to the inhibition of the Human Epithelial Receptor type 2 (HER2), impairing the cell signaling in cardiomyocytes; and the inhibition of programmed cell death proteins (PD-1) causing inflammatory infiltrates in the heart tissue (8–10). This cardiotoxicity can lead to bradycardia (paclitaxel and thalidomide), promote QT interval prolongation and arrhythmias (amsacrine and anthracyclines), evoke myocardial ischemia via coronary vasospasm (anti-metabolites and 5-fluorouracil), impair the left ventricle function (anthracyclines, tyrosine kinase inhibitors, alkylating agents, and cisplatin), and evoke myocarditis, pericarditis, and heart failure (immunotherapy) (6, 11, 12).

The objective of cardioprotection is to limit cardiac damage while maintaining antineoplastic efficacy (8). In the clinics, combinations with drugs like statins, antiarrhythmic, beta-blockers, calcium-channel inhibitors, and ACE (angiotensin-converting enzyme) inhibitors are some of the strategies (13). Interestingly, preclinical and clinical studies show that nanotechnology can also lead to cardioprotection in cancer treatment (14).

The basic concept of nanomedicine is to alter both pharmacokinetics and biodistribution of nanoencapsulated drugs, increasing their accumulation in the tumor site and decreasing their delivery to non-target organs, such as the heart. Passive and active targeting mechanisms can enable nanocarriers to reach the tumor site efficiently. The passive mechanism is based on the Enhanced Permeability and Retention (EPR) effect, which leads to the accumulation of nanostructures in the tumor site due to the characteristic leaky vasculature and absence of lymphatic drainage in the tumor microenvironment (**Figure 1A**) (15). In turn, active targeting involves the attachment of high-affinity ligands to tumor cells on the surface of the nanocarriers. The idea is to use ligands for which cancer cells express a high number of specific receptors, whereas normal cells express very few. A wide variety of ligands have been used for this purpose, including folic acid, hyaluronic acid, transferrin, among others (**Figure 1B**) (15, 16). Another interesting approach to evoke cardioprotection through nanotechnology is the co-delivery of antineoplastic drugs and cardioprotective agents (17). For example, the co-encapsulation of DOX with curcumin, quercetin, or docosahexaenoic acid within the same nanocarrier has been proposed in several nanoscale systems (18–20).

In 1995, Doxil® (pegylated liposomal DOX) was the first nanocarrier approved for clinical use (21, 22). This formulation was designed to reduce DOX toxicity while preserving its antitumor efficacy by altering its tissue distribution and pharmacokinetics (23). Several randomized controlled trials have demonstrated a reduction in the risk of clinical cardiotoxicity for liposomal DOX-based chemotherapy compared to free DOX (24, 25). At present, various commercial formulations of nanocarriers have been approved or are under clinical trial for cancer therapy. These nanocarriers deliver classic chemotherapeutics, such as isolated paclitaxel, irinotecan, the synergistic combination of daunorubicin and cytarabine, and recent innovative treatments for T-cell cancer immunotherapy (26, 27).

CONSIDERATIONS ABOUT PRECLINICAL STUDIES OF NANOCARRIERS

The evaluation of the cardiotoxicity of nanostructures can be performed both *in vitro* and *in vivo*. Human pluripotent stem cell-derived cardiomyocytes (hiPSC-CM) emerge as a practical approach for the early *in vitro* screening of cardiotoxicity of new drugs (28–30). However, investigations on animal models are still required to develop their use in clinical practice despite some limitations. Nonetheless, some characteristics of these models, such as age, gender, drug doses, and tumor models, are often not correctly considered (**Figure 2A**). We will discuss these aspects in the following sections.

Age and Gender

Most cancer patients are more than 60 years old, with aging being a critical predisposition factor for cancer and CVD (5). Despite these predictions, many preclinical cancer studies use mice whose age correlates with that of adolescents (**Figure 2A**), a period of life when cancer and cardiovascular events are fortunately rare. The physiological differences between young and old animals are significant, and one example is related to the EPR effect. Tumor-bearing young animals may exhibit a more pronounced EPR effect than older animals since older subjects present a lower tumor angiogenesis rate (31). This issue makes less probable the formation of blood vessels with fenestrations allowing the higher permeation of nanocarriers by tumor tissues in young animals compared to older subjects (32). Cardiovascular adverse effects of therapeutics can also be underestimated in young animals since the hearts of these animals have a higher regenerative potential

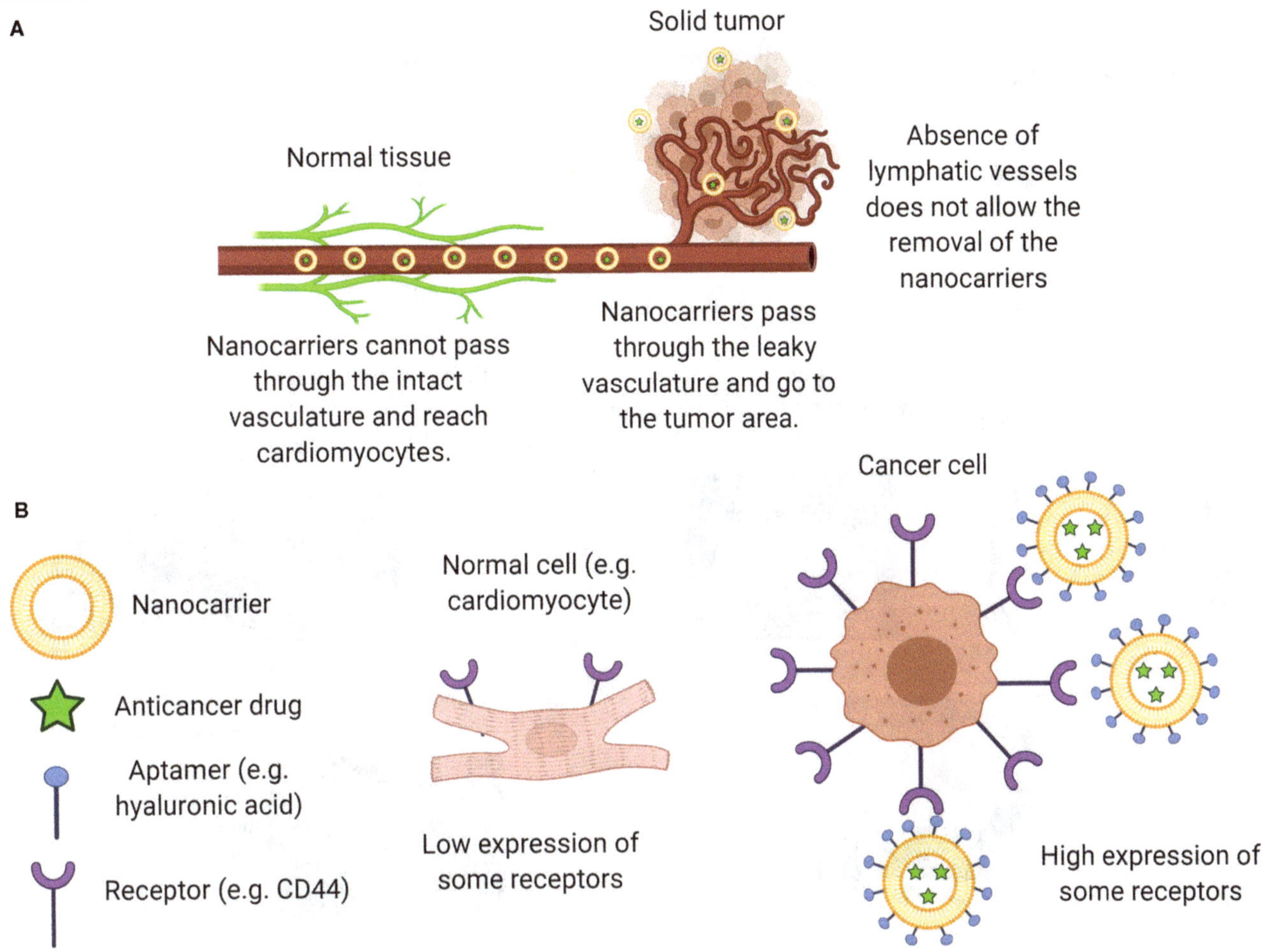

FIGURE 1 | (A) Representation of the EPR effect with the nanocarriers accumulating within the solid tumor and not within the cardiomyocytes; **(B)** Nanocarriers with active targeting, favoring the specificity for cancer cells instead of cardiomyocytes. EPR effect, enhanced permeability and retention effect.

than the hearts of old animals (33, 34). Therefore, the widespread use of very young animals is a serious flaw that impairs the translation of the results from preclinical to clinical studies.

Regarding gender, men are the most affected by almost all types of cancer, with a few exceptions, such as anorectal, gallbladder, thyroid, and breast cancer. However, we expect the number of women affected by neoplasms to increase. Therefore, it is essential to evaluate some risk factors affecting women when they are gender-specific or affect women more intensely, such as menopause, smoking, diabetes, and pregnancy (35). Additionally, drug treatments for CVD may not be the same due to physiological differences between the sexes (36). As an example, anthracyclines-induced cardiotoxicity can be less pronounced in women due to some benefits provided by estrogens (37). Despite all this, most studies use only male animals (**Figure 2A**), which does not reveal whether a particular cancer treatment works in the same way in women or whether its side effects are the same. Overall, preclinical cancer research should include sex as a biological variable in all investigations (35) (**Figure 2B**).

Tumor Models

Regarding the formation of tumors in animal models, there are issues such as their location and size. The orthotopic localization provides the appropriate microenvironment to mimic metastases caused by a specific tumor (38). However, the establishment of orthotopic tumors is an exception, and most studies involve subcutaneous inoculation of tumor cells in the flank of the animals. In addition, the sizes of the tumors implanted subcutaneously are generally substantial to allow their measurements through calipers. Consequently, the relationship between tumor weight/animal weight becomes much higher than that observed in humans, leading to errors when interpreting the results. Human tumors treated with nanomedicine are usually in the order of a few grams, so the tumor/body weight relationship is insignificant. In mice, on the other hand, tumors can reach up to 10% of the animal's weight. Large size is one factor that causes the EPR effect of nanomedicines to be overestimated in animals, as larger tumors can promote higher colloidal buildup (39). Ideally, the tumors should not exceed few millimeters to respect better the relationship between tumor and body weight

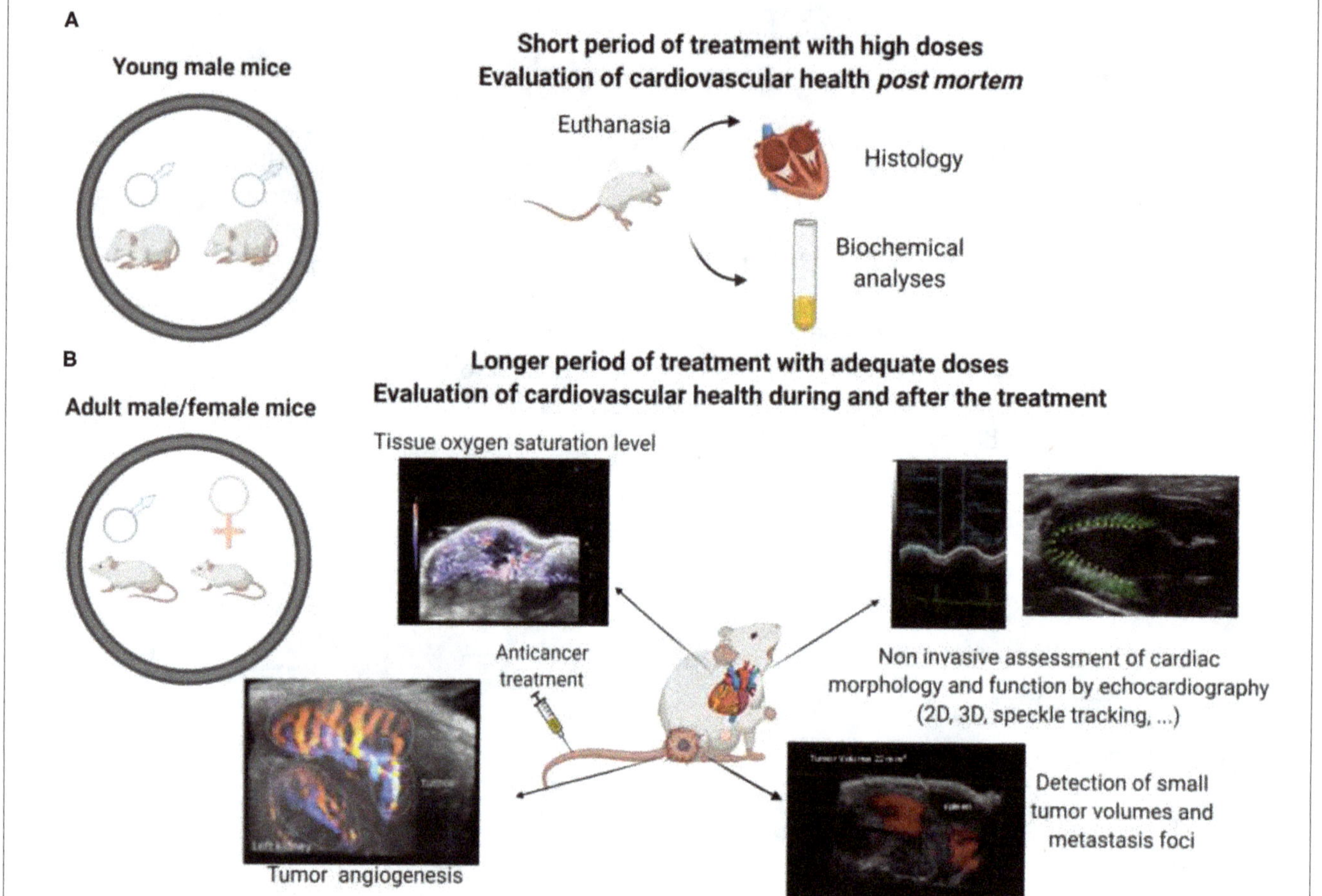

FIGURE 2 | (A) Representation of how anticancer animal studies are generally conducted up to now, with cardiotoxicity evaluation being conducted only after euthanasia of the animals, with high doses administered of the nanocarriers and the use of only male and very young animals; **(B)** Suggestion of how to conduct animal studies with nanocarriers using both female and male older mice; evaluation of cardiotoxicity during and after the treatment administered with lower doses of the nanocarriers. The ultrasound-based techniques allow the simultaneous evaluation of antitumor activity and cardiotoxicity.

observed in humans. Additionally, small tumors allow more prolonged treatment and animal monitoring periods, as animals must be euthanized when the tumors reach high volumes.

Administered Doses of Nanomedicines

It is essential to administer, to the animals, doses related to the plasma blood concentrations found in the clinics (40). However, the choice of dosage in efficacy and toxicity preclinical studies is often neglected, compromising the success of these therapies in humans. First, very high doses are often utilized in animal studies to reduce large volume tumors. Therefore, the use of lower doses relies on the inoculation of smaller volume tumors in the animals. In addition, the maximum tolerated doses in mice are generally higher than in humans (40). Thus, the doses used in animal models can sometimes not be applied to human studies, making the clinical translation of these formulations limited. In the specific case of nanocarriers, their reduced systemic toxicity allows the administration of even higher doses to the animals (41). Nonetheless, one should stress that reduced acute toxicity does not always mean reduced chronic toxicity (42, 43).

Evaluation of Chronic Cardiotoxic Events

An important concept to apply in preclinical studies with nanocarriers is the follow-up of animals after anticancer treatment. Many significant cardiac side effects often occur later, even years after antineoplastic therapy (44). However, animals are often euthanized rapidly after the treatment is completed (39). Additionally, most preclinical studies using nanotechnology for the treatment of cancer only perform post-mortem cardiovascular assessments. These analyses are based mainly on the biochemical quantification of certain enzymes and the histology of the heart. Although the information obtained by these methods is valid, this does not reflect an oncocardiology approach, as they do not monitor cardiovascular health during cancer treatment, as practiced in human patients. Moreover, studies that focus on cardiovascular toxicity are usually done in healthy animals rather than in animals with tumors, with some drawbacks because the toxic effects may differ in non-tumor subjects and tumor carriers (45).

The following of laboratory animals through more extensive periods, although desirable, can be costly and laborious for the researchers. One exciting option is the use of domestic animals such as dogs and cats. These species spontaneously develop tumors, and the owners maintain their pets through the years after the diagnosis. These animals can participate in experimental therapies, close to clinical trials, evaluating tumor regression and cardiovascular health in partnership with veterinaries (46, 47).

Simultaneous Evaluation of Antitumor and Cardiotoxic Effects

Anticancer activity and cardiotoxicity should, when possible, be considered simultaneously (**Figure 2B**). A holistic approach could help in the exploitation of divergent results. For example, the combination of DOX, trastuzumab, and taxanes is very effective in treating breast cancer, but it produces severe synergistic cardiotoxic events in female patients (48, 49). Additionally, premature aging induced by cancer treatment may contribute to chronic health problems in cancer survivors (7). Moreover, the nanocarriers can evoke cardiotoxicity *per se*. One example is the immune reactions to polyethylene glycol molecules attached to the surface of nanocarriers, known as complement activation-related pseudoallergy, which can even lead to a patient's death due to arrhythmias, ventricular fibrillation, and cardiac arrest (50). Moreover, oncolytic viruses, an increasingly used drug delivery vehicle, can replicate themselves in non-targeted tissues, evoking inflammation of the heart, leading to myocarditis (51).

Few preclinical studies have monitored both antitumor activity and cardiac function, in the same animal model, during and after the treatment with nanocarriers. To the best of our knowledge, the three studies presented below are the only ones to have evaluated both simultaneously, all of them using DOX-loaded nanocarriers. DOX loaded in folate-coated liposomes, injected intravenously in breast tumor-bearing mice, showed higher antitumor activity than free DOX and reduced cardiotoxicity (52). Similar findings were found after administering a liposomal formulation loading DOX to colon tumor-bearing mice (53). In addition, polymeric magnetic nanoparticles co-encapsulating DOX and verapamil (a calcium channel blocker) with active targeting of RGD (arginyl glycyl aspartic acid) peptide improved antitumor activity and decreased cardiotoxicity compared to free DOX (54). All these studies evaluated cardiotoxicity during treatment by analysis of the ECG and the QT interval. Imaging techniques have not been used, although they can provide essential data. To monitor smaller and orthotopic tumors and cardiotoxicity more precisely, during and after treatment, the use of non-invasive imaging techniques should be encouraged (**Figure 2B**).

Ultrasound Techniques to Assess the Antitumor Activity and Cardiotoxicity of Nanomedicines

Different imaging techniques such as magnetic resonance imaging (MRI), positron emission tomography (PET), SPECT (single photon emission tomography), and computed tomography (X - computer tomography) can simultaneously assess antitumor activity and cardiotoxicity evoked by anticancer treatments (55–57). These imaging techniques allow the early detection and monitoring of a wide range of cardiotoxic events, including systolic and diastolic dysfunction, morphological changes, coronary artery, valve, and pericardial diseases resulting from cancer treatment (56). However, the significant problems with these techniques are their high cost, long scanning time (30–60 min/animal), and radiation exposure (PET, SPECT, and CT) (58).

Real-time image acquisition, ease of data interpretation, and low cost make ultrasound imaging a promising and suitable approach, compared to other techniques, to monitor cardiotoxic events in preclinical studies (59–63). Ultrasound allows rapid longitudinal monitoring (<10 min/animal for each control) of tumor and cardiac function before, during, and after anticancer treatment. This opportunity is of particular interest for monitoring tumor growth, as it is possible to monitor the animals for more extended periods (64, 65) and to assess the volume of implanted orthotopic tumors (66). This approach also makes it possible, on a practical level, to homogenize the different study groups as a function of a reference tumor volume. This possibility reduces the number of animals used while minimizing the variability in the distribution within each experimental group.

Finally, photoacoustic imaging (PAI) is another promising ultrasound-based technique. It is a relatively new hybrid modality that combines optical imaging contrast with the spatial resolution of ultrasound (67, 68). PAI provides high-resolution images of optical absorption in deep tissues, allowing visualization of angiogenesis, tissue oxygen saturation, and metabolic or inflammatory parameters (69–71). In addition, PAI has shown promise in detecting, diagnosing, and guiding cancer treatment due to its ability to detect or activate specific nanostructures to enhance contrast (72, 73).

CONCLUDING REMARKS

Clinics have widely demonstrated the concept that nanomedicines improve the therapeutic index of anticancer drugs (15, 74). The advances in nanoscale delivery systems offer great hope to increase the efficacy of drugs in a targeted manner and overcome the toxicity limitations associated with conventional free drug delivery. Translating the results from preclinical studies to more clinically relevant models is an urgent demand and a significant challenge to alleviate the burden of the undesirable cardiotoxic effects of anticancer drugs (41, 75). Considering the advantages and limitations of animal models and the peculiarities of nanoformulations, appropriate techniques for monitoring antitumor efficacy and cardiovascular health will be essential to practice the best oncocardiology approach.

AUTHOR CONTRIBUTIONS

All authors contributed to the writing and editing of the manuscript.

FUNDING

GB and EL thank CAPES (Coordenação de Aperfeiçoamento de Pessoal de Nível Superior, Brazil) and FAPEMIG (Fundação de Amparo à Pesquisa do Estado de Minas Gerais, Brazil) for the scolarhips provided. SR, PS, and LF acknowledge CAPES-COFECUB for supporting a bilateral research collaboration program (no. 978/20) between Brazil (UFMG; Prof. Mônica Cristina De Oliveira) and France (Université de Montpellier; SR).

ACKNOWLEDGMENTS

The figures of this manuscript were made with the aid of Biorender.com.

REFERENCES

Cautela J, Lalevée N, Ammar C, Ederhy S, Peyrol M, Debourdeau P, et al. Management and research in cancer treatment-related cardiovascular toxicity: challenges and perspectives. *Int J Cardiol.* (2016) 224:366–75. doi: 10.1016/j.ijcard.2016.09.046

Curigliano G, Cardinale D, Dent S, Criscitiello C, Aseyev O, Lenihan D, et al. Cardiotoxicity of anticancer treatments: epidemiology, detection, and management. *CA Cancer J Clin.* (2016) 66:309–25. doi: 10.3322/caac.21341

Masoudkabir F, Sarrafzadegan N, Gotay C, Ignaszewski A, Krahn AD, Davis MK, et al. Cardiovascular disease and cancer: evidence for shared disease pathways and pharmacologic prevention. *Atherosclerosis.* (2017) 263:343–51. doi: 10.1016/j.atherosclerosis.2017.06.001

Moslehi J, Fujiwara K, Guzik T. Cardio-oncology: a novel platform for basic and translational cardiovascular investigation driven by clinical need. *Cardiovasc Res.* (2019) 115:819–23. doi: 10.1093/cvr/cvz048

Okura Y, Takayama T, Ozaki K, Tanaka H, Kikuchi A, Saito T, et al. Future projection of cancer patients with cardiovascular disease in Japan by the year 2039: a pilot study. *Int J Clin Oncol.* (2019) 24:983–94. doi: 10.1007/s10147-019-01426-w

Lenneman Carrie G., Sawyer Douglas B. Cardio-oncology. *Circ Res.* (2016) 118:1008–20. doi: 10.1161/CIRCRESAHA.115.303633

Abe J-I, Martin JF, Yeh ETH. The future of onco-cardiology: we are not just "Side Effect Hunters." *Circ Res.* (2016) 119:896–9. doi: 10.1161/CIRCRESAHA.116.309573

Witteles RM, Bosch X. Myocardial protection during cardiotoxic chemotherapy. *Circulation.* (2015) 132:1835–45. doi: 10.1161/CIRCULATIONAHA.114.010486

Yeh ETH, Chang H-M. Oncocardiology-past, present, and future: a review. *JAMA Cardiol.* (2016) 1:1066–72. doi: 10.1001/jamacardio.2016.2132

Manolis AA, Manolis TA, Mikhailidis DP, Manolis AS. Cardiovascular safety of oncologic agents: a double-edged sword even in the era of targeted therapies - Part 2. *Expert Opin Drug Saf.* (2018) 17:893–915. doi: 10.1080/14740338.2018.1513489

Bansal N, Amdani S, Lipshultz ER, Lipshultz SE. Chemotherapy-induced cardiotoxicity in children. *Expert Opin Drug Metab Toxicol.* (2017) 13:817–32. doi: 10.1080/17425255.2017.1351547

Ganatra S, Parikh R, Neilan TG. Cardiotoxicity of immune therapy. *Cardiol Clin.* (2019) 37:385–97. doi: 10.1016/j.ccl.2019.07.008

Herrmann J. Adverse cardiac effects of cancer therapies: cardiotoxicity and arrhythmia. *Nat Rev Cardiol.* (2020) 17:474–502. doi: 10.1038/s41569-020-0348-1

Monahan DS, Almas T, Wyile R, Cheema FH, Duffy GP, Hameed Towards the use of localised delivery strategies to counteract cancer therapy-induced cardiotoxicities. *Drug Deliv Transl Res.* (2021) doi: 10.1007/s13346-020-00885-3. [Epub ahead of print].

Wicki A, Witzigmann D, Balasubramanian V, Huwyler J. Nanomedicine in cancer therapy: challenges, opportunities, and clinical applications. *J Control Release.* (2015) 200:138–57. doi: 10.1016/j.jconrel.2014.12.030

Tran S, DeGiovanni P-J, Piel B, Rai P. Cancer nanomedicine: a review of recent success in drug delivery. *Clin Transl Med.* (2017) 6:44. doi: 10.1186/s40169-017-0175-0

Yan T, Li D, Li J, Cheng F, Cheng J, Huang Y, et al. Effective co- delivery of doxorubicin and curcumin using a glycyrrhetinic acid-modified chitosan-cystamine-poly(ε-caprolactone) copolymer micelle for combination cancer chemotherapy. *Colloids Surf B Biointerfaces.* (2016) 145:526–38. doi: 10.1016/j.colsurfb.2016.05.070

Tahover E, Patil YP, Gabizon AA. Emerging delivery systems to reduce doxorubicin cardiotoxicity and improve therapeutic index: focus on liposomes. *Anticancer Drugs.* (2015) 26:241–58. doi: 10.1097/CAD.0000000000000182

Dou X-Q, Wang H, Zhang J, Wang F, Xu G-L, Xu C-C, et al. Aptamer-drug conjugate: targeted delivery of doxorubicin in a HER3 aptamer-functionalized liposomal delivery system reduces cardiotoxicity. *Int J Nanomedicine.* (2018) 13:763–76. doi: 10.2147/IJN.S149887

Lages EB, Fernandes RS, Silva J de O, de Souza ÂM, Cassali GD, de Barros ALB, et al. Co-delivery of doxorubicin, docosahexaenoic acid, and α-tocopherol succinate by nanostructured lipid carriers has a synergistic effect to enhance antitumor activity and reduce toxicity. *Biomed Pharmacother.* (2020) 132:110876. doi: 10.1016/j.biopha.2020.110876

Okada H, Toguchi H. Biodegradable microspheres in drug delivery. *Crit Rev Ther Drug Carrier Syst.* (1995) 12:1–99. doi: 10.1615/critrevtherdrugcarriersyst.v12.i1.10

Park J, Fong PM, Lu J, Russell KS, Booth CJ, Saltzman WM, et al. PEGylated PLGA nanoparticles for the improved delivery of doxorubicin. *Nanomedicine.* (2009) 5:410–8. doi: 10.1016/j.nano.2009.02.002

Barenholz Y. DoxilQR -the first FDA-approved nano-drug: lessons learned. *J Control Release.* (2012) 160:117–34. doi: 10.1016/j.jconrel.2012. 03.020

Rafiyath SM, Rasul M, Lee B, Wei G, Lamba G, Liu D. Comparison of safety and toxicity of liposomal doxorubicin vs. conventional anthracyclines: a meta-analysis. *Exp Hematol Oncol.* (2012) 1:10. doi: 10.1186/2162-3619-1-10

Xing M, Yan F, Yu S, Shen P. Efficacy and cardiotoxicity of liposomal doxorubicin-based chemotherapy in advanced breast cancer: a meta-analysis of ten randomized controlled trials. *PLoS ONE.* (2015) 10:e0133569. doi: 10.1371/journal.pone.0133569

Anselmo AC, Mitragotri S. Nanoparticles in the clinic: an update. *Bioeng Transl Med.* (2019) 4:e10143. doi: 10.1002/btm2.10143

Gong N, Sheppard NC, Billingsley MM, June CH, Mitchell MJ. Nanomaterials for T-cell cancer immunotherapy. *Nat Nanotechnol.* (2021) 16:25–36. doi: 10.1038/s41565-020-00822-y

Golforoush PA, Narasimhan P, Chaves-Guerrero PP, Lawrence E, Newton G, Yan R, et al. Selective protection of human cardiomyocytes from anthracycline cardiotoxicity by small molecule inhibitors of MAP4K4. *Sci Rep.* (2020) 10:12060. doi: 10.1038/s41598-020-68907-1

Lyra-Leite DM, Burridge PW. Pluripotent stem cell modeling of anticancer therapy-induced cardiotoxicity. *Curr Cardiol Rep.* (2020) 22:56. doi: 10.1007/s11886-020-01325-x

Schwach V, Slaats RH, Passier R. Human pluripotent stem cell-derived cardiomyocytes for assessment of anticancer drug-induced cardiotoxicity. *Front Cardiovasc Med.* (2020) 7:50. doi: 10.3389/fcvm.2020.00050

Bojovic B, Crowe DL. Chronologic aging decreases tumor angiogenesis and metastasis in a mouse model of head and neck cancer. *Int J Oncol.* (2010) 36:715–23. doi: 10.3892/ijo_00000547

Andriyanov AV, Portnoy E, Koren E, Inesa S, Eyal S, Goldberg SN, et al. Therapeutic efficacy of combined PEGylated liposomal doxorubicin and radiofrequency ablation: comparing single and combined therapy in young and old mice. *J Control Release.* (2017) 257:2–9. doi: 10.1016/j.jconrel.2017.02.018

Dai D-F, Rabinovitch PS. Cardiac aging in mice and humans: the role of mitochondrial oxidative stress. *Trends Cardiovasc Med.* (2009) 19:213–20. doi: 10.1016/j.tcm.2009.12.004

Chiao YA, Rabinovitch PS. The aging heart. *Cold Spring Harb Perspect Med.* (2015) 5:a025148. doi: 10.1101/cshperspect.a025148

Rubin JB, Lagas JS, Broestl L, Sponagel J, Rockwell N, Rhee G, et al. Sex differences in cancer mechanisms. *Biol Sex Differ.* (2020) 11:17. doi: 10.1186/s13293-020-00291-x

Maas AHEM, Appelman YEA. Gender differences in coronary heart disease. *Neth Heart J.* (2010) 18:598–602. doi: 10.1007/s12471-010-0841-y

Cadeddu Dessalvi C, Pepe A, Penna C, Gimelli A, Madonna R, Mele D, et al. Sex differences in anthracycline-induced cardiotoxicity: the benefits of estrogens. *Heart Fail Rev.* (2019) 24:915–25. doi: 10.1007/s10741-019-09 820-2

Lwin TM, Hoffman RM, Bouvet M. Advantages of patient-derived orthotopic mouse models and genetic reporters for developing fluorescence- guided surgery. *J Surg Oncol.* (2018) 118:253–64. doi: 10.1002/jso. 25150

Nichols JW, Bae YH. EPR: evidence and fallacy. *J Control Release.* (2014) 190:451–64. doi: 10.1016/j.jconrel.2014.03.057

Day C-P, Merlino G, Van Dyke T. Preclinical mouse cancer models: a maze of opportunities and challenges. *Cell.* (2015) 163:39–53. doi: 10.1016/j.cell.2015.08.068

Hare JI, Lammers T, Ashford MB, Puri S, Storm G, Barry ST. Challenges and strategies in anticancer nanomedicine development: an industry perspective. *Adv Drug Deliv Rev.* (2017) 108:25–38. doi: 10.1016/j.addr.2016.04.025

Yemm KE, Alwan LM, Malik AB, Salazar LG. Renal toxicity with liposomal doxorubicin in metastatic breast cancer. *J Oncol Pharm Pract.* (2019) 25:1738–42. doi: 10.1177/1078155218798157

Savani M, Woerner K, Bu L, Birkenbach M, Skubitz KM. Pegylated liposomal doxorubicin-induced renal toxicity in retroperitoneal liposarcoma: a case report and literature review. *Cancer Chemother Pharmacol.* (2021) 87:289–94. doi: 10.1007/s00280-020-04203-z

Dong J, Chen H. Cardiotoxicity of anticancer therapeutics. *Front Cardiovasc Med.* (2018) 5:9. doi: 10.3389/fcvm.2018.00009

Wang F, Iskra B, Kleinerman E, Alvarez-Florez C, Andrews T, Shaw A, et al. Aerobic exercise during early murine doxorubicin exposure mitigates cardiac toxicity. *J Pediatr Hematol Oncol.* (2018) 40:208–15. doi: 10.1097/MPH.0000000000001112

Khanna C, Lindblad-Toh K, Vail D, London C, Bergman P, Barber L, et al. The dog as a cancer model. *Nat Biotechnol.* (2006) 24:1065–6. doi: 10.1038/nbt0906-1065b

Rossa C, D'Silva NJ. Non-murine models to investigate tumor-immune interactions in head and neck cancer. *Oncogene.* (2019) 38:4902–14. doi: 10.1038/s41388-019-0776-8

Gianni L, Salvatorelli E, Minotti G. Anthracycline cardiotoxicity in breast cancer patients: synergism with trastuzumab and taxanes. *Cardiovasc Toxicol.* (2007) 7:67–71. doi: 10.1007/s12012-007-0013-5

El-Sherbeny WS, Sabry NM, Sharbay RM. Prediction of trastuzumab- induced cardiotoxicity in breast cancer patients receiving anthracycline-based chemotherapy. *J Echocardiogr.* (2019) 17:76–83. doi: 10.1007/s12574-018-0394-4

Szebeni J. Complement activation-related pseudoallergy: a stress reaction in blood triggered by nanomedicines and biologicals. *Mol Immunol.* (2014) 61:163–73. doi: 10.1016/j.molimm.2014.06.038

Hazini A, Pryshliak M, Brückner V, Klingel K, Sauter M, Pinkert S, et al. Heparan sulfate binding coxsackievirus B3 strain PD: a novel avirulent oncolytic agent against human colorectal carcinoma. *Hum Gene Ther.* (2018) 29:1301–14. doi: 10.1089/hum.2018.036

de Oliveira Silva J, Fernandes RS, Ramos Oda CM, Ferreira TH, Machado Botelho AF, Martins Melo M, et al. Folate-coated, long-circulating and pH-sensitive liposomes enhance doxorubicin antitumor effect in a breast cancer animal model. *Biomed Pharmacother.* (2019) 118:109323. doi: 10.1016/j.biopha.2019.109323

Razavi-Azarkhiavi K, Jafarian AH, Abnous K, Razavi BM, Shirani K, Zeinali M, et al. The comparison of biodistribution, efficacy and toxicity of two PEGylated liposomal doxorubicin formulations in mice bearing c-26 colon carcinoma: a preclinical study. *Drug Res.* (2016) 66:330–6. doi: 10.1055/s-0035-1569447

Shen J-M, Gao F-Y, Yin T, Zhang H-X, Ma M, Yang Y-J, et al. cRGD- functionalized polymeric magnetic nanoparticles as a dual-drug delivery system for safe targeted cancer therapy. *Pharmacol Res.* (2013) 70:102–15. doi: 10.1016/j.phrs.2013.01.009

Thuny F, Huttin O, Ederhy S. Cardio-oncology: Clinical and imaging perspectives for optimal cardiodetection and cardioprotection in patients with cancer. *Arch Cardiovasc Dis.* (2019) 112:550–8. doi: 10.1016/j.acvd.2019.07.001

Biersmith MA, Tong MS, Guha A, Simonetti OP, Addison D. Multimodality cardiac imaging in the era of emerging cancer therapies. *J Am Heart Assoc.* (2020) 9:e013755. doi: 10.1161/JAHA.119.013755

López-Fernández T. Cardiac imaging in oncology patients in Europe: a model for advancement of CV safety and development of comprehensive CV care. *J Cardiovasc Transl Res.* (2020) 13:490–4. doi: 10.1007/s12265-020-10028-1

Moran CM, Thomson AJW, Rog-Zielinska E, Gray GA. High- resolution echocardiography in the assessment of cardiac physiology and disease in preclinical models. *Exp Physiol.* (2013) 98:629–44. doi: 10.1113/expphysiol.2012.068577

Branquinho RT, Roy J, Farah C, Garcia GM, Aimond F, Le Guennec J-Y, et al. Biodegradable polymeric nanocapsules prevent cardiotoxicity of anti-trypanosomal lychnopholide. *Sci Rep.* (2017) 7:44998. doi: 10.1038/srep44998

Sicard P, Jouitteau T, Andrade-Martins T, Massad A, Rodrigues de Araujo G, David H, et al. Right coronary artery ligation in mice: a novel method to investigate right ventricular dysfunction and biventricular interaction. *Am J Physiol Heart Circ Physiol.* (2019) 316:H684–92. doi: 10.1152/ajpheart.00573.2018

Moreira Souza AC, Grabe-Guimarães A, Cruz JDS, Santos-Miranda A, Farah C, Teixeira Oliveira L, et al. Mechanisms of artemether toxicity on single cardiomyocytes and protective effect of nanoencapsulation. *Br J Pharmacol.* (2020) 177:4448–63. doi: 10.1111/bph.15186

Ader I, Gstalder C, Bouquerel P, Golzio M, Andrieu G, Zalvidea S, et al. Neutralizing S1P inhibits intratumoral hypoxia, induces vascular remodelling and sensitizes to chemotherapy in prostate cancer. *Oncotarget.* (2015) 6:13803–21. doi: 10.18632/oncotarget.3144

Ogier C, Colombo P-E, Bousquet C, Canterel-Thouennon L, Sicard P, Garambois V, et al. Targeting the NRG1/HER3 pathway in tumor cells and cancer-associated fibroblasts with an anti-neuregulin 1 antibody inhibits tumor growth in pre-clinical models of pancreatic cancer. *Cancer Lett.* (2018) 432:227–36. doi: 10.1016/j.canlet.2018.06.023

Graham KC, Wirtzfeld LA, MacKenzie LT, Postenka CO, Groom AC, MacDonald IC, et al. Three-dimensional high-frequency ultrasound imaging for longitudinal evaluation of liver metastases in preclinical models. *Cancer Res.* (2005) 65:5231–7. doi: 10.1158/0008-5472.CAN-05-0440

McVeigh LE, Wijetunga I, Ingram N, Marston G, Prasad R, Markham AF, et al. Development of orthotopic tumour models using ultrasound-guided intrahepatic injection. *Sci Rep.* (2019) 9:9904. doi: 10.1038/s41598-019-46410-6

Pigula M, Huang H-C, Mallidi S, Anbil S, Liu J, Mai Z, et al. Size- dependent tumor response to photodynamic therapy and irinotecan monotherapies revealed by longitudinal ultrasound monitoring in an orthotopic pancreatic cancer model. *Photochem Photobiol.* (2019) 95:378–86. doi: 10.1111/php.13016

Raes F, Sobilo J, Le Mée M, Rétif S, Natkunarajah S, Lerondel S, et al. High resolution ultrasound and photoacoustic imaging of orthotopic lung cancer in mice: new perspectives for onco-pharmacology. *PLoS ONE.* (2016) 11:e0153532. doi: 10.1371/journal.pone.0153532

Wang S, Zhao Y, Xu Y. Recent advances in applications of multimodal ultrasound-guided photoacoustic imaging technology. *Vis Comput Ind Biomed Art.* (2020) 3:24. doi: 10.1186/s42492-020-00061-x

Mukaddim RA, Rodgers A, Hacker TA, Heinmiller A, Varghese T. Real-time *in vivo* photoacoustic imaging in the assessment of myocardial dynamics in murine model of myocardial ischemia. *Ultrasound Med Biol.* (2018) 44:2155– 64. doi: 10.1016/j.ultrasmedbio.2018.05.021

Karlas A, Fasoula N-A, Paul-Yuan K, Reber J, Kallmayer M, Bozhko D, et al. Cardiovascular optoacoustics: from mice to men - a review. *Photoacoustics.* (2019) 14:19–30. doi: 10.1016/j.pacs.2019.03.001

David H, Ughetto A, Gaudard P, Plawecki M, Paiyabhroma N, Zub E, et al. Experimental myocardial infarction elicits time-dependent patterns of vascular hypoxia in peripheral organs and in the brain. *Front Cardiovasc Med.* (2021) 7:615507. doi: 10.3389/fcvm.2020.615507

Weber J, Beard PC, Bohndiek SE. Contrast agents for molecular photoacoustic imaging. *Nat Methods.* (2016) 13:639–50. doi: 10.1038/nmeth.3929

Nishio N, van den Berg NS, Martin BA, van Keulen S, Fakurnejad S, Rosenthal EL, et al. Photoacoustic molecular imaging for the identification of lymph node metastasis in head and neck cancer using an anti-EGFR antibody- dye conjugate. *J Nucl Med.* (2020) 62:648–55. doi: 10.2967/jnumed.120.2 45241

Bobo D, Robinson KJ, Islam J, Thurecht KJ, Corrie SR. Nanoparticle-based medicines: a review of FDA-approved materials and clinical trials to date. *Pharm Res.* (2016) 33:2373–87. doi: 10.1007/s11095-016-1958-5

Shi J, Kantoff PW, Wooster R, Farokhzad OC. Cancer nanomedicine: progress, challenges and opportunities. *Nat Rev Cancer.* (2017) 17:20–37. doi: 10.1038/nrc.2016.108

16

Nanoparticles for Stem Cell Tracking and the Potential Treatment of Cardiovascular Diseases

Huihua Huang[1,2], Xuejun Du[1], Zhiguo He[3], Zifeng Yan[3] and Wei Han[1]*

[1] Emergency Department, Shenzhen University General Hospital, Shenzhen University, Shenzhen, China, [2] Guangdong Key Laboratory for Biomedical Measurements and Ultrasound Imaging, School of Biomedical Engineering, Shenzhen University, Health Science Center, Shenzhen, China, [3] Advanced Materials Institute, Graduate School at Shenzhen, Tsinghua University, Shenzhen, China

***Correspondence:**
Wei Han
sugh_hanwei@szu.edu.cn

Stem cell-based therapies have been shown potential in regenerative medicine. In these cells, mesenchymal stem cells (MSCs) have the ability of self-renewal and being differentiated into different types of cells, such as cardiovascular cells. Moreover, MSCs have low immunogenicity and immunomodulatory properties, and can protect the myocardium, which are ideal qualities for cardiovascular repair. Transplanting mesenchymal stem cells has demonstrated improved outcomes for treating cardiovascular diseases in preclinical trials. However, there still are some challenges, such as their low rate of migration to the ischemic myocardium, low tissue retention, and low survival rate after the transplantation. To solve these problems, an ideal method should be developed to precisely and quantitatively monitor the viability of the transplanted cells *in vivo* for providing the guidance of clinical translation. Cell imaging is an ideal method, but requires a suitable contrast agent to label and track the cells. This article reviews the uses of nanoparticles as contrast agents for tracking MSCs and the challenges of clinical use of MSCs in the potential treatment of cardiovascular diseases.

Keywords: nanoparticles, stem cell therapy, mesenchymal stem cell, cardiovascular diseases, imaging technique

INTRODUCTION

In the medical world, stem cell-based therapies have emerged and expanded as a potentially promising therapeutic treatment (Heslop et al., 2015). In such a treatment process, stem cells, possessing properties of self-renewal and potency, play a significant role, and under appropriate conditions, these cells can be differentiated into a variety of cells (Srivastava and Ivey, 2006; Maumus et al., 2011; Hao et al., 2014; Aly, 2020). Compared with direct transplantation of tissue or organ for patients, stem cell-based therapies are more promising and potential because these cells can be feasibly and readily obtained avoiding donor shortage and immune incompatibility (Diekman and Guilak, 2013; Lilly et al., 2016). In general, stem cells can be divided into two major types, embryonic stem cells (ESCs) and adult stem cells (ASCs) (Lv et al., 2014). The transplantation of ESCs derived from the early embryo has been demonstrated to be effective in the treatment of many diseases, due to their being highly undifferentiated cells and having the ability of evolving into all tissues and organs (Krebsbach and Robey, 2002; Hao et al., 2009). However, the research for ESCs is controversial, being difficult to accepted by common people (Li et al., 2010). Compared with ESCs, ASCs, which originated from tissues, are easily accepted and have been widely applied in preclinical and clinical trials, but leads to low capacity of differentiation (Young and Black, 2004; Ye et al., 2006; Alison and Islam, 2009). For example, the hematopoietic stem cells (bone marrow), originated from ASCs in the blood, can differentiate into various types of mature blood cells, and their transplantation has been used to treat all kinds of blood diseases (Carella et al., 2000; Schmitz et al., 2002; Mikkola and Orkin, 2006; DiPersio et al., 2009; Jaiswal et al., 2009). Neural stem cells, possessing the ability of differentiating into neurons and astroglia, are also derived from ASCs, and their transplantation may treat diseases of the nervous systems (Temple, 2001; Lee et al., 2005, 2009; Andres et al., 2008; Stenudd et al., 2015). In 1970, Friedenstein discovered a rare type of stromal cells in human bone marrow that are now known as mesenchymal stem cells (MSCs) (Friedenstein et al., 1970). Although MSCs have similar abilities to ASCs, there is still a lot of debate about their origin. Moreover, some researchers claimed that the name of MSCs should be changed to medicinal signaling cells in order to accurately reflect the fact that these cells play the role of constructing new tissues (Caplan, 2017). At present, MSCs are found in many tissues beyond the bone marrow, including adipose tissue, lung tissue, synovial membrane, endometrium, and peripheral blood. In different tissues, MSCs exhibit differences in immunophenotype, differentiation potential, and immunomodulatory. The researches show that the transplantation of MSCs is an effectively promising and potentially therapeutic treatment for various diseases including wound healing, ischemic encephalopathy, and ischemic heart disease (Grauss et al., 2007; Wu et al., 2007; Uccelli et al., 2008; Kim et al., 2015a; Xie et al., 2016).

To date, stem cell-based therapies have been intensively employed in the treatment of wounds, blood and cardiovascular diseases, cartilage defect, diabetes, etc. (Goradel et al., 2018; Vagnozzi et al., 2020). However, there are still much to be further explored for stem cell-based therapies, in order to identify therapeutic efficacy and further dosage (Yi et al., 2017). For these purposes, it is necessary to track stem cells *in vitro* and *in vivo* with high temporal and spatial resolution in a real-time manner during a prolonged period, which involves monitoring stem cells' behavior *in vivo*, identifying if they are capable of surviving, integrating with the host tissue, undertaking the desired cellular differentiation, and finally unveiling the responses and behaviors of transplanted cells upon exposure to various diseased environments.

THE MEANS OF TRACKING STEM CELLS AND THE IMPORTANCE OF NANOPARTICLES

For tracking stem cells, non-invasive cell imaging is currently a very hot field of research (Kircher et al., 2011). Compared with traditional histopathological techniques, non-invasive cell imaging can monitor the behaviors of the transplanted cells over time *in vivo* for further treatment offering detailed information, thus, showing more efficient therapeutic effects (Cahill et al., 2004; Walczak and Bulte, 2007; Bulte, 2017; Meir and Popovtzer, 2018; Peng et al., 2018). Only by using non-invasive means can the viability of the transplanted cells be estimated in the clinical setting, showing potential prospects (Shang et al., 2017; Tkaczyk, 2017). Non-invasive cell tracking can be divided into direct and indirect labeling techniques. Compared with direct labeling, which can directly label cells, possessing easy operation but being unable to track daughter cells due to fast signal decay, indirect labeling obtains the ability of labeling cells by implanting an indicator into cells (Li et al., 2008; Kraitchman and Bulte, 2009; Kim et al., 2016a,b). Although indirect labeling is complex and expensive, it is more effective and stable for tracking the differentiation of the transplanted cells (Davis, 1972; Akins and Dubey, 2008; Hong et al., 2010). In general, indirect labeling can be divided into two major classes, gene modification and external label. Gene modification is suitable for long-term tracking because the labeled genes can be steadily expressed in the next generation (Chan et al., 2017; Su et al., 2019). However, the imaging technique of gene modification is single and only being detected by a tracking fluorophore leading to the limitation of tissue penetration (Herschman, 2004; Loewen et al., 2004). In addition, the labeled genes are derived from exosomes, leading to immune incompatibility (Zheng et al., 2017). Another indirect labeling method, external label, can overcome the obstacle of the foreign gene by introducing additional contrast agents, but it still has some limitations (Crabbe et al., 2010; Li et al., 2013; Hachani et al., 2017). Because the introduction of contrast agents brings some new problems, including the reduction effect of photo-signal over time, optical interference is induced by tissue autofluorescence, incompatibility, cytotoxicity, and low labeling efficiency (Bellin, 2006; Cosgrove, 2006; Lusic and Grinstaff, 2013). Thus, an appropriate contrast agent should be developed and utilized to break through these limitations.

Nanoparticles (NPs), the diameter of which ranges from 1 to 100 nm, cover a diverse range of chemical composition with an equally diverse number of applications (Khan et al., 2019). Due to their nanoscale dimensions, NPs can easily transport across cell membrane and reach the crucial organelles including the endoplasmic reticulum, mitochondria, and nucleus (McNamara and Tofail, 2017). Moreover, a high surface area-over-volume ratio augments their interaction with cellular components (Bhirde et al., 2011; Edmundson et al., 2013). Furthermore, the morphology and size of NPs determine their physicochemical properties leading to the differences in cellular uptake and interaction with biological tissues, which could not be achieved by bulk materials (Barua and Mitragotri, 2014). As a result, NPs have been regarded as a promising contrast agent. Nowadays, nanotechnology in medical science has been regarded as a great breakthrough in this century (Zhang et al., 2008; Lin, 2015). Importantly, some special NPs have unique magnetic and/or optical properties, which can offer real-time imaging *in vivo* for tracking the transplanted stem cells, showing a strong potential in breaking through the obstacle of external label (Rhyner et al., 2006; Hahn et al., 2011). These NPs for tracking stem cells include organic, inorganic, and composite NPs, and the representative examples have magnetic NPs and photoacoustic NPs (Van Den Bos et al., 2003; Ferreira, 2009; Wang et al., 2012b; Gao et al., 2013; Accomasso et al., 2016; Riera et al., 2019).

The transplanted stem cells labeled by these NPs can be detected by multiple imaging methods, such as magnetic resonance imaging (MRI), nuclear imaging [including single-photon emission computed tomography imaging (SPECT) and positron emission tomography-computed tomography (PET-CT)], and photoacoustic imaging (Sutton et al., 2008; Andreas et al., 2012; Cheng et al., 2016; Guo et al., 2019b; Patrick et al., 2020). However, there are still many problems to be addressed in the actual application process for NPs. First, NPs for tracking stem cells *in vivo* always require good cellular uptake and efficient internalization. Therefore, the surface chemistry of NPs should be importantly considered (Accomasso et al., 2016). In most cases, NPs with positive charge have the improvement of cellular uptake due to electrostatic interaction, leading to an accelerated internalization (Saha et al., 2013; Behzadi et al., 2017). Certainly, NPs with positive charge also may delay their internalization process, due to the influence on the adsorption of some specific proteins (Jambhrunkar et al., 2014). Second, importantly, before use, NPs should be comprehensively characterized for their composition and purity under different conditions, in order to evaluate their toxic effects on cells and ensure safety *in vivo* (Chandran et al., 2017). The reasons are that their toxic effects on cells may highly depend on the unique characteristics of NPs themselves. What is more, compared with bulk material, NPs have higher surface area-to-volume ratio and surface reactivity, which are more susceptible to the environment, so they should be modestly employed (Alkilany and Murphy, 2010; Lankoff et al., 2012). In addition, close attention should be paid to the agglomeration of NPs, which may lead to bad cellular uptake and further induced cytotoxicity (Gliga et al., 2014).

The internalization of NPs is influenced by their charge, size, shape, and the ability of cellular uptake, due to the force of their internalization driven by endocytosis. After internalization by endocytosis, NPs will pass environments of lysosomes and peroxisomes where the acidic material and oxidative substance could entirely degrade them. Possibly, a part of them may undergo exocytosis or escape to other intracellular locations (Chen et al., 2013; Calero et al., 2014).

NANOPARTICLES FOR TRACKING MSCS AND THE POTENTIAL TREATMENT OF CARDIOVASCULAR DISEASES

Cardiovascular diseases (CVDs), with high incident, are one of the major causes of human deaths worldwide and responsible for more than 17.7 million deaths in 2015, according to the World Health Organization (Zampelas and Magriplis, 2020). Therefore, developing an effective means for treating CVDs is of paramount urgency (Behlke et al., 2020). Currently, the means for treating CVDs include, but are not limited to, surgical treatment, delivering the targeted drug, and the repair and regeneration of the cardiac tissues (Godin et al., 2010; Cui et al., 2016; Deng et al., 2020). However, surgical treatment and targeted drug delivery only can delay and relieve the progression of CVDs but are unable to solve the inherent problems due to the deficiency of the regeneration for dead heart cells. In regenerative medicine, adult stem cell-based therapies have been shown as a promising potential for treating cardiovascular diseases in preclinical trials because the repair and regeneration of the cardiac tissues can be expected to solve the differentiation of stem cells into heart cells, thereby, offering improved efficacy (Kastrup, 2011). In these cells, MSCs play an important role in the therapy of CVDs, due to their ability of self-renewal and differentiating into various types of cells, including cardiovascular cells (Caplan, 2009; Ye et al., 2014). Moreover, after transplantation of MSCs, they can generate a structure resembling cardiac myocytes and exert anti-inflammatory effects, which can protect the myocardium, further improving the repair of the cardiovascular system. Notably, MSCs have been demonstrated by preclinical studies to have a strong ability to generate blood vessels with minimal adverse effects on the tissues near the injected region. Therefore, the transplantation of MSCs is potentially promising to improve the treatment of CVDs (Trivedi et al., 2010; Goradel et al., 2018; Guo et al., 2020). Despite its great potential for CVD treatment, MSC-based therapies still face some challenges, for example, the real-time tracking for MSC fate after their transplantation, which can provide information such as cell differentiation, the role that MSCs play in vascular repair, and mechanisms of cardiovascular regeneration to guide therapy process and improve therapeutic effect.

Cell imaging is an ideal method for real-time tracking of MSCs, but requires a suitable contrast agent to label MSCs. NPs are a group of contrast agent, which have been widely applied in MSC tracking (Zhang and Wu, 2007; Fu et al., 2011; Liang et al., 2013; Santoso and Yang, 2016; Yi et al., 2017; Guo et al., 2019a). Especially, MSCs labeled by magnetic and/or optical NPs can directly be imaged to offer a real-time tracking *in vivo* (Jing et al., 2008; Betzer et al., 2014; Wu et al., 2014; Perez et al., 2017). These NPs include superparamagnetic iron oxide (SPIO) NPs, gadolinium (Gd)-based NPs, gold (Au)-based NPs, quantum dots (QDs)-based NPs, upconversion (UC)-based NPs, silicon-based NPs, and several other classes of NPs. Here, we will summarize and discuss in detail NPs for labeling and tracking MSCs *in vivo*, shown in **Table 1**.

Superparamagnetic Iron Oxide Nanoparticles

Generally, SPIO NPs are a kind of NPs with a core–shell structure, in which the core is composed of an iron oxide and then is covered by a coating layer as the shell. The coatings layer alters the surface properties of SPIO NPs, and the iron oxide core provides its magnetic properties (Singh et al., 2010; Mahmoudi et al., 2011). Due to unique magnetic properties, SPIO NPs have the ability to generate a strong inhomogeneous field leading to the contraction of T2 relaxation time, thereby, generating obvious contrast in T2-weighted MRI, and are generally used as a T2-contrast agent (Andreas et al., 2012; Li et al., 2013; Bull et al., 2014; Santoso and Yang, 2016; Jiang et al., 2019). So far, SPIOs are the only commercial NPs, several formulations of which have already been approved by the Food and Drug Administration and have been regulated for clinical applications (Wang et al., 2013). MSCs labeled by SPIO NPs can be tracked by MRI, providing a

TABLE 1 | Comparison between nanoparticles for tracking mesenchymal stem cells (MSCs).

Example	Types of nanoparticles (NPs)	Preparation	Imaging modality	Types of MSCs	Advantages	Disadvantages	Main results
Lu et al., 2007; Andreas et al., 2012	Superparamagnetic iron oxide (SPIO) NPs	Easy	T2-weighted magnetic resonance imaging (MRI)	Human MSCs	Obvious contrast	Low cell-labeling efficiency for MSCs; necessary to functionalize SPIO NPs	No apparent influences on viability of MSCs
Babic et al., 2008; Kim et al., 2011; Szpak et al., 2013; Lewandowska-Łańcucka et al., 2014; Park et al., 2014; Liao et al., 2016; Rawat et al., 2019; Gu et al., 2018; Lee et al., 2020	SPIO NPs	Complex	T2-weighted MRI	Human MSCs; mouse MSCs	Obvious contrast; enhancement of cellular internalization	Induce precipitation of NPs; perturb the cell membrane	No apparent influences on viability of MSCs
Zhang et al., 2010	SPIO NPs	Easy	Proton (^{1}H) MRI images	Human MSCs	High sensitivity of cell detection	Difficult to accurately quantify cell population	No apparent influences on viability of MSCs
Sehl et al., 2019	SPIO NPs	Complex	Proton (^{1}H) MRI images	Mouse MSCs	High sensitivity of cell detection; quantify the persistence of transplanted MSCs		No apparent influences on viability of MSCs
Sherry et al., 1988; Ratzinger et al., 2010	Gd-based NPs	Easy	T1-weighted	Human MSCs	Distinguish some similar low signal	Low cellular uptake for MSCs	No apparent influences on viability of MSCs
Kim et al., 2015b; Santelli et al., 2018	Gd-based NPs	Easy	T1-weighted MRI	Human MSCs	Distinguish some similar low signal; long-term tracking		No apparent influences on viability of MSCs
Huang et al., 2020	Au-based NPs	Easy	Photoacoustic imaging and CT imaging	Mouse MSCs	Detected in deep tissue at a high resolution; directly labeled; excellent biocompatibility		No apparent influences on viability of MSCs
Chen G. et al., 2015; Li et al., 2016	QD-based NPs	Complex	Fluorescence imaging	Human MSCs	Longer lifetime than traditional fluorescence dye; photochemical stability	Unsatisfied cytotoxicity and stochastic blinking; the contradiction of sensitivity and definition	No apparent influences on viability of MSCs
Idris et al., 2009; Ang et al., 2011; Zhao et al., 2013; Chen X. et al., 2015; Ma et al., 2016	UC-based NPs	Complex	UC luminescence imaging	Human MSCs	Detected in deeper tissue; more stable and higher definition	Poor biocompatibility; low uptake for cellular	No apparent influences on viability of MSCs
Huang et al., 2005; Chen and Jokerst, 2020; Yao et al., 2020	Silicon-based NPs	Complex	Fluorescence imaging	Human MSCs	Excellent biocompatibility and chemical inertness; easily modified by bioconjugation; good cellular uptake		No apparent influences on viability of MSCs
Chen et al., 2019	Silicon-based NPs	Complex	Photoacoustic imaging	Human MSCs	Good biocompatible and cells tracking capacity; long time		No apparent influences on viability of MSCs
Gao et al., 2016	Other-based NPs	Complex	Aggregation-induced emission imaging	Mouse bone marrow-derived MSCs	Possessing long-term tracking and strong anti-photobleaching ability		No apparent influences on viability of MSCs
Yin et al., 2018	Other-based NPs	Complex	Photoacoustic imaging	Human MSCs	High signal-to-noise; deeper tissue imaging		No apparent influences on viability of MSCs

non-invasive method to monitor the fate of transplanted MSCs *in vivo* (Li et al., 2013; Bull et al., 2014; Guldris et al., 2017; Xie et al., 2019; Elkhenany et al., 2020).

However, MSCs lack phagocytic capacity, and the surface charge of SPIO NPs are negative, which is a similar charge to that of the cellular membrane. Therefore, the internalization of SPIO NPs is limited, leading to a low efficiency of cell labeling. In order to solve these problems, it is necessary to functionalize SPIO NPs by introducing positive charges or other cell membrane-penetrating moieties on the surface (Lu et al., 2007; Andreas et al., 2012). Moreover, these unique functionalized surfaces also increase the stability of SPIO NPs in hydrophilic conditions, as well as are used as a coating layer for delaying the degradation of the iron oxide core (Barrow et al., 2015). For example, the uses of cationic polymers such as poly-L-lysine (PLL) and chitosan have commonly been utilized to improve the cellular internalization of SPIO NPs and protect them from being easily degraded *in vivo* (Babic et al., 2008; Szpak et al., 2013; Lewandowska-Łańcucka et al., 2014; Park et al., 2014). As an MRI probe for tracking MSCs, PLL-SPIONs were more efficient and safer than naked iron oxide NPs, which was in accordance with the fact that their R_2 value was higher than that of uncoated nanoparticles. However, the highly positive charge of PLL induced the precipitation of NPs and perturbed the cell membrane. Liu et al. (2011) used polyethylenimine with a low molecular weight (2 kDa) to wrap SPIO NPs and obtain PEI–SPIO NPs, which could be readily internalized by MSCs for long-term tracking (19 days). Compared with single SPIO NPs, the modified SPIO NPs hold a controlled clustering structure, leading to much higher T2 relaxivity. Moreover, Lewin et al. (2000) used a short HIV-Tat peptide to functionalize SPIO NPs, which could be effectively engulfed by hematopoietic and neural progenitor cells. The results suggested that the cellular uptake of iron can reach an extremely high level (10–30 pg per cell) showing effective cell labeling and MRI tracking. However, NPs functionalized by cationic polymer or molecules may cause a certain level of toxicity, although it would drastically enhance cellular uptake of NPs. Therefore, some researchers (Kim et al., 2011; Liao et al., 2016) utilized 2-aminoethyl-trimethyl ammonium (TMA) to modified SPIO NPs. It was found that TMA–SPIO NPs could easily and efficiently label MSCs to monitor their fate *in vivo*, and the labeled MSCs showed low cytotoxicity. In another work, Gu et al. (2018) synthesized PA–SPIO NPs using a self-assembled lipopeptide amphiphile (PA) to modify the surfaces of SPIO NPs for labeling mouse MSCs. The modified NPs showed the enhancement of labeling efficiencies and the improvement of their contrast by shortening the relaxation time. In addition, these NPs exhibited excellent dispersibility and stability in water. More importantly, MSCs labeled by the PA–SPIO NPs were transplanted into mouse, showing no adverse effects on the osteogenic and adipogenic differentiation. Rawat et al. (2019) synthesized SPIO NPs and then used them to label MSCs. The labeled MSCs could be tracked by MRI to understand their fate *in vivo*. Moreover, these labeled MSCs still maintained differentiation potential. Lee et al. (2020) used poly lactic-co-glycolic acid (PLGA) to modify SPIO NPs, and then utilized fluorescent dye Cy5.5 to functionalize the prepared NPs for labeling and tracking MSCs to investigate the interactions between PLGA–SPIO NPs and MSCs. The results showed that the prepared NPs had no apparent influences on the survival and differentiation of MSCs when the concentration was at 40 μg/ml for more than 96 h, demonstrating that the internalization pathway of MSCs is via endocytosis.

In proton (^{1}H) MRI images, SPIO NP-labeled cells appear as signal void regions (Miguel et al., 2007). This effect gives rise to enhance the sensitivity of cell detection, but poses challenges for accurate quantification of the cell population as well. Another limitation for SPIO NP-based cell tracking is the lack of specificity in some tissues. It is ambiguous to identify these cells *in vivo*, as other regions in anatomic MRI appear as dark as well (Zhang et al., 2010). To overcome these limitations, Sehl et al. (2019) utilized the combination of iron-based MRI, ^{19}F MRI, and MPI cellular imaging technologies to monitor and quantify the persistence of the transplanted MSCs and infiltrate macrophages *in vivo*, shown in **Figure 1**. First, MSCs were labeled with iron oxide NPs (ferumoxytol) and then implanted into the hind limb muscle of 10 C578/6 mice. Finally, a perfluorocarbon agent was administered intravenously for uptake by phagocytic macrophages *in situ*. The ferumoxytol-labeled MSCs were detected by proton (H^1) MRI and magnetic particle imaging (MPI). Perfluorocarbon-labeled macrophages were detected by fluorine-19 (19F) MRI. These three modalities are complementary and provide integrated information (specificity, sensitivity, and quantification of cell number). They proposed that these cellular imaging techniques could be used to monitor MSC engraftment over time and detect the infiltration of macrophages at transplant sites.

Gadolinium-Based Nanoparticles

T1-weighted sequences are often collected before and after infusion of T1-shortening MR contrast agents, so as to reduce the T1 relaxation times of ^{1}H atoms in water molecules and produce hyperintensities in T1-weighted images appearing white (Na and Hyeon, 2009). Currently, Gd-based NPs are the most widely used T1-contrast agent for labeling and tracking stem cells (Ni and Chen, 2015). Compared with T2-contrast agent of SPIO NPs, T1-contrast agent of Gd-based NPs can distinguish some similar low signal resulting from intrinsic signal in tissue or hemorrhage, due to their capability of generating a bright positive signal. Therefore, a T1-contrast agent generally is predominately employed as a probe in detecting the transplanted stem cells in a low-signal region (Na and Hyeon, 2009; Zhu et al., 2013; Robert et al., 2015).

Gd-based NPs usually are complex NPs, being composed of Gd^{3+} and their chelating ligand of which diethylenetriamine pentaacetic acid (DTPA) is the most common (Sherry et al., 1988; Ratzinger et al., 2010). Modified by DTPA, GD-based NPs reduced cytotoxicity due to the enhancement of hydrophilicity, but also weakened the interaction with the cell membrane leading to low cellular uptake for MSCs. Furthermore, their labeling efficiency was low resulting from the poor targeting ability of MSCs. Considering these problems, Tseng et al. (2010) prepared Gd-based NPs used as an MRI contrast agent to label and track human MSCs. Due to the modification of hexanedione, the

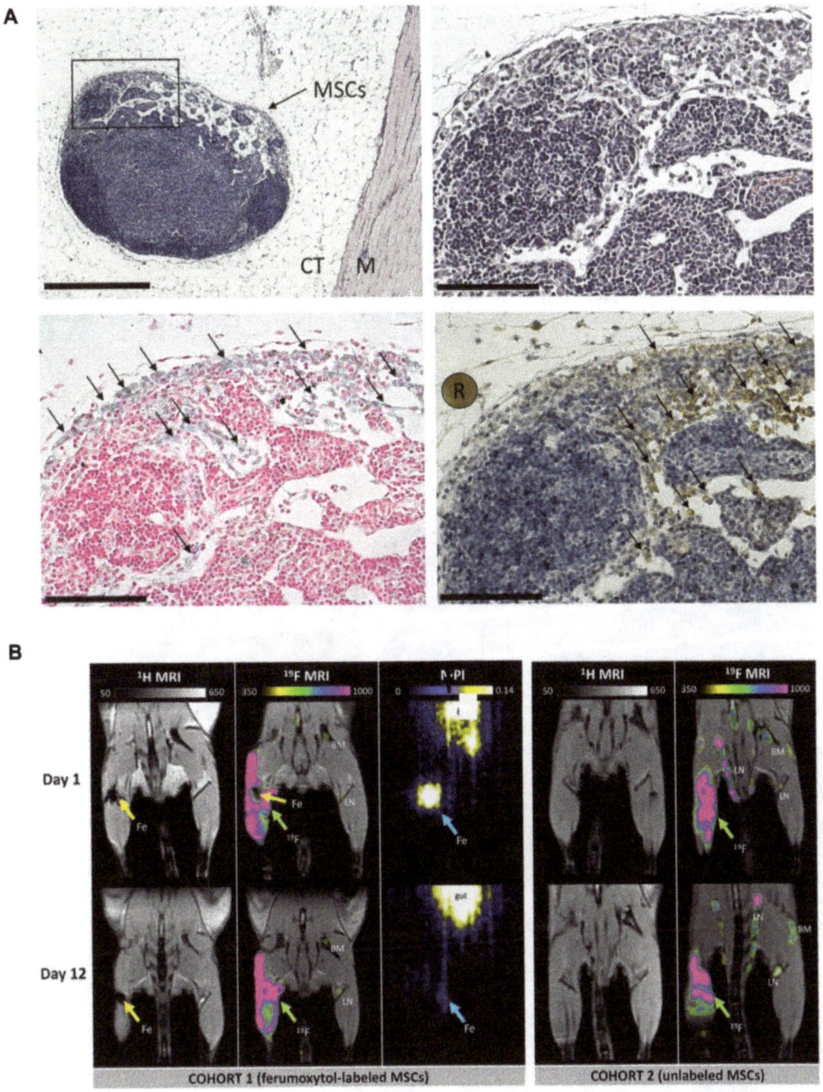

FIGURE 1 | (A) Histological validation showing the presence of MSCs surrounded in connective tissue (CT) and muscle (M) in hematoxylin and eosin at × 10 magnification (scale bar 500 μm). **(B)** *In vivo* proton (^{1}H)/fluorine 19 (^{19}F) magnetic resonance imaging (MRI) and magnetic particle imaging (MPI) (adapted Sehl et al., 2019).

biocompatibility of the prepared Gd-based NPs was improved. Moreover, compared with Gd-based NPs modified by DPTA, the prepared Gd-based NPs showed more excellent cellular uptake for MSCs and could be easily detected *in vivo* due to the shortening of T1 relaxation times. In another work, Kim et al. (2015b) reported a Gd-based NP to label MSCs, in which Gd^{3+} was chelated with a pullulan derivative ligand. It was found that the prepared Gd-based NPs could dramatically enhance cellular uptake for MSCs, leading to the enhancement of internalization efficiency from 32 ± 2 to 98 ± 4 pg Gd/cell. Moreover, the labeled MSCs achieved a long-term tracking of 21 days *in vivo*, due low signal attenuation. Cai et al. (2017) fabricated Gd-based NPs of 7 nm for tracking MSCs by utilizing melanin to modify Gd^{3+}. The results showed that Gd-based NPs modified by melanin increased the stability of MRI contrast agent and shorten T1 relaxation time, compared with traditional Gd-based NPs modified by DTPA. The labeled MSCs achieved long-term tracking for more than 4 weeks, due to the enhancement of labeling efficiency. Importantly, the labeled MSCs had no apparent cytotoxicity at a proper concentration of 800 μg/ml. However, preclinical studies suggested that for tracking MSCs *in vitro* and *in vivo*, the single-imaging technique was difficult to complete, and the integration of multiple labeling means often was required. Consequently, Santelli et al. (2018) developed multimodality imaging to track MSCs labeled by Gd-based NPs, shown in **Figure 2**. The GD-based NPs composed of spherical europium-doped gadolinium oxysulfide ($Gd_2O_2S:Eu^{3+}$) could be detected by MRI, X-ray imaging, and photoluminescence imaging. In the *in vitro* test, the number of MSCs labeled by $Gd_2O_2S:Eu^{3+}$ was up to 2,500, showing feasible cell tracking.

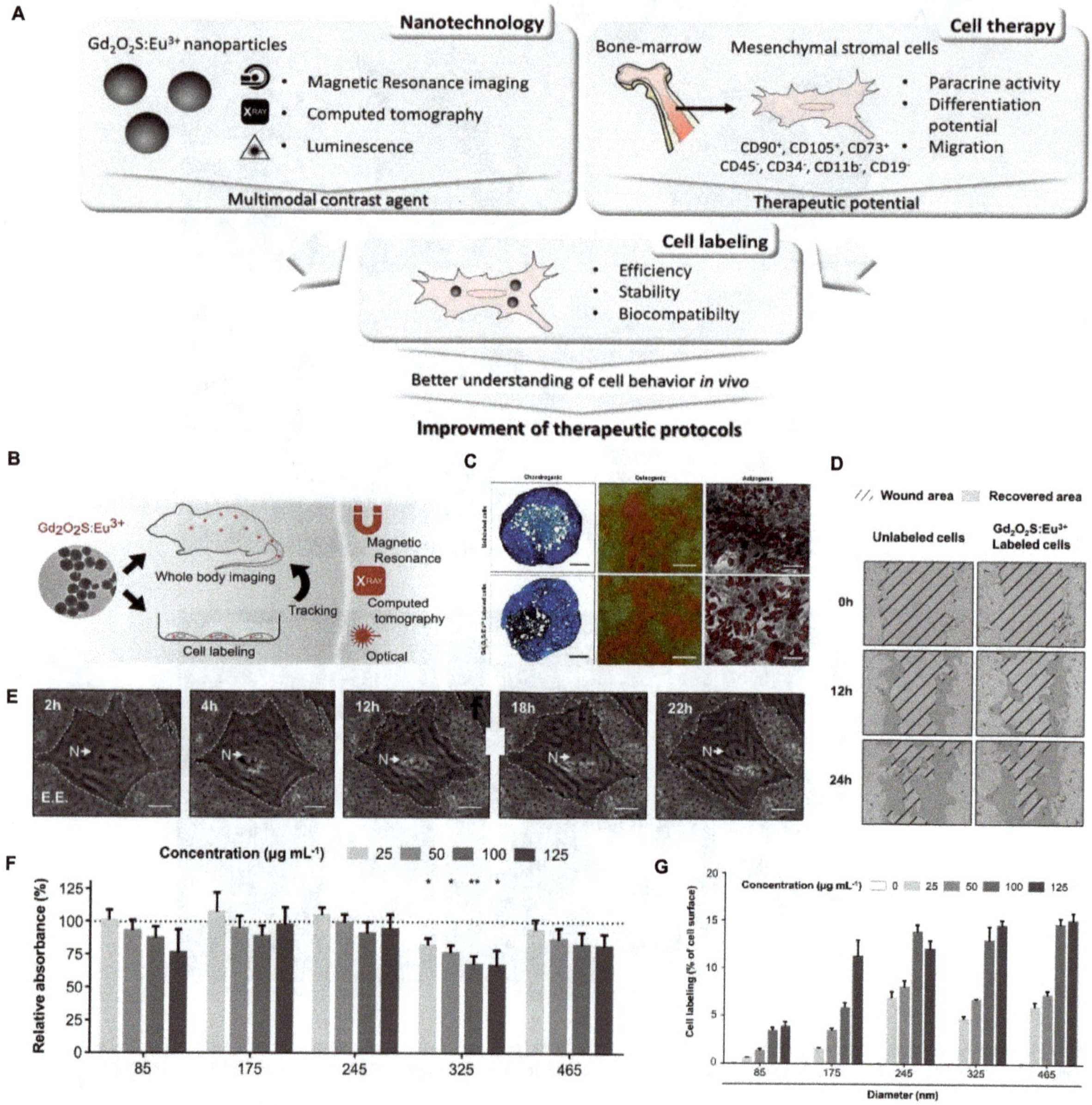

FIGURE 2 | (A) Schematic representation of nanoparticle potential in cell therapy and future impact. **(B)** Multimodality imaging for tracking mesenchymal stem cells (MSCs). **(C)** Differentiation of MSCs (scale bar 150 μm). **(D)** Representative phase-contrast images of wound closing. **(E)** Time-lapse of labeling extracted from video microscopy acquisition. **(F)** Viability of MSCs after 24-h $Gd_2O_2S:Eu^{3+}$ labeling evaluated by MTT. **(G)** Quantification of MSC labeling with $Gd_2O_2S:Eu^{3+}$ expressed as the percentage of cell surface area occupied by NPs (adapted by Santelli et al., 2018).

Moreover, the results suggested that the effects of the NPs on viability, proliferation, migration, and differentiation of the transplanted MSCs were innocuousness.

Gold-Based Nanoparticles

Due to their cytocompatibility and strong optical absorption in the near-infrared region, Au-based NPs are potential contrast agents of photoacoustic imaging. In addition, Au-based NPs can be detected in deep tissue at 2 cm at a high resolution of 100 μm, so they are emerging as an alternative method for tracking cells *in vivo* (Murphy et al., 2008; Giljohann et al., 2010). More importantly, MSCs can be directly labeled by Au-based NPs, so their differentiation after transplantation *in vivo* can be detected using photoacoustic imaging *in vivo* (Turjeman et al., 2015). Donnelly et al. (2018) utilized Au-based NPs as a photoacoustic contrast agent for real-time tracking MSCs to guide their delivery. It was found that the labeled MSCs could be detected by ultrasound/photoacoustic imaging in the spinal cord. In another work, Dhada et al. (2019) prepared Au-based NPs to label and track MSCs by photoacoustic imaging, which was composed of gold nanorods and IR775. The results suggested that cell death also could be detected because IR775 was sensitive

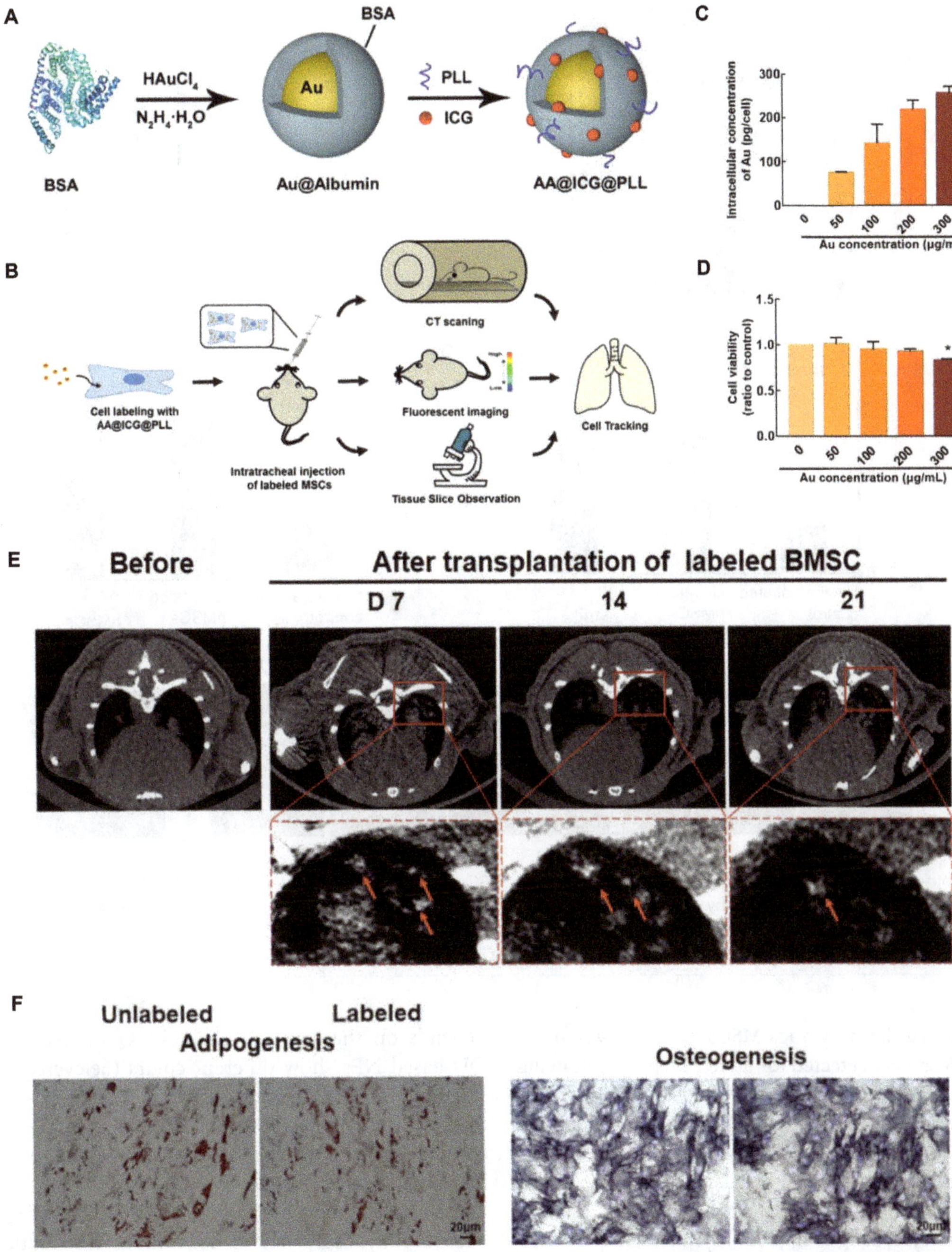

FIGURE 3 | (A) Schematic illustration of the synthesis of AA@ICG@PLL gold (Au)-based nanoparticles (NPs). **(B)** Experimental design for tracking AA@ICG@PLL-labeled MSCs in a silica-induced PF mouse model. **(C)** Intracellular Au content measured by ICP-MS. **(D)** Relative viability of BMSCs labeled with AA@ICG@PLL NPs at various Au concentrations. **(E)** *In vivo* computed tomography (CT) images of AA@ICG@PLL-labeled BMSCs at 7, 14, and 21 days after transplantation. **(F)** Bright-field images of Oil Red O staining and ALP staining of NP-loaded and unloaded BMSCs. Scale bar = 20 mm (adapted by Huang et al., 2020). *$p < 0.05$ compared with the unlabeled group.

to reactive oxygen species (ROS). Therefore, the viability of the transplanted MSCs *in vivo* was quantificationally measured. Moreover, Laffey et al. (2020) studied the viability of MSCs labeled by Au-based NPs in a frozen environment. The results showed that the labeled MSCs undergoing the process of freeing, storing, and thawing for 2 months still could be detected by photoacoustic imaging, and their differential ability also had no apparent difference with the unlabeled MSCs.

Certainly, Au-based NPs also can be detected by computed tomography (CT), due to the high X-ray absorption. Thus, they are used as a CT maker to label and track MSCs. For example, Betzer et al. (2017) used Au-based NPs as labeling agents to

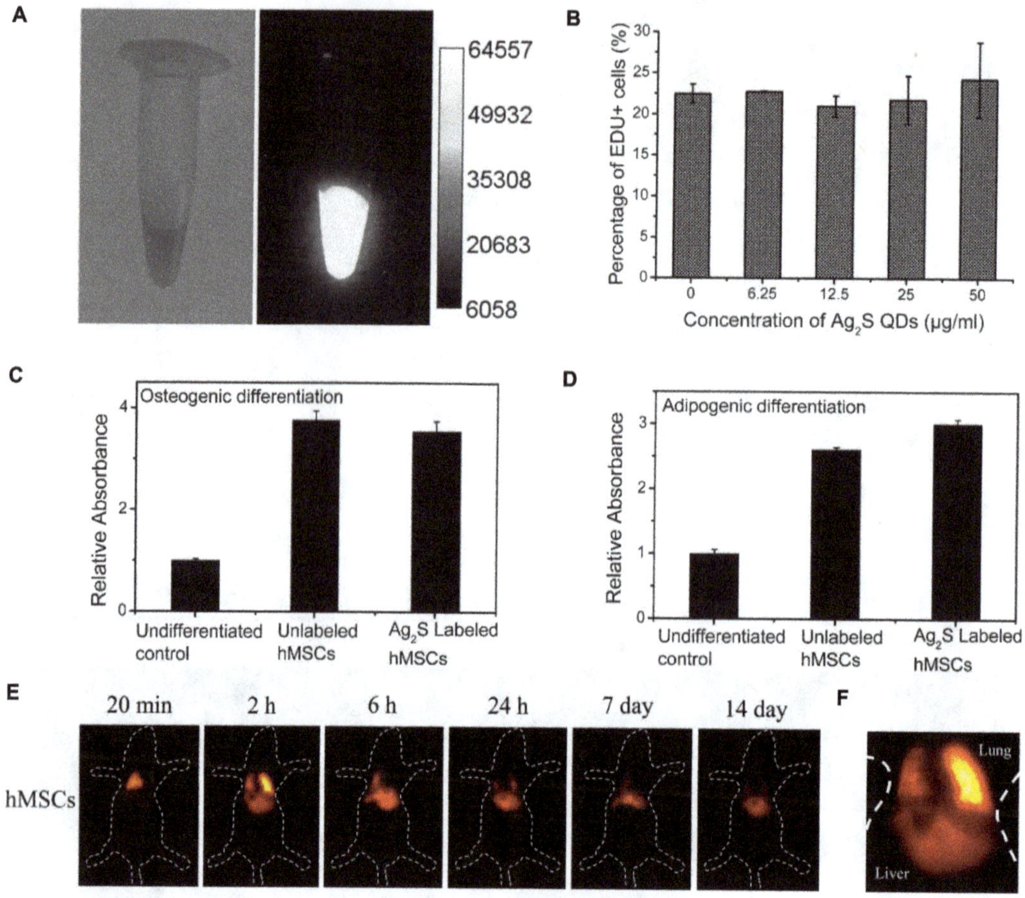

FIGURE 4 | (A) A photoluminescence image (PA) of the Ag_2S QD-labeled human MSC solution at a density of 4×10^6 cell ml^{-1}. **(B)** Cell proliferation. Quantification of **(C)** osteogenic and **(D)** adipogenic differentiation by measuring the absorbance of Oil-Red O and alizarin red extracted from cell lysates at 404 nm, respectively. **(E)** The time course of the *in vivo* near-infrared (NIR) PL images of a healthy mouse after transplantation of Ag_2S QD-labeled human MSCs. **(F)** Higher magnification NIR PL image of mice transplanted with human MSCs only after 2 h (adapted from Chen G. et al., 2015).

longitudinally and quantitatively track MSCs *in vivo*. It was found that the labeled MSCs were detected for up to 24 h by CT, showing a long-term tracking. Nafiujjaman and Kim (2020) reported a biocompatible Au-based NPs used as a CT maker, in which Au NPs were modified by poly-L-lysine (PLL) to change the charge properties of surface enhancing the cellular uptake. The MSCs labeled by Au-based NPs could be detected by CT and showed high labeling efficiency. Huang et al. (2020) synthesized Au-based NPs (AA@ICG@PLL) with dual-modal imaging (CT and near-infrared fluorescence) to label and track MSCs of mice *in vivo*, shown in **Figure 3**. Due to modification by indocyanine green (ICG) and poly-L-lysine (PLL), AA@ICG@PLL showed excellent cellular uptake for MSCs and biocompatibility. It was found that the labeled MSCs could be tracked via dual-modal imaging for more than 21 days, and importantly, the prepared NPs had anti-inflammatory properties.

Quantum Dot-Based Nanoparticles

QD-based NPs are semiconductor NPs with II–VI or III–V elements, which can emit particular frequency light after being stimulated (Jaiswal et al., 2004). The emitted light frequency depends on the size and shape of QD-based NPs. Therefore, QD-based NPs show different colors (Seleverstov et al., 2006). In general, the fluorescence lifetime of QD-based NPs is longer than traditional fluorescence dye (Bailey et al., 2004). In addition, compared with fluorescent dye, QD-based NPs are easier to be detected due to the non-overlapping of absorption and emission (Mazumder et al., 2009). Specifically, QD-based NPs have broad absorption of continuous distribution, but show narrow and symmetrical properties (Yukawa and Baba, 2017). More importantly, they have the advantage of photochemical stability. As a result, QD-based NPs have been used as contrast agents for long-term tracking of MSCs *in vivo*. However, QD-based NPs also have some disadvantages, such as unsatisfied cytotoxicity and stochastic blinking. Moreover, the augmentation of QD-based NPs in dosage increases the sensitivity of cell imaging, but may decrease their definition (Shah et al., 2007; Liang et al., 2013).

Hsieh et al. (2006) reported a QD-based NP to label human MSCs, in which CdSe was used as the core, and the shell was covered by ZnS. In addition, the commercial QD-based NPs also were developed and utilized as contrast

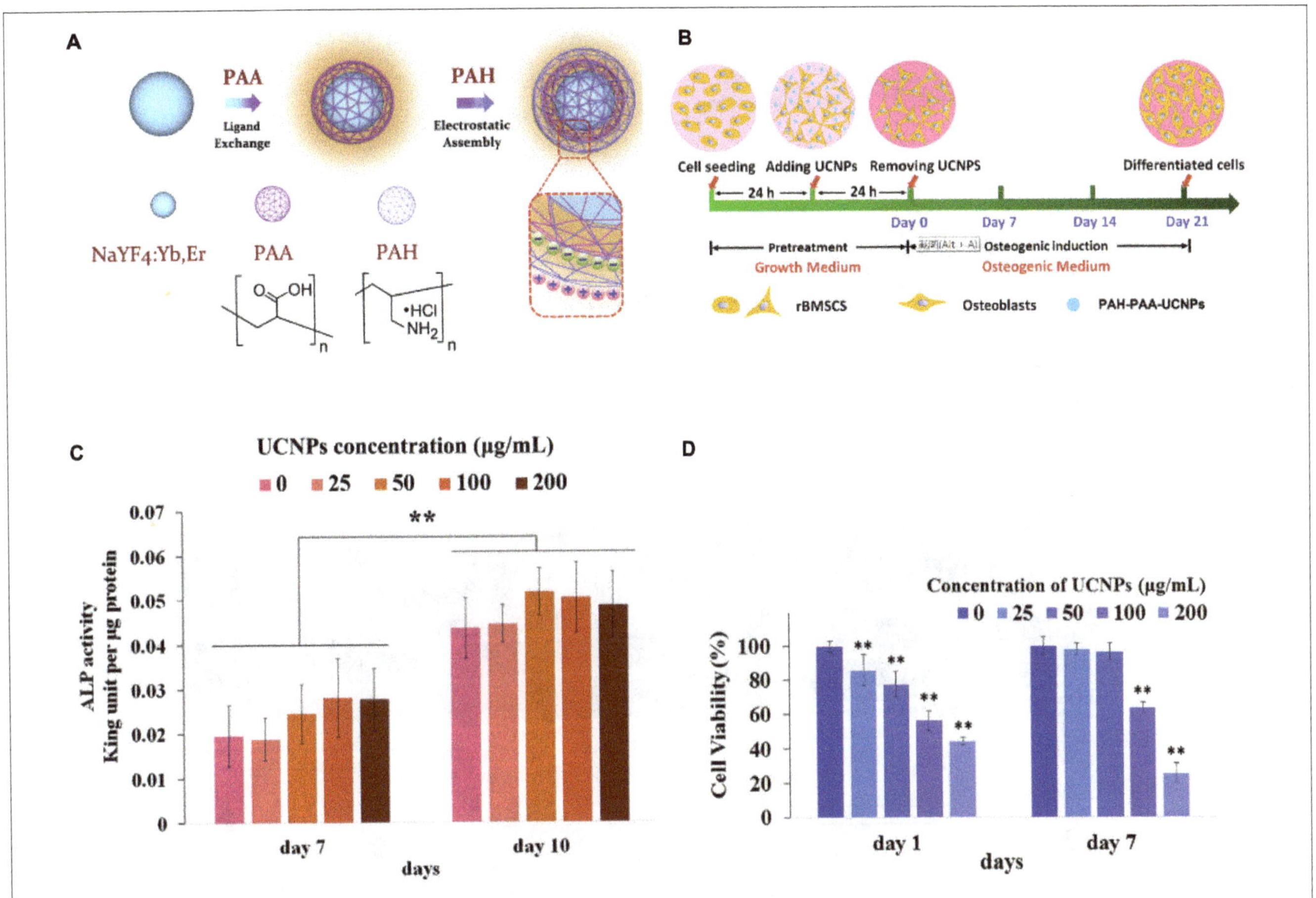

FIGURE 5 | (A) Upconversion (UC)-based NPs synthesis. **(B)** Cell pretreatment and osteogenic differentiation process. **(C)** Normalized alkaline phosphatase activity expression by MSCs. **(D)** Cell viability (adapted by Ma et al., 2016). $^{**}p$ < 0.01 compared with control group.

agents to label and track the cell distributions. However, these QD-based NPs showed unsatisfied biocompatibility and cytotoxicity, so they had to be modified before use. In recent years, Li et al. (2016) prepared QDs-based NPs (RGD-β-CD-QDs) to label and track human MSCs, which were composed of QDs, β-cyclodextrin (β-CD), and Cys-Lys-Lys-ArgGly-Asp (CKKRGD) peptide. The QDs modified by β-CD enhanced the cellular uptake and facilitated the differentiation of MSCs, due to the small molecule dexamethasone and siRNA carried by β-CD. More importantly, the labeled MSCs could be detected for up to 3 weeks. Chen G. et al. (2015) reported a AgS_2 QD-based NP for tracking human MSCs *in vivo* by utilizing fluorescence imaging, shown in **Figure 4**. It was found that the prepared NPs with good biocompatibility could be detected in the second near infrared, and the stability of fluorescence reached up to 30 days. Furthermore, the labeled MSCs was dynamically visualized at high resolution of 100 ms for more than 14 days. Chetty et al. (2019) prepared $CuInS_2$-ZnS QD-based NPs to label umbilical cord-derived MSCs, and the labeling efficiency reached 98% due to the prepared QD-based NPs displaying high photoluminescence quantum yield of 88%. In addition, the labeled MSCs showed no apparent influences on stemness and had the ability of long-term tracking.

Upconversion-Based Nanoparticles

UC-based NPs, usually being lanthanide-doped nanocrystals, can undergo a photon UC process in which the sequential absorption of two or more photons leads to anti-Stokes type emission of a single higher-energy photon (Wang et al., 2010). Due to the unique properties of being sensitive to the near-infrared light, UC-based NPs can be detected in deeper tissue compared with traditional contrast agents with fluorescence. More importantly, the imaging of UC-based NPs is more stable and has higher definition (Ang et al., 2011; Chen X. et al., 2015).

Idris et al. (2009) reported a contrast agent of UC-based NPs to label and track MSCs, which was composed of $NaYF_4$:Yb, Er NPs, and silicon. The labeled MSCs could directly be imaged *in vivo* to dynamically visualize their behaviors, but the region imaged by confocal microscopy was small. Wang et al. (2012a) fabricated UC-based NPs to label MSCs, which was modified by polyethylene glycol (PEG) and oligo-arginine. MSCs labeled by the UC-based NPs were detected by fluorescence imaging *in vivo*, and the introduction of oligo-arginine improved the cellular uptake of the NPs, showing excellent labeling efficiency and high sensitivity of 10 cells. In another work, Cheng et al. (2013) developed a multifunctional UC-based NP, integrating magnetic properties into UC luminescence NPs. Utilizing the

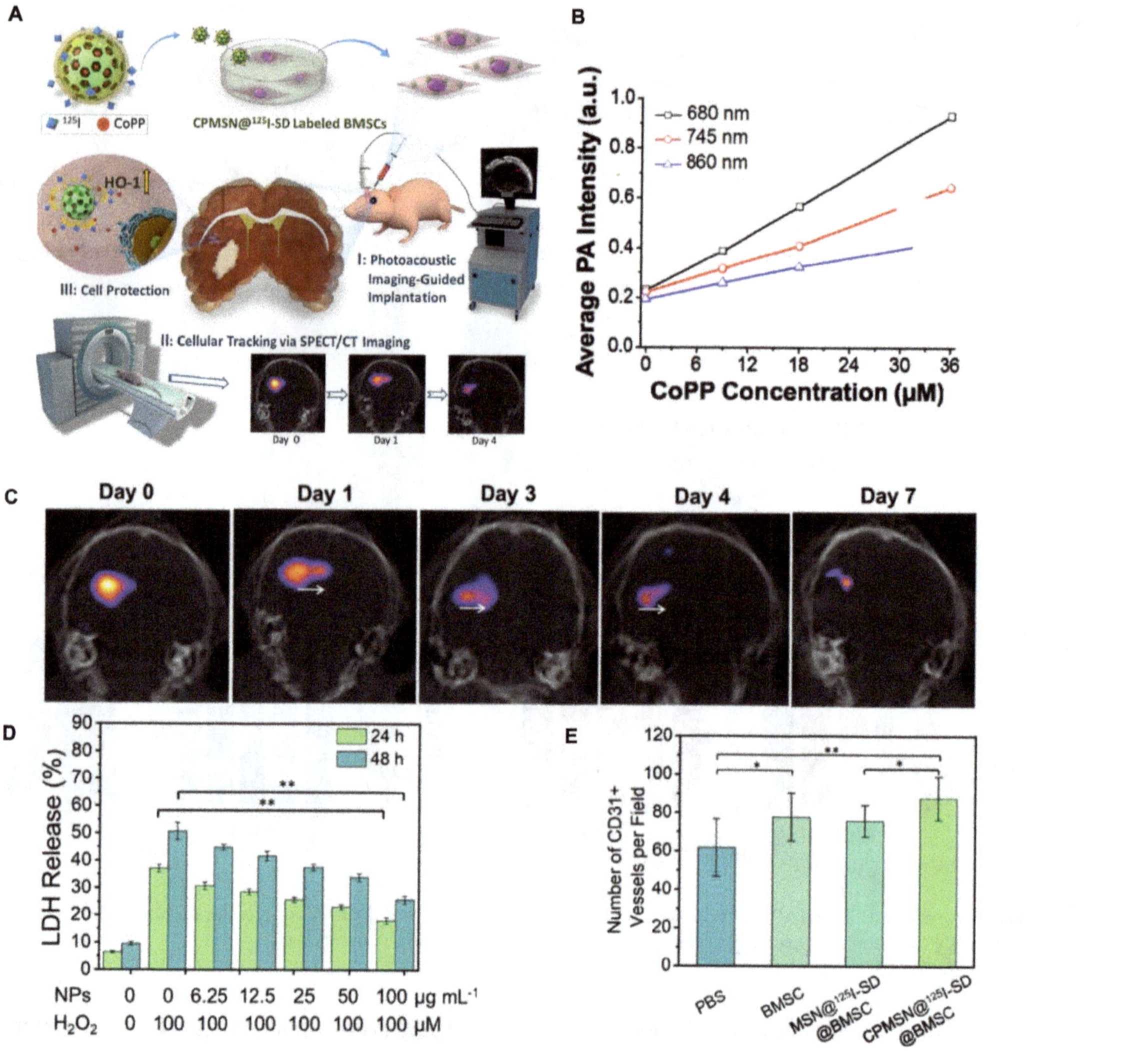

FIGURE 6 | (A) Schematic illustrating the triple functionality of CPMSN@125I-SD for stem cell therapy of brain ischemia. **(B)** Corresponding average intensities of CPMSN@125I-SD with various cobalt protoporphyrin IX (CoPP) concentrations in the NIR region. **(C)** Single-photon emission computed tomography imaging (SPECT)/CT images of ischemic mouse brain tissue on different days (0–7 days) after intracerebral injection of the labeled BMSCs (500,000 cells). **(D)** Cell death assessment for MSCs after treatment with different concentrations of CPMSN@125I-SD (0–100 μg ml^{-1}) and exposure to 100 μM H_2O_2 for 24 and 48 h. **(E)** Bar graph showing the quantification of the number of CD^{31+} cells (adapted from Yao et al., 2020). *$p < 0.05$; **$p < 0.01$.

prepared NPs, the labeled MSCs can be tracked via fluorescence imaging and MRI, possessing highly effective sensitivity of 10 cells in mouse *in vivo*. Zhao et al. (2013) prepared a UC-based NP for labeling mouse MSCs, which was composed of polyethylenimine (PEI) and (α-$NaYbF_4$:Tm^{3+})/CaF_2, enhancing the detective depth *in vivo* due to absorption and emission for near-infrared light.

In recent years, Ma et al. (2016) reported a UC-based NP, which was composed of $NaYF_4$:Yb^{3+}, Er^{3+} NPs, poly (acrylic acid) (PAA), and poly (allylamine hydrochloride) (PAH), as a fluorescence maker for tracking bone marrow MSCs *in vitro*, shown in **Figure 5**. The biocompatibility and cellular uptake of $NaYF_4$:Yb^{3+}, Er^{3+} NPs were highly enhanced, due to electrostatic interaction. Moreover, it was found that the effects of cellular uptake of UC-based NPs ($\leq$50 μg/ml) on the osteogenic differentiation had no apparent difference by tracking the MSCs. Kang et al. (2018) prepared a UC-based NP with NIR-controllable properties to label MSCs. By a remote-controllable way, the stem cell differentiation was regulated. Furthermore, Ren et al. (2020) used ligand-free NaYF4:Yb/Er UC-based NPs to label and track mouse bone MSCs, demonstrating that the UC-based NPs at a proper concentration could enhance osteogenic differentiation.

Silicon-Based Nanoparticles

Recently, silicon-based NPs have been demonstrated as a good contrast agent to label cells because they can be easily modified by bioconjugation (Shin et al., 2019). Furthermore, it has excellent biocompatibility and chemical inertness, thus, being able to serve as a probe for tracking cells *in vivo* (Huang et al., 2005; Hsiao et al., 2008). Silicon-based NPs, being simply divided into

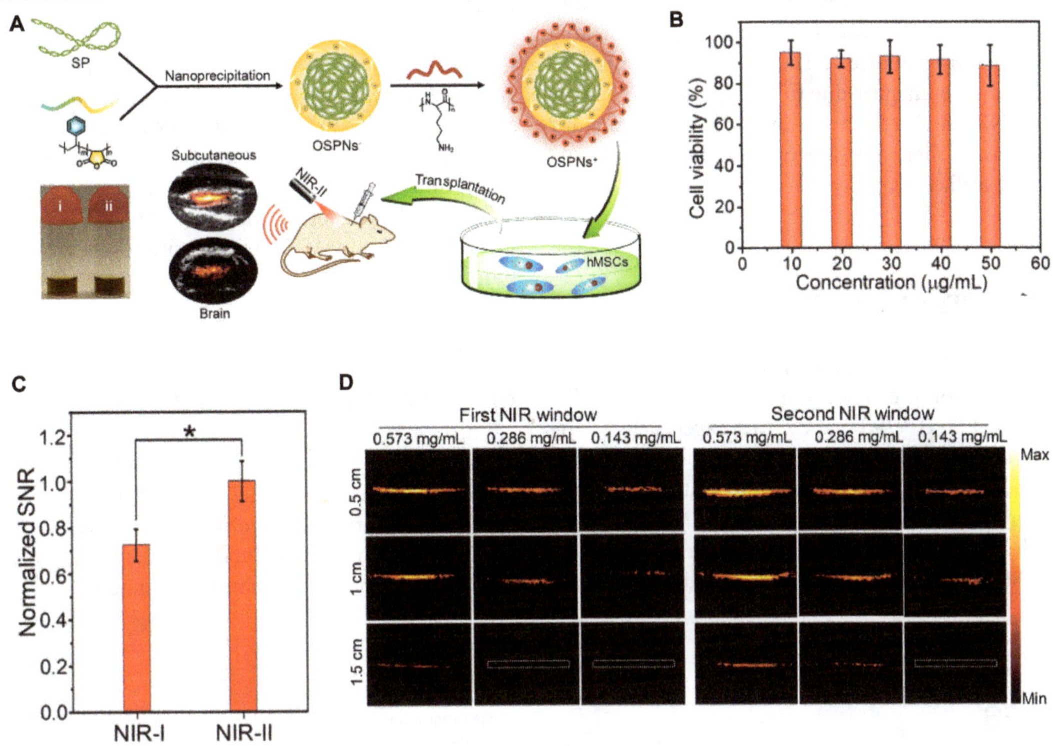

FIGURE 7 | (A) Illustration of the preparation procedure of $OSPNs^+$ and the photoacoustic labeling of human MSCs after transplantation. **(B)** The MTT assay of human MSCs treated by $OSPNs^+$ for 12 h under various concentrations. **(C)** Normalized PA SNR of $OSPNs^+$-labeled hMSCs implanted into mice brain under NIR-I (860 nm) or NIR-II (1,064 nm) light excitation ($^*p < 0.05$). **(D)** PA imaging of aqueous $OSPNs^+$ solutions (0.573, 0.286, and 0.143 mg/ml) (adapted from Yin et al., 2018).

silica NPs and silicon carbide NPs, not only contain fluorescent properties but also are used as ultrasound agents (Chen and Jokerst, 2020; Yao et al., 2020).

Huang et al. (2005) prepared a mesoporous silica NP modified by fluorescein isothiocyanate, and the labeled MSCs could be detected by imaging to track their viability *in vivo*. Due to clathrin-mediated endocytosis, the NPs could be internalized into MSCs and showed good cellular uptake. In addition, the highly efficient labeling had no apparent influences on the viability of MSCs. In another work, Chen and Jokerst (2020) used silica NPs to label MSCs and then track the MSCs *in vivo* by ultrasound imaging. The results showed that silica NPs could significantly increase the ultrasound signal of MSCs *in vivo*. Yao et al. (2020) reported a unique core–shell NP in which the core is composed of cobalt protoporphyrin IX (CoPP)-loaded mesoporous silica NPs, and the shell is a ^{125}I-conjugated/spermine-modified dextran polymer, to label and guide the transplantation of MSCs by PA imaging and SPCT nuclear imaging, shown in **Figure 6**. The obtained NPs not only could instantly image the transplantation of MSCs but also quantitatively tracked their migrations for a long time. Significantly, the NPs steadily released CoPP to increase the survival of MSCs in ischemic mice.

Another type of silicon-based NPs is silicon carbide NPs, which are commonly used as protecting layer due to their unique properties of being durable and chemically inert. Moreover, typically, silicon carbide NPs ($\leq$10 nm) are utilized as contrast agents to label and track cells *in vivo* because of their photoluminescence resulting from quantum confinement effects. Chen et al. (2019) used three sizes of silicon carbide NPs to label MSCs, showing dual modality imaging (photoluminescence and photoacoustic imaging). When the size of the NPs is 620 nm, the labeled MSCs could be detected *in vitro* for more than 20 days. Moreover, the NPs also exhibited good biocompatibility and the capacity of cell tracking because the differentiated cells also could be imaged.

Other Nanoparticles

Gao et al. (2016) prepared an aggregation-induced emission NP, the surface of which is modified by Tat peptide. The obtained NPs had highly efficient ability of labeling mouse bone marrow-derived MSCs, and the red emission could be detected for more than 12 passages, which were not achieved by traditional fluorescence, possessing long-term tracking and strong anti-photobleaching ability. More importantly, MSCs labeled by the NPs showed low cytotoxicity, and their viability and differentiation had no apparent influences. Lim et al. (2019) developed bicyclo nonyne (BCN)-conjugated glycol chitosan NPs (BCN-NPs) as a delivery system of dual-modal stem cell imaging probes. Yin et al. (2018) reported an organic semiconducting polymer NP ($OSPN^+$) as a PA contrast agent for tracking MSCs, utilizing a second near-infrared (NIR-II) adsorption to broaden the limitation of conventional inorganic PA contrast agents and the narrow range of the wavelength in the first near-infrared (NIR-I) window, shown in **Figure 7**. The prepared cationic NPs showed the deeper tissue imaging due to the significantly higher signal-to-noise (SNR) and enhanced the cellular uptake for human MSCs because of their good biocompatibility, appropriate size, and optimized surface property.

PROBLEMS AND PROSPECTS

Mesenchymal stem cell transplantation has been shown to be a strong potential for the treatment of CVDs. Many NPs have been fabricated and used as contrast agents by non-invasive imaging to track and monitor the transplanted MSCs, for providing more information to guide further therapy. However, one big issue associated with NPs for labeled MSCs is that NPs released from dead cells will be uptaken by macrophages, which give false-positive information *in vivo*. Maybe, we can label dead cells with other methods to exclude the false-positive information. Moreover, the single-imaging technique can be inefficient to meet all needs for tracking, and each of those has its own disadvantages. Although there are some multimodal imaging techniques, more multimodal labeling agent-based NPs should be developed in the future to optimize MSC dose and delivery route for the treatment of CVDs. Importantly, the poor targeted migration and low survival rate of MSCs transplanted into the cardiovascular should be solved.

AUTHOR CONTRIBUTIONS

HH completed the first draft of the manuscript. XD, ZH, and ZY offered the excellent advices and perfected the first draft. WH improved the first draft and finally finished the manuscript and provided the support of funds. All authors contributed to the article and approved the submitted version.

REFERENCES

Accomasso, L., Gallina, C., Turinetto, V., and Giachino, C. J. (2016). Stem cell tracking with nanoparticles for regenerative medicine purposes: an overview. *Stem Cells Int.* 2016:7920358.

Akins, E. J., and Dubey, P. (2008). Noninvasive imaging of cell-mediated therapy for treatment of cancer. *J. Nucl. Med.* 49, 180S–195S.

Alison, M., and Islam, S. (2009). Attributes of adult stem cells. *J. Pathol.* 217, 144–160. doi: 10.1002/path.2498

Alkilany, A. M., and Murphy, C. J. (2010). Toxicity and cellular uptake of gold nanoparticles: what we have learned so far? *J. Nanopart Res.* 12, 2313–2333. doi: 10.1007/s11051-010-9911-8

Aly, R. M. (2020). Current state of stem cell-based therapies: an overview. *Stem Cell Investig.* 7:8. doi: 10.21037/sci-2020-001

Andreas, K., Georgieva, R., Ladwig, M., Mueller, S., Notter, M., Sittinger, M., et al. (2012). Highly efficient magnetic stem cell labeling with citrate-coated superparamagnetic iron oxide nanoparticles for MRI tracking. *Biomaterials* 33, 4515–4525. doi: 10.1016/j.biomaterials.2012.02.064

Andres, R. H., Choi, R., Steinberg, G. K., and Guzman, R. (2008). Potential of adult neural stem cells in stroke therapy. *Regen. Med.* 3, 893–905. doi: 10.2217/17460751.3.6.893

Ang, L. Y., Lim, M. E., Ong, L. C., and Zhang, Y. J. N. (2011). Applications of upconversion nanoparticles in imaging, detection and therapy. *Nanomedicine (Lond)* 6, 1273–1288. doi: 10.2217/nnm.11.108

Babic, M., Horák, D., Trchová, M., Jendelová, P., Glogarová, K., Lesný, P., et al. (2008). Poly (L-lysine)-modified iron oxide nanoparticles for stem cell labeling. *Bioconjug Chem.* 19, 740–750. doi: 10.1021/bc700410z

Bailey, R. E., Smith, A. M., and Nie, S. (2004). Quantum dots in biology and medicine. *Physica E: Low-dimensional Systems Nanostruct.* 25, 1–12.

Barrow, M., Taylor, A., Murray, P., Rosseinsky, M. J., and Adams, D. J. (2015). Design considerations for the synthesis of polymer coated iron oxide nanoparticles for stem cell labelling and tracking using MRI. *Chem. Soc. Rev.* 44, 6733–6748. doi: 10.1039/c5cs00331h

Barua, S., and Mitragotri, S. (2014). Challenges associated with penetration of nanoparticles across cell and tissue barriers: a review of current status and future prospects. *Nano Today* 9, 223–243. doi: 10.1016/j.nantod.2014.04.008

Behlke, L. M., Lenze, E. J., and Carney, R. M. (2020). The cardiovascular effects of newer antidepressants in older adults and those with or at high risk for cardiovascular diseases. *CNS Drugs* 34, 1133–1147. doi: 10.1007/s40263-020-00763-z

Behzadi, S., Serpooshan, V., Tao, W., Hamaly, M. A., Alkawareek, M. Y., Dreaden, E. C., et al. (2017). Cellular uptake of nanoparticles: journey inside the cell. *Chem. Soc. Rev.* 46, 4218–4244. doi: 10.1039/c6cs00636a

Bellin, M.-F. (2006). MR contrast agents, the old and the new. *Eur. J. Radiol.* 60, 314–323. doi: 10.1016/j.ejrad.2006.06.021

Betzer, O., Meir, R., Motiei, M., Yadid, G., and Popovtzer, R. (2017). "Gold nanoparticle-cell labeling methodology for tracking stem cells within the brain," in *Proceedings of the Nanoscale Imaging, Sensing, and Actuation for Biomedical Applications XIV: International Society for Optics and Photonics*, (Bellingham, DC: SPIE).

Betzer, O., Shwartz, A., Motiei, M., Kazimirsky, G., Gispan, I., Damti, E., et al. (2014). Nanoparticle-based CT imaging technique for longitudinal and quantitative stem cell tracking within the brain: application in neuropsychiatric disorders. *ACS Nano* 8, 9274–9285. doi: 10.1021/nn503131h

Bhirde, A., Xie, J., Swierczewska, M., and Chen, X. J. N. (2011). Nanoparticles for cell labeling. *Nanoscale* 3, 142–153.

Bull, E., Madani, S. Y., Sheth, R., Seifalian, A., Green, M., and Seifalian, A. M. (2014). Stem cell tracking using iron oxide nanoparticles. *Int. J. Nanomed.* 9:1641. doi: 10.2147/ijn.s48979

Bulte, J. W. J. R. (2017). Science to practice: can MR imaging cell tracking of macrophage infiltration be used as a predictive imaging biomarker for transplanted stem cell rejection? *Radiology* 284, 307–309. doi: 10.1148/radiol.2017170536

Cahill, K. S., Gaidosh, G., Huard, J., Silver, X., Byrne, B. J., and Walter, G. A. J. T. (2004). Noninvasive monitoring and tracking of muscle stem cell transplants. *Transplantation* 78, 1626–1633. doi: 10.1097/01.tp.0000145528.51525.8b

Cai, W. W., Wang, L. J., Li, S. J., Zhang, X. P., Li, T. T., Wang, Y. H., et al. (2017). Effective tracking of bone mesenchymal stem cells in vivo by magnetic resonance imaging using melanin-based gadolinium3+ nanoparticles. *J. Biomed. Mater. Res. A* 105, 131–137. doi: 10.1002/jbm.a.35891

Calero, M., Gutiérrez, L., Salas, G., Luengo, Y., Lázaro, A., Acedo, P., et al. (2014). Efficient and safe internalization of magnetic iron oxide nanoparticles: two fundamental requirements for biomedical applications. *Nanomedicine* 10, 733–743. doi: 10.1016/j.nano.2013.11.010

Caplan, A. I. (2009). Why are MSCs therapeutic? new data: new insight. *J. Pathol.* 217, 318–324. doi: 10.1002/path.2469

Caplan, A. I. (2017). Mesenchymal stem cells: time to change the name! *Stem Cells Transl. Med.* 6, 1445–1451. doi: 10.1002/sctm.17-0051

Carella, A. M., Cavaliere, M., Lerma, E., Ferrara, R., Tedeschi, L., Romanelli, A., et al. (2000). Autografting followed by nonmyeloablative immunosuppressive chemotherapy and allogeneic peripheral-blood hematopoietic stem-cell transplantation as treatment of resistant Hodgkin's disease and non-Hodgkin's lymphoma. *J. Clin. Oncol.* 18, 3918–3924. doi: 10.1200/jco.2000.18.23.3918

Chan, K. Y., Jang, M. J., Yoo, B. B., Greenbaum, A., Ravi, N., Wu, W.-L., et al. (2017). Engineered AAVs for efficient noninvasive gene delivery to the central and peripheral nervous systems. *Nat. Neurosci.* 20, 1172–1179. doi: 10.1038/nn.4593

Chandran, P., Riviere, J. E., and Monteiro-Riviere, N. A. J. N. (2017). Surface chemistry of gold nanoparticles determines the biocorona composition impacting cellular uptake, toxicity and gene expression profiles in human endothelial cells. *Nanotoxicology* 11, 507–519. doi: 10.1080/17435390.2017.1314036

Chen, F., and Jokerst, J. V. (2020). Stem cell tracking with nanoparticle-based ultrasound contrast agents. *Methods Mol. Biol.* 2126, 141–153. doi: 10.1007/978-1-0716-0364-2_13

Chen, F., Zhao, E. R., Hu, T., Shi, Y., Sirbuly, D. J., and Jokerst, J. V. (2019). Silicon carbide nanoparticles as a photoacoustic and photoluminescent dual-imaging contrast agent for long-term cell tracking. *Nanoscale Adv.* 1, 3514–3520. doi: 10.1039/c9na00237e

Chen, G., Tian, F., Li, C., Zhang, Y., Weng, Z., Zhang, Y., et al. (2015). In vivo real-time visualization of mesenchymal stem cells tropism for cutaneous regeneration using NIR-II fluorescence imaging. *Biomaterials* 53, 265–273. doi: 10.1016/j.biomaterials.2015.02.090

Chen, X., Peng, D., Ju, Q., and Wang, F. J. (2015). Photon upconversion in core–shell nanoparticles. *Chem. Soc. Rev.* 44, 1318–1330.

Chen, X., Tian, F., Zhang, X., and Wang, W. J. (2013). Internalization pathways of nanoparticles and their interaction with a vesicle. *Soft Matter.* 9, 7592–7600. doi: 10.1039/c3sm50931a

Cheng, L., Wang, C., Ma, X., Wang, Q., Cheng, Y., Wang, H., et al. (2013). Multifunctional upconversion nanoparticles for dual-modal imaging-guided stem cell therapy under remote magnetic control. *Adv. Functional. Mater.* 23, 272–280. doi: 10.1002/adfm.201201733

Cheng, S.-H., Yu, D., Tsai, H.-M., Morshed, R. A., Kanojia, D., Lo, L.-W., et al. (2016). Dynamic in vivo SPECT imaging of neural stem cells functionalized with radiolabeled nanoparticles for tracking of glioblastoma. *J. Nucl. Med.* 57, 279–284. doi: 10.2967/jnumed.115.163006

Chetty, S. S., Praneetha, S., Govarthanan, K., Verma, R. S., and Vadivel Murugan, A. J. (2019). Noninvasive tracking and regenerative capabilities of transplanted human umbilical cord-derived mesenchymal stem cells labeled with I-III-IV semiconducting nanocrystals in liver-injured living mice. *ACS Appl. Mater. Interfaces* 11, 8763–8778. doi: 10.1021/acsami.8b19953

Cosgrove, D. J. (2006). Ultrasound contrast agents: an overview. *Eur. J. Radiol.* 60, 324–330. doi: 10.1016/j.ejrad.2006.06.022

Crabbe, A., Vandeputte, C., Dresselaers, T., Sacido, A. A., Verdugo, J. M. G., Eyckmans, J., et al. (2010). Effects of MRI contrast agents on the stem cell phenotype. *Cell Transplant* 19, 919–936. doi: 10.3727/096368910x494623

Cui, Z., Yang, B., and Li, R.-K. (2016). Application of biomaterials in cardiac repair and regeneration. *Engineering* 2, 141–148. doi: 10.1016/j.eng.2016.01.028

Davis, W. C. (1972). H-2 antigen on cell membranes: an explanation for the alteration of distribution by indirect labeling techniques. *Science* 175, 1006–1008. doi: 10.1126/science.175.4025.1006

Deng, Y., Zhang, X., Shen, H., He, Q., Wu, Z., Liao, W., et al. (2020). Application of the nano-drug delivery system in treatment of cardiovascular diseases. *Front. Bioeng. Biotechnol.* 7:489. doi: 10.3389/fbioe.2019.00489

Dhada, K. S., Hernandez, D. S., and Suggs, L. J. (2019). In vivo photoacoustic tracking of mesenchymal stem cell viability. *ACS Nano* 13, 7791–7799. doi: 10.1021/acsnano.9b01802

Diekman, B. O., and Guilak, F. J. (2013). Stem cell-based therapies for osteoarthritis: challenges and opportunities. *Curr. Opin. Rheumatol.* 25:119. doi: 10.1097/bor.0b013e32835aa28d

DiPersio, J. F., Stadtmauer, E. A., Nademanee, A., Micallef, I. N., Stiff, P. J., Kaufman, J. L., et al. (2009). Plerixafor and G-CSF versus placebo and G-CSF to mobilize hematopoietic stem cells for autologous stem cell transplantation in patients with multiple myeloma. *Blood* 113, 5720–5726. doi: 10.1182/blood-2008-08-174946

Donnelly, E. M., Kubelick, K. P., Dumani, D. S., and Emelianov, S. Y. (2018). Photoacoustic image-guided delivery of plasmonic-nanoparticle-labeled mesenchymal stem cells to the spinal cord. *Nano Lett.* 18, 6625–6632. doi: 10.1021/acs.nanolett.8b03305

Edmundson, M., Thanh, N. T., and Song, B. J. T. (2013). Nanoparticles based stem cell tracking in regenerative medicine. *Theranostics* 3, 573–582. doi: 10.7150/thno.5477

Elkhenany, H., Abd Elkodous, M., Ghoneim, N. I., Ahmed, T. A., Ahmed, S. M., Mohamed, I. K., et al. (2020). Comparison of different uncoated and starch-coated superparamagnetic iron oxide nanoparticles: implications for stem cell tracking. *Int. J. Biol. Macromol.* 143, 763–774. doi: 10.1016/j.ijbiomac.2019.10.031

Ferreira, L. J. (2009). Nanoparticles as tools to study and control stem cells. *J. Cell Biochem.* 108, 746–752. doi: 10.1002/jcb.22303

Friedenstein, A., Chailakhjan, R., and Lalykina, K. (1970). The development of fibroblast colonies in monolayer cultures of guinea-pig bone marrow and spleen cells. *Cell Prolif.* 3, 393–403. doi: 10.1111/j.1365-2184.1970.tb00347.x

Fu, Y., Azene, N., Xu, Y., and Kraitchman, D. L. (2011). Tracking stem cells for cardiovascular applications in vivo: focus on imaging techniques. *Imag. Med.* 3, 473–486. doi: 10.2217/iim.11.33

Gao, M., Chen, J., Lin, G., Li, S., Wang, L., Qin, A., et al. (2016). Long-term tracking of the osteogenic differentiation of mouse BMSCs by aggregation-induced emission nanoparticles. *ACS Appl. Mater.* 8, 17878–17884. doi: 10.1021/acsami.6b05471

Gao, Y., Cui, Y., Chan, J. K., and Xu, C. J. (2013). Stem cell tracking with optically active nanoparticles. *Am. J. Nucl. Med. Mol. Imag.* 3, 232–246.

Giljohann, D. A., Seferos, D. S., Daniel, W. L., Massich, M. D., Patel, P. C., and Mirkin, C. A. (2010). Gold nanoparticles for biology and medicine. *Angew Chem. Int. Ed Engl.* 49, 3280–3294.

Gliga, A. R., Skoglund, S., Wallinder, I. O., Fadeel, B., and Karlsson, H. L. (2014). Size-dependent cytotoxicity of silver nanoparticles in human lung cells: the role of cellular uptake, agglomeration and Ag release. *Part Fibre Toxicol.* 11:11. doi: 10.1186/1743-8977-11-11

Godin, B., Sakamoto, J. H., Serda, R. E., Grattoni, A., Bouamrani, A., and Ferrari, M. J. (2010). Emerging applications of nanomedicine for the diagnosis and treatment of cardiovascular diseases. *Trends Pharmacol. Sci.* 31, 199–205. doi: 10.1016/j.tips.2010.01.003

Goradel, N. H., Hour, F. G., Negahdari, B., Malekshahi, Z. V., Hashemzehi, M., Masoudifar, A., et al. (2018). Stem cell therapy: a new therapeutic option for cardiovascular diseases. *J. Cell Biochem.* 119, 95–104. doi: 10.1002/jcb.26169

Grauss, R. W., Winter, E. M., van Tuyn, J., Pijnappels, D. A., Steijn, R. V., Hogers, B., et al. (2007). Mesenchymal stem cells from ischemic heart disease patients improve left ventricular function after acute myocardial infarction. *Am. J. Physiol. Heart Circ. Physiol.* 293, H2438–H2447.

Gu, L., Li, X., Jiang, J., Guo, G., Wu, H., Wu, M., et al. (2018). Stem cell tracking using effective self-assembled peptide-modified superparamagnetic nanoparticles. *Nanoscale* 10, 15967–15979. doi: 10.1039/c7nr07618e

Guldris, N., Argibay, B. R., Gallo, J., Iglesias-Rey, R. N., Carbo-Argibay, E., Kolen'ko, Y. V., et al. (2017). Magnetite nanoparticles for stem cell labeling with high efficiency and long-term in vivo tracking. *Bioconjugate Chem.* 28, 362–370. doi: 10.1021/acs.bioconjchem.6b00522

Guo, B., Chen, J., Chen, N., Middha, E., Xu, S., Pan, Y., et al. (2019a). High-Resolution 3D NIR-II photoacoustic imaging of cerebral and tumor vasculatures using conjugated polymer nanoparticles as contrast agent. *Adv. Mater.* 31:1808355. doi: 10.1002/adma.201808355

Guo, B., Feng, Z., Hu, D., Xu, S., Middha, E., Pan, Y., et al. (2019b). Precise deciphering of brain vasculatures and microscopic tumors with dual NIR-II fluorescence and photoacoustic imaging. *Adv. Mater.* 31:1902504. doi: 10.1002/adma.201902504

Guo, Y., Yu, Y., Hu, S., Chen, Y., and Shen, Z. J. (2020). The therapeutic potential of mesenchymal stem cells for cardiovascular diseases. *J. Mol. Endocrinol.* 11, R109–R120.

Hachani, R., Birchall, M. A., Lowdell, M. W., Kasparis, G., Tung, L. D., Manshian, B. B., et al. (2017). Assessing cell-nanoparticle interactions by high content imaging of biocompatible iron oxide nanoparticles as potential contrast agents for magnetic resonance imaging. *Sci. Rep.* 7:7850.

Hahn, M. A., Singh, A. K., Sharma, P., Brown, S. C., and Moudgil, B. M. (2011). Nanoparticles as contrast agents for in-vivo bioimaging: current status and future perspectives. *Anal. Bioanal. Chem.* 399, 3–27. doi: 10.1007/s00216-010-4207-5

Hao, J., Zhu, W., Sheng, C., Yu, Y., and Zhou, Q. J. (2009). Human parthenogenetic embryonic stem cells: one potential resource for cell therapy. *Sci. China C Life Sci.* 52, 599–602. doi: 10.1007/s11427-009-0096-2

Hao, L., Zou, Z., Tian, H., Zhang, Y., Zhou, H., and Liu, L. J. (2014). Stem cell-based therapies for ischemic stroke. *Biomed. Res. Int.* 2014:468748.

Herschman, H. R. (2004). PET reporter genes for noninvasive imaging of gene therapy, cell tracking and transgenic analysis. *Crit. Rev. Oncol. Hematol.* 51, 191–204. doi: 10.1016/j.critrevonc.2004.04.006

Heslop, J. A., Hammond, T. G., Santeramo, I., Tort Piella, A., Hopp, I., Zhou, J., et al. (2015). Concise review: workshop review: understanding and assessing the risks of stem cell-based therapies. *Stem Cells Transl. Med.* 4, 389–400.

Hong, H., Yang, Y., Zhang, Y., and Cai, W. J. (2010). Non-invasive cell tracking in cancer and cancer therapy. *Curr. Top Med. Chem.* 10, 1237–1248. doi: 10.2174/156802610791384234

Hsiao, J. K., Tsai, C. P., Chung, T. H., Hung, Y., Yao, M., Liu, H. M., et al. (2008). Mesoporous silica nanoparticles as a delivery system of gadolinium for effective human stem cell tracking. *Small* 4, 1445–1452. doi: 10.1002/smll.200701316

Hsieh, S.-C., Wang, F.-F., Lin, C.-S., Chen, Y.-J., Hung, S.-C., and Wang, Y.-J. (2006). The inhibition of osteogenesis with human bone marrow mesenchymal stem cells by CdSe/ZnS quantum dot labels. *Biomaterials* 27, 1656–1664. doi: 10.1016/j.biomaterials.2005.09.004

Huang, D. M., Hung, Y., Ko, B. S., Hsu, S. C., Chen, W. H., Chien, C. L., et al. (2005). Highly efficient cellular labeling of mesoporous nanoparticles in human mesenchymal stem cells: implication for stem cell tracking. *FASEB J.* 19, 2014–2016. doi: 10.1096/fj.05-4288fje

Huang, J., Ning, X., Luo, W., Chen, M., Wang, Z., Zhang, W., et al. (2020). CT/NIRF dual-modal imaging tracking and therapeutic efficacy of transplanted mesenchymal stem cells labeled with Au nanoparticles in silica-induced pulmonary fibrosis. *J. Mater. Chem. B* 8, 1713–1727. doi: 10.1039/c9tb02652e

Idris, N. M., Li, Z., Ye, L., Sim, E. K. W., Mahendran, R., Ho, P. C.-L., et al. (2009). Tracking transplanted cells in live animal using upconversion fluorescent nanoparticles. *Biomaterials* 30, 5104–5113. doi: 10.1016/j.biomaterials.2009.05.062

Jaiswal, J. K., Goldman, E. R., Mattoussi, H., and Simon, S. M. (2004). Use of quantum dots for live cell imaging. *Nat. Methods* 1, 73–78. doi: 10.1038/nmeth1004-73

Jaiswal, S., Jamieson, C. H., Pang, W. W., Park, C. Y., Chao, M. P., Majeti, R., et al. (2009). CD47 is upregulated on circulating hematopoietic stem cells and leukemia cells to avoid phagocytosis. *Cell* 138, 271–285. doi: 10.1016/j.cell.2009.05.046

Jambhrunkar, S., Qu, Z., Popat, A., Yang, J., Noonan, O., Acauan, L., et al. (2014). Effect of surface functionality of silica nanoparticles on cellular uptake and cytotoxicity. *Mol. Pharm.* 11, 3642–3655. doi: 10.1021/mp500385n

Jiang, R., Liao, Y., Yang, F., Cheng, Y., Dai, X., and Chao, J. J. (2019). SPIO nanoparticle-labeled bone marrow mesenchymal stem cells inhibit pulmonary EndoMT induced by SiO2. *Exp. Cell Res.* 383:111492. doi: 10.1016/j.yexcr.2019.07.005

Jing, X.-H., Yang, L., Duan, X.-J., Xie, B., Chen, W., Li, Z., et al. (2008). In vivo MR imaging tracking of magnetic iron oxide nanoparticle labeled, engineered, autologous bone marrow mesenchymal stem cells following intra-articular injection. *Joint Bone Spine* 75, 432–438. doi: 10.1016/j.jbspin.2007.09.013

Kang, H., Zhang, K., Pan, Q., Lin, S., Wong, D. S. H., Li, J., et al. (2018). Remote control of intracellular calcium using upconversion nanotransducers regulates stem cell differentiation in vivo. *Adv. Funct. Mater.* 28:1802642. doi: 10.1002/adfm.201802642

Kastrup, J. J. (2011). Stem cells therapy for cardiovascular repair in ischemic heart disease: how to predict and secure optimal outcome? *EPMA J.* 2, 107–117. doi: 10.1007/s13167-011-0062-5

Khan, I., Saeed, K., and Khan, I. J. (2019). Nanoparticles: Properties, applications and toxicities. *Arabian J. Chem.* 12, 908–931. doi: 10.1016/j.arabjc.2017.05.011

Kim, H., Dae, H.-M., Park, C., Kim, E. O., Kim, D., Kim, I.-H., et al. (2011). A highly sensitive magnetite nanoparticle as a simple and rapid stem cell labelling agent for MRI tracking. *J. Mater. Chem.* 21, 7742–7747. doi: 10.1039/c1jm10247h

Kim, J., Shapiro, L., and Flynn, A. J. (2015a). The clinical application of mesenchymal stem cells and cardiac stem cells as a therapy for cardiovascular disease. *Pharmacol Ther.* 151, 8–15. doi: 10.1016/j.pharmthera.2015.02.003

Kim, K. S., Park, W., and Na, K. J. B. (2015b). Gadolinium-chelate nanoparticle entrapped human mesenchymal stem cell via photochemical internalization for cancer diagnosis. *Biomaterials* 36, 90–97. doi: 10.1016/j.biomaterials.2014.09.014

Kim, M. H., Lee, Y. J., and Kang, J. H. (2016a). Stem cell monitoring with a direct or indirect labeling method. *Nucl. Med. Mol. Imag.* 50, 275–283. doi: 10.1007/s13139-015-0380-y

Kim, S. J., Lewis, B., Steiner, M. S., Bissa, U. V., Dose, C., Frank, J. A., et al. (2016b). Superparamagnetic iron oxide nanoparticles for direct labeling of stem cells and in vivo MRI tracking. *Contrast Media Mol. Imag.* 11, 55–64. doi: 10.1002/cmmi.1658

Kircher, M. F., Gambhir, S. S., and Grimm, J. J. (2011). Noninvasive cell-tracking methods. *Nat. Rev. Clin. Oncol.* 8:677.

Kraitchman, D. L., and Bulte, J. W. J. A. (2009). In vivo imaging of stem cells and beta cells using direct cell labeling and reporter gene methods. *Arterioscler Thromb Vasc. Biol.* 29, 1025–1030. doi: 10.1161/atvbaha.108.165571

Krebsbach, P. H., and Robey, P. G. (2002). Dental and skeletal stem cells: potential cellular therapeutics for craniofacial regeneration. *J. Dent Educ.* 66, 766–773. doi: 10.1002/j.0022-0337.2002.66.6.tb03557.x

Laffey, M. K., Kubelick, K. P., Donnelly, E. M., and Emelianov, S. Y. (2020). Effects of freezing on mesenchymal stem cells labeled with gold nanoparticles. *Tissue Eng. Part C Methods* 26, 1–10. doi: 10.1089/ten.tec.2019.0198

Lankoff, A., Arabski, M., Wegierek-Ciuk, A., Kruszewski, M., Lisowska, H., Banasik-Nowak, A., et al. (2012). Effect of surface modification of silica nanoparticles on toxicity and cellular uptake by human peripheral blood lymphocytes in vitro. *Nanotoxicology* 7, 235–250. doi: 10.3109/17435390.2011.649796

Lee, H., Park, I., Kim, H., and Kim, S. J. (2009). Human neural stem cells overexpressing glial cell line-derived neurotrophic factor in experimental cerebral hemorrhage. *Gene Ther.* 16, 1066–1076. doi: 10.1038/gt.2009.51

Lee, S. H., Park, D. J., Yun, W. S., Park, J.-E., Choi, J. S., Key, J., et al. (2020). Endocytic trafficking of polymeric clustered superparamagnetic iron oxide nanoparticles in mesenchymal stem cells. *J. Control. Release* 326, 408–418. doi: 10.1016/j.jconrel.2020.07.032

Lee, S.-T., Chu, K., Park, J.-E., Lee, K., Kang, L., Kim, S. U., et al. (2005). Intravenous administration of human neural stem cells induces functional recovery in Huntington's disease rat model. *Neurosci. Res.* 52, 243–249. doi: 10.1016/j.neures.2005.03.016

Lewandowska-Łańcucka, J., Staszewska, M., Szuwarzyński, M., Kępczyński, M., Romek, M., Tokarz, W., et al. (2014). Synthesis and characterization of the superparamagnetic iron oxide nanoparticles modified with cationic chitosan and coated with silica shell. *J. Alloys Compounds* 586, 45–51. doi: 10.1016/j.jallcom.2013.10.039

Lewin, M., Carlesso, N., Tung, C.-H., Tang, X.-W., Cory, D., Scadden, D. T., et al. (2000). Tat peptide-derivatized magnetic nanoparticles allow in vivo tracking and recovery of progenitor cells. *Nat. Biotechnol.* 18, 410–414. doi: 10.1038/74464

Li, J., Lee, W. Y., Wu, T., Xu, J., Zhang, K., Li, G., et al. (2016). Multifunctional quantum dot nanoparticles for effective differentiation and long-term tracking of human mesenchymal stem cells in vitro and in vivo. *Adv. Healthc. Mater.* 5, 1049–1057. doi: 10.1002/adhm.201500879

Li, L., Jiang, W., Luo, K., Song, H., Lan, F., Wu, Y., et al. (2013). Superparamagnetic iron oxide nanoparticles as MRI contrast agents for non-invasive stem cell labeling and tracking. *Theranostics* 3, 595–615. doi: 10.7150/thno.5366

Li, Y., He, J., Wang, F., Ju, Z., Liu, S., Zhang, Y., et al. (2010). Differentiation of embryonic stem cells in adult bone marrow. *J. Genet. Genomics* 37, 431–439.

Li, Y., Song, Y., Zhao, L., Gaidosh, G., Laties, A. M., and Wen, R. J. (2008). Direct labeling and visualization of blood vessels with lipophilic carbocyanine dye DiI. *Nat. Protoc.* 3, 1703–1708. doi: 10.1038/nprot.2008.172

Liang, C., Wang, C., and Liu, Z. J. P. (2013). Stem cell labeling and tracking with nanoparticles. *Stem Cells Int.* 30, 1006–1017.

Liao, N., Wu, M., Pan, F., Lin, J., Li, Z., Zhang, D., et al. (2016). Poly (dopamine) coated superparamagnetic iron oxide nanocluster for noninvasive labeling, tracking, and targeted delivery of adipose tissue-derived stem cells. *Sci. Rep.* 6:18746.

Lilly, M. A., Davis, M. F., Fabie, J. E., Terhune, E. B., and Gallicano, G. I. (2016). Current stem cell based therapies in diabetes. *Am. J. Stem Cells* 5, 87–98.

Lim, S., Yoon, H. Y., Jang, H. J., Song, S., Kim, W., Park, J., et al. (2019). Dual-modal imaging-guided precise tracking of bioorthogonally labeled mesenchymal stem cells in mouse brain stroke. *ACS Nano* 13, 10991–11007. doi: 10.1021/acsnano.9b02173

Lin, W. (2015). *Introduction: Nanoparticles in Medicine.* Washington, DC: ACS Publications.

Liu, G., Wang, Z., Lu, J., Xia, C., Gao, F., Gong, Q., et al. (2011). Low molecular weight alkyl-polycation wrapped magnetite nanoparticle clusters as MRI probes for stem cell labeling and in vivo imaging. *Biomaterials* 32, 528–537. doi: 10.1016/j.biomaterials.2010.08.099

Loewen, N., Fautsch, M. P., Teo, W.-L., Bahler, C. K., Johnson, D. H., Poeschla, E. M., et al. (2004). Long-term, targeted genetic modification of the aqueous humor outflow tract coupled with noninvasive imaging of gene expression in vivo. *Invest. Ophthalmol. Vis. Sci.* 45, 3091–3098. doi: 10.1167/iovs.04-0366

Lu, C.-W., Hung, Y., Hsiao, J.-K., Yao, M., Chung, T.-H., Lin, Y.-S., et al. (2007). Bifunctional magnetic silica nanoparticles for highly efficient human stem cell labeling. *Nano Lett.* 7, 149–154. doi: 10.1021/nl0624263

Lusic, H., and Grinstaff, M. W. (2013). X-ray-computed tomography contrast agents. *Chem. Rev.* 113, 1641–1666. doi: 10.1021/cr200358s

Lv, F.-J., Tuan, R. S., Cheung, K. M., and Leung, V. Y. (2014). Concise review: the surface markers and identity of human mesenchymal stem cells. *Stem Cells* 32, 1408–1419. doi: 10.1002/stem.1681

Ma, Y., Ji, Y., You, M., Wang, S., Dong, Y., Jin, G., et al. (2016). Labeling and long-term tracking of bone marrow mesenchymal stem cells in vitro using NaYF4: Yb3+, Er3+ upconversion nanoparticles. *Acta Biomater.* 42, 199–208. doi: 10.1016/j.actbio.2016.07.030

Mahmoudi, M., Sant, S., Wang, B., Laurent, S., and Sen, T. J. (2011). Superparamagnetic iron oxide nanoparticles (SPIONs): development, surface modification and applications in chemotherapy. *Adv. Drug Delivery Rev.* 63, 24–46. doi: 10.1016/j.addr.2010.05.006

Maumus, M., Guérit, D., Toupet, K., Jorgensen, C., and Noël, D. J. (2011). Mesenchymal stem cell-based therapies in regenerative medicine: applications in rheumatology. *Stem Cells Res. Ther.* 2:14. doi: 10.1186/scrt55

Mazumder, S., Dey, R., Mitra, M., Mukherjee, S., and Das, G. J. (2009). Biofunctionalized quantum dots in biology and medicine. *J. Nanomaterials* 2009:815734.

McNamara, K., and Tofail, S. A. (2017). Nanoparticles in biomedical applications. *Adv. Phys.* 2, 54–88.

Meir, R., and Popovtzer, R. J. (2018). Cell tracking using gold nanoparticles and computed tomography imaging. Wiley Interdiscip. *Rev. Nanomed. Nanobiotechnol.* 10:e1480. doi: 10.1002/wnan.1480

Miguel, O. B., Gossuin, Y., Morales, M., Gillis, P., Muller, R., and Veintemillas-Verdaguer, S. J. (2007). Comparative analysis of the 1H NMR relaxation enhancement produced by iron oxide and core-shell iron–iron oxide nanoparticles. *Magn. Reson. Imaging* 25, 1437–1441. doi: 10.1016/j.mri.2007.04.006

Mikkola, H. K., and Orkin, S. H. J. D. (2006). The journey of developing hematopoietic stem cells. *Development* 133, 3733–3744. doi: 10.1242/dev.02568

Murphy, C. J., Gole, A. M., Stone, J. W., Sisco, P. N., Alkilany, A. M., Goldsmith, E. C., et al. (2008). Gold nanoparticles in biology: beyond toxicity to cellular imaging. *Acc. Chem. Res.* 41, 1721–1730. doi: 10.1021/ar800035u

Na, H. B., and Hyeon, T. J. (2009). Nanostructured T1 MRI contrast agents. *J. Mater. Chem.* 19, 6267–6273. doi: 10.1039/b902685a

Nafiujjaman, M., and Kim, T. (2020). Gold nanoparticles as a computed tomography marker for stem cell tracking. *Methods Mol. Biol.* 2126, 155–166. doi: 10.1007/978-1-0716-0364-2_14

Ni, Z., and Chen, R. (2015). Transcranial magnetic stimulation to understand pathophysiology and as potential treatment for neurodegenerative diseases. *Transl. Neurodegener.* 4:22. doi: 10.1186/s40035-015-0045-x

Park, W., Yang, H. N., Ling, D., Yim, H., Kim, K. S., Hyeon, T., et al. (2014). Multi-modal transfection agent based on monodisperse magnetic nanoparticles for stem cell gene delivery and tracking. *Biomaterials* 35, 7239–7247. doi: 10.1016/j.biomaterials.2014.05.010

Patrick, P. S., Kolluri, K. K., Thin, M. Z., Edwards, A., Sage, E. K., Sanderson, T., et al. (2020). Lung delivery of MSCs expressing anti-cancer protein TRAIL visualised with 89 Zr-oxine PET-CT. *Stem Cell Res. Ther.* 11:256.

Peng, X., Li, C., Bai, Y., Wang, X., Zhang, Y., An, Y., et al. (2018). Noninvasive evaluation of the migration effect of transplanted endothelial progenitor cells in ischemic muscle using a multimodal imaging agent. *Int. J. Nanomed.* 13, 1819–1829. doi: 10.2147/ijn.s152976

Perez, J. R., Ybarra, N., Chagnon, F., Serban, M., Lee, S., Seuntjens, J., et al. (2017). Tracking of mesenchymal stem cells with fluorescence endomicroscopy imaging in radiotherapy-induced lung injury. *Sci. Rep.* 7:40748.

Ratzinger, G., Agrawal, P., Körner, W., Lonkai, J., Sanders, H. M., Terreno, E., et al. (2010). Surface modification of PLGA nanospheres with Gd-DTPA and Gd-DOTA for high-relaxivity MRI contrast agents. *Biomaterials* 31, 8716–8723. doi: 10.1016/j.biomaterials.2010.07.095

Rawat, S., Gupta, S., Bhat, M., Dinda, A. K., and Mohanty, S. (2019). Efficient labeling of human mesenchymal stem cells using iron oxide nanoparticles. *Methods Mol. Biol.* 2150, 113–120. doi: 10.1007/7651_2019_265

Ren, N., Liang, N., Yu, X., Wang, A., Xie, J., and Sun, C. J. N. (2020). Ligand-free upconversion nanoparticles for cell labeling and their effects on stem cell differentiation. *Nanotechnology* 31:145101. doi: 10.1088/1361-6528/ab62cc

Rhyner, M. N., Smith, A. M., Gao, X., Mao, H., Yang, L., and Nie, S. (2006). Quantum dots and multifunctional nanoparticles: new contrast agents for tumor imaging. *Nanomedicine* 1, 209–217. doi: 10.2217/17435889.1.2.209

Riera, R., Feiner-Gracia, N., Fornaguera, C., Cascante, A., Borrós, S., and Albertazzi, L. J. N. (2019). Tracking the DNA complexation state of PBAE polyplexes in cells with super resolution microscopy. *Nanoscale* 11, 17869–17877. doi: 10.1039/c9nr02858g

Robert, P., Lehericy, S., Grand, S., Violas, X., Fretellier, N., Idée, J.-M., et al. (2015). T1-weighted hypersignal in the deep cerebellar nuclei after repeated administrations of gadolinium-based contrast agents in healthy rats: difference between linear and macrocyclic agents. *Invest. Radiol.* 50, 473–480. doi: 10.1097/rli.0000000000000181

Saha, K., Kim, S. T., Yan, B., Miranda, O. R., Alfonso, F. S., Shlosman, D., et al. (2013). Surface functionality of nanoparticles determines cellular uptake mechanisms in mammalian cells. *Small* 9, 300–305. doi: 10.1002/smll.201201129

Santelli, J., Lechevallier, S., Baaziz, H., Vincent, M., Martinez, C., Mauricot, R., et al. (2018). Multimodal gadolinium oxysulfide nanoparticles: a versatile contrast agent for mesenchymal stem cell labeling. *Nanoscale* 10, 16775–16786. doi: 10.1039/c8nr03263g

Santoso, M. R., and Yang, P. C. (2016). Magnetic nanoparticles for targeting and imaging of stem cells in myocardial infarction. *Stem Cells Int.* 2016:4198790.

Schmitz, N., Pfistner, B., Sextro, M., Sieber, M., Carella, A. M., Haenel, M., et al. (2002). Aggressive conventional chemotherapy compared with high-dose chemotherapy with autologous haemopoietic stem-cell transplantation for relapsed chemosensitive Hodgkin's disease: a randomised trial. *Lancet* 359, 2065–2071. doi: 10.1016/S0140-6736(02)08938-9

Sehl, O. C., Makela, A. V., Hamilton, A. M., and Foster, P. J. (2019). Trimodal cell tracking in vivo: combining iron-and fluorine-based magnetic resonance imaging with magnetic particle imaging to monitor the delivery of mesenchymal stem cells and the ensuing inflammation. *Tomography* 5, 367–376. doi: 10.18383/j.tom.2019.00020

Seleverstov, O., Zabirnyk, O., Zscharnack, M., Bulavina, L., Nowicki, M., Heinrich, J.-M., et al. (2006). Quantum dots for human mesenchymal stem cells labeling. a size-dependent autophagy activation. *Nano Lett.* 6, 2826–2832. doi: 10.1021/nl0619711

Shah, B. S., Clark, P. A., Moioli, E. K., Stroscio, M. A., and Mao, J. J. (2007). Labeling of mesenchymal stem cells by bioconjugated quantum dots. *Nano Lett.* 7, 3071–3079. doi: 10.1021/nl071547f

Shang, Y., Li, T., and Yu, G. J. (2017). Clinical applications of near-infrared diffuse correlation spectroscopy and tomography for tissue blood flow monitoring and imaging. *Physiol. Meas.* 38, R1–R26. doi: 10.1088/1361-6579/aa60b7

Sherry, A. D., Cacheris, W. P., and Kuan, K. T. (1988). Stability constants for Gd3+ binding to model DTPA-conjugates and DTPA-proteins: implications for their use as magnetic resonance contrast agents. *Magn. Reson. Med.* 8, 180–190. doi: 10.1002/mrm.1910080208

Shin, T. H., Lee, D. Y., Ketebo, A. A., Lee, S., Manavalan, B., Basith, S., et al. (2019). Silica-coated magnetic nanoparticles decrease human bone marrow-derived mesenchymal stem cell migratory activity by reducing membrane fluidity and impairing focal adhesion. *Nanomaterials* 9:1475. doi: 10.3390/nano9101475

Singh, N., Jenkins, G. J., Asadi, R., and Doak, S. H. (2010). Potential toxicity of superparamagnetic iron oxide nanoparticles (SPION). *Nano Rev.* 1:5358. doi: 10.3402/nano.v1i0.5358

Srivastava, D., and Ivey, K. N. (2006). Potential of stem-cell-based therapies for heart disease. *Nature* 441, 1097–1099. doi: 10.1038/nature04961

Stenudd, M., Sabelström, H., and Frisén, J. J. (2015). Role of endogenous neural stem cells in spinal cord injury and repair. *JAMA Neurol.* 72, 235–237. doi: 10.1001/jamaneurol.2014.2927

Su, X., Shen, Y., Weintraub, N. L., and Tang, Y. (2019). Imaging and tracking stem cell engraftment in ischemic hearts by near-infrared fluorescent protein (iRFP) labeling. *Methods Mol. Biol.* 2150, 121–129. doi: 10.1007/7651_2019_226

Sutton, E. J., Henning, T. D., Pichler, B. J., Bremer, C., and Daldrup-Link, H. E. (2008). Cell tracking with optical imaging. *Eur. Radiol.* 18, 2021–2032. doi: 10.1007/s00330-008-0984-z

Szpak, A., Kania, G., Skórka, T., Tokarz, W., Zapotoczny, S., and Nowakowska, M. J. (2013). Stable aqueous dispersion of superparamagnetic iron oxide nanoparticles protected by charged chitosan derivatives. *J. Nanopart. Res.* 15:1372. doi: 10.1007/s11051-012-1372-9

Temple, S. J. (2001). The development of neural stem cells. *Nature* 414, 112–117. doi: 10.1038/35102174

Tkaczyk, E. R. (2017). Innovations and developments in dermatologic non-invasive optical imaging and potential clinical applications. *Acta Derm. Venereol.* 128, 5–13. doi: 10.2340/00015555-2717

Trivedi, P., Tray, N., Nguyen, T., Nigam, N., and Gallicano, G. I. (2010). Mesenchymal stem cell therapy for treatment of cardiovascular disease: helping people sooner or later. *Stem Cells Dev.* 19, 1109–1120. doi: 10.1089/scd.2009.0465

Tseng, C.-L., Shih, I.-L., Stobinski, L., and Lin, F.-H. (2010). Gadolinium hexanedione nanoparticles for stem cell labeling and tracking via magnetic resonance imaging. *Biomaterials* 31, 5427–5435. doi: 10.1016/j.biomaterials.2010.03.049

Turjeman, K., Bavli, Y., Kizelsztein, P., Schilt, Y., Allon, N., Katzir, T. B., et al. (2015). Nano-Drugs based on nano sterically stabilized liposomes for the treatment of inflammatory neurodegenerative diseases. *PLoS One* 10:e0130442. doi: 10.1371/journal.pone.0130442

Uccelli, A., Moretta, L., and Pistoia, V. J. (2008). Mesenchymal stem cells in health and disease. *Nat. Rev. Immunol.* 8, 726–736. doi: 10.1038/nri2395

Vagnozzi, R. J., Maillet, M., Sargent, M. A., Khalil, H., Johansen, A. K. Z., Schwanekamp, J. A., et al. (2020). An acute immune response underlies the benefit of cardiac stem cell therapy. *Nature* 577, 405–409. doi: 10.1038/s41586-019-1802-2

Van Den Bos, E. J., Wagner, A., Mahrholdt, H., Thompson, R. B., Morimoto, Y., Sutton, B. S., et al. (2003). Improved efficacy of stem cell labeling for magnetic resonance imaging studies by the use of cationic liposomes. *Cell Transplant.* 12, 743–756. doi: 10.3727/000000003108747352

Walczak, P., and Bulte, J. W. (2007). The role of noninvasive cellular imaging in developing cell-based therapies for neurodegenerative disorders. *Neurodegener. Dis.* 4, 306–313. doi: 10.1159/000101887

Wang, C., Cheng, L., Xu, H., and Liu, Z. J. B. (2012a). Towards whole-body imaging at the single cell level using ultra-sensitive stem cell labeling with oligo-arginine modified upconversion nanoparticles. *Biomaterials* 33, 4872–4881. doi: 10.1016/j.biomaterials.2012.03.047

Wang, C., Ma, X., Ye, S., Cheng, L., Yang, K., Guo, L., et al. (2012b). Protamine functionalized single-walled carbon nanotubes for stem cell labeling and in vivo raman/magnetic resonance/photoacoustic triple-modal imaging. *Adv. Funct. Mater.* 22, 2363–2375. doi: 10.1002/adfm.201200133

Wang, F., Banerjee, D., Liu, Y., Chen, X., and Liu, X. J. A. (2010). Upconversion nanoparticles in biological labeling, imaging, and therapy. *Analyst* 135, 1839–1854. doi: 10.1039/c0an00144a

Wang, Y., Xu, C., and Ow, H. J. T. (2013). Commercial nanoparticles for stem cell labeling and tracking. *Theranostics* 3:544. doi: 10.7150/thno.5634

Wu, C., Li, J., Pang, P., Liu, J., Zhu, K., Li, D., et al. (2014). Polymeric vector-mediated gene transfection of MSCs for dual bioluminescent and MRI tracking in vivo. *Biomaterials* 35, 8249–8260. doi: 10.1016/j.biomaterials.2014.06.014

Wu, Y., Chen, L., Scott, P. G., and Tredget, E. E. (2007). Mesenchymal stem cells enhance wound healing through differentiation and angiogenesis. *Stem Cells* 25, 2648–2659. doi: 10.1634/stemcells.2007-0226

Xie, B., Gu, P., Wang, W., Dong, C., Zhang, L., Zhang, J., et al. (2016). Therapeutic effects of human umbilical cord mesenchymal stem cells transplantation on hypoxic ischemic encephalopathy. *Am. J. Transl. Res.* 8:3241.

Xie, Y., Liu, W., Zhang, B., Wang, B., Wang, L., Liu, S., et al. (2019). Systematic intracellular biocompatibility assessments of superparamagnetic iron oxide nanoparticles in human umbilical cord mesenchyme stem cells in testifying its reusability for inner cell tracking by MRI. *J. Biomed. Nanotechnol.* 15, 2179–2192. doi: 10.1166/jbn.2019.2845

Yao, M., Shi, X., Zuo, C., Ma, M., Zhang, L., Zhang, H., et al. (2020). Engineering of SPECT/Photoacoustic imaging/antioxidative stress triple-function nanoprobe for advanced mesenchymal stem cell therapy of cerebral ischemia. *ACS Appl. Mater. Interfaces* 12, 37885–37895. doi: 10.1021/acsami.0c10500

Ye, L., Chang, Y.-H., Xiong, Q., Zhang, P., Zhang, L., Somasundaram, P., et al. (2014). Cardiac repair in a porcine model of acute myocardial infarction with human induced pluripotent stem cell-derived cardiovascular cells. *Cell Stem Cell* 15, 750–761. doi: 10.1016/j.stem.2014.11.009

Ye, L., Haider, H. K., and Sim, E. K. (2006). Adult stem cells for cardiac repair: a choice between skeletal myoblasts and bone marrow stem cells. *Exp. Biol. Med.* 231, 8–19. doi: 10.1177/153537020623100102

Yi, D. K., Nanda, S. S., Kim, K., and Selvan, S. T. (2017). Recent progress in nanotechnology for stem cell differentiation, labeling, tracking and therapy. *J. Mater. Chem. B* 5, 9429–9451. doi: 10.1039/C7TB02532G

Yin, C., Wen, G., Liu, C., Yang, B., Lin, S., Huang, J., et al. (2018). Organic semiconducting polymer nanoparticles for photoacoustic labeling and tracking of stem cells in the second near-infrared window. *ACS Nano* 12, 12201–12211. doi: 10.1021/acsnano.8b05906

Young, H. E., and Black, A. C. (2004). Adult stem cells. *Anat. Rec. A Discov. Mol. Cell Evol. Biol.* 276, 75–102. doi: 10.1002/ar.a.10134

Yukawa, H., and Baba, Y. J. A. C. (2017). In vivo fluorescence imaging and the diagnosis of stem cells using quantum dots for regenerative medicine. *Anal. Chem.* 89, 2671–2681. doi: 10.1021/acs.analchem.6b04763

Zampelas, A., and Magriplis, E. J. (2020). Dietary patterns and risk of cardiovascular diseases: a review of the evidence. *Proc. Nutr. Soc.* 79, 68–75. doi: 10.1017/S0029665119000946

Zhang, L., Gu, F., Chan, J., Wang, A., Langer, R., Farokhzad, O. J., et al. (2008). Nanoparticles in medicine: therapeutic applications and developments. *Clin. Pharmacol. Ther.* 83, 761–769. doi: 10.1038/sj.clpt.6100400

Zhang, S. J., and Wu, J. C. (2007). Comparison of imaging techniques for tracking cardiac stem cell therapy. *J. Nucl. Med.* 48, 1916–1919. doi: 10.2967/jnumed.107.043299

Zhang, Z., Hancock, B., Leen, S., Ramaswamy, S., Sollott, S. J., Boheler, K. R., et al. (2010). Compatibility of superparamagnetic iron oxide nanoparticle labeling for 1H MRI cell tracking with 31P MRS for bioenergetic measurements. *NMR Biomed.* 23, 1166–1172. doi: 10.1002/nbm.1545

Zhao, L., Kutikov, A., Shen, J., Duan, C., Song, J., and Han, G. J. T. (2013). Stem cell labeling using polyethylenimine conjugated (α-NaYbF4: Tm3+)/CaF2 upconversion nanoparticles. *Theranostics* 3, 249–257. doi: 10.7150/thno.5432

Zheng, Y., Huang, J., Zhu, T., Li, R., Wang, Z., Ma, F., et al. (2017). Stem cell tracking technologies for neurological regenerative medicine purposes. *Stem Cells Int.* 2017:2934149. doi: 10.1155/2017/2934149

Zhu, D., Liu, F., Ma, L., Liu, D., and Wang, Z. J. (2013). Nanoparticle-based systems for T1-weighted magnetic resonance imaging contrast agents. *Int. J. Mol. Sci.* 14, 10591–10607. doi: 10.3390/ijms140510591

17

New Forms of Electrospun Nanofibers Applied in Cardiovascular Field

Weimin Huang [1,2], Mengen Huo [3], Nan Cheng [2] and Rong Wang [2]*

[1] Baotou Clinical Medical College, Inner Mongolia Medical University, Hohhot, China, [2] Department of Cardiac Surgery, Chinese PLA General Hospital, Beijing, China, [3] Institute of Poisons and Drugs, Beijing Academy of Military Medical Sciences, Beijing, China

***Correspondence:**
Rong Wang
wangrongd@126.com

Cardiovascular disease (CVD) is one of the leading causes of death worldwide. In recent years, regenerative medicine, tissue engineering and the development of new materials have become the focus of attention this field, and electrospinning technology to prepare nanofibrous materials for the treatment of cardiovascular diseases has attracted people's attention. Unlike previous reviews, this research enumerates the experimental methods and applications of electrospinning technology combined with nanofibrous materials in the directions of myocardial infarction repair, artificial heart valves, artificial blood vessels and cardiovascular patches from the perspective of cardiovascular surgery. In the end, this review also summarizes the limitations, unresolved technical challenges, and possible future directions of this technology for cardiovascular disease applications.

Keywords: electrospinning (ES), nanofibers (NFs), cardiac patch, vascular transplantation, tissue engineering

INTRODUCTION

In 1985, Weinstein and Stason (1) have reported that coronary heart disease (CHD) is the leading cause of death and disability in the United States. One in five Americans develops CHD on their sixtieth birthday. Of these, 11% did die suddenly and another 44% suffered a non-fatal myocardial infarction, with an economic burden of well-over $100 billion.

In today's society, cardiovascular disease is still the leading cause of death throughout the world, causing more than 17.9 million deaths each year (2). According to the American Heart Association (AHA) estimates, by 2035, 46.1% of the US population will have some form of cardiovascular disease, when the total cost associated with cardiovascular disease will be 1.1 trillion dollars (3), which is enough to see the great harm and burden of cardiovascular disease to humans.

Myocardial infarction is usually due to the lack of oxygen and nutrients in the myocardium, resulting in the death of cardiomyocytes (4). The myocardial tissue after infarction lacks the ability of regeneration. Implanting tissue-engineered myocardium into diseased heart seems to be the simplest way to repair infarcted myocardium. At present, the limitations of myocardial tissue regeneration include the inability to fully summarize the structure and mechanical environment of natural heart tissue (5). Scaffolds made of electrospinning nanofibers have been actively explored for myocardial tissue regeneration.

As shown in the **Figure 1**, in order to improve the survival rate of stem cells in repairing myocardial injury, electrospinning scaffolds are used to mechanically support and mimic extracellular matrix structure to improve cell adhesion, viability, and regeneration (6).

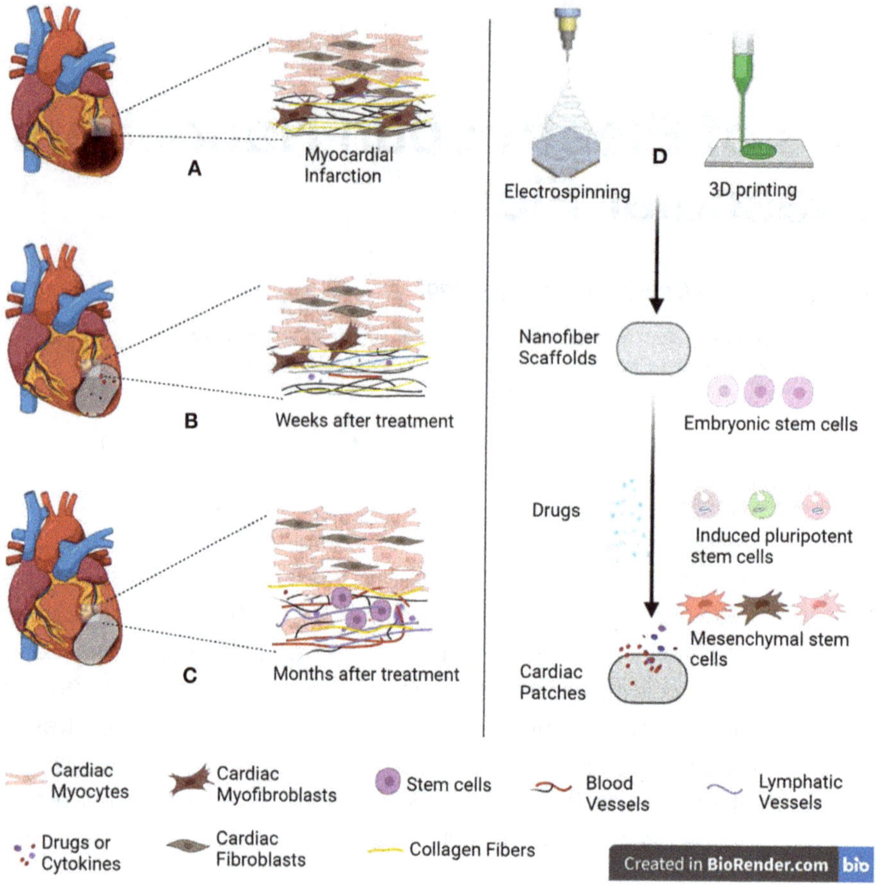

FIGURE 1 | Schematic diagram of cardiac patch repairing myocardial infarction. **(A)** When myocardial infarction occurs, collagen fibers proliferate and form scar tissue. **(B)** Several weeks after treatment. **(C)** Several months after treatment. **(D)** Cardiac patch is made by electrospinning combined with 3D printing technology. The patch simulates extracellular matrix (ECM) to provide mechanical support for cells. Created with BioRender.com.

More than 50% of all deaths caused by CVD are attributed to vascular injury induced by vascular plaque aggregation, which leads to vascular obstruction and sclerosis (7). People have been trying to develop appropriate alternative vessels from autologous vascular transplantation, allografts and synthetic grafts. However, these sources could not meet the needs of alternative vessels, especially the long-term patency rate of small-diameter vascular transplantation has always been a difficult problem in the world (8).

For more than 50 years, conventional coronary artery bypass grafting (CABG) has been the gold standard for the treatment of coronary heart disease (9). There are hundreds of thousands of coronary artery bypass procedures in the world each year, for small diameter grafts (<6 mm), these synthetic grafts often failed due to rapid occlusion and thrombosis, so there is still no effective alternative to autologous vascular grafting (10, 11).

The patency and biocompatibility of small-diameter vascular grafts synthesized by traditional tissue engineering strategies are poor (32), and their clinical transformation is seriously limited by high cost and long production time (20). In recent years, tissue engineering using rapidly degradable materials can induce the regeneration potential of the host, and summarize natural tissue regeneration through reasonable graft design, including structural optimization (30, 33) and functionalization (5, 34).

It is not only required that the small-diameter vascular stent should have the characteristics of maintaining the blood flow in the lumen without leakage, but also that it should have anticoagulant and antithrombotic ability in function to prevent stenosis and occlusion (35). Therefore, many researchers are engaged in electrospinning technology to prepare grafts with different materials, and study the methods to promote the proliferation of vascular intimal endothelial cells and control the proliferation of smooth muscle cells (SMCs). The general method is to fold the electrospinning membrane into a tubular structure through a rolling rod collector, and load heparin (22), growth factors (36) and other active substances (37) on its surface for the study of vascular tissue regeneration. As shown in the **Table 1**, Animal models, included rat abdominal aorta (19, 20, 29), rabbit carotid artery (21–23, 29), sheep carotid artery (31) and canine femoral artery (38), are often used to test the performance of vascular stents, ranging from several weeks to months.

TABLE 1 | Construction strategies and *vivo/vitro* experiments of electrospun fiber membrane in the reviews.

Nanofiber materials	Diameter/Aperture	Thickness (μm)	Drugs or cells	Animals	Experiments	Time (weeks)	References
PCL	Inner: 300 ± 100 nm Out: 2.8 ± 0.13 μm	100 μm	Cardiomyocytes /fibroblasts	Mice	*In vitro*	1	(12)
PLGA	N/A	110 ± 10μm	Endothelial cells, VEGF granules, dexamethasone	Mice	Cardiac patch	2	(13)
PCL-Gelatin	578 ± 184 nm	115 ± 11 μm	hiPSC-CMs	N/A	*In vitro*	2	(6)
PCL	200–5,500 nm	50 μm	Bone marrow and heart stem cells	Mice	LAD in rats (suture)	3	(14)
β-PVDF	N/A	N/A	TiO2	N/A	*In vitro*	6*	(15)
AuNRs	500 nm/20–60 nm	60–80/100–120 μm	Left ventricular cardiomyocytes	Mice	Cardiac patch (Near IR)	1	(16)
PCL/GelMA-Ppy nanoparticles	948 ± 153 nm	N/A	Cardiomyocytes/fibroblasts	Mice	Cardiac patch 1.5 × 1.5cm	4	(17)
PCL/NO	690 nm/3.4 μm	600 μm	NO_2	Mice	Cardiac patch 0.4 × 0.6cm	4	(18)
PCL/Heparin coating	-/21.2 ± 0.79 μm	295 ± 5.52 μm	Heparin	Mice	Aortic replacement	3	(19)
PLCL	6 μm/300 nm	500 μm	Hyaluronan	Mice	Aortic replacement	24	(20)
PELCL/chitosan-hydrogel	Inner: 754 ± 385 nm Out: 1,087 ± 526 nm	N/A	Inner: VEGF Out: PDGF	Rabbits	Carotid artery transplantation	4	(21)
PLCL	821 ± 102.87 nm	300 ± 17 μm	Heparin / Silk Fibroin	Rabbits	Carotid artery transplantation	32	(22)
PCL	263.1 ± 90.2 nm	N/A	KSNO	Rabbits	Carotid artery transplantation	4	(23)
PLA-PCL	N/A	40 ± 7/175 ± 4 μm	Human fibroblast	N/A	*In vitro*	8	(24)
ADF4(C16)	1.6 ± 0.2 μm	N/A	N/A	Mice	Arteriovenous loop model	4	(25)
ESM/TPU	435.86 ± 173.27 nm	50–70 μm	HUVEC	N/A	*In vitro*	1	(26)
CS-PVA-CNT	255 ± 3.5 nm	N/A	MSCs	N/A	*In vitro*	3	(11)
CS/PLCL	110.09 ± 16.33nm	50 μm	Dextran Sulfate	Mice	*In vivo*	4	(27)
SF/TPU	N/A	100–500 μm	SF (Silk Fibroin)	Dogs	Aortic wall repair 2 × 1 cm	12	(28)
SF/PU	1.32 ± 0.78 μm	100 μm	SF (Silk Fibroin)	Mice	Aortic wall repair, 0.3 × 0.6 cm	24	(29)
PLA/PCL PU/PCL	N/A	15.47 ± 1.31 μm 127.87 ± 2.38 μm 19.96 ± 1.18 μm	HUVCEs/VSMCs	N/A	*In vitro* evaluation, 0.6 cm	1	(30)
PCL/collagen scaffolds	4.45 ± 0.81 μm	400 μm	ECs/SMCs	Sheep	Carotid artery, 4.75 mm × 5 cm	24	(31)
PELCL/chitosan hydrogel	754 ± 385 nm 1,124 ± 529 nm	N/A	VEGF/PDGF	Rabbits	Carotid artery, 2.2mm	4	(21)

PCL, polycaprolactone; PLCL, poly(L-Lactide-co-caprolactone); PLGA, poly-lactic-co-glycolic acid; β-PVDF, β-polyvinylidene fluoride; AuNRs, albumin electrospinning fibers and gold nanorods; GelMA-Ppy, methacrylic anhydride-gelatin-polypyrrole; PELCL, poly-(ethylene glycol)-b-poly(L-lactide-co-caprolactone); PLA-PCL, poly-L-lactide-co-poly-ε-caprolactone; KSNO, NO donor of S-nitrosated keratin; ADF4(C16), one of the spider silk protein; ESM/TPU, double-layered eggshell membrane/thermoplastic polyurethane; CS-PVA-CNT, chitosan, polyvinyl alcohol, carbon nanotube; HUVEC, human umbilical vein endothelial cell; MSCs, mesenchymal stem cells; VEGF, vascular endothelial growth factor; PDGF, platelet-derived growth factor; ECs, endothelial cells; SMCs, smooth cells.
The "" symbol represents the unit of data mentioned in the literature as hours, not weeks. The "N/A" symbol is not available which means that the data cannot be extracted or not mentioned in this article.*

With the development of tissue engineering technologies in recent years, a series of nanofibrous materials based on electrospinning technology have attracted much attention of researchers (39).

In the field of cardiovascular tissue regeneration, compared with traditional regeneration technology, electrospinning technology has the following advantages:

1. The cardiac patches loaded with stem cells can repair the infarcted myocardial region without limiting the later cardiac systolic activity.
2. Simulating the unique physical structure of natural cardiac leaflets, the leaflet structure with the same anisotropy and mechanical strength is provided.

3. The vascular scaffold can be used to match the proliferation of vascular endothelial cells with the degradation of the material, so as to ensure a higher patency rate.
4. It can provide intelligent health monitoring function, which can early evaluate and prevent acute and chronic cardiovascular diseases.

In this study, we would focus on nanofibers, introduce the progress of different electrospinning technologies in the field of heart and vessel-related tissue engineering, compare the effect of some nanofiber materials, and forecast the development of electrospinning technology in the field of cardiovascular medicine and the problems to be broken through.

Myocardial Infarction Repair

From the microstructure,Sharon Fleischer (12) divided the myocardium into three fiber groups with specific effect and different sizes: nanoscale endomysial fibers, perimysial fibers with a diameter of 1 μm and epimysium fibers with a diameter of several microns. He also reported that the electrospinning fiber stent with spring-like coiled fiber structure was conducive to cardiac tissue engineering. Later, the team (13) designed a cage structure with microgrooves and sidewall microchannel albumin stent to arrange the cardiac tissue and accommodate the growth of endothelial cells. This cage structure can also accommodate the particle system, control the release of VEGF, promote vascularization, and even load dexamethasone drugs to achieve the effect. In addition, Zhu et al. (18) mixed the polymer caprolactone with caprolactone NO_2 to prepare nitric acid-functionalized cardiac patches to implant the site of myocardial infarction using the electrospinning method. The results showed that NO was gradually released from the patch under ischemic microenvironment, and the effect of NO patch group was significant. What attracts our attention is an aligned polycaprolactone (PCL) -Gelatin coaxial nanofiber patch was fabricated by Kuma (6) using electrospinning. The results show that cells on cardiac patches exhibit synchronous contraction and exhibit a rapid response to cardiac drugs. The patches could be scaled to serve as an *in vitro* drug screening platform for cardiotoxicity studies.

Despite some success with cell-loading techniques, many scaffolds have limited cell infiltration and low cell survival (40). In order to overcome the limited cell infiltration of cardiac patches and also consider the supporting mechanical properties of these patches, Chen and Kan (14) designed the thickness of the patches to about 50 μm. Both bone marrow and human cardiac stem cells cultured on these patches had good survival and infiltration (~30 μm). In addition, the tensile strength of the patch could withstand the severe pumping effect of myocardium, confirming that the material prepared by this method has the potential to be used as a scaffold for cardiomyocyte repair and application. Unlike the above ideas, the glycosaminoglycan (GAG) mimetic peptide nanofiber gel synthesized by Rufaihah et al. (41) was injected into the infarct site, emphasizing its approach of repairing the myocardium and inducing neovascularization without adding any biologically derived factors or stem cells. This predicts the possibility of electrospinning technology combined with nanofibrous hydrogels in tissue engineering.

In order to avoid the problem of additional damage caused by suturing the patch to the heart using surgical means in the past, Malki et al. (16) developed a nanocomposite scaffold composed of albumin electrospinning fibers and gold nanorods (AuNRs), which was positioned and irradiated with a near-infrared laser (808 nm), and AuNRs were able to absorb light and convert it into thermal energy, locally change the molecular structure of the fibrous scaffold, eventually attach it strongly but safely to the heart wall. Subsequently, He et al. (17) were inspired by mussels to design conductive nanofibrous membranes to repair myocardial infarction by enhancing cardiac function and revascularization. The result showed that 4 weeks after patch transplantation on the infarcted heart, the infarct size was reduced by about 50%, the percentage of left ventricular fraction was increased by about 20%, and the density of neovascularization in the infarcted area was significantly increased by about 9-fold compared with the control group.

In order for the patches to exhibit mechanical and conductive properties similar to those of autologous myocardium, Walker et al. (42) developed cardiac gaskets, first of which was gelatin methacryloyl (GelMA), followed by highly adhesive fibrous scaffolds modified with conjugated choline-based biological ionic liquids (bio-IL), based on the formation of ionic bonds between Bio-IL and native tissue, and the engineered patches adhered strongly to rat myocardium without suturing.

In order to establish a model for evaluating the performance of engineered heart *in vitro*, Polylactic acid (PLA) and poly-ε-caprolactone (PCL) were used to fabricate the porous scaffold via 3D printing and electrospinning, and then cardiomyocytes from neonatal Sprague Dawley (SD) rats were cultured on the PLA/PCL scaffold to construct the engineered cardiac tissue (ECT). The strength and biocompatibility of the scaffold were verified via evaluating the cell viability and mechanical beating status (43). This work provides a new approach for evaluating ECT, which is expected to be applied to pharmaceutical studies.

Tissue Engineering of Heart Valves

At present, biological valves also have some limitations, especially in young patients, so it is critical to continue to develop new materials. But heart valve tissue engineering still faces challenges, for example, the valve component has three layers, which are circumferential, random and radial, respectively, which increases the difficulty of material preparation. Wu et al. (44) began to believe that the hydrogel system of methacrylic hyaluronic acid (Me-HA) and methacrylate gelatin (Me-Gel) mixed with each other can simulate the unique 3D physiological microenvironment of the ECM of native aortic valve leaflets, but it was later found that these hydrogel materials lacked macroscopic anisotropic structure and had weak extension ability, so it was thought to compensate for the disadvantages of hydrogels by adding fibrous components.

In order to better simulate the direction, Jana and Lerman (45) from Mayo Clinic firstly designed three new collectors to fabricate three nanofiber layers with these directions from polymeric biomaterials in electrospinning systems.

Cardiac Surgeries

In order to develop a new generation of biomaterials for closure of atrial septal defect, Kaiser firstly designed chamber-deficient patches using medical grade polyurethane loaded with bioactive agents chitosan nanoparticles and collagen, followed by coating with heparin (46). In the postoperative aspect of cardiac surgery, sternal and epicardial adhesions increase the risk and complexity of cardiac reoperation, which is a significant challenge for the later rehabilitation of all patients who underwent cardiac surgery again. Feng et al. (47) fabricated a bioabsorbable GT/PCL composite membrane to prevent adhesions in cardiac surgery in a rabbit model and proposed its use as a novel pericardial substitute for cardiac surgery.

Small-Caliber Vascular Grafts

At present, there are practical non-tissue engineered grafts for large vessels in clinical practice, but doctors often face failure in front of small-caliber vascular grafts due to the easy thrombosis. To prevent thrombosis, Zhang et al. (21) developed two modified coaxial electrospinning techniques, which are to achieve vascular compliance. Interestingly, previous studies have been observed in vascular transplantation experiments for a maximum of 3 months (19), while Qin et al. (20) reported the time up to 6 months. They agreed that the vascular smooth muscle layer is essential for maintaining the mechanical strength and vasoactive reactivity of blood vessels, so hyaluronic acid was loaded on rapidly biodegradable vascular grafts in the study and concluded that it promotes vascular smooth muscle regeneration.

However, Kuang et al. (22) considered that smooth muscle cells (SMCs) are prone to excessive proliferation and cause restenosis at the late stage of implantation. In order to develop a safe and unobstructed artificial blood vessel, they prepared a small-caliber artificial blood vessel with composite nanofiber nucleocapsid structure by a combination of conjugated electrospinning and lyophilization technology. The inner layer provides mechanical support during vascular reconstruction. The shell, heparin/silk fibroin layer, enhances the biocompatibility of the graft, and the release of heparin at the early stage after transplantation can regulate the microenvironment, promote endothelial cell growth and inhibit smooth muscle proliferation. This animal experiment showed that the graft patency time remained more than 8 months, which far exceeded 3 months which Wu has reported (19).

In order to better promote the endo-thelialization of transplanted vessels and simulate the extracellular matrix, hyaluronic acid oligosaccharide-modified collagen was fabricated into nanofibers by electrospinning technique in Kang et al. (48) from Shandong University. The *in vitro* experimental results supported that it promoted endothelial cell proliferation and had antithrombotic properties. Lee et al. (39) of Seoul University encapsulated human ASC spheres in alginate-based scaffolding structures by a combined 3D printing/electrospinning system. In order to treat peripheral arterial occlusive disease, Dorati preliminarily explored the replacement of artificial blood vessels in damaged peripheral arteries, which showed that the electrospinning technique was suitable for obtaining grafts $<6\,\text{mm}$ in diameter and between 140 ± 7 and $175 \pm 4\,\mu\text{m}$ in thickness. Finally, vascular grafts with the best mechanical properties similar to natural bovine blood vessels were designed (24).

In order to reduce the toxicity of transplanted blood vessels, Li et al. (23) synthesized a low-toxic NO donor of S-nitrosated keratin (KSNO) and then co-electrospinning with poly-ε-caprolactone to obtain NO-releasing small-diameter vascular grafts. In order to improve the biocompatibility of transplantation, Yan et al. (26) reported a wavy structure of small-diameter, double-layered eggshell membrane/thermoplastic polyurethane (ESM/TPU) vascular graft.

It is not easy to maintain good supporting performance of transplanted blood vessels and make their cell adhesion strong. To obtain vascular graft with stronger mechanical properties and cell-guided growth ability, Liu has developed a biomimetic three-layer vascular graft with strong mechanical properties and cell-guided growth ability (30).

Of course, the strategy of vascular tissue engineering is eventually to combine autologous vascular cells with tubular biodegradable scaffolds, and Ju et al. did manufacture vascular substitutes (31). This study demonstrates that electrospinning double-layer vascular scaffolds combined with autologous vascular cells may be a clinically applicable alternative to conventional graft substitutes.

Vascular Patches

Vascular patches currently used in cardiovascular surgery have several disadvantages, including material degeneration, calcification, and pseudointimal hyperplasia leading to hemodynamic disturbances (28). Initially Chantawong et al. (29) created three patches of different composition using an electrospinning method, all of which were made of a combination of silk fibroin (SF) and a synthetic polymer thermoplastic polyurethane (TPU). They implanted each type of patch ($n = 18$) into the abdominal aorta of rats and assessed histopathology at 1, 3, and 6 months after implantation, and concluded that the increase in SF concentration in SF/PU patches had a positive effect on vascular remodeling. Later, Shimada et al. (28) in the team replaced part of the descending aortic wall of the dog with SF/TPU patches for this experiment, and the patches were removed 3 months later for histological examination.

Surgical Induction of Angiogenesis

Although encouraging results have now been achieved with tissue engineering, the short-term integration of tissue-engineered constructs with the host vasculature remains one of the major obstacles (25). In addition to integrating endothelial cells (49) or angiogenic growth factors (50), surgery-induced angiogenesis appears to be a promising strategy to improve vascularization. In 1980, Erol and Sira (51) demonstrated that neovascularization of the skin through arteriovenous fistula is possible. A vascular bed can be created by use of long inter-positional vein grafts. In 2019, Steiner conducted a similar experiment which resulted that spider silk proteins have good biocompatibility and slow biodegradation, thinner electrospinning fibers showed faster biodegradation and vascularization (25).

DISCUSSION

Limitations and Challenges

In the past two decades, through electrospinning technology, cell-loaded nanofiber scaffolds have been widely studied in wound healing (52), drug delivery (53), and cardiac patches (14, 15, 46, 54–56) have shown good performance in preclinical studies of cardiac repair, there are still many problems before clinical implementation (57), such as cardiac patch therapy currently requiring open-heart surgery, which causes anxiety in most patients with myocardial infarction (58), low degree of cell infiltration and cell survival on electrospinning scaffolds (40, 59), insufficient mechanical support performance (60), and biocompatibility that cannot meet clinical needs (61).

The current nanofiber scaffold technology is plagued by some limitations that must be overcome in order to produce highly functional and treatment-related functional engineered cardiac tissues (fECTs), including: (1) Low porosity hinders the deep penetration of seed cells, (2) When cardiomyocytes are cultured on a rigid substrate mimicking a post-infarct fibrotic scar, they lose their synchronized beating, and (3) It is difficult to expand the technology currently used in human applications (62, 63).

In terms of small vessel tissue engineering, Kuang et al. transplanted composite nanofibrous small vessel grafts prepared by a combination of conjugated electrospinning and lyophilization techniques into rabbit carotid arteries (22). Although this team considers matching the degradation rate of vascular stents with the rate of tissue remodeling, it remains a challenge to synchronize the stent degradation rate and new tissue formation rate over a period of time (64, 65).

Potential Development Direction of Electrospinning

The primary goal of electrospinning technology in cardiovascular tissue regeneration is to prepare good biomimetic scaffolds *in vitro* to regenerate myocardium or vascular tissue and restore their function, and then study their biocompatibility and specific function *in vivo* tests (11, 27).

We may try to do the combination of electrospinning with nanofiber hydrogels (66) to improve their mechanical properties. We can also continue to develop more 3D printed scaffolds as templates to promote cardiomyocyte infiltration (67).

The continuously updated electrospinning technology will certainly promote the development of cardiovascular tissue engineering, such as the melt electrospinning fabricated sinusoidal fibers showing great potential in cardiac tissue regeneration (68, 69).

AUTHOR CONTRIBUTIONS

WH wrote the text of this review paper with guidance from RW. NC and MH made valuable suggestions. All authors have reviewed the final version and approved of the content in this manuscript.

ACKNOWLEDGMENTS

All authors hereby thank Professor Yunze Long and his student Yuan Gao from Qingdao University for their constructive suggestions and great help in this paper.

REFERENCES

Weinstein MC, Stason WB. Cost-effectiveness of interventions to prevent or treat coronary heart disease. *Annu Rev Public Health.* (1985) 6:41– 63. doi: 10.1146/annurev.pu.06.050185.000353

Roth GA, Johnson C, Abajobir A, Abd-Allah F, Abera SF, Abyu G, et al. Global, regional, and national burden of cardiovascular diseases for 10 causes, 1990 to 2015. *J Am Coll Cardiol.* (2017) 70:1–25. doi: 10.1016/j.jacc.2017.04.052

Benjamin EJ, Virani SS, Callaway CW, Chamberlain AM, Chang AR, Cheng S, et al. Heart disease and stroke statistics-2018 update: a report from the american heart association. *Circulation.* (2018) 137:e67– 492. doi: 10.1161/CIR.0000000000000573

Lodrini AM, Goumans MJ. Cardiomyocytes cellular phenotypes after myocardial infarction. *Front Cardiovasc Med.* (2021) 8:750510. doi: 10.3389/fcvm.2021.750510

Weinberger F, Mannhardt I, Eschenhagen T. Engineering cardiac muscle tissue: a maturating field of research. *Circ Res.* (2017) 120:1487–500. doi: 10.1161/CIRCRESAHA.117.310738

Kumar N, Sridharan D, Palaniappan A, Dougherty JA, Czirok A, Isai DG, et al. Scalable biomimetic coaxial aligned nanofiber cardiac patch: a potential model for "clinical trials in a dish". *Front Bioeng Biotechnol.* (2020) 8:567842. doi: 10.3389/fbioe.2020.567842

Gui L, Dash BC, Luo J, Qin L, Zhao L, Yamamoto K, et al. Implantable tissue-engineered blood vessels from human induced pluripotent stem cells. *Biomaterials.* (2016) 102:120–9. doi: 10.1016/j.biomaterials.2016.06.010

Navarro RS, Jiang L, Ouyang Y, Luo J, Liu Z, Yang Y, et al. Biomimetic tubular scaffold with heparin conjugation for rapid degradation in in situ regeneration of a small diameter neoartery. *Biomaterials.* (2021) 274:120874. doi: 10.1016/j.biomaterials.2021.120874

Alasnag M, Yaqoub L, Saati A, Al-Shaibi K. Left main coronary artery interventions. *Interv Cardiol.* (2019) 14:124–30. doi: 10.15420/icr.2019.10.R2

Tara S, Kurobe H, Maxfield MW, Rocco KA, Yi T, Naito Y, et al. Evaluation of remodeling process in small-diameter cell-free tissue-engineered arterial graft. *J Vasc Surg.* (2015) 62:734–43. doi: 10.1016/j.jvs.2014.03.011

Mombini S, Mohammadnejad J, Bakhshandeh B, Narmani A, Nourmohammadi J, Vahdat S, et al. Chitosan-PVA-CNT nanofibers as electrically conductive scaffolds for cardiovascular tissue engineering. *Int J Biol Macromol.* (2019) 140:278–87. doi: 10.1016/j.ijbiomac.2019.08.046

Fleischer S, Miller J, Hurowitz H, Shapira A, Dvir T. Effect of fiber diameter on the assembly of functional 3D cardiac patches. *Nanotechnology.* (2015) 26:291002. doi: 10.1088/0957-4484/26/29/291002

Fleischer S, Shapira A, Feiner R, Dvir T. Modular assembly of thick multifunctional cardiac patches. *Proc Natl Acad Sci U S A.* (2017) 114:1898– 903. doi: 10.1073/pnas.1615728114

Chen WL, Kan CD. Using cell-seeded electrospun patch for myocardial injury: *in-vitro* and in rat model. *Annu Int Conf IEEE Eng Med Biol Soc.* (2018) 2018:5338–41. doi: 10.1109/EMBC.2018.8513557

Arumugam R, Srinadhu ES, Subramanian B, Nallani S. β-PVDF based electrospun nanofibers - a promising material for developing cardiac patches. *Med Hypotheses.* (2019) 122:31–4. doi: 10.1016/j.mehy.2018.10.005

Malki M, Fleischer S, Shapira A, Dvir T. Gold nanorod-based engineered cardiac patch for suture-free engraftment by near IR. *Nano Letters.* (2018) 18:4069–73. doi: 10.1021/acs.nanolett.7b04924

He Y, Ye G, Song C, Li C, Xiong W, Yu L, et al. Mussel-inspired conductive nanofibrous membranes repair myocardial infarction by enhancing cardiac function and revascularization. *Theranostics.* (2018) 8:5159–77. doi: 10.7150/thno.27760

Zhu D, Hou J, Qian M, Jin D, Hao T, Pan Y, et al. Nitrate- functionalized patch confers cardioprotection and improves heart repair after myocardial infarction via local nitric oxide delivery. *Nat Commun.* (2021) 12:4501. doi: 10.1038/s41467-021-24804-3

Wu W, Allen RA, Wang Y. Fast-degrading elastomer enables rapid remodeling of a cell-free synthetic graft into a neoartery. *Nat Med.* (2012) 18:1148–53. doi: 10.1038/nm.2821

Qin K, Wang F, Simpson RML, Zheng X, Wang H, Hu Y, et al. Hyaluronan promotes the regeneration of vascular smooth muscle with potent contractile function in rapidly biodegradable vascular grafts. *Biomaterials.* (2020) 257:120226. doi: 10.1016/j.biomaterials.2020.120226

Zhang H, Jia X, Han F, Zhao J, Zhao Y, Fan Y, et al. Dual-delivery of VEGF and PDGF by double-layered electrospun membranes for blood vessel regeneration. *Biomaterials.* (2013) 34:2202–12. doi: 10.1016/j.biomaterials.2012. 12.005

Kuang H, Wang Y, Shi Y, Yao W, He X, Liu X, et al. Construction and performance evaluation of Hep/silk-PLCL composite nanofiber small-caliber artificial blood vessel graft. *Biomaterials.* (2020) 259:120288. doi: 10.1016/j.biomaterials.2020.120288

Li P, Jin D, Dou J, Wang L, Wang Y, Jin X, et al. Nitric oxide- releasing poly(ε-caprolactone) /S-nitrosylated keratin biocomposite scaffolds for potential small-diameter vascular grafts. *Int J Biol Macromol.* (2021) 189:516–27. doi: 10.1016/j.ijbiomac.2021.08.147

Dorati R, Pisani S, Chiesa E, Genta I, Bruni G, Modena T, et al. Electrospun tubular vascular grafts to replace damaged peripheral arteries: a preliminary formulation study. *Int J Pharm.* (2021) 596:120198. doi: 10.1016/j.ijpharm.2021.120198

Steiner D, Lang G, Fischer L, Winkler S, Fey T, Greil P, et al. Intrinsic vascularization of recombinant eadf4(c16) spider silk matrices in the arteriovenous loop model. *Tissue Eng Part A.* (2019) 25:1504– 13. doi: 10.1089/ten.tea.2018.0360

Yan S, Napiwocki B, Xu Y, Zhang J, Zhang X, Wang X, et al. Wavy small-diameter vascular graft made of eggshell membrane and thermoplastic polyurethane. *Mater Sci Eng C Mater Biol Appl.* (2020) 107:110311. doi: 10.1016/j.msec.2019.110311

Du H, Tao L, Wang W, Liu D, Zhang Q, Sun P, et al. Enhanced biocompatibility of poly(llactidecoepsiloncaprolactone) electrospun vascular grafts via self-assembly modification. *Mater Sci Eng C Mater Biol Appl.* (2019) 100:845–54. doi: 10.1016/j.msec.2019.03.063

Shimada R, Konishi H, Ozawa H, Katsumata T, Tanaka R, Nakazawa Y, et al. Development of a new surgical sheet containing both silk fibroin and thermoplastic polyurethane for cardiovascular surgery. *Surg Today.* (2018) 48:486–94. doi: 10.1007/s00595-017-1615-6

Wang Z, Mithieux SM, Weiss AS. Fabrication techniques for vascular and vascularized tissue engineering. *Adv Healthc Mater.* (2019) 8:e1900742. doi: 10.1002/adhm.2019 00742

Wang Z, Cui Y, Wang J, Yang X, Wu Y, Wang K, et al. The effect of thick fibers and large pores of electrospun poly(epsilon-caprolactone) vascular grafts on macrophage polarization and arterial regeneration. *Biomaterials.* (2014) 35:5700–10. doi: 10.1016/j.biomaterials.2014.03.078

Issa Bhaloo S, Wu Y, Le Bras A, Yu B, Gu W, Xie Y, et al. Binding of dickkopf-3 to CXCR7 enhances vascular progenitor cell migration and degradable graft regeneration. *Circ Res.* (2018) 123:451– 66. doi: 10.1161/CIRCRESAHA.118.312945

Badv M, Bayat F, Weitz JI, Didar TF. Single and multi-functional coating strategies for enhancing the biocompatibility and tissue integration of blood-contacting medical implants. *Biomaterials.* (2020) 258:120291. doi: 10.1016/j.biomaterials.2020.120291

Han F, Jia X, Dai D, Yang X, Zhao J, Zhao Y, et al. Performance of a multilayered small-diameter vascular scaffold dual- loaded with VEGF and PDGF. *Biomaterials.* (2013) 34:7302– 13. doi: 10.1016/j.biomaterials.2013.06.006

Strobel HA, Qendro EI, Alsberg E, Rolle MW. Targeted delivery of bioactive molecules for vascular intervention and tissue engineering. *Front Pharmacol.* (2018) 9:1329. doi: 10.3389/fphar.2018.01329

Xue J, Wu T, Dai Y, Xia Y. Electrospinning and electrospun nanofibers: methods, materials, and applications. *Chem Rev.* (2019) 119:5298–415. doi: 10.1021/acs.chemrev.8b00593

Lee JS, Chae S, Yoon D, Yoon D, Chun W, Kim GH. Angiogenic factors secreted from human ASC spheroids entrapped in an alginate-based hierarchical structure via combined 3D printing/electrospinning system. *Biofabrication.* (2020) 12:045028. doi: 10.1088/1758-5090/abaf9a

Lin W, Chen M, Qu T, Li J, Man Y. Three-dimensional electrospun nanofibrous scaffolds for bone tissue engineering. *J Biomed Mater Res Part B Appl Biomater.* (2020) 108:1311–21. doi: 10.1002/jbm.b.34479

Rufaihah AJ, Yasa IC, Ramanujam VS, Arularasu SC, Kofidis T, Guler MO, et al. Angiogenic peptide nanofibers repair cardiac tissue defect after myocardial infarction. *Acta Biomater.* (2017) 58:102–12. doi: 10.1016/j.actbio.2017.06.009

Walker BW, Lara RP, Yu CH, Sani ES, Kimball W, Joyce S, et al. Engineering a naturally-derived adhesive and conductive cardiopatch. *Biomaterials.* (2019) 207:89–101. doi: 10.1016/j.biomaterials.2019.03.015

Wei X, Gao Q, Xie C, Gu C, Liang T, Wan H, et al. Extracellular recordings of bionic engineered cardiac tissue based on a porous scaffold and microelectrode arrays. *Analytical Methods.* (2019) 11:5872– 9. doi: 10.1039/C9AY01888C

Wu S, Duan B, Qin X, Butcher JT. Living nano-micro fibrous woven fabric/hydrogel composite scaffolds for heart valve engineering. *Acta Biomater.* (2017) 51:89–100. doi: 10.1016/j.actbio.2017.01.051

Jana S, Lerman A. Behavior of valvular interstitial cells on trilayered nanofibrous substrate mimicking morphologies of heart valve leaflet. *Acta Biomater.* (2019) 85:142–56. doi: 10.1016/j.actbio.2018.12.005

Kaiser E, Jaganathan SK, Supriyanto E, Ayyar M. Fabrication and characterization of chitosan nanoparticles and collagen-loaded polyurethane nanocomposite membrane coated with heparin for atrial septal defect (ASD) closure. *3 Biotech.* (2017) 7:174. doi: 10.1007/s13205-017-0830-6

Feng B, Wang S, Hu D, Fu W, Wu J, Hong H, et al. Bioresorbable electrospun gelatin/polycaprolactone nanofibrous membrane as a barrier to prevent cardiac postoperative adhesion. *Acta Biomater.* (2019) 83:211– 20. doi: 10.1016/j.actbio.2018.10.022

Kang L, Jia W, Li M, Wang Q, Wang C, Liu Y, et al. Hyaluronic acid al. Silk fibroin-PellethaneOR cardiovascular patches: Effect of silk fibroin oligosaccharide-modified collagen nanofibers as vascular tissue-engineered\ concentration on vascular remodeling in rat model. *J Mater Sci Mater Med.* (2017) 28:191. doi: 10.1007/s10856-017-5999-z

Liu K, Wang N, Wang W, Shi L, Li H, Guo F, et al. A bio-inspired high strength three-layer nanofiber vascular graft with structure guided cell growth. *J Mater Chem B.* (2017) 5:3758–64. doi: 10.1039/C7TB00465F

Ju YM, Ahn H, Arenas-Herrera J, Kim C, Abolbashari M, Atala A, et al. Electrospun vascular scaffold for cellularized small diameter blood vessels: a preclinical large animal study. *Acta Biomater.* (2017) 59:58– 67. doi: 10.1016/j.actbio.2017.06.027

Chantawong P, Tanaka T, Uemura A, Shimada K, Higuchi A, Tajiri H, et scaffold for promoting endothelial cell proliferation. *Carbohydr Polym.* (2019) 223:115106. doi: 10.1016/j.carbpol.2019.115106

Strassburg S, Nienhueser H, Bjorn Stark G, Finkenzeller G, Torio-Padron N. Co-culture of adipose-derived stem cells and endothelial cells in fibrin induces angiogenesis and vasculogenesis in a chorioallantoic membrane model. *J Tissue Eng Regen Med.* (2016) 10:496–506. doi: 10.1002/term .1769

Arkudas A, Pryymachuk G, Hoereth T, Beier JP, Polykandriotis E, Bleiziffer O, et al. Dose-finding study of fibrin gel-immobilized vascular endothelial growth factor 165 and basic fibroblast growth factor in the arteriovenous loop rat model. *Tissue Eng Part A.* (2009) 15:2501–11. doi: 10.1089/ten.tea.2008.0477

Erol OO, Sira M. New capillary bed formation with a surgically constructed arteriovenous fistula. *Plast Reconstr Surg.* (1980) 66:109– 15. doi: 10.1097/00006534-198007000-00021

Pezeshki-Modaress M, Mirzadeh H, Zandi M, Rajabi-Zeleti S, Sodeifi N, Aghdami N, et al. Gelatin/chondroitin sulfate nanofibrous scaffolds for stimulation of wound healing: *In-vitro* and *in-vivo* study. *J Biomed Mater Res A.* (2017) 105:2020–34. doi: 10.1002/jbm.a. 35890

Chen S, Li R, Li X, Xie J. Electrospinning: an enabling nanotechnology platform for drug delivery and regenerative medicine. *Adv Drug Deliv Rev.* (2018) 132:188–213. doi: 10.1016/j.addr.2018.05.001

Rolph D, Das H. Generation of Myocardial Ischemic Wounds and

Healing with Stem Cells. *Methods Mol Biol.* (2021) 2193:141– 7. doi: 10.1007/978-1-0716-0845-6_14

Sharma D, Ferguson M, Kamp TJ, Zhao F. Constructing biomimetic cardiac tissues: a review of scaffold materials for engineering cardiac patches. *Emerg Mater.* (2019) 2:181–91. doi: 10.1007/s42247-019-00046-4

Qian Z, Sharma D, Jia W, Radke D, Kamp T, Zhao F. Engineering stem cell cardiac patch with microvascular features representative of native myocardium. *Theranostics.* (2019) 9:2143–57. doi: 10.7150/thno.29552

Kitsara M, Agbulut O, Kontziampasis D, Chen Y, Menasche P. Fibers for hearts: a critical review on electrospinning for cardiac tissue engineering. *Acta Biomater.* (2017) 48:20–40. doi: 10.1016/j.actbio.2016.11.014

Sax H, Bloemberg G, Hasse B, Sommerstein R, Kohler P, Achermann Y, et al. Prolonged outbreak of mycobacterium chimaera infection after open-chest heart surgery. *Clin Infect Dis.* (2015) 61:67–75. doi: 10.1093/cid/civ198

Wu J, Hong Y. Enhancing cell infiltration of electrospun fibrous scaffolds in tissue regeneration. *Bioact Mater.* (2016) 1:56–64. doi: 10.1016/j.bioactmat.2016.07.001

Khorshidi S, Solouk A, Mirzadeh H, Mazinani S, Lagaron JM, Sharifi S, et al. A review of key challenges of electrospun scaffolds for tissue-engineering applications. *J Tissue Eng Regen Med.* (2016) 10:715– 38. doi: 10.1002/term.1978

Ding H, Cheng Y, Niu X, Hu Y. Application of electrospun nanofibers in bone, cartilage and osteochondral tissue engineering. *J Biomater Sci Polym Ed.* (2021) 32:536–61. doi: 10.1080/09205063.2020.1849922

Kharaziha M, Nikkhah M, Shin SR, Annabi N, Masoumi N, Gaharwar AK, et al. PGS:Gelatin nanofibrous scaffolds with tunable mechanical and structural properties for engineering cardiac tissues. *Biomaterials.* (2013) 34:6355–66. doi: 10.1016/j.biomaterials.2013.04.045

Pomeroy JE, Helfer A, Bursac N. Biomaterializing the promise of cardiac tissue engineering. *Biotechnol Adv.* (2020)42:107353. doi: 10.1016/j.biotechadv.2019.02.009

Pan Y, Zhou X, Wei Y, Zhang Q, Wang T, Zhu M, et al. Small-diameter hybrid vascular grafts composed of polycaprolactone and polydioxanone fibers. *Sci Rep.* (2017) 7:3615. doi: 10.1038/s41598-017-03851-1

Bergmeister H, Seyidova N, Schreiber C, Strobl M, Grasl C, Walter I, et al. Biodegradable, thermoplastic polyurethane grafts for small diameter vascular replacements. *Acta Biomater.* (2015) 11:104–13. doi: 10.1016/j.actbio.2014.09.003

Li J, Celiz AD, Yang J, Yang Q, Wamala I, Whyte W, et al. Tough adhesives for diverse wet surfaces. *Science.* (2017) 357:378–81. doi: 10.1126/science.aah6362

Sridharan D, Palaniappan A, Blackstone BN, Powell HM, Khan M. Electrospun aligned coaxial nanofibrous scaffold for cardiac repair. *Methods Mol. Biol.* (2021) 2193:129–40. doi: 10.1007/978-1-0716-0845-6_13

Castilho M, Feyen D, Flandes-Iparraguirre M, Hochleitner G, Groll J, Doevendans PAF, et al. Melt electrospinning writing of poly-hydroxymethylglycolide-co-epsilon-caprolactone-based scaffolds for cardiac tissue engineering. *Adv Healthc Mater.* (2017) 6:18. doi: 10.1002/adhm.201700311

Zhao YT, Zhang J, Gao Y, Liu XF, Liu JJ, Wang XX, et al. Self-powered portable melt electrospinning for in situ wound dressing. *J Nanobiotechnology.* (2020) 18:111. doi: 10.1186/s12951-020-00671-w

18

Anti-Inflammatory Nanomedicine for Cardiovascular Disease

Shunsuke Katsuki[1,2], Tetsuya Matoba[1], Jun-ichiro Koga[1,3], Kaku Nakano[3] and Kensuke Egashira[1,3]*

[1] *Department of Cardiovascular Medicine, Kyushu University Graduate School of Medical Sciences, Fukuoka, Japan,* [2] *Center for Excellence in Vascular Biology, Division of Cardiovascular Medicine, Department of Medicine, Brigham and Women's Hospital, Harvard Medical School, Boston, MA, United States,* [3] *Department of Cardiovascular Research, Development, and Translational Medicine, Center for Cardiovascular Disruptive Innovation, Kyushu University, Fukuoka, Japan*

Correspondence:
Tetsuya Matoba
matoba@cardiol.med.kyushu-u.ac.jp

Coronary artery disease, in the development of which inflammation mediated by innate immune cells plays a critical role, is one of the leading causes of death worldwide. The 3-hydroxy-3-methylglutaryl coenzyme A reductase inhibitors (statins) are a widely used lipid-lowering drug that has lipid-independent vasculoprotective effects, such as improvement of endothelial dysfunction, antioxidant properties, and inhibitory effects on inflammation. Despite recent advances in lipid-lowering therapy, clinical trials of statins suggest that anti-inflammatory therapy beyond lipid-lowering therapy is indispensible to further reduce cardiovascular events. One possible therapeutic option to the residual risk is to directly intervene in the inflammatory process by utilizing a nanotechnology-based drug delivery system (nano-DDS). Various nano-sized materials are currently developed as DDS, including micelles, liposomes, polymeric nanoparticles, dendrimers, carbon nanotubes, and metallic nanoparticles. The application of nano-DDS to coronary artery disease is a feasible strategy since the inflammatory milieu enhances incorporation of nano-sized materials into mononuclear phagocytic system and permeability of target lesions, which confers nano-DDS on "passive-targeting" property. Recently, we have developed a polymeric nanoparticle-incorporating statin to maximize its anti-inflammatory property. This statin nanoparticle has been tested in various disease models, including plaque destabilization and rupture, myocardial ischemia-reperfusion injury, and ventricular remodeling after acute myocardial infarction, and its clinical application is in progress. In this review, we present current development of DDS and future perspective on the application of anti-inflammatory nanomedicine to treat life-threatening cardiovascular diseases.

Keywords: coronary artery disease, inflammation, nanomedicine, monocytes, macrophages

ANTI-INFLAMMATORY THERAPEUTICS FOR CORONARY ARTERY DISEASE

Coronary artery disease is the leading cause of death worldwide and can be life threatening especially when it develops into acute myocardial infarction (AMI), the most severe type of atherosclerotic cardiovascular disease. The 3-hydroxy-3-methylglutaryl coenzyme A (HMG-CoA) reductase inhibitors (statins) are potent inhibitors of cholesterol synthesis and established therapies for the prevention of coronary artery disease. The first randomized trial to demonstrate that cholesterol-lowering therapy with statins improves prognosis in patients with high cholesterol and coronary artery disease, the Scandinavian Simvastatin Survival Study (4S), was reported in 1994 (1). Since then, lipid-lowering therapy with statins has become the mainstay for the prevention of coronary artery disease. The subsequent studies for the secondary prevention such as the CARE (Cholesterol and Recurrent Events) (2) and LIPID (Long Term Intervention with Pravastatin in Ischemic Disease) trials (3) further extended that the benefits of statins to the majority of patients whose cholesterol levels were in the normal range. The WOSCOPS (West of Scotland Coronary Prevention Study) (4) and the AFCAPS/TexCAPS (Air Force/Texas Coronary Atherosclerosis Prevention Study) (5) also extended the benefits for the primary prevention of atherosclerotic cardiovascular diseases. A decade after 4S, Ridker et al. demonstrated in the JUPITER (Justification for the Use of Statins in Primary Prevention: an Intervention Trial Evaluating Rosuvastatin) trial that high-intensity cholesterol-lowering therapy with statins reduced high-sensitivity C-reactive protein levels to lower than 2 mg/L and then achieved further risk reduction of cardiovascular events even among patients with normal cholesterol levels (6). Statins have a wide range of lipid-independent cardiovascular protective effects (so called "pleiotropic effects"), such as improvement of endothelial dysfunction, antioxidant properties, and inhibitory effects on inflammation (7) This landmark study suggested that anti-inflammatory therapy beyond lipid-lowering therapy is needed to further reduce cardiovascular events. At present, plaque erosion appears on the rise as a cause of acute coronary syndrome (ACS) in this statin era (8), but plaque rupture of unstable plaques with macrophage accumulation, fibrous cap thinning, and lipid deposition, followed by arterial occlusive thrombosis remains the primary mechanisms of ACS. Despite recent advances in lipid-lowering therapy by the emergence of Niemann-Pick C1-Like 1 inhibitor (ezetimibe) (9, 10) and proprotein convertase subtilisin/kexin type 9 inhibitors (11), there are still residual risks of cardiovascular events. One possible approach to the residual risks is to directly intervene in the inflammatory process during atherogenesis. Current medicinal therapy, including statins, has limitation of bioavailability in the diseased organs. Most small molecule drugs are absorbed from the intestines, metabolized in the liver, delivered to the bloodstream, and excreted from the kidneys, that is, drugs need to overcome the physiological barriers to achieve effective concentration in the blood and tissue. Adverse effects that any drugs possess may also limit their maximum dose in terms of safety. Recent innovation in nanomedicine can achieve effective drug delivery to targeted organs and cells, and spare undesirable adverse effects. In the first part of this review, we summarize recent advances in nanotechnology-based drug delivery system (nano-DDS). In the second part, we demonstrate the data of nano-DDS of statins in coronary artery disease for maximizing its anti-inflammatory effects.

VARIOUS NANO-SIZED MATERIALS AS DRUG DELIVERY SYSTEMS

Currently, various nano-sized materials (nanomaterials) have been tested and approved in clinical settings: lipid nanoparticles such as micelles or liposomes (12), polymeric nanoparticles (13), dendrimers (14), carbon nanotubes, and metallic nanoparticles. The characteristics of these materials and clinical applications are as follows (**Table 1**).

Micelles

Micelles consist of lipids and other amphiphilic artificial molecules, such as polymers. Micelles are self-assembling in aqueous solution to form a monolayer with a hydrophobic phase inside so that they can incorporate hydrophobic therapeutic agents. The diameter of micelles is usually 10–100 nm and the enclosed space is more confined than that of liposomes.

Liposomes

Since United States Food and Drug Administration (FDA) approved liposomal formulations of doxorubicin and amphotericin B in the mid-1990s (15), liposomes have been investigated most extensively in nanomedicine with approval due to less toxicity for *in vivo* application and capacity to deliver a variety of payloads. Liposomes mainly consist of phospholipids to form bilayers with an aqueous phase inside, which confer superior biocompatibility on liposomes. They can not only incorporate hydrophilic therapeutic agents inside but also hydrophobic agents in the liposomal membrane. Macromolecular drugs, including nucleic acid and crystalline metals, can be also incorporated in liposomes.

TABLE 1 | Characteristics of various nano-sized materials as drug delivery systems.

	Micelle	Liposome	Polymer nanoparticle	Dendrimer	Carbon nanotube	Metallic nanoparticle
Geometry	Spherical vesicles composed of a monolayer of lipids or synthetic amphiphiles	Spherical vesicles composed of phospholipids bilayers	An assembly of macromolecular polymers	Highly branched monodisperse macromolecules from a central core	Single or multi-walled tubular form of graphite sheets	A magnetic core coated with hydrophilic polymers
Size (nm)	10–100	40–1,000	20–1,000	3–20	0.5–3.0 × 20–1,000	60–150 (core 4–5)
Features	Encapsulation of hydrophobic agents inside	Encapsulation of hydrophilic agents inside, embedding hydrophobic agents in the membrane	Incorporation of hydrophilic and hydrophobic agents, controlled release of incorporated agents	Multivalent properties by exterior funciton groups	Encapsulation of agents into its inner space with chemically modified external surface	Contrast agents for biological imaging, photothermal properties

The diameter of liposomes is usually 40–1,000 nm. Liposomes obtain specific characteristics through modification of its surface with polymers, antibodies, and protein. PEGylated liposomal doxorubicin (Doxil®) is the first FDA-approved nanomedicine and enhanced the drug concentration in malignant effusions by 4-fold to 16-fold, while reducing cardiotoxic side effects (16).

Polymeric Nanoparticle

Food and Drug Administration-approved polymers, polylactic acid (PLA), polyglycolic acid (PGA), and poly lactic-co-glycolic acid (PLGA), are widely used for the synthesis of polymeric biodegradable nano-DDS, because they are eliminated from the body in the form of water and carbon dioxide. PLGA is a copolymer of PLA and PGA, the most frequently used constitution among these polymers, and is being tested for a DDS for intractable diseases, including cardiovascular disease. PLA is more hydrophobic, whereas PGA is more hydrophilic; the degradation speed of PLGA can be adjusted by the PLA:PGA ratio and their molecular weights, which achieves controlled release of incorporated drugs. PLGA polymers incorporate hydrophilic and hydrophobic therapeutic agents, including chemicals and nucleotides by emulsion solvent diffusion methods. The diameter of polymeric nanoparticles widely ranges from 20 to 1,000 nm. FDA-approved PLGA nanoparticle utilizing these advantages is leuprolide acetate (a testosterone inhibitor)-incorporated nanoparticle for prostate cancer (Eligard®). PLGA achieves slow and sustained leuprolide acetate release after subcutaneous injection.

Dendrimer

Dendrimers are dendritically expanded macromolecules with monodisperse structure that consist of a central core, branching interior, and exterior functional groups (14). Dendrimers can incorporate therapeutic agents in their three-dimensional branching interior voids and work as a drug delivery carrier. The number of repeating branching cycles is called generations. Exterior function groups increase exponentially as generation increases, which confer multivalent properties on dendrimers. This multivalent effect has the advantage of enhancing the binding capacity when its exterior surface is modified with some ligands or antibodies as an active targeting (17).

Carbon Nanotube

Carbon nanotubes are a subfamily of fullerenes and consist of graphite sheets rolled up into tubular form. As drug carriers, they can incorporate drugs into its inner space and have a chemically modified external surface with biomolecules, such as proteins and nucleotides, for selective targeting. Carbon nanotube-based anticancer therapy such as cisplatin-incorporated carbon nanohorn is currently being investigated (18).

Metallic Nanoparticle

Metallic nanoparticles include iron oxide and gold nanoparticles. Iron oxide nanoparticles consist of a magnetic core (4–5 nm) and hydrophilic polymers such as dextran or poly(ethyleneglycol)s. Superparamagnetic iron oxide (SPIO) (60–150 nm) has been investigated as a contrast agent for magnetic resonance imaging (MRI). Ferumoxytol (Feraheme®), caraboxymethydextran-coated iron oxide, is the only FDA-approved SPIO. The clinical use of ferumoxytol is limited to iron replacement therapy for patients with chronic kidney disease and is under investigation as an imaging agent. Resovist®, carboxydextran-coated iron oxide, has been withdrawn from FDA-approved drugs due to lack of clinical users, and is currently available in limited countries including Japan (19). Gold nanoparticles has unique photothermal properties, tunable size and shape, and easily modified surface. No gold nanoparticles have been clinically approved to date, but they are actively investigated especially in research fields targeting cancer (20).

Although micro-sized particles are considered to be biologically inert, nano-sized materials could activate innate immune sensors. In fact, nano-sized inorganic metal oxides, such as silica dioxide (SiO_2) and titanium dioxide (TiO_2) (21), and silver nanoparticle (22) have been reported to activate the NLR pyrin domain containing 3 (NLRP3) inflammasome in human macrophages. Since carbon nanotubes are fiber-shaped material, the morphology of which is similar to that of asbestos, the concern for the toxicity of carbon nanotubes has been raised (23). In animal models, intratracheal exposure with the above-mentioned nanomaterials demonstrated airway inflammation (21, 24). The activation of inflammasome is mediated by potassium efflux (25), lysosome degradation that results in cathepsin B leakage, generation of reactive oxygen species (ROS) (26), and production of adenosine (27). These data suggested that greater caution might be needed to these widely produced nanomaterials.

IN VIVO KINETICS OF NANOPARTICLE-MEDIATED DRUG DELIVERY SYSTEM

Although there are numerous determinants to affect *in vivo* kinetics of nano-DDS other than geometry as previously discussed, the size and surface modification of nanoparticles are the most important in the physiological behaviors of nano-DDS. Large-sized nanomaterials (>1,000 nm in diameter) tend to accumulate in the liver and lungs, and sometimes can be the cause of microemboli in capillaries, while small-sized nanomaterials (<10 nm) tend to be excreted from the kidneys. Middle-sized nanomaterials (10–1,000 nm) remain in circulation for longer time avoiding renal excretion. These circulating nanomaterials are generally incorporated by the mononuclear phagocytic system (MPS) in the liver, spleen, lymph nodes, and bone marrow (28). A surface modification with polyethylene glycol (PEG) serves as a hydrophilic shield that reduces protein absorption and undesirable non-specific interaction with MPS, which is preferable for nano-DDS in cancer. However, incorporation of nanomaterials into MPS itself is one of the intended mechanisms of drug delivery, especially when targeting inflammatory diseases including atherosclerosis. On the other hand, accumulation of nanomaterials depends on the permeability of target lesions. In tumor blood vessels, inflammatory atherosclerotic lesions, and ischemic myocardium, nanomaterials extravasate from blood vessels due to enhanced permeability. Tumors lack functional lymphatic vessels in their tumor microenvironment, which enhances the accumulation of nanomaterials. These phenomena are referred to as "enhanced permeability and retention effects" (29) or "passive-targeting" (**Figure 1**).

By contrast, "active-targeting" strategy employs target-specific structures, such as antibodies and proteins on nanomaterials, which bind to the target molecule that is specific for a certain disease process. "Active-targeting" strategy is being developed in cancer therapeutics targeting molecules associated with angiogenesis and cell proliferation (30). Adhesion molecules are one of the candidates for cardiovascular imaging as described later in this review, and innovative cardiovascular imaging using "active-targeting" strategy is being investigated. Regardless of the benefits of "active targeting," only a few clinically validated nanomaterials utilize this strategy. Engineered protein combining IL-2 and diphtheria toxin (Ontak®) is the only FDA-approved "active-targeting" nanomaterial to date (15).

THE ROLE OF MONOCYTES/ MACROPHAGES IN CORONARY ARTERY DISEASE

Monocytes/macrophages play a key role in the inflammatory hypothesis of atherothrombosis (31). Atherogenesis starts with endothelial dysfunction caused by oxidative, hemodynamic, or biochemical stimuli (from smoking, hypertension, or

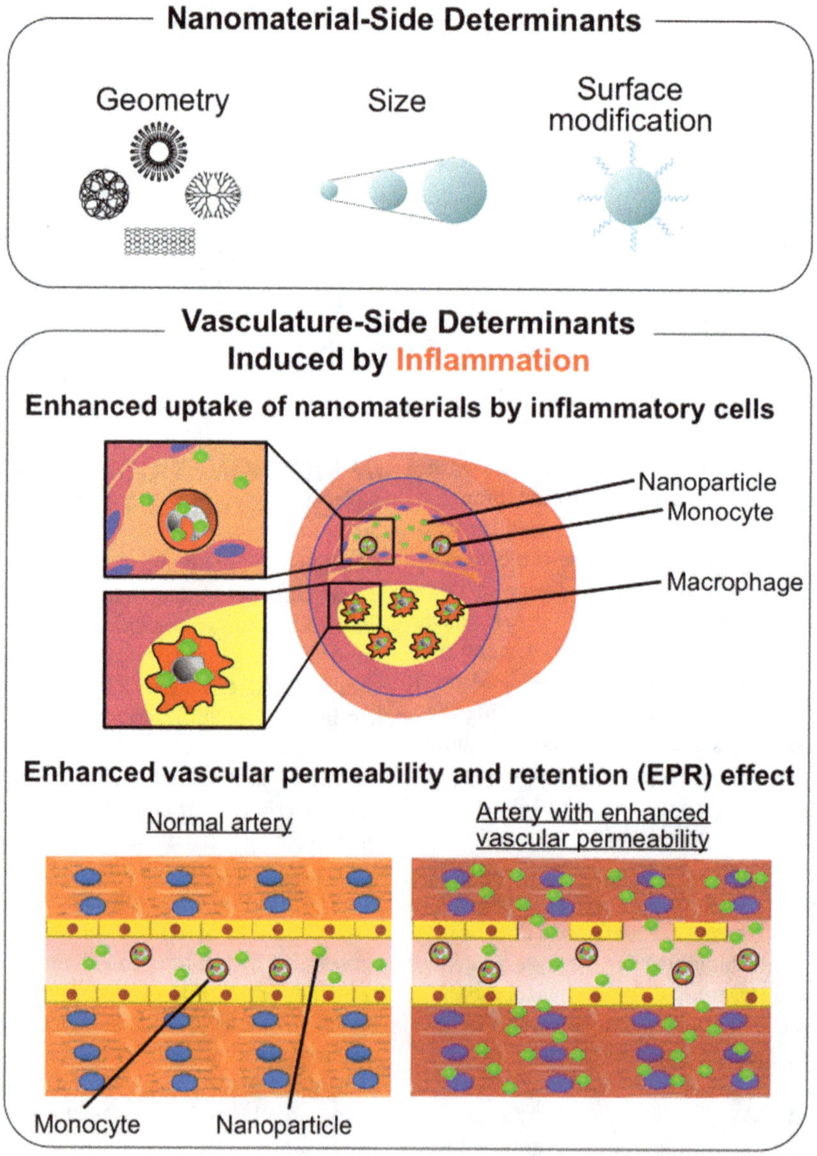

FIGURE 1 | Schematic description of determinants of physiological behavior of nanomaterials. (Upper panel) Nanomaterial-side determinants: geometry, size, and surface modification. (Lower panel) Vasculature-side determinants induced by inflammation: enhanced uptake of nanomaterials by inflammatory cells and enhanced vascular permeability and retention (EPR) effect.

dyslipidemia) and inflammatory factors. Endothelial dysfunction leads to enhanced permeability for cholesterol-containing low-density lipoprotein (LDL) particles and the expression of adhesion molecules to promote adhesion of circulating monocytes. Adhesive monocytes migrate into subendothelial space by chemoattractant proteins including monocyte chemoattractant protein-1 (MCP-1), where monocytes are differentiated into macrophages by macrophage-colony stimulating factor and activated through phagocytosis of oxidized lipid components to become foam cells. Activated macrophages secrete inflammatory cytokines to trigger positive feedback loop between cytokines and immune cells and matrix metalloproteinases (MMPs) leading to fibrous cap thinning. Rupture-prone plaques are characterized by the abundant accumulation of innate immune cells (mainly monocytes/macrophages), lipid core formation, and induction of several proteinases that catabolize the extracellular matrix (32).

Monocytes are functionally heterogeneous and are classified into at least two major subsets in mice: inflammatory monocytes (Ly-6C^{high}CCR2^{+}CX3CR1^{low}) and non-inflammatory monocytes (Ly-6C^{low}CCR2^{-}CX3CR1^{high}) (33). Previously, we developed a mouse model of "plaque rupture" utilizing a high-fat diet and angiotensin II infusion in apolipoprotein E (ApoE)-deficient mice and reported that adoptive transfer of Ly-6C^{high}CCR2^{+} inflammatory monocytes increases buried fibrous caps in the brachiocephalic arteries (34), suggesting a critical role for inflammatory monocytes in plaque destabilization. Although their functional similarities have not been fully determined, CD14^{++}CD16^{-} classical monocytes and CD14^{+}CD16^{++} non-classical monocytes are described as their respective counterparts of Ly-6C^{high} and Ly-6C^{low} monocytes according to their chemokine receptor expression in humans, and intermediate monocytes (CD14^{++}CD16^{+}) have been recently identified as not only a transitory state but also likely to possess unique features (35). There were not any significant differences in the peak levels of circulating CD14^{++}CD16^{-} monocytes among the patients with AMI, unstable angina pectoris (UAP), and stable angina pectoris (SAP), but that of circulating CD14^{+}CD16^{+} monocytes (defined as CD14^{++}CD16^{+} plus CD14^{+}CD16^{++} monocytes) were significantly decreased in AMI patients compared with those in patients with UAP or SAP (36). A conventional paradigm proposed two subpopulations in macrophages corresponding to the monocyte heterogeneity: "classically activated or inflammatory M1 macrophages" and "alternatively activated or anti-inflammatory M2 macrophages." Although the balance between "M1" and "M2" subpopulations may contribute to the development of cardiovascular disease, emerging evidence suggests that heterogeneity of macrophage subpopulation seems much more complex than "M1" and "M2" dichotomy (37). "M2" macrophages are divided into at least three subpopulations according to the stimulus they are activated; "M2a," "M2b," and "M2c." All "M2" macrophages have anti-inflammatory properties to secrete IL-10 and TGF-β. "M2b" is an exception because they additionally secrete pro-inflammatory cytokines, such as IL-1β, IL-6, and TNFα. The tissue microenvironment in atherosclerotic plaques can affect macrophage population (38). Oxidized phospholipids induce "Mox" and intraplaque hemorrhage induces "Mhem (HA-mac)" or "M(Hb)." Although localization of "Mox" in human atherosclerotic lesions remains to be elucidated, the population was detected in approximately 30% of macrophages in advanced atherosclerotic plaque of LDL receptor-deficient mice. "Mox" not only shows an pro-inflammatory phenotype by producing cyclooxygenase-2 and IL-1β but also control redox status by inducing redox-regulating genes such as heme oxygenase-1 (HO-1), sufiredoxin-1 (Srnx1), and thioredoxin reductase 1 *via* nuclear factor erythroid 2-like 2 (NFE2L2). They also display reduced chemotactic and phagocytic capacities, which might contribute to perpetuation of inflammation and tissue damage (39). "Mhem" (previously named as "HA-mac" by the same investigators), originally defined as CD163^{high} human leukocyte antigen-DR^{low}, was detected in human hemorrhaged atherosclerotic plaque. "Mhem" is an atheroprotective subpopulation that drives adaptation to intraplaque hemorrhage through activation transcription factor 1-mediated induction of HO-1 by heme (40). Another investigators named this population "M(Hb)" and further demonstrated that "M(Hb)" has high expression of "M2 markers" mannose receptor and CD163, and reduces ROS production and promotes LXRα-mediated reverse cholesterol transport (41). Platelet chemokine CXCL4 induces "M4" macrophages. They lack CD163 and are unable to increase HO-1 production in response to hemoglobin or hemoglobin–haptoglobin complexes. Co-expression of MMP7 and S100 calcium-binding protein A8 (S100A8) in "M4" in human atherosclerotic plaques might lead to plaque destabilization by increased expression of MMP7 and affect lesion progression through decreased macrophage proliferation (42). In this way, the description of macrophage activation has been expanded and confusing, and then a group of scientists proposed the updated nomenclature to define the activator, i.e., M(IFNγ), M(LPS), M(IL-4), and M(IL-10), instead of the current complex nomenclature in *in vitro* experiments. This helps researchers to avoid using different definitions of activated macrophages. They also provide the framework within which researchers place a given population for *in vivo* experiments (37).

Macrophage is also a protagonist in myocardial ischemia-reperfusion (IR) injury and wound healing process of ischemic heart disease following AMI. In patients with ST-segment elevation acute MI (STEMI), early reperfusion is a standard therapy to salvage viable myocardium and limit MI size. Regardless of significant reductions in door-to-balloon time in the last decade, the mortality of patients with MI has not improved as shown in recent cohort studies. It is well recognized that the reperfusion of coronary arteries can paradoxically induce cardiomyocyte death, called "myocardial IR injury." The major contributing factors in myocardial IR include ROS, calcium overload, and the rapid restoration of physiological PH at reperfusion, which induces the opening of the mitochondrial permeability transition pore that leads to the necrosis and apoptosis of cardiomyocytes in the first several minutes of reperfusion. Over several hours after reperfusion, myocardial inflammation contributes to cardiomyocyte apoptosis and the healing of infarcted myocardium (43, 44). The recruitment of neutrophils and inflammatory monocytes is an established phenomenon after myocardial injury. Uncontrolled macrophage infiltration following MI results in ischemic heart failure. We and another group demonstrated that infarcted myocardium sequentially recruits Ly-6C^{hi} monocytes and Ly-6C^{lo}

monocytes in murine MI model (45) and IR injury model (46); Ly-6C^{hi} monocyte dominates in early phase to exhibit inflammatory functions including phagocytic and proteolytic activity, while Ly-6C^{low} monocyte dominates in later phase to resolute inflammation and promote angiogenesis. In consistent with this preclinical data, circulating CD14^{++}CD16^{-} and CD14^{+}CD16^{+} monocytes sequentially increase in patients with AMI. The peak levels of circulating CD14^{++}CD16^{-} monocytes were negatively correlated with the degree of myocardial salvage, suggesting that manipulating classical inflammatory monocyte could be a therapeutic target for salvaging for ischemic myocardial damage after MI (36).

Monocyte chemoattractant protein-1 belongs to the CC chemokine subfamily and its primary receptor CCR2 is highly expressed on a subpopulation of monocytes (Ly-6C^{high} monocytes in mice and CD14^{++}CD16^{-} monocytes in humans). These inflammatory monocytes depend on CCR2 to migrate into the injured tissue. We previously demonstrated that systemic gene therapy with plasmids encoding 7ND, a deletion mutant of MCP-1, limits atherogenesis associated with increased lesional extracellular matrix content, one of characteristics of stable plaques, without any effects on serum lipid concentration (47). Furthermore, this gene therapy not only limits progression of established preexisting atheroma but also leads to plaque stabilization (48). We then utilized the 7ND-incorporated PLGA nanoparticle for interfering with MCP-1/CCR2 signaling and demonstrated inhibition of macrophage accumulation in the atherosclerotic plaque, followed by amelioration of morphological characteristics similar to human destabilized/ruptured plaque in the brachiocephalic artery of ApoE-deficient mice (34). Leuschner et al. demonstrated that inhibition of monocyte CCR2 with siCCR2-incorporated lipid nanoparticle inhibits macrophage accumulation in sites of inflammation and reduces atherosclerotic formation and infarct size in myocardial IR injury (49). Another group reported that blockade of CCR2 markedly reduced macrophage infiltration in ischemic lesions that results in attenuation of myocardial IR injury in mice *via* inhibition of macrophage-related oxidative stress and MMPs (50) They also demonstrated that macrophage infiltration into infarcted tissue was impaired in CCR2$^{-/-}$ mice after coronary ligation and the CCR2 deficiency ameliorates post-MI left ventricular (LV) remodeling *via* inhibition of macrophage-related MMPs (51). These data suggested that inflammatory subpopulations of monocytes/macrophages are feasible therapeutic targets for coronary artery disease.

Other immune cells, including dendritic cells (DCs), T cells, and B cells, also play important roles in atherosclerosis. A predominant subpopulation of T cells in atherosclerotic lesion is CD4^{+} T cells. CD8^{+} T cells and natural killer T cells are minor T cell subpopulations. Antigen-presenting cells such as macrophages and DCs process the disease-related antigens including oxidized LDL, heat-shock proteins and microbes, and present them to CD4^{+} T cells as fragments loaded onto major-histocompatibility-complex class II molecules, which translates innate to adaptive immunity and is one of the therapeutic targets in adaptive immunity. In fact, vaccination targeting oxidized LDL-immuned DCs ameliorates atherosclerosis in LDL receptor-deficient mice (52). Activated T cells subsequently produce the type 1 helper T (Th1) cytokines (e.g., interferon γ) to initiate pro-inflammatory responses. Atherosclerotic lesions usually contain Th1 cytokines rather than the type 2 helper T (Th2) cytokines. In contrast, regulatory T cells modulate the process by producing anti-inflammatory cytokines, such as IL-10 and transforming growth factor-β (TGF-β) (53). The role of B cells in the progression of atherosclerosis still remains poorly understood, but it has recently gained more attention. B cells have two main subsets in mice based on their origin; B1 and B2. The role of the majority subset B2 cells in atherosclerotic lesion is controversial, while B1 cells seem to be atheroprotective (54). The corresponding B cell subsets in humans have not been clearly demonstrated. Nanomedicine can be applied to those atherosclerosis-regulating immune cells. However, the application of nanomedicine to atherosclerotic disease is extremely limited so far. A previous study demonstrated that intranasal immunization with chitosan/pCETP nanoparticles inhibits atherosclerosis in rabbit, in which the nanoparticulation enabled an efficient delivery of the antigen peptide to antigen presenting cells while sparing mucociliary clearance (55). Further studies are needed for the development of nanomedicine targeting adaptive immunity by utilizing nanoparticles as antigen delivery carriers of vaccination.

NANOMATERIALS FOR IMAGING OF MACROPHAGES

We have described that macrophage-mediated inflammation plays a crucial role in coronary artery disease. Hence, imaging of macrophages provides insight for future therapeutic options for cardiovascular diseases, in which several nanomaterials are being investigated as new imaging modalities. Developing those modalities for imaging macrophages is also indispensable in terms of quantitative analysis of therapeutic effects of anti-inflammatory drugs. Computed tomography (CT) is widely used for imaging of coronary artery in clinical setting. Nanomaterials for CT are limited because it requires high concentrations of absorbent nanomaterials to detect macrophages with X-ray. N1177, a crystalline iodined aroyloxy ester covered with a polymer, can detect macrophage-rich arterial walls in rabbits by CT (56). Macrophage-targeted gold high-density lipoprotein (HDL) nanoparticle can be localized in the macrophages of atherosclerotic plaque in the aorta of ApoE-deficient mice (57). MRI has high soft tissue contrast resolution and can detect plaque morphology non-invasively without radiation exposure. SPIO nanoparticle and ultrasmall superparamagnetic iron oxide (USPIO) are nanomaterial developed as the negative contrast for MRI. SPIO- and USPIO-based contrast agents consist of iron oxide core with hydrophilic polymeric coating, such as dextran-coated monocrystalline iron oxide nanoparticle-47 (MION-47) and dextran-crosslinked iron oxides. High-resolution MRI after administration of MION-47 can assess macrophage burden in atheromata induced by balloon injury of cholesterol-fed New Zealand White rabbits (58). In clinical setting, ATHEROMA trial has been conducted to examine USPIO-related signal change in patients with carotid stenosis >40%, but USPIO-enhanced MRI did not predict cardiovascular events significantly (59). On the other hand, USPIO-based contrast, ferumoxytol, has succeeded in characterizing infarcted myocardium mainly by detecting infiltrating macrophages (60). There are some reagents that adopt "active-targeting" strategy to image lesional macrophages. One good example is that iron oxide nanoparticle conjugated with ligand of vascular cell adhesion molecule 1 (VCAM-1) visualized VCAM-1-expressing endothelial cells and macrophages in ApoE-deficient mice (61). Nano-sized probes for near infrared fluorescence (NIRF) are used in animal studies. The excitation and emission wavelengths of NIRF probes range from 600 to 900 nm. In that range, the absorbance and scattering of biological tissues are relatively low. These probes are designed to be activated when target protease cleaves protease-specific peptide substrates linked to quenched fluorescent dyes. MMP (62, 63) and cathepsin are used as the substrates to image macrophage burden (64).

ANTI-INFLAMMATORY THERAPEUTICS WITH NANOMATERIALS FOR CORONARY ARTERY DISEASE

Atherosclerosis

We have recently developed an innovative nano-DDS utilizing polymeric PLGA nanoparticle-incorporating pitavastatin (Pitava-NP) without PEGylation to enhance the anti-inflammatory effects of statin on monocyte/macrophage-mediated inflammation of coronary artery disease. The average diameter of polymeric nanoparticles is 200 nm. Fluorescence-labeled nanoparticle (FITC-NP) was incorporated mainly Lineage (CD90/B220/CD49b/NK1.1/Ly-6G)$^-$CD11b$^+$ monocytes in blood and Lineage$^-$CD11b$^+$ monocytes/macrophages in aorta by intravenous injection (**Figure 2A**). Fluorescence microscopic images demonstrated that FITC signal was observed in atherosclerotic plaque of brachiocephalic artery 24 h after intravenous injection of FITC-NP, suggesting that FITC-NP was passively delivered to atherosclerotic lesion with enhanced permeability (**Figure 2B**). Time course analysis of FITC signal in peripheral and aortic leukocytes by flow cytometry revealed that the delivery of FITC-NP to peripheral monocytes was followed by its delivery to aortic macrophages over 2–7 days after injection, suggesting a direct delivery of intravenous PLGA nanoparticles to blood monocytes, which gradually migrate to the atherosclerotic aorta. Weekly intravenous treatment with Pitava-NPs reduced circulating inflammatory Ly-6C^{high} monocytes, macrophage accumulation in the atherosclerotic lesions of the aortic root, and ameliorated morphological characteristics similar to human destabilized/ruptured plaque in the brachiocephalic arteries of ApoE-deficient mice (**Figures 2C,D**) (34). In consistent with these data, a preclinical study from other investigators reported that a statin-loaded reconstituted HDL (rHDL) nanoparticle inhibits atherosclerotic formation. Using dual gadolinium and fluorescent dye-labeled rHDL nanoparticle, they demonstrated that intravenously administered rHDL was incorporated into lesional monocytes and macrophages, and inhibits plaque formation with reduced macrophage content in the aortic root (65).

Myocardial IR Injury

Several pharmacological agents, including statins and erythropoietin analogs, have been shown to reduce MI size in preclinical studies (44). However, several clinical trials on pharmacological cardioprotection for myocardial IR injury have failed to demonstrate a positive impact on clinical outcome, and there is no effective therapy for preventing myocardial reperfusion injury in STEMI patients (44, 67). One possible explanation for the failure of current clinical trials is an insufficient drug delivery during a limited interventional time window, while administered at the time of reperfusion. Therefore, from a clinical perspective, it is feasible to apply an effective DDS that facilitates delivery to the sites of IR injury during reperfusion, a clinically feasible time point. In addition to macrophage-mediated inflammation, the activation of pro-survival kinases including PI3K/Akt and Erk1/2 that are known as reperfusion injury salvage kinases (RISK) in ischemic myocardium is another potential therapeutic target to reduce reperfusion-induced necrosis and apoptosis, and then limits MI size. Statins are known to afford cardioprotection from IR injury in animals (68). The cardioprotection of statins on infarct size is mediated partly by activating the RISK pathway. Intravenously injected nanoparticles accumulate not only in MPS but also in injured tissues, including IR myocardium, where vascular permeability is enhanced (13). Thus, nano-DDS may be a feasible for myocardial IR injury targeting both inflammatory monocytes/macrophages and ischemic myocardium. Therefore, we examined the efficacy of Pitava-NP as a DDS for myocardial IR injury. In a rat model of myocardial 30-min IR, PLGA nanoparticles were found exclusively in the ischemic myocardium (**Figure 3A**). Flow cytometric analysis showed the incorporation of FITC-NPs in CD11b$^+$ leukocytes in blood and IR heart. Intravenous treatment with Pitava-NPs at the time of myocardial reperfusion significantly reduced infarct size 24 h after reperfusion (**Figure 3B**). The therapeutic effect of Pitava-NP derived from the inhibition of MCP-1/CCR2 pathway by inactivation of NF-κB, which resulted in reduced macrophage-mediated inflammation (**Figure 3C**) and the activation of RISK pathway in ischemic myocardium (69). To establish preclinical proof-of-concept, we also demonstrated the therapeutic efficiency of Pitava-NPs in a preclinical conscious pig IR injury model (70). These data suggested that nano-DDS of statin to inflammatory cells and ischemic myocardium is a feasible strategy for the treatment of myocardial IR injury. Other nanomaterials can be applied as a nano-DDS for myocardial IR injury. PEGylated liposomes also showed the prolonged circulating time in blood and the specific accumulation in ischemic/reperfused myocardium. The liposomes encapsulating adenosine demonstrated the enhanced cardioprotection effects of adenosine against myocardial IR injury in rats (71). Dendrimer nanoparticles might be another candidate for the nano-DDS due to selective localization in ischemic myocardium (72). Further studies are needed to assess the therapeutic effects of a dendrimer–drug conjugate in myocardial IR injury.

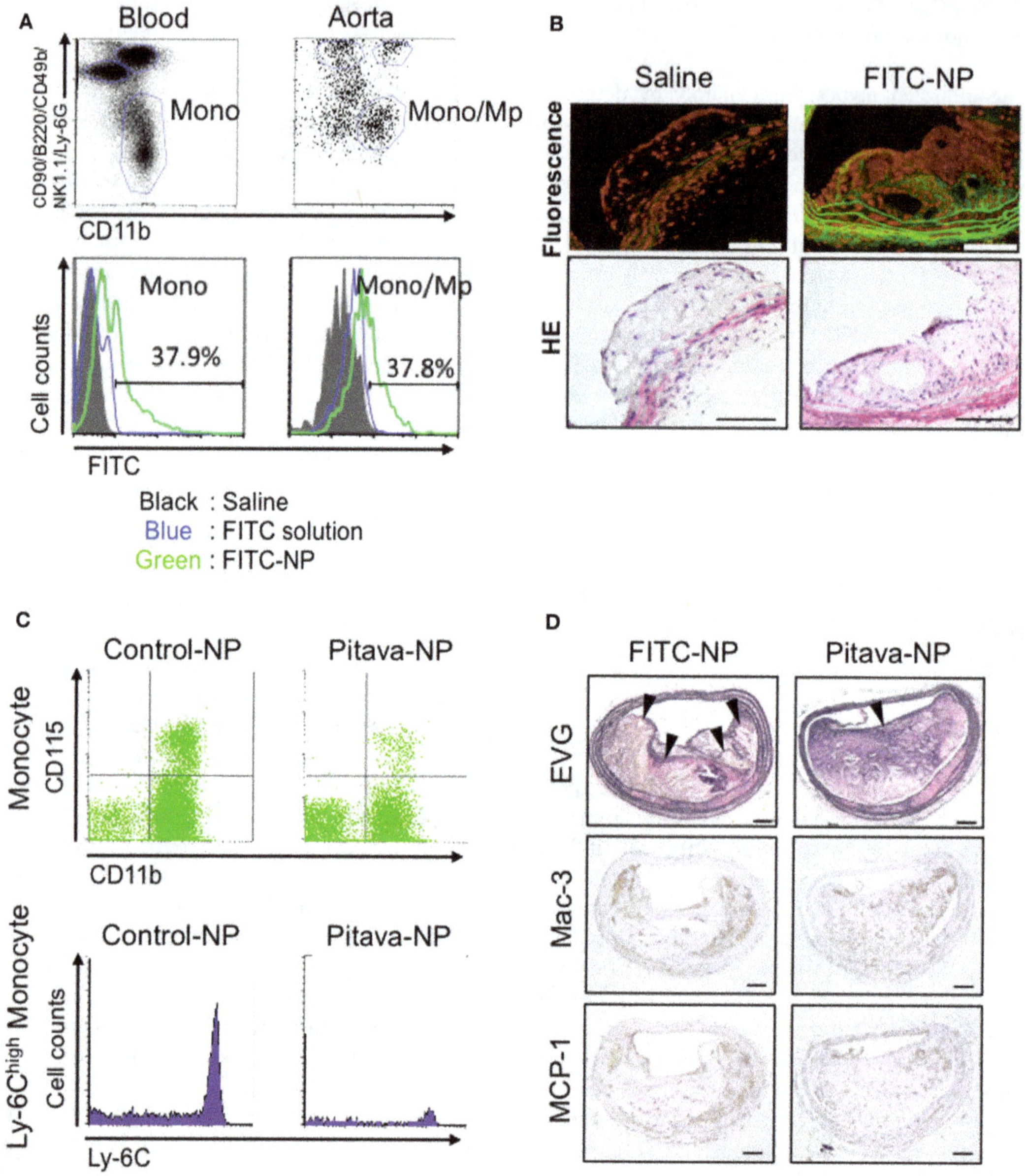

FIGURE 2 | Efficacy of pitavastatin-nanoparticle in atherosclerotic mice. **(A)** Flow cytometry of circulating leukocytes 2 days after intravenous injection of poly lactic-co-glycolic acid nanoparticles encapsulated with FITC (FITC-NP). The histograms demonstrate FITC uptake by monocytes in the blood and the aorta. **(B)** Fluorescent and light micrographs of brachiocephalic arteries 24 h after intravenous injection of saline or FITC-NP. **(C)** Flow cytometric dot plots and histograms of leukocytes from mice injected intravenously with control (empty)-NPs or pitavastatin-NPs (Pitava-NP). **(D)** Weekly intravenous injection of Pitava-NP increased fibrous cap thickness and decreased the number of buried fibrous caps in the atherosclerotic plaques with reduced macrophage accumulation (Mac-3) and monocyte chemoattractant protein-1 (MCP-1) expression. Arrows indicate disrupted/buried fibrous caps.

Post-MI LV Remodeling

Recent advances in therapeutic strategy including coronary intervention and optimal medication decreased the acute phase mortality of MI, but the prevalence of chronic heart failure in MI survivors is increasing (73). Intractable heart failure due to LV remodeling (dilatation and remodeling) associated with increased fibrosis and wall thinning after MI remains a major clinical concern. Therefore, there is also an unmet need for cardioprotective modalities to ameliorate post-infarct LV remodeling. The infarcts show high inflammatory response with the recruitment of innate immune cells including macrophages and monocytes derived from extramedullary hematopoiesis such as spleen (74). We have examined the efficacy of PLGA nanoparticles as a DDS for post-infarct LV remodeling. After permanent left anterior descending coronary artery (LAD) ligation, Pitava-NP was intravenously administered for three consecutive days. Intravenously injected

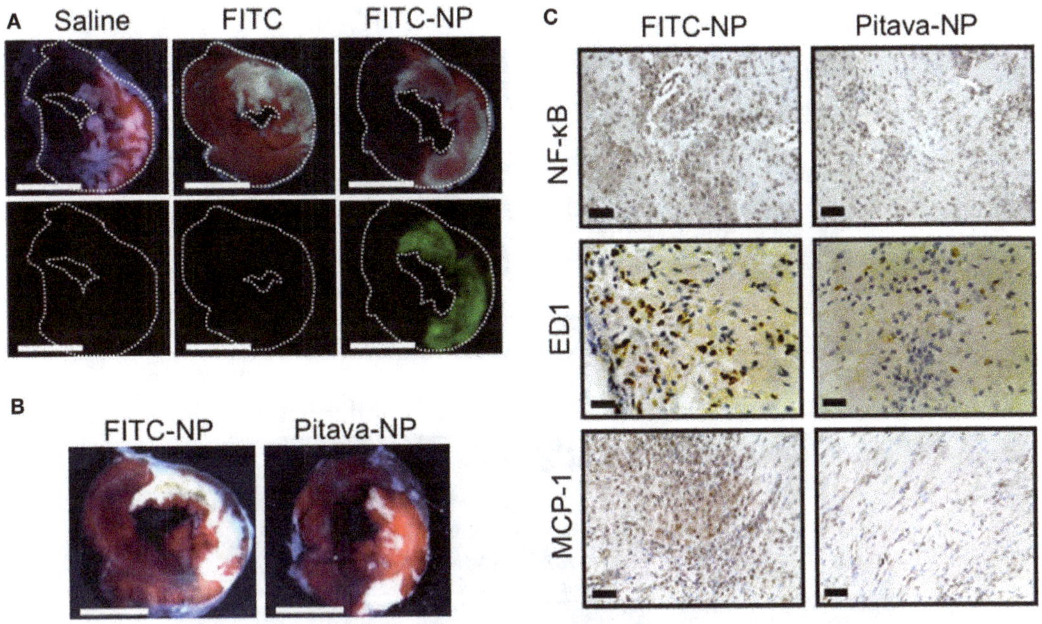

FIGURE 3 | Efficacy of pitavastatin-nanoparticle in myocardial ischemia-reperfusion injury. **(A)** Representative light (upper) and fluorescence (lower) stereomicrographs of cross-section of the ischemia-reperfusion (IR) hearts 3 h after intravenous injection of saline, FITC alone, or FITC-NP. **(B)** Intravenous treatment with Pitava-NP at the time of reperfusion reduced infarct size 24 h after reperfusion. **(C)** Cross-sections from IR myocardium stained with NF-κB, ED-1, and monocyte chemoattractant protein-1 (MCP-1).

FITC-NPs were delivered to Lineage$^-$CD11b$^+$ monocytes in the blood, spleen, and heart, but not in non-infarcted myocardium within the area at risk due to coronary ligation (**Figure 4A**), suggesting that the beneficial effects of Pitava-NPs on post-infarct LV remodeling can be predominantly derived from those on inflammatory cells. Actually, Pitava-NP decreased macrophage accumulation in the heart by inhibiting not only angiotensin II-mediated monocyte mobilization from the spleen (**Figure 4B**) but also monocyte mobilization from the bone marrow that is supposed to be mediated by CCR2 (75). Intravenous treatment with Pitava-NPs after MI induced by permanent LAD ligation attenuated post-infarct LV remodeling associated with reduced monocyte/macrophage accumulation in the heart (**Figure 4C**) (76). A delayed transition from inflammatory to anti-inflammatory macrophages by prolonged recruitment of classical inflammatory monocytes to myocardium may also interfere with post-infarct LV remodeling (77). Other investigators have intervened a transcription factor that shifts macrophages to inflammatory subsets by utilizing siRNA lipid nanoparticles targeting interferon regulatory factor 5 (IRF5). They demonstrated that siIRF5 improves post-infarct LV remodeling by reprogramming macrophages toward anti-inflammatory subsets (78).

SUMMARY AND CLINICAL PERSPECTIVE

In this review, we have summarized a series of evidence including (1) the anti-inflammatory therapeutics for coronary artery disease, (2) a variety of nanomaterials for drug delivery systems, (3) the role and imaging of monocytes/macrophages in coronary artery disease, and (4) application of nano-DDS based on PLGA nanoparticle to coronary artery disease, such as plaque destabilization, IR injury, and post-MI LV remodeling. Applications of nano-DDS for coronary artery disease is a feasible strategy by utilizing increased incorporation of nanomaterials by MPS and enhanced permeability of inflammatory vasculature (**Figure 1**). In addition to the therapeutic effects of nano-DDS on coronary artery disease, there are a wide variety of opportunities to combine nano-DDS and various therapeutic agents, including chemical, nucleotide, peptide, and others, which may extend the possibility of current pharmacotherapy for several cardiovascular diseases. Possible application of nano-DDS in other cardiovascular diseases may include, pulmonary hypertension (79, 80), vein graft disease (81), and coronary artery stents (82). The clinical application of nano-DDS utilizing Good Manufacturing Practice-compliant Pitava-NPs in this review is in progress. We have already completed phase I/IIa investigators' initiated clinical trial testing the efficacy of Pitava-NP in patients with critical limb ischemia in the Kyushu University Hospital (UMIN000008011). We have also completed a phase I clinical trial testing the safety of an intravenous administration of Pitava-NP in healthy volunteers (UMIN000014940). Recently, phase III CANTOS trial targeting interleukin-1β with human anti-IL-1β monoclonal antibody, canakinumab, has demonstrated that the inhibition of systemic inflammation may reduce cardiovascular risk even in the absence of concomitant lipid lowering (83). This trial has proved the concept that anti-inflammatory therapeutics targeting innate immunity pathway can be applicable in humans, and our novel DDS utilizing PLGA polymer-based nanotechnology might be one of promising therapeutic strategies for various cardiovascular diseases in the near future.

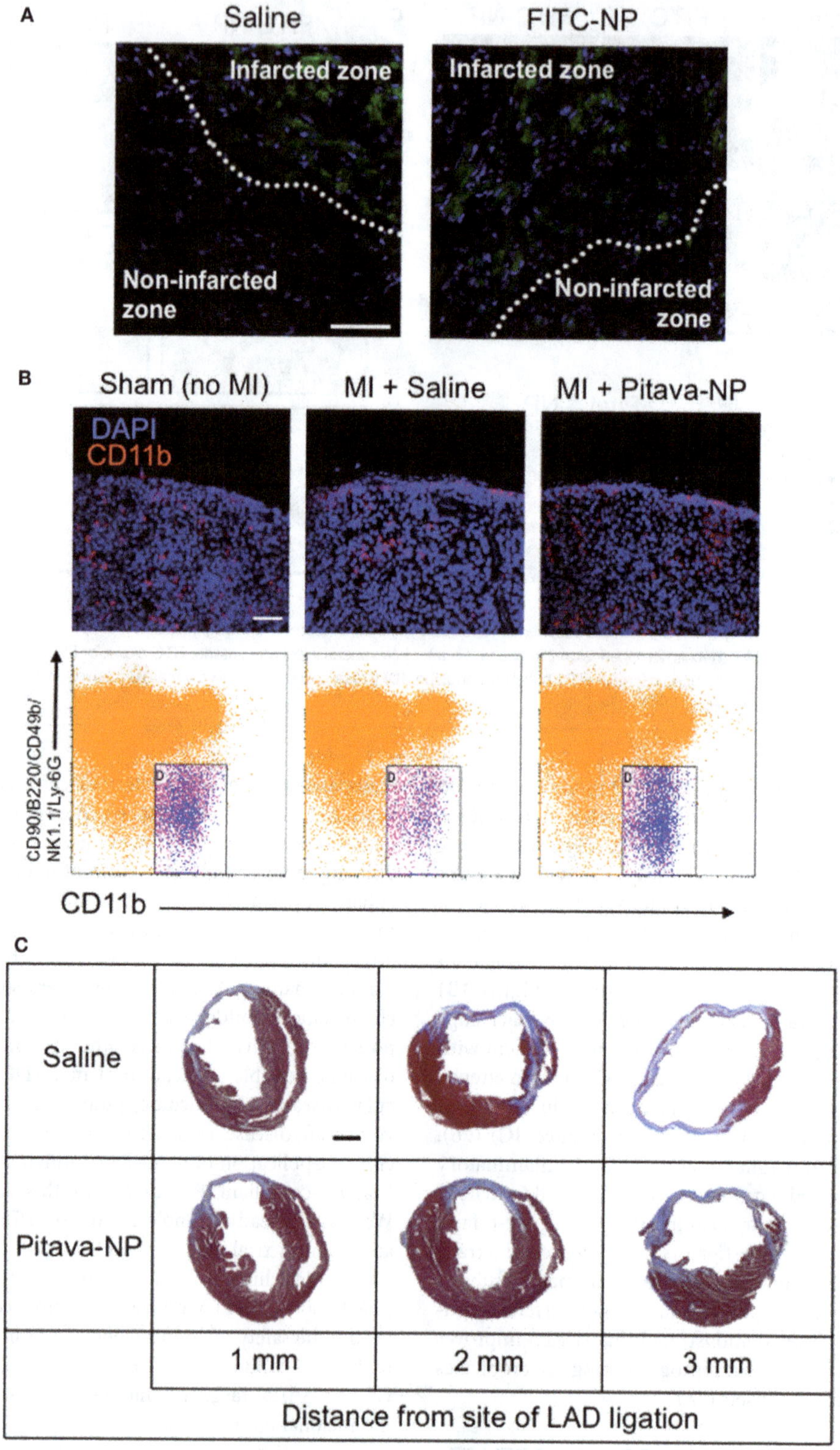

FIGURE 4 | Efficacy of pitavastatin-nanoparticle in post-myocardial infarction left ventricular (LV) remodeling. **(A)** Cross sectional pictures of the infarcted myocardium observed under fluorescent microscope 3 days after LAD ligation. Saline or FITC-NP were injected for three consecutive days after ligation. Weak fluorescent signals observed in infarcted zones are auto-fluorescence from dead cardiomyocytes. **(B)** (Upper panel) Splenic sections stained with anti-CD11b antibody (red) and DAPI (blue) showing the subcapsular red pulp. (Lower panel) Dot plots of flow cytometric analysis of spleen samples. Treatment with Pitava-NPs inhibited MI-induced Lineage (CD90/B220/CD49b/NK1.1/Ly-6G)$^{-}$CD11b^{+} monocyte reduction in the spleen. **(C)** Intravenous treatment with Pitava-NPs for three consecutive days ameliorated LV remodeling 4 weeks after myocardial infarction.

AUTHOR CONTRIBUTIONS

SK, TM, J-iK, KN, and KE make substantial contributions to conception and design and acquisition, analysis, and interpretation of data.

ACKNOWLEDGMENTS

This work was supported by Grants-in-Aid for Scientific Research from the Ministry of Education, Culture, Sports, Science and Technology, Tokyo, Japan (25860607 to SK, 17K09590 to TM, 22390160 and 25293185 to KE), the Translational Research Network Program from the Japan Agency for Medical Research and Development, Tokyo, Japan (to KE) and Health Science Research Grants (Translational Research, Research on Intractable Diseases, and Research on Nanomedicine) from the Ministry of Health, Labour and Welfare, Tokyo, Japan (to KE). The authors thank Kazuhiro Nagaoka, Yajing Mao, Soichi Nakashiro, and Yasuhiro Nakano for their excellent works demonstrated in this review.

REFERENCES

Randomised trial of cholesterol lowering in 4444 patients with coronary heart disease: the Scandinavian Simvastatin Survival Study (4S). *Lancet* (1994) 344:1383–9.

Sacks FM, Pfeffer MA, Moye LA, Rouleau JL, Rutherford JD, Cole TG, et al. The effect of pravastatin on coronary events after myocardial infarction in patients with average cholesterol levels. Cholesterol and Recurrent Events Trial investigators. *N Engl J Med* (1996) 335:1001–9. doi:10.1056/NEJM199610033351401

Long-term intervention with pravastatin in ischaemic disease (LIPID) study group. Prevention of cardiovascular events and death with pravastatin in patients with coronary heart disease and a broad range of initial cholesterol levels. *N Engl J Med* (1998) 339:1349–57. doi:10.1056/NEJM199811053391902

Shepherd J, Cobbe SM, Ford I, Isles CG, Lorimer AR, MacFarlane PW, et al. Prevention of coronary heart disease with pravastatin in men with hypercholesterolemia. West of Scotland Coronary Prevention Study Group. *N Engl J Med* (1995) 333:1301–7. doi:10.1056/NEJM199511163332001

Downs JR, Clearfield M, Weis S, Whitney E, Shapiro DR, Beere PA, et al. Primary prevention of acute coronary events with lovastatin in men and women with average cholesterol levels: results of AFCAPS/TexCAPS. Air Force/Texas Coronary Atherosclerosis Prevention Study. *JAMA* (1998) 279:1615–22. doi:10.1001/jama.279.20.1615

Ridker PM, Danielson E, Fonseca FA, Genest J, Gotto AM, Kastelein JJ, et al. Reduction in C-reactive protein and LDL cholesterol and cardiovascular event rates after initiation of rosuvastatin: a prospective study of the JUPITER trial. *Lancet* (2009) 373:1175–82. doi:10.1016/S0140-6736(09)60447-5

Takemoto M, Liao JK. Pleiotropic effects of 3-hydroxy-3-methylglutaryl coenzyme A reductase inhibitors. *Arterioscler Thromb Vasc Biol* (2001) 21:1712–9. doi:10.1161/hq1101.098486

Libby P, Pasterkamp G. Requiem for the 'vulnerable plaque'. *Eur Heart J* (2015) 36:2984–7. doi:10.1093/eurheartj/ehv349

Cannon CP, Blazing MA, Giugliano RP, McCagg A, White JA, Theroux P, et al. Ezetimibe added to statin therapy after acute coronary syndromes. *N Engl J Med* (2015) 372:2387–97. doi:10.1056/NEJMoa1410489

Takase S, Matoba T, Nakashiro S, Mukai Y, Inoue S, Oi K, et al. Ezetimibe in combination with statins ameliorates endothelial dysfunction in coronary arteries after stenting: the CuVIC Trial (effect of cholesterol absorption inhibitor usage on target vessel dysfunction after coronary stenting), a multicenter randomized controlled trial. *Arterioscler Thromb Vasc Biol* (2016) 37(2):350–8. doi:10.1161/ATVBAHA.116.308388

Sabatine MS, Giugliano RP, Keech AC, Honarpour N, Wiviott SD, Murphy SA, et al. Evolocumab and clinical outcomes in patients with cardiovascular disease. *N Engl J Med* (2017) 376:1713–22. doi:10.1056/NEJMoa1615664

Mulder WJM, Strijkers GJ, van Tilborg GAF, Cormode DP, Fayad ZA, Nicolay K. Nanoparticulate assemblies of amphiphiles and diagnostically active materials for multimodality imaging. *Acc Chem Res* (2009) 42:904–14. doi:10.1021/ar800223c

Acharya S, Sahoo SK. PLGA nanoparticles containing various anticancer agents and tumour delivery by EPR effect. *Adv Drug Deliv Rev* (2011) 63: 170–83. doi:10.1016/j.addr.2010.10.008

Morgan MT, Carnahan MA, Finkelstein S, Prata CAH, Degoricija L, Lee SJ, et al. Dendritic supramolecular assemblies for drug delivery. *Chem Commun* (2005) 97:4309–4303. doi:10.1039/b502411k

Bobo D, Robinson KJ, Islam J, Thurecht KJ, Corrie SR. Nanoparticle-based medicines: a review of FDA-approved materials and clinical trials to date. *Pharm Res* (2016) 33:2373–87. doi:10.1007/s11095-016-1958-5

Gabizon A, Catane R, Uziely B, Kaufman B, Safra T, Cohen R, et al. Prolonged circulation time and enhanced accumulation in malignant exudates of doxorubicin encapsulated in polyethylene-glycol coated liposomes. *Cancer Res* (1994) 54:987–92.

Thomas TP, Joice M, Sumit M, Silpe JE, Kotlyar A, Bharathi S, et al. Design and in vitro validation of multivalent dendrimer methotrexates as a folate-targeting anticancer therapeutic. *Curr Pharm Des* (2013) 19:6594–605. doi:10.2174/1381612811319370004

Ajima K, Yudasaka M, Murakami T, Maigné A, Shiba K, Iijima S. Carbon nanohorns as anticancer drug carriers. *Mol Pharm* (2005) 2:475–80. doi:10.1021/mp0500566

Wang Y-XJ, Idée J-M. A comprehensive literatures update of clinical researches of superparamagnetic resonance iron oxide nanoparticles for magnetic resonance imaging. *Quant Imaging Med Surg* (2017) 7:88–122. doi:10.21037/qims.2017.05.05

Jain S, Hirst DG, O'Sullivan JM. Gold nanoparticles as novel agents for cancer therapy. *BJR* (2012) 85:101–13. doi:10.1259/bjr/59448833

Yazdi AS, Guarda G, Riteau N, Drexler SK, Tardivel A, Couillin I, et al. Nanoparticles activate the NLR pyrin domain containing 3 (Nlrp3) inflam- masome and cause pulmonary inflammation through release of IL-1α and IL-1β. *Proc Natl Acad Sci U S A* (2010) 107:19449–54. doi:10.1073/pnas. 1008155107

Murphy A, Casey A, Byrne G, Chambers G, Howe O. Silver nanoparticles induce pro-inflammatory gene expression and inflammasome activation in human monocytes. *J Appl Toxicol* (2016) 36:1311–20. doi:10.1002/jat.3315

Seaton A, Tran L, Aitken R, Donaldson K. Nanoparticles, human health hazard and regulation. *J R Soc Interface* (2009) 7:S119–29. doi:10.1098/rsif.2009.0252.focus

Kim BG, Lee PH, Lee SH, Park MK, Jang AS. Effect of TiO2 nanoparticles on inflammasome-mediated airway inflammation and responsiveness. *Allergy Asthma Immunol Res* (2017) 9:257–64. doi:10.4168/aair.2017.9.3.257

Pétrilli V, Papin S, Dostert C, Mayor A, Martinon F, Tschopp J. Activation of the NALP3 inflammasome is triggered by low intracellular potassium concentration. *Cell Death Differ* (2007) 14:1583–9. doi:10.1038/sj.cdd.4402195

Hornung V, Bauernfeind F, Halle A, Samstad EO, Kono H, Rock KL, et al. Silica crystals and aluminum salts activate the NALP3 inflammasome through phagosomal destabilization. *Nat Immunol* (2008) 9:847–56. doi:10.1038/ni.1631

Baron L, Gombault A, Fanny M, Villeret B, Savigny F, Guillou N, et al. The NLRP3 inflammasome is activated by nanoparticles through ATP, ADP and adenosine. *Cell Death Dis* (2015) 6:e1629–1615. doi:10.1038/cddis.2014.576

Weissleder R, Nahrendorf M, Pittet MJ. Imaging macrophages with nanopar- ticles. *Nat Mater* (2014) 13:125–38. doi:10.1038/nmat3780

Asai T. Nanoparticle-mediated delivery of anticancer agents to tumor angiogenic vessels. *Biol Pharm Bull* (2012) 35(11):1855–61. doi:10.1248/bpb.b212013

Byrne JD, Betancourt T, Brannon-Peppas L. Active targeting schemes for nanoparticle systems in cancer therapeutics. *Adv Drug Deliv Rev* (2008) 60:1615–26. doi:10.1016/j.addr.2008.08.005

Ross R. Atherosclerosis—an inflammatory disease. *New Engl J Med* (1999) 340(2):115–26. doi:10.1056/NEJM199901143400207

Libby P. Inflammation in atherosclerosis. *Nature* (2002) 420:868–74. doi:10.1038/nature01323

Gordon S. Macrophage heterogeneity and tissue lipids. *J Clin Invest* (2007) 117:1–4. doi:10.1172/JCI30992

Katsuki S, Matoba T, Nakashiro S, Sato K, Koga J-I, Nakano K, et al. Nanoparticle-mediated delivery of pitavastatin inhibits atherosclerotic plaque destabilization/rupture in mice by regulating the recruitment of inflammatory monocytes. *Circulation* (2014) 129:896–906. doi:10.1161/ CIRCULATIONAHA.113.002870

Ziegler-Heitbrock L, Hofer TPJ. Toward a refined definition of monocyte subsets. *Front Immunol* (2013) 4:1–5. doi:10.3389/fimmu.2013.00023

Tsujioka H, Imanishi T, Ikejima H, Kuroi A, Takarada S, Tanimoto T, et al. Impact of heterogeneity of human peripheral blood monocyte subsets on myocardial salvage in patients with primary acute myocardial infarction. *J Am Coll Cardiol* (2009) 54:130–8. doi:10.1016/j.jacc.2009.04.021

Murray PJ, Allen JE, Biswas SK, Fisher EA, Gilroy DW, Goerdt S, et al. Macrophage activation and polarization: nomenclature and experimental guidelines. *Immunity* (2014) 41:14–20. doi:10.1016/j.immuni.2014.06.008

Chinetti-Gbaguidi G, Colin S, Staels B. Macrophage subsets in atherosclerosis. *Nat Rev Cardiol* (2014) 12:10–7. doi:10.1038/nrcardio.2014.173

Kadl A, Meher AK, Sharma PR, Lee MY, Doran AC, Johnstone SR, et al. Identification of a novel macrophage phenotype that develops in response to atherogenic phospholipids via Nrf2. *Circ Res* (2010) 107:737–46. doi:10.1161/ CIRCRESAHA.109.215715

Boyle JJ, Harrington HA, Piper E, Elderfield K, Stark J, Landis RC, et al. Coronary intraplaque hemorrhage evokes a novel atheroprotective macrophage phenotype. *Am J Pathol* (2009) 174:1097–108. doi:10.2353/ ajpath.2009.080431

Finn AV, Nakano M, Polavarapu R, Karmali V, Saeed O, Zhao X, et al. Hemoglobin directs macrophage differentiation and prevents foam cell formation in human atherosclerotic plaques. *J Am Coll Cardiol* (2012) 59:166–77. doi:10.1016/j.jacc.2011.10.852

Erbel C, Tyka M, Helmes CM, Akhavanpoor M, Rupp G, Domschke G, et al. CXCL4-induced plaque macrophages can be specifically identified by co-expression of MMP7 +S100A8 +in vitroand in vivo. *Innate Immun* (2014) 21:255–65. doi:10.1177/1753425914526461

Hausenloy DJ, Yellon DM. Myocardial ischemia-reperfusion injury: a neglected therapeutic target. *J Clin Invest* (2013) 123:92–100. doi:10.1172/ JCI62874

Yellon DM, Hausenloy DJ. Myocardial reperfusion injury. *N Engl J Med* (2007) 357:1121–35. doi:10.1056/NEJMra071667

Nahrendorf M, Swirski FK, Aikawa E, Stangenberg L, Wurdinger T, Figueiredo JL, et al. The healing myocardium sequentially mobilizes two monocyte subsets with divergent and complementary functions. *J Exp Med* (2007) 204:3037–47. doi:10.1084/jem.20070885

Nakano Y, Matoba T, Tokutome M, Funamoto D, Katsuki S, Ikeda G, et al. Nanoparticle-mediated delivery of irbesartan induces cardioprotection from myocardial ischemia-reperfusion injury by antagonizing monocyte-mediated inflammation. *Sci Rep* (2016) 6:e6–14. doi:10.1038/srep29601

Ni W, Egashira K, Kitamoto S, Kataoka C, Koyanagi M, Inoue S, et al. New anti-monocyte chemoattractant protein-1 gene therapy attenuates atherosclerosis in apolipoprotein E-knockout mice. *Circulation* (2001) 103:2096–101. doi:10.1161/01.CIR.103.16.2096

Inoue S, Egashira K, Ni W, Kitamoto S, Usui M, Otani K. Anti-monocyte chemoattractant protein-1 gene therapy limits progression and destabilization of established atherosclerosis in apolipoprotein E-knockout mice. *Circulation* (2002) 106:2700–6. doi:10.1161/01.CIR.0000038140.80105.AD

Leuschner F, Dutta P, Gorbatov R, Novobrantseva TI, Donahoe JS, Courties G, et al. Therapeutic siRNA silencing in inflammatory monocytes in mice. *Nat Biotechnol* (2011) 29:1005–10. doi:10.1038/nbt.1989

Hayasaki T, Kaikita K, Okuma T, Yamamoto E, Kuziel WA, Ogawa H, et al. CC chemokine receptor-2 deficiency attenuates oxidative stress and infarct size caused by myocardial ischemia-reperfusion in mice. *Circ J* (2006) 70:342–51. doi:10.1253/circj.70.342

Kaikita K, Hayasaki T, Okuma T, Kuziel WA, Ogawa H, Takeya M. Targeted deletion of CC chemokine receptor 2 attenuates left ventricular remodeling after experimental myocardial infarction. *Am J Pathol* (2004) 165:439–47. doi:10.1016/S0002-9440(10)63309-3

Habets KLL, van Puijvelde GHM, van Duivenvoorde LM, van Wanrooij EJA, de Vos P, Tervaert J-WC, et al. Vaccination using oxidized low-density lipoprotein-pulsed dendritic cells reduces atherosclerosis in LDL receptor-de- ficient mice. *Cardiovasc Res* (2009) 85:622–30. doi:10.1093/cvr/cvp338

Hansson GK. Inflammation, atherosclerosis, and coronary artery disease. *N Engl J Med* (2005) 352:1685–95. doi:10.1056/NEJMra043430

Tsiantoulas D, Diehl CJ, Witztum JL, Binder CJ. B cells and humoral immunity in atherosclerosis. *Circ Res* (2014) 114:1743–56. doi:10.1161/ CIRCRESAHA.113.301145

Yuan X, Yang X, Cai D, Mao D, Wu J, Zong L, et al. Intranasal immunization with chitosan/pCETP nanoparticles inhibits atherosclerosis in a rabbit model of atherosclerosis. *Vaccine* (2008) 26:3727–34. doi:10.1016/j.vaccine.2008.04.065

Hyafil F, Cornily J-C, Feig JE, Gordon R, Vucic E, Amirbekian V, et al. Noninvasive detection of macrophages using a nanoparticulate contrast agent for computed tomography. *Nat Med* (2007) 13:636–41. doi:10.1038/nm1571

Cormode DP, Roessl E, Thran A, Skajaa T, Gordon RE. Atherosclerotic plaque composition: analysis with multicolor CT and targeted gold nanoparticles. *Radiology* (2010) 256(3):774–82. doi:10.1148/radiol.10092473

Morishige K, Kacher DF, Libby P, Josephson L, Ganz P, Weissleder R, et al. High-resolution magnetic resonance imaging enhanced with superparamag- netic nanoparticles measures macrophage burden in atherosclerosis. *Circulation* (2010) 122:1707–15. doi:10.1161/CIRCULATIONAHA.109.891804

Degnan AJ, Patterson AJ, Tang TY, Howarth SPS, Gillard JH. Evaluation of ultrasmall superparamagnetic iron oxide-enhanced MRI of carotid atherosclerosis to assess risk of cerebrovascular and cardiovascular events: follow-up of the ATHEROMA trial. *Cerebrovasc Dis* (2012) 34:169–73. doi:10.1159/000339984

Yilmaz A, Dengler MA, van der Kuip H, Yildiz H, Rösch S, Klumpp S, et al. Imaging of myocardial infarction using ultrasmall superparamagnetic iron oxide nanoparticles: a human study using a multi-parametric cardiovascular magnetic resonance imaging approach. *Eur Heart J* (2012) 34:462–75. doi:10.1093/eurheartj/ehs366

Nahrendorf M, Jaffer FA, Kelly KA, Sosnovik DE, Aikawa E, Libby P, et al. Noninvasive vascular cell adhesion molecule-1 imaging identifies inflammatory activation of cells in atherosclerosis. *Circulation* (2006) 114:1504–11. doi:10.1161/CIRCULATIONAHA.106.646380

Deguchi J-O, Aikawa M, Tung C-H, Aikawa E, Kim D-E, Ntziachristos V, et al. Inflammation in atherosclerosis: visualizing matrix metalloproteinase action in macrophages in vivo. *Circulation* (2006) 114:55–62. doi:10.1161/ CIRCULATIONAHA.106.619056

Koga J-I, Nakano T, Dahlman JE, Figueiredo J-L, Zhang H, Decano J, et al. Macrophage notch ligand delta-like 4 promotes vein graft lesion development: implications for the treatment of vein graft failure. *Arterioscler Thromb Vasc Biol* (2015) 35:2343–53. doi:10.1161/ATVBAHA.115.305516

Jaffer FA, Kim DE, Quinti L, Tung CH, Aikawa E, Pande AN, et al. Optical visualization of cathepsin K activity in atherosclerosis with a novel, protease-activatable fluorescence sensor. *Circulation* (2007) 115:2292–8. doi:10.1161/ CIRCULATIONAHA.106.660340

Duivenvoorden R, Tang J, Cormode DP, Mieszawska AJ, Izquierdo-Garcia D, Ozcan C, et al. A statin-loaded reconstituted high-density lipoprotein nanoparticle inhibits atherosclerotic plaque inflammation. *Nat Commun* (2014) 5:227–212. doi:10.1038/ncomms4065

Nakashiro S, Matoba T, Umezu R, Koga JI, Tokutome M, Katsuki S, et al. Pioglitazone-incorporated nanoparticles prevent plaque destabilization and rupture by regulating monocyte/macrophage differentiation in ApoE-/- mice. *Arterioscler Thromb Vasc Biol* (2016) 36:491–500. doi:10.1161/ATVBAHA. 115.307057

Hausenloy DJ, Yellon DM. Targeting myocardial reperfusion injury – the searchcontinues.*NEnglJ Med*(2015)373:1073–5.doi:10.1056/NEJMe1509718

Bell RM, Yellon DM. Atorvastatin, administered at the onset of reperfusion, and independent of lipid lowering, protects the myocardium by up-regulating a pro-survival pathway. *J Am Coll Cardiol* (2003) 41:508–15. doi:10.1016/ S0735-1097(02)02816-4

Nagaoka K, Matoba T, Mao Y, Nakano Y, Ikeda G, Egusa S, et al. A new therapeutic modality for acute myocardial infarction: nanoparticle-mediated delivery of pitavastatin induces cardioprotection from ischemia-reperfusion injury via activation of PI3K/Akt pathway and anti-inflammation in a rat model. *PLoS One* (2015) 10:e132451. doi:10.1371/journal.pone.0132451

Ichimura K, Matoba T, Nakano K, Tokutome M, Honda K, Koga JI, et al. A translational study of a new therapeutic approach for acute myocardial infarction: nanoparticle-mediated delivery of pitavastatin into reperfused myocardium reduces ischemia-reperfusion injury in a preclinical porcine model. *PLoS One* (2016) 11:e162425. doi:10.1371/journal.pone.0162425

Takahama H, Minamino T, Asanuma H, Fujita M, Asai T, Wakeno M, et al. Prolonged targeting of ischemic/reperfused myocardium by liposomal adenosine augments cardioprotection in rats. *J Am Coll Cardiol* (2009) 53:709–17. doi:10.1016/j.jacc.2008.11.014

Magruder JT, Crawford TC, Lin YA, Zhang F, Grimm JC, Kannan RM, et al. Selective localization of a novel dendrimer nanoparticle in myocardial ischemia-reperfusion injury. *Ann Thorac Surg* (2017) 104:891–8. doi:10.1016/j. athoracsur.2016.12.051

Nahrendorf M, Pittet MJ, Swirski FK. Monocytes: protagonists of infarct inflammation and repair after myocardial infarction. *Circulation* (2010) 121:2437–45. doi:10.1161/CIRCULATIONAHA.109.916346

Swirski FK, Nahrendorf M, Etzrodt M, Wildgruber M, Cortez- Retamozo V, Panizzi P, et al. Identification of splenic reservoir monocytes and their deployment to inflammatory sites. *Science* (2009) 325:612–6. doi:10.1126/ science.1175202

Jia T, Pamer EG. Dispensable but not irrelevant. *Science* (2009) 325:549–50. doi:10.1126/science.1178329

Mao Y, Koga JI, Tokutome M, Matoba T, Ikeda G, Nakano K, et al. Nanoparticle-mediated delivery of pitavastatin to monocytes/macrophages inhibits left ventricular remodeling after acute myocardial infarction by inhibiting monocyte-mediated inflammation. *Int Heart J* (2017) 58:615–23. doi:10.1536/ihj.16-457

Panizzi P, Swirski FK, Figueiredo JL, Waterman P, Sosnovik DE, Aikawa E, et al. Impaired infarct healing in atherosclerotic mice with Ly-6chi monocytosis. *J Am Coll Cardiol* (2010) 55:1629–38. doi:10.1016/j.jacc.2009. 08.089

Courties G, Heidt T, Sebas M, Iwamoto Y, Jeon D, Truelove J, et al. In vivo silencing of the transcription factor IRF5 reprograms the macrophage phe- notype and improves infarct healing. *J Am Coll Cardiol* (2014) 63:1556–66. doi:10.1016/j.jacc.2013.11.023

Kimura S, Egashira K, Chen L, Nakano K, Iwata E, Miyagawa M, et al. Nanoparticle- mediated delivery of nuclear factor kappaB decoy into lungs ameliorates monocrotaline-induced pulmonary arterial hypertension. *Hypertension* (2009) 53:877–83. doi:10.1161/HYPERTENSIONAHA.108.121418

Chen L, Nakano K, Kimura S, Matoba T, Iwata E, Miyagawa M, et al. Nanoparticle-mediated delivery of pitavastatin into lungs ameliorates the development and induces regression of monocrotaline-induced pulmonary artery hypertension. *Hypertension* (2011) 57(2):343–50. doi:10.1161/HYPERTENSIONAHA.110.157032

Kimura S, Egashira K, Nakano K, Iwata E, Miyagawa M, Tsujimoto H, et al. Local delivery of imatinib mesylate (STI571)-incorporated nanoparticle ex vivo suppresses vein graft neointima formation. *Circulation* (2008) 118: S65–70. doi:10.1161/CIRCULATIONAHA.107.740613

Ridker PM, Everett BM, Thuren T, Macfadyen JG, Chang WH, Ballantyne C, et al. Antiinflammatory therapy with canakinumab for atherosclerotic disease. *N Engl J Med* (2017) 377:1119–31. doi:10.1056/NEJMoa1707914

19

A Bibliometric Analysis of Reactive Oxygen Species Based Nanotechnology for Cardiovascular Diseases

Yun Liang[1,2]*, Shenjie Liao*[1] *and Xiaoshen Zhang*[1*]

[1] *Department of Cardiovascular Surgery, The First Affiliated Hospital, Jinan University, Guangzhou, China,* [2] *Academician Workstation, Affiliated Hospital of North Sichuan Medical College, Nanchong, China*

Correspondence:
Xiaoshen Zhang
178399881@qq.com

Cardiovascular diseases (CVDs) continue to be the leading cause of health problems around the world. Because of its unique properties, reactive oxygen species (ROS)-based nanotechnology offers novel solutions to the diagnosis and treatment of CVDs. In order to identify and further promote the development of ROS-based nanotechnology in CVDs, we here provide a bibliometric analysis. 701 eligible articles about the ROS–based nanotechnology for CVD up to May 26th, 2022, were taken from the Web of Science Core Collection database. The VOSviewer was used to analyze annual publications, countries/institutions, funding agencies, journals and research category, and the research hotspots. From the publication of the first article in 2005 to 2021, the output and the number of citations of articles are on the rise. Based on the bibliometric analysis, we found that the current research focuses on the correlation between diagnosis (sensors and), treatment (oxidative stress, inflammation, and drug delivery) and safety (toxicity). Since 2019, research on nanomedicine and drug delivery has become a hotspot. So, more research in chemistry, materials, biology, and medicine is required to further develop and construct ROS-based nanomaterials.

Keywords: nanotechnology, reactive oxygen species, bibliometric analysis, cardiovascular disease, CVD risk assessment, CVD risk prediction, data visualization analysis

INTRODUCTION

According to World Health Organization (WHO) estimates, cardiovascular diseases (CVDs) are one of the most important causes affecting health status and the leading cause of death worldwide (1).

Cardiovascular diseases are a broad term for any condition that affects the heart or blood vessels, such as high blood pressure, stroke, coronary heart disease, myocardial infarction, etc (2). However, accumulating evidences demonstrated that some patients' CVDs may due to oxidative stress injury caused by excessive production of reactive oxygen species (ROS) (3). ROS are a group of highly reactive molecules and free radicals that are made by the metabolism of molecular oxygen (4). Under normal circumstances, ROS are produced at low levels in all cells *via* the electron-transport chain during aerobic respiration and by a variety of constitutively active oxidases (5). However, in the presence of CVDs, the excessive production of ROS that cannot be neutralized by antioxidants in cells [such as superoxide dismutase (SOD) and catalase] and results in oxidative stress may aggravate myocardial damage and impair cell components such as membrane lipids, proteins, and DNA (6). In other words, this also provides an efficient approach for dealing with and preventing CVDs *via* the regulation of ROS. However, current medical methods, leading to ineffective or excessive treatment, cannot take advantage of the changes in ROS concentration in the microenvironment of diseased tissues (7). Nanotechnology has the potential to bring up new avenues for assisting or overcoming constraints in CVD diagnosis and treatment due to its unique features. ROS-based nanotechnology focuses on the ROS-related nano chemistry interface (ROS generation, ROS transition, and ROS scavenging) for improved reaction efficiencies, as well as the ROS-related nanobiology interactions (bioavailability, biodegradability, and biocompatibility) for improved therapeutic outcomes. In recent years, various advanced ROS-based nanotechnologies have been developed and applied to the diagnosis and treatment of cardiovascular illnesses in response to the growing interest of scholars (8). Inspired by the vast advances in the field of ROS-based nanotechnology for CVD, we present this article regarding ROS-based nanotechnology for CVD *via* the aid of bibliometric analysis, with the aim of identifying current research advances and further promoting the development of this important field. In this work, the Web of Science(WoS) innate function and bibliometric methods are used to identify annual publication trends, the most productive countries/institutions, publication-related journals, and research hotspots in the field. Based on the macroscopic and objective results obtained from this analysis, we further proposed a prospects for future research directions and clinical translations of the applications of ROS-base nanotechnology for CVDs. This paper may serve as a reference, not only for researchers, but also for doctors who work in the field of nanotechnology in CVD.

MATERIALS AND METHODS

All publications relating to ROS-based nanotechnology for CVD were retrieved from Clarivate analysis's Web of Science Core collection Database including editions of SCI-EXPANDED (2003–present), SSCI (2003–present), A & HCI (2003–present), ESCI (2015–present), CCR-EXPANDED (1985–present), and IC (1993–present) (9, 10). The data was obtained on May 26th, 2022 and the following search query was developed to extract the total number of published items.

TS = (nanoparticle* or nanomaterial* or nanodot* or "quantum dot*" or nanosphere* or nanorod* or nanofiber* or nanotube* or nanosheet* or nanocomposite* or nanodevice* or nanocluster* or nanotech* or nanocarrier* or nanowire* or nanoliposome* or nanoemulsion* or nanocrystal* or nanogels* or nanoconjugate* or nanodiamond*) (11) and TS = ("high blood pressure" or hypertension* or "peripheral arter*" disease* or "atrial fibrillar*" or tachycardia* or endocarditis* or pericard* or ischem* or arrhythmia* or thrombo* or cardio* or cardiac* or "heart failure" or "heart beat" or "heart rate*" or "heart val*" or coronary* or angina* or ventric* or myocard*) (11) and TS = ("reactive oxygen species" or "ROS" or "H2O2" or "hydrogen peroxide") (12).

Additional, the language was limited to "English." We extracted the following information about the studies: year of publication, distribution of articles by countries or institutions, funding agencies, authors, keywords, and major journals' published articles. VOSviewer was employed to conduct the data visualization.

RESULTS

Search Results

A total of 713 publications were retrieved (**Supplementary Figure 1**). These included 616 articles, 85 reviews, 6 meeting abstracts and other types of papers. Document types such as corrections, meeting abstracts, and editorial materials do not share the same citation rates, therefore, only document types including original articles and reviews were utilized (in total 701 publications) in our following analysis (**Supplementary Table 1**).

The Annual Trend of Paper Publication Quantity

Figure 1 illustrates the annual publications and citations growth of literatures regarding ROS-based nanotechnology for CVD. It displayed an upward trend from 2 documents published in 2005 to 131 documents published in 2021. The period from 2013 to 2021 was a rapid development period. Citation analysis is a simple and objective way to evaluate the quality of published articles, journals, research organizations and even individual researchers; The times of an articles cited reflect its scientific impact (13). Among all the retrieved articles, there were 18,474 citing documents including 279 self-citations and 18,195 without self-citation (accounted for 98.49% of all citing documents). Sum of the times cited was 22,032 including 21,360 without self-cited which accounted for 96.95%.

Most Productive Countries/Regions and Institutions

Of these 701 documents, 60 countries and regions contributed to this research field. China was the most productive country which published the maximum number of related studies (n = 324, accounted for 41.45% of all). It was followed by the United States (n = 138, 19.686%), India (n = 66, 9.415%), South Korea (n = 41, 5.849%) and Germany (n = 20, 2.853%). In addition, the average citations and h-index of the top 7 most productive and influential countries are also presented (**Figure 2**). With this, China, the United States, and India rank in top three positions in terms of the h-index, reflecting a relatively high number of publications and associated citations from these countries. Japan topped the list with the highest average citations (47.05), followed by the United States (45.79) and India (35.35). When it comes to institution rankings (**Figure 3**), the Chinese Academy of Sciences takes the first rank position in terms of publication numbers, with 39 publications, while League of European Research Universities occupies the leading institution in terms of the h-index (14).

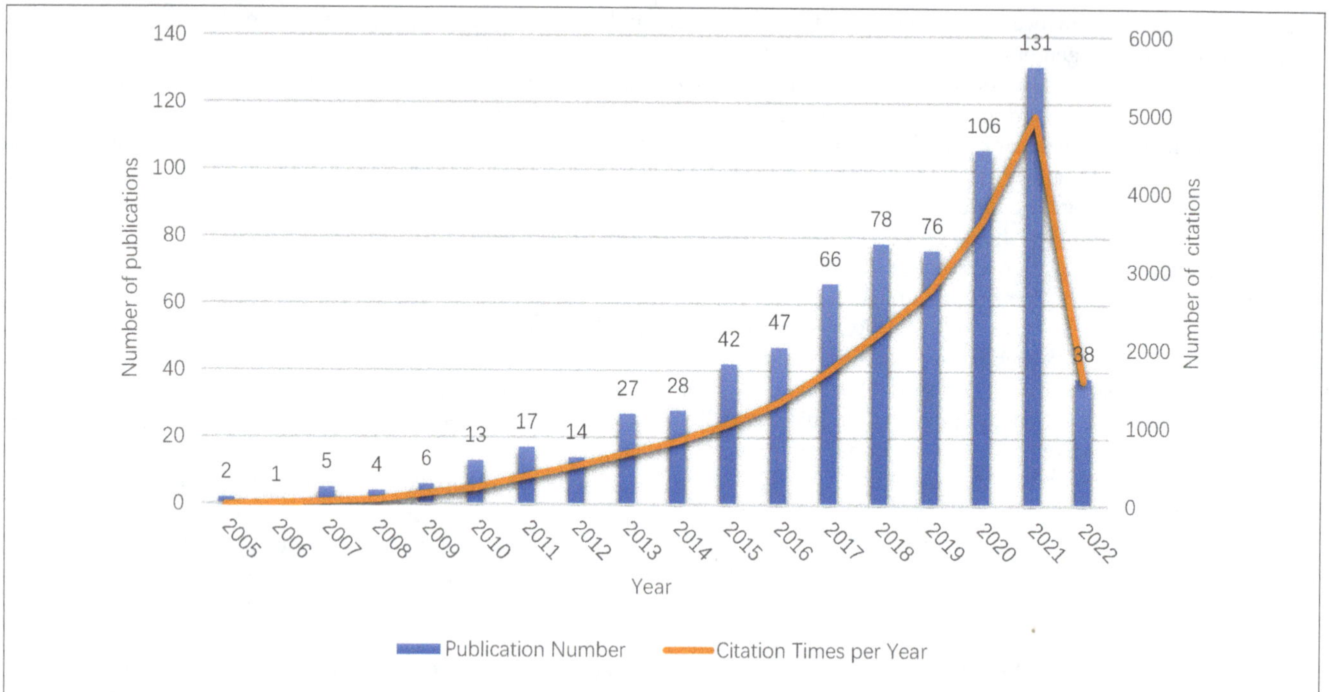

FIGURE 1 | The annual publication and citation growth of literature.

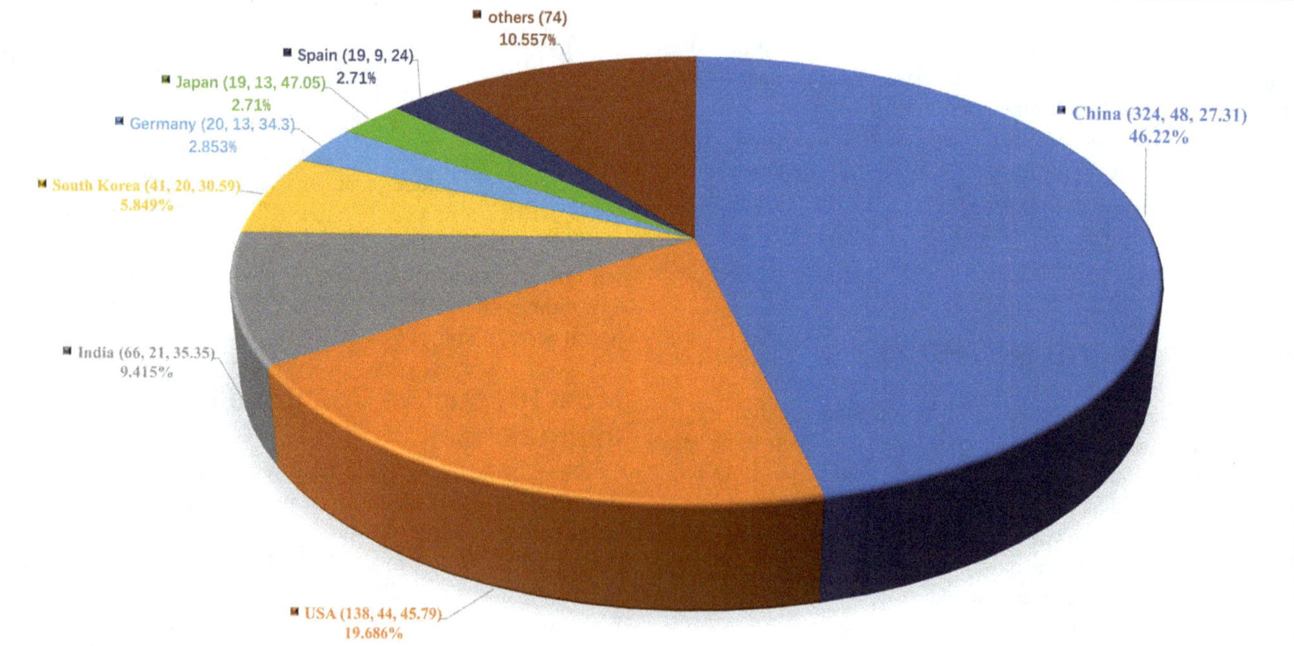

FIGURE 2 | Distribution of publications in countries/regions. The number in the brackets goes: (publication numbers, h-index, average citations). Percentage indicates the proportion of the publication number in global scale.

Furthermore, the Council of Scientific Industrial Research ranked the first position in terms of the average citations (49.18).

Productivity by Funding Agencies

Based on the selection criteria, the top 10 funding agencies are represented in **Figure 4**. Among these funding agencies, the National Natural Science Foundation of China (NSFC) ranked first, accounting for 242 funded projects. The United States Department of Health Human Services and National Institutes of Health in the United States ranked second and third, with 81 funded projects and 80 funded projects, respectively. However, 100 articles, which

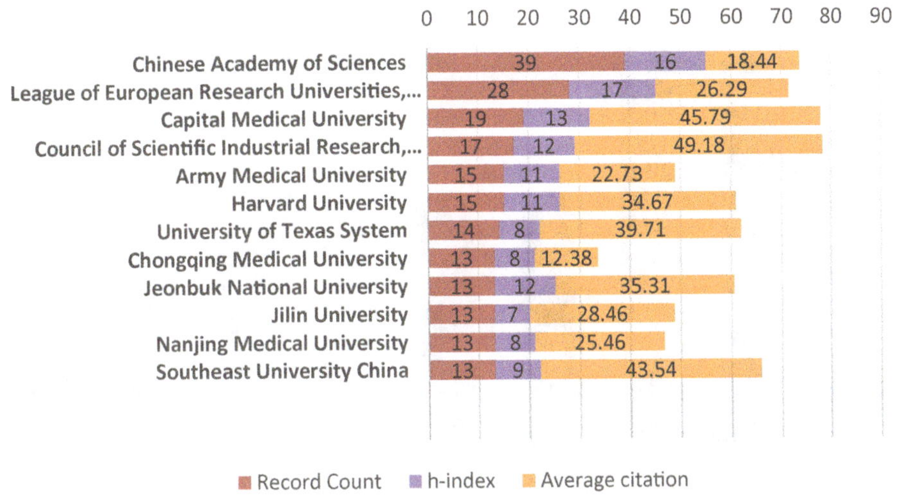

FIGURE 3 | The most contributing institutes in the field of ROS based nanotechnology for cardiovascular diseases.

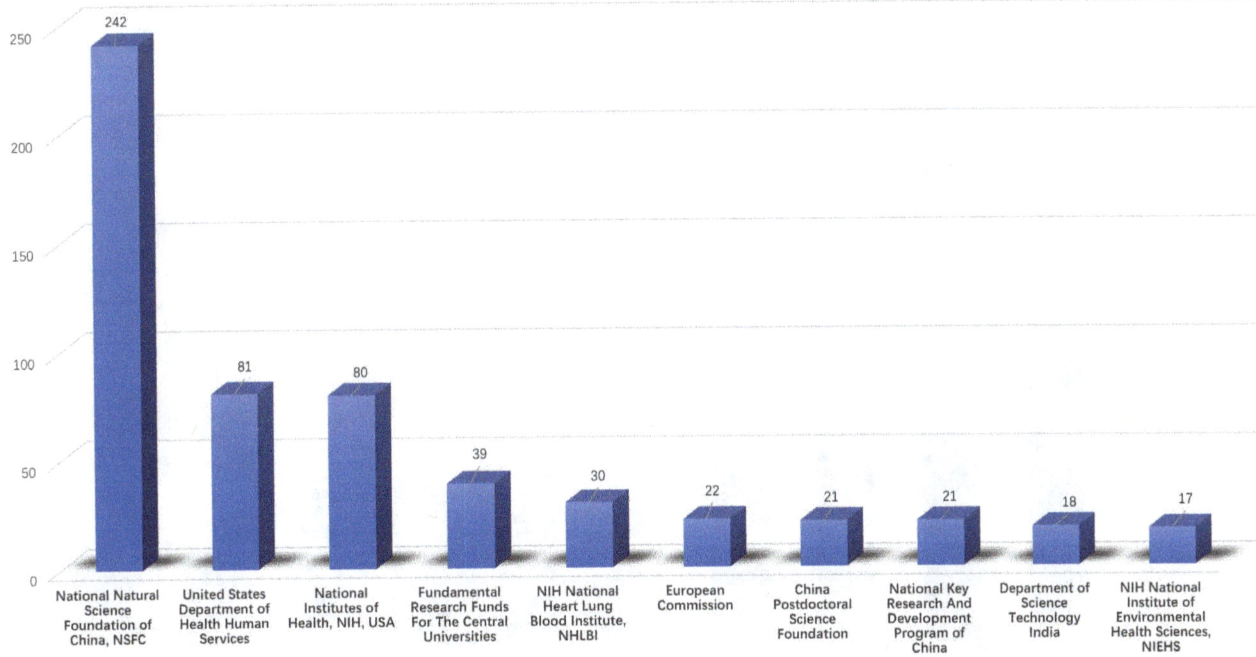

FIGURE 4 | Distribution of articles by funding agencies (top 10 funding agencies).

accounted for nearly 14.265% of the total, were without any funding support.

Journals and Research Category Analysis

These 701 documents were published in 296 kinds of journals. The top 10 most productive journals in this area were shown on **Figure 5**. These top 10 journals published a 157 total of documents, accounting for 22.40% of all. Biosensors Bioelectronics published the most document (n = 25). The second most popular journal was Biomaterials which has 23 publications. International Journal of Nanomedicine ranked No. 3 ($n = 22$) and was followed by ACS Applied Materials Interfaces ($n = 15$) and ACS Nano ($n = 14$).

In terms of research categories, a total of 74 research categories were involved. Based on the quantity of publications, the top 10 research categories are demonstrated in **Figure 6**. " Nanoscience Nanotechnology " (167 publications), " Pharmacology Pharmacy " (107 publications), " Chemistry Multidisciplinary " (104 publications), " Materials Science Multidisciplinary " (91 publications) and " Materials Science Biomaterials " (81

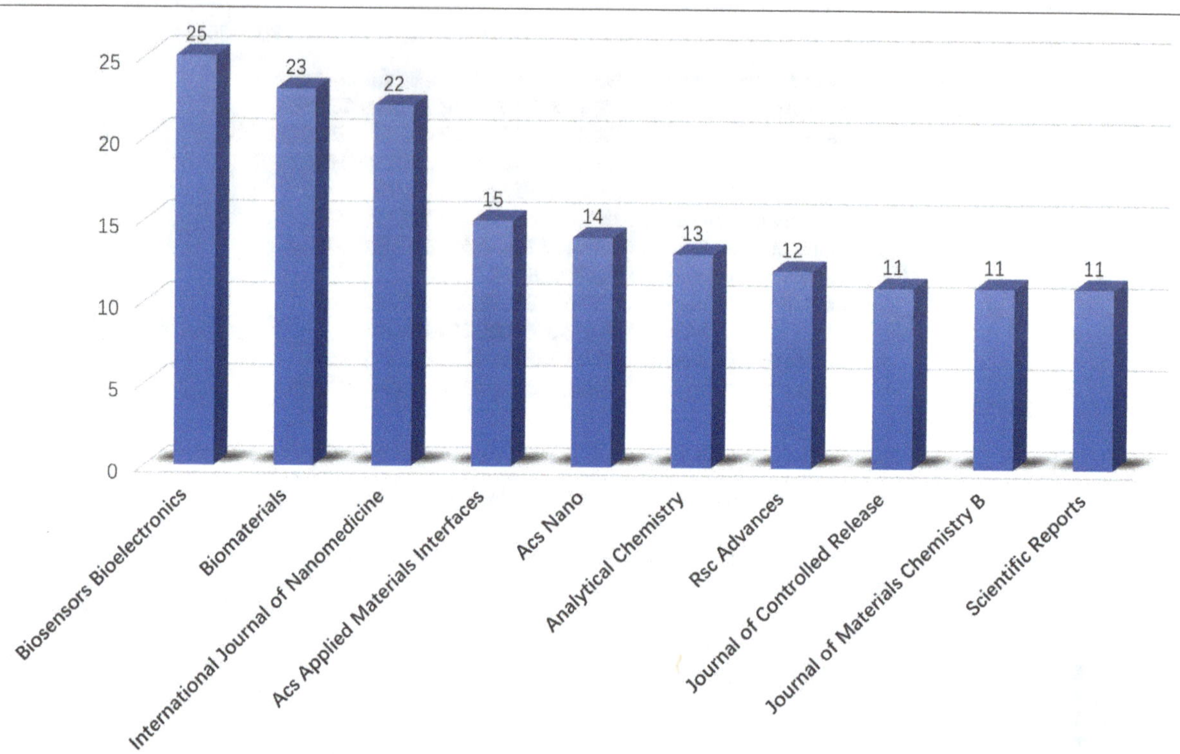

FIGURE 5 | Productivity of journals (top 10 journals).

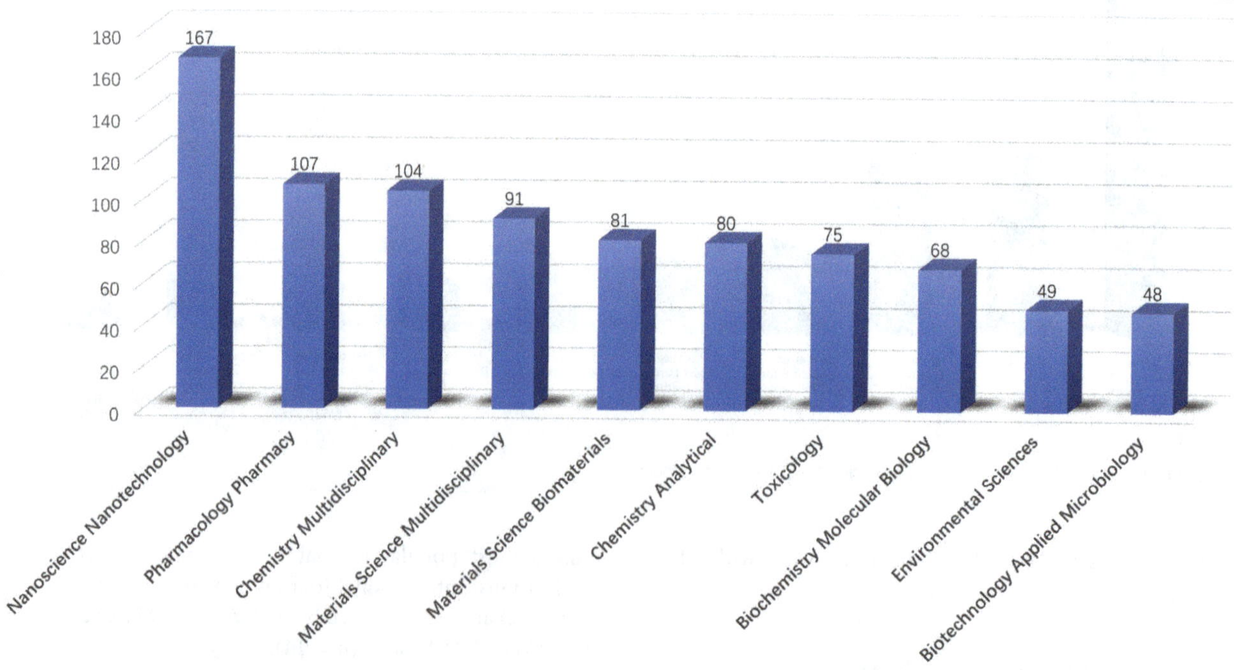

FIGURE 6 | The top 10 research categories.

publications) are ranked in top 5 positions. As for the publisher, the most represented publishers based on the number of the publications were " Elsevier " (225 publications), " Springer Nature " (80 publications), " Amer Chemical Soc " (74 publications), " Wiley " (58 publications), and " Royal Soc Chemistry " (45 publications).

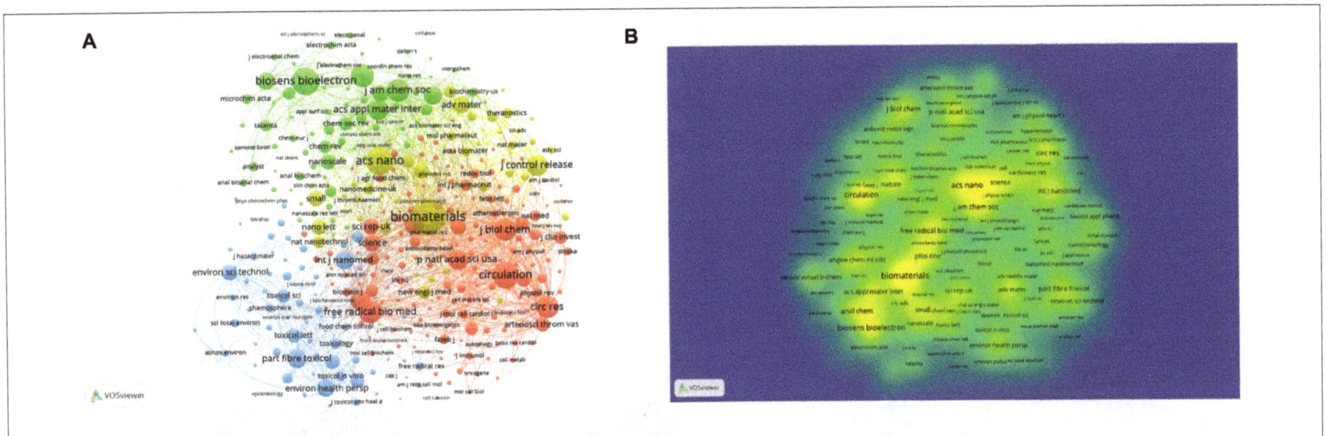

FIGURE 7 | Co-citation analysis of citated sources. Node size suggests the citation amount. Settings in VOSviewer Analysis:Minimum number of citations of a source: 20 (of the 4,772 sources, 378 meet the threshold) Method: Association strength; Layout: Attractions 6, Repulsion −1. Clustering: Resolution 1.00, Min.cluster.size 1. **(A)** Network mapping of citated sources (four clusters). **(B)** Density mapping according to the citation amount of a source (yellow means more of a source).

Co-citation Analysis of Cited Journals

A co-citation analysis of cited journals identifies the most relevant sources cited by publications in the specified topic (15). This analysis can identify the leading journals in the field of CVD that cover ROS-based nanotechnology. In addition, it can also offer information with regard to research topics in the field of ROS-based nanotechnology in CVD, as indicated by journal titles. With an analysis by means of the VOSviewer, 4,772 cited journals were referred by the 701 publications. 378 journals with employed the threshold at 20 citations were used for co-citation analysis and presented in **Figure 7**. The top 5 cited journals are Biomaterials (994 citations), ACS nano (687 citations), Biosensors Bioelectronics (662 citations), Circulation (617 citations) and Anal Chem (494 citations). Most of the journals are associated with nanoscience while cardiovascular-focused journals such as Circulation, J Clin Invest, Circ Res, J Am Coll Cardiol or Cardiovasc Res. were also recognized in our database. As can be inferred from the clusters, the major fields of ROS-based nanotechnology in CVD application lie in biomedicine (red color)-, biosensor (green)-, toxicology (blue)- and biomaterials/nanomaterials (yellow)-related science.

Research Hotspots in Reactive Oxygen Species–Based Nanotechnology for Cardiovascular Diseases Applications

In order to obtain a general understanding of the research focuses of the ROS-based nanotechnology in CVD field, a co-occurrence analysis of keywords was conducted by using VOS viewer (**Figure 8**). A keyword co-occurrence landscape of 93 keywords, acquired from 701 publications, with a minimum occurrence of 12 times, is presented. The top 10 most frequently occurring keywords are oxidative stress (occurred 237 times), nanoparticles (215 times), apoptosis (101 times), ROS (85 times), inflammation (80 times), *in vitro* (72 times), toxicity (67 times), hydrogen-peroxide (65 times), mechanisms (58 times), and gold nanoparticles (56 times). Such high-frequency keywords indicate that the major application of ROS–based nanotechnology in CVD lies in oxidative stress, apoptosis, inflammation, mechanisms and other theragnostic-related fields. In addition, three clusters in different colors indicating different research fields were identified and adjusted by the innate function of the VOSviewer. As indicated, the largest red cluster, which is related to the regulation of oxidative stress, was the most significant application of ROS–based nanotechnology in CVD. The second biggest cluster was colored in green, demonstrating the mechanism and toxicity of nanomaterials for CVD. In addition, the third biggest cluster was colored in blue, demonstrating the construction and functional verification of novel nano materials based on ROS. Likewise, it can be inferred from this result that ROS–based nanotechnology in CVD is targeted mainly at diagnosis (sensor and), therapy (oxidative stress, inflammatory and drug delivery) and safety (toxicity) studies. Meanwhile, through the analysis of **Figure 8B**, we also see that since 2019, the research on nanomedicine and drug delivery has become a hotspot.

DISCUSSION

With the help of bibliometric analysis, this paper was given about ROS-based nanotechnology for CVDs. Up to May 26th, 2020, the total number of documents on this topic was 713. Finally, only 701 documents, including original articles and reviews, were used for bibliometric analysis. The publication output was rich in the period from 2013 to 2021 and displayed an upward trend. It is explicit that research on ROS-based nanotechnology for CVD has advanced rapidly over the last decade. ROS-based nanotechnology for CVD is predicted to remain a research hotspot in the future. Among all the retrieved 701 articles, a total of 22,032 citations was received with an average time cited per document of 31.43. It was seen that the number of citations has increased 4983-fold since 2005 to 2021, reflecting the rising importance of this research area.

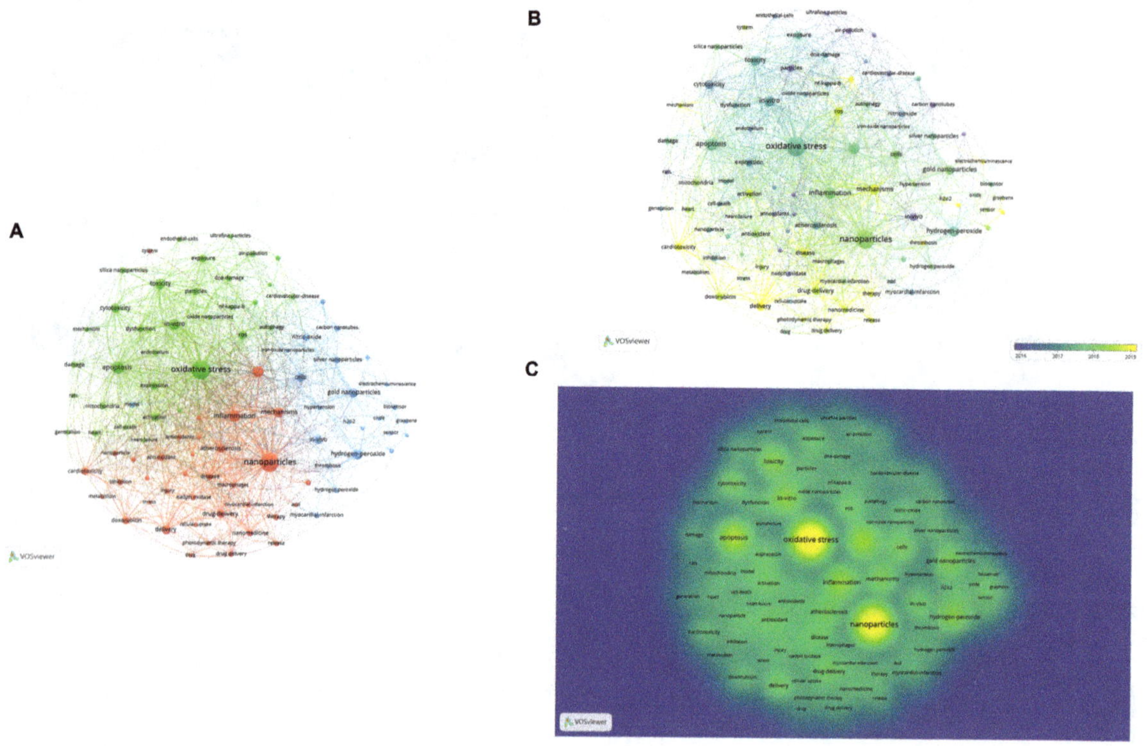

FIGURE 8 | Co-occurrence analysis of all keywords with an occurrence frequency more than 12 (of the 3,922 keywords, 93 meet the threshold). Colors are used to indicate clusters. Circle size is based on the number of occurrence. Settings in VOSviewer Analysis: Method: Lin Log/modularity; Resolution: 1.0; Minimum cluster size: 2; Attractions:1; Repulsion:-1. **(A)** Network mapping of keywords of related studies (three clusters). **(B)** Overlay mapping of keywords according to average publication year (blue means earlier, yellow means later). **(C)** Density mapping of keywords according to the frequency of appearance (yellow means more frequent).

In total, 41.45% of all these articles were from China, and the Chinese Academy of Sciences takes the first rank position in terms of publication numbers. Through analysis, we note that China was also the leading country with the maximum average citations. Additionally, India ranks third in the world in terms of article output and h-index. In terms of institutional contribution, the Chinese Academy of Sciences ranks first with the highest document output. However, the League of European Research Universities in the United States leads in terms of the h-index, while the Council of Scientific Industrial Research in India leads in terms of average citations. The achievements of two developing countries with large populations (China and India) in this field have greatly encouraged the innovation of global CVD prevention and treatment technology.

Based on the funding source for these articles, we found that China and the United States have the most funded projects in this field. Accordingly, it also explains why China and the United States have made great achievements in this field. We speculate that nanotechnology has become a priority for government funding in the two countries as a means of safeguarding healthcare. It is admirable that Indian scholars have received relatively few fund-supported projects, but their literature output and quality are high. However, about 14.265% of the articles were not funded by any funding agency. It is clear that the significance of ROS-based nanotechnology for CVD is still underappreciated in many countries.

Among the top 10 most productive journals out of 296 kinds of journal involved, 7 of them were categorized in " Chemistry" or " Materials," while the remaining 3 were, respectively, listed in "medicine" ($n = 2$), and "Comprehensive" ($n = 1$). Of the top 10 research categories, 8 categories belong to the categories of "chemistry or materials science," while 2 categories belong to the categories of "medicine." From this analysis result, we can infer that the application of ROS based nanotechnology in the field of CVD is more reflected in innovation in the field of chemistry and materials.

The top 5 journals with the largest number of articles accounted for 68.76% of all the publications. Among them, journals belonging to Elsevier publishers accounted for 32.097%. "Amer chemical SOC" and "Royal SOC chemistry" are the top journals in the professional field, and the number of papers included accounts for 16.98% of the total. Through further co-citation analysis of cited journals, we found that the application of ROS based nanotechnology in CVD mainly focuses on biomedicine, biosensors, toxicology, and biomaterials/nanomaterials related science. So far, the analysis results have proved that nanotechnology combines materials science, chemistry, and biology and is involved in the diagnosis and treatment of CVDs by sensing and regulating ROS levels (16).

Then, using keyword co-occurrence analysis, the research focuses of ROS-based nanotechnology in the CVD field were determined. The result shows that ROS-based nanotechnology

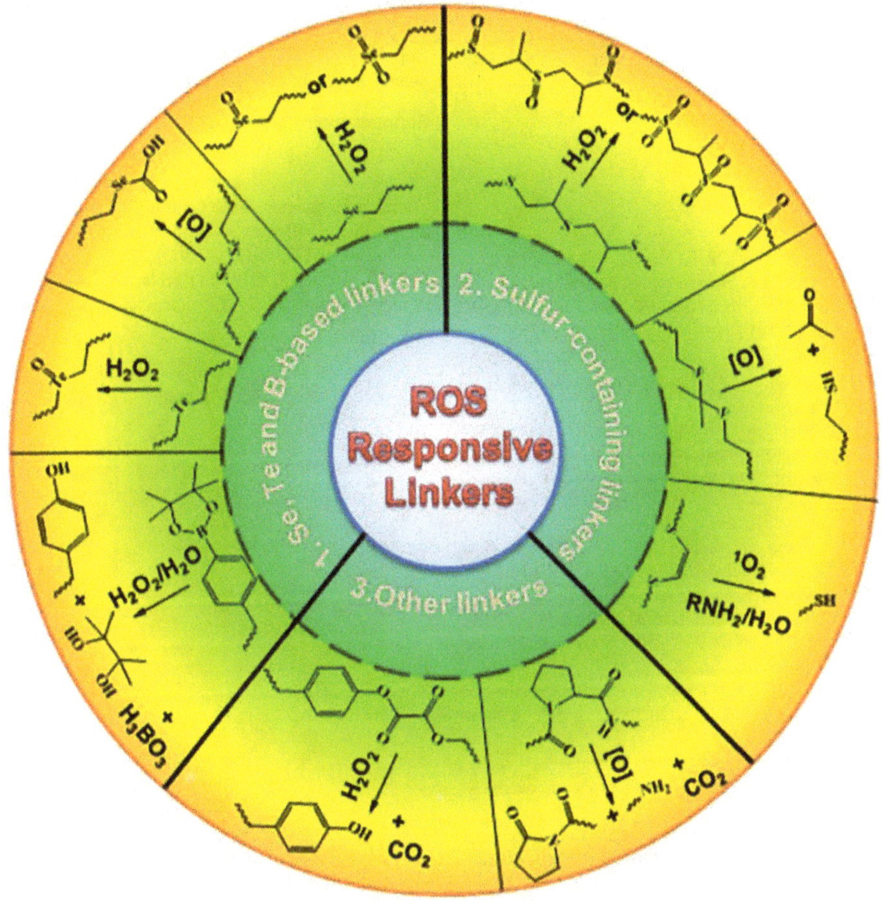

FIGURE 9 | Representative ROS-responsive linkers that have employed for the design of ROS-responsive drug carriers.

in CVD is targeted mainly at diagnosis (sensor and), therapy (oxidative stress, inflammatory, and drug delivery) and safety (toxicity) studies. Additionally, the research on nanomedicine and drug delivery has become a hotspot since 2019. Current studies have demonstrated that oxidative stress is the key mechanisms of CVDs (17). As one of the application means of ROS-based nanotechnology, the drug delivery system acts on cardiovascular lesions by targeting, thus more effectively reducing oxidative damage and eliminating inflammation (18). This abnormal biochemical change in CVDs has prompted researchers to use unbalanced ROS levels to develop target-specific drug delivery systems (14). ROS-based drug delivery and nanomedicine will primarily focus on polymeric nanoparticles, hydrogels, inorganic nanoparticles, and activatable prodrugs integrated with diverse ROS-responsive moieties for spatiotemporally controlled drug release for effective therapy (19). The design goal of ROS-based nanomaterial is to match the degradation rate and dynamic ROS concentration of the material itself, which is very important for timely detection of signal molecules, releasing drug loading as needed, and regulating the growth and growth of transfer cells (20). By utilizing ROS-responsive materials and linkers (**Figure 9**), various ROS-responsive drug delivery systems have been developed and investigated for therapeutic purposes. So, more research in chemistry, materials, biology, and medicine is required to further develop and construct ROS-based nanomaterials (21).

CONCLUSION

China, the United States, and India, 60 countries or regions dominated by these three countries, have made outstanding contributions to research in the field of ROS based nanotechnology applied to CVDs. From the publication of the first article in 2005 to 2021, the output and the number of citations of articles are on the rise. The current research focuses on the correlation between diagnosis (sensors and), treatment (oxidative stress, inflammation, and drug delivery) and safety (toxicity). Since 2019, research on nanomedicine and drug delivery has become a hotspot. To further develop and construct ROS-based nanomaterials, more research in chemistry, materials, biology, and medicine is required.

AUTHOR CONTRIBUTIONS

YL: formal analysis, data curation, and writing – original draft. SL: data curation. XZ: supervision and writing – review and editing. All authors contributed to manuscript revision, read, and approved the submitted version.

ACKNOWLEDGMENTS

We thank those individuals who provided software's usage guidance, language help, writing assistance, and proofreading of the manuscript.

SUPPLEMENTARY MATERIAL

Supplementary Figure 1 | The retrieval strategy and results of publications. The search was conducted in the WoS core collection database on May 26th, 2022.

Supplementary Table 1 | The 701 analyzed papers.

REFERENCES

Nowbar AN, Gitto M, Howard JP, Francis DP, Al-Lamee R. Mortality from ischemic heart disease: analysis of data from the world health organization and coronary artery disease risk factors from NCD risk factor collaboration. *Circ Cardiovasc Qual Outcomes.* (2019) 12:1–11.

Zhao D, Liu J, Wang M, Zhang X, Zhou M. Epidemiology of cardiovascular disease in China: current features and implications. *Nat Rev Cardiol.* (2019) 16:203–12. doi: 10.1038/s41569-018-0119-4

Zhao T, Wu W, Sui L, Huang Q, Nan Y, Liu J, et al. Reactive oxygen species- based nanomaterials for the treatment of myocardial ischemia reperfusion injuries. *Bioact Mater.* (2022) 7:47–72. doi: 10.1016/j.bioactmat.2021.06.006

Li R, Jia Z, Trush MA. Defining ROS in biology and medicine. *React Oxyg Species (Apex).* (2016) 1:9. doi: 10.20455/ros.2016.803

Xu Q, He C, Xiao C, Chen X. Reactive oxygen species (ROS) responsive polymers for biomedical applications. *Macromol Biosci.* (2016) 16:635–46. doi: 10.1002/mabi.201500440

Joshi-Barr S, de Gracia Lux C, Mahmoud E, Almutairi A. Exploiting oxidative microenvironments in the body as triggers for drug delivery systems. *Antioxid Redox Signal.* (2013) 21:730–54. doi: 10.1089/ars.2013.5754

Chen W, Li D. Reactive oxygen species (ROS)-responsive nanomedicine for solving ischemia-reperfusion injury. *Front Chem.* (2020) 8:732. doi: 10.3389/fchem.2020.00732

Sabir F, Barani M, Mukhtar M, Rahdar A, Cucchiarini M, Zafar MN, et al. Nanodiagnosis and nanotreatment of cardiovascular diseases: an overview. *Chemosensors.* (2021) 9:67.

Ahmad T, Murad MA, Baig M, Hui J. Research trends in COVID-19 vaccine: a bibliometric analysis. *Hum Vaccines Immunother.* (2021) 17:2367–72. doi: 10.1080/21645515.2021.1886806

Khan M, Ahmad T, Khan MM, Murad MA, Baig M, Ali A, et al. Research trends in polio during the last 50 years: a bibliometric analysis. *J Univ Med Dent Coll.* (2022) 13:341–6.

Zheng Z, Zhu S, Lv M, Gu Z, Hu H. Harnessing nanotechnology for cardiovascular disease applications - a comprehensive review based on bibliometric analysis. *Nano Today.* (2022) 44:101453. doi: 10.1016/j.nantod.2022.101453

Zhang Z, Dalan R, Hu Z, Wang J, Chew NWS, Poh K, et al. Reactive oxygen species scavenging nanomedicine for the treatment of ischemic heart disease. *Adv Mater.* (2022) 8:2202169. doi: 10.1002/adma.202202169

Sevinc A. Web of science: a unique method of cifed reference searching. *J Natl Med Assoc.* (2004) 96:980–3.

Yao Y, Zhang H, Wang Z, Ding J, Wang S, Huang B, et al. Reactive oxygen species (ROS)-responsive biomaterials mediate tissue microenvironments and tissue regeneration. *J Mater Chem B.* (2019) 7:5019–37. doi: 10.1039/c9tb00847k

Liu Y, Zhu S, Gu Z, Zhao Y. A bibliometric analysis: research progress and prospects on transition metal dichalcogenides in the biomedical field. *Chin Chem Lett.* (2021) 32:3762–70.

Purcell BP, Lobb D, Charati MB, Dorsey SM, Wade RJ, Zellars KN, et al. Injectable and bioresponsive hydrogels for on-demand matrix metalloproteinase inhibition. *Nat Mater.* (2014) 13:653–61. doi: 10.1038/nmat3922

González-Montero J, Brito R, Gajardo AI, Rodrigo R. Myocardial reperfusion injury and oxidative stress: therapeutic opportunities. *World J Cardiol.* (2018) 10:74–86. doi: 10.4330/wjc.v10.i9.74

Hajipour MJ, Mehrani M, Abbasi SH, Amin A, Kassaian SE, Garbern JC, et al. Nanoscale technologies for prevention and treatment of heart failure: challenges and opportunities. *Chem Rev.* (2019) 119:11352–90. doi: 10.1021/acs.chemrev.8b00323

Saravanakumar G, Kim J, Kim WJ. Reactive-oxygen-species-responsive drug delivery systems: promises and challenges. *Adv Sci.* (2017) 4:1600124. doi: 10.1002/advs.201600124

Agrahari V, Agrahari V. Facilitating the translation of nanomedicines to a clinical product: challenges and opportunities. *Drug Discov Today.* (2018) 23:974–91. doi: 10.1016/j.drudis.2018.01.047

Pelaz B, Alexiou C, Alvarez-Puebla RA, Alves F, Andrews AM, Ashraf S, et al. Diverse applications of nanomedicine. *ACS Nano.* (2017) 11:2313–81.

20

Nanotechnology for Targeted Therapy of Atherosclerosis

Seyedmehdi Hossaini Nasr[1,2]* *and Xuefei Huang*[1,2,3]*

[1]Department of Chemistry, Michigan State University, East Lansing, MI, United States, [2]Institute for Quantitative Health Science and Engineering, Michigan State University, East Lansing, MI, United States, [3]Department of Biomedical Engineering, Michigan State University, East Lansing, MI, United States

***Correspondence:**
Xuefei Huang
huangxu2@msu.edu
Seyedmehdi Hossaini Nasr
hossain5@msu.edu

Atherosclerosis is the major cause of heart attack and stroke that are the leading causes of death in the world. Nanomedicine is a powerful tool that can be engineered to target atherosclerotic plaques for therapeutic and diagnosis purposes. In this review, advances in designing nanoparticles with therapeutic effects on atherosclerotic plaques known as atheroprotective nanomedicine have been summarized to stimulate further development and future translation.

Keywords: atherosclerosis, nanomedicine, drug delivery, inflammation, statins

INTRODUCTION

Atherosclerosis is the thickening of artery vessel walls that can develop in arteries supplying blood to various organs such as heart, brain, and kidneys. It is a major cause of heart attack and stroke (Weber and Noels, 2011), the leading causes of death in the world. The majority of patients who experience cardiac arrests have atherosclerosis (Chelly et al., 2012). It has been estimated that by 2030, the global cost of cardiovascular diseases would reach a staggering number, $1,044 billion (Benjamin et al., 2017).

To better understand atherosclerosis pathology, it is important to know the structure of arterial walls, which consist of three different parts, i.e., tunica intima, tunica media and tunica externa (**Figure 1**). Squamous endothelial cells line the tunica intima and internal elastic lamina separates it from the tunica media. The tunica media contains elastic lamellae and elastic fibers alternating with layers of smooth muscle cells. Proteoglycans and reticular fibers are the other components of the media. Finally, connective tissues consisting of collagen and elastic fibers form the tunica externa (Mescher, 2016).

Atherosclerosis is a chronic inflammatory condition (Weber and Noels, 2011). One important trigger for the formation of atherosclerotic plaques is hypercholesterolemia. Cholesterol is transported in the plasma through lipoproteins. Among them, apolipoprotein B is responsible for carrying cholesterol and fat molecule around the body generally packed in particles known as low density lipoprotein (LDL). High levels of cholesterol in plasma results in the accumulation of lipids into the arterial wall. This accrual is mediated mostly through LDL particles together with changes in endothelial cell permeabilities. Overexpression of receptors such as vascular adhesion molecule 1 (VCAM-1) and selectins enhances their interactions with LDL and mediates LDL entrance into the arterial wall (Sakakura et al., 2013). In addition, oxidized LDL (oxLDL) favors the intracellular accumulation of cholesterol esters (Maiolino et al., 2013). Moreover, oxLDL is a potent inducer of inflammatory molecules and mediates monocyte binding to endothelial cells (Berliner et al., 1995).

Both innate and adaptive immunity play roles in pathophysiology of atherosclerosis (Herrero-Fernandez et al., 2019). As mentioned above, monocytes and macrophages, as the main contributors of innate immune response, initiate the progression of atherosclerosis. Following this step, the adaptive immune system can get activated and promote the plaque formation (Miteva et al., 2018).

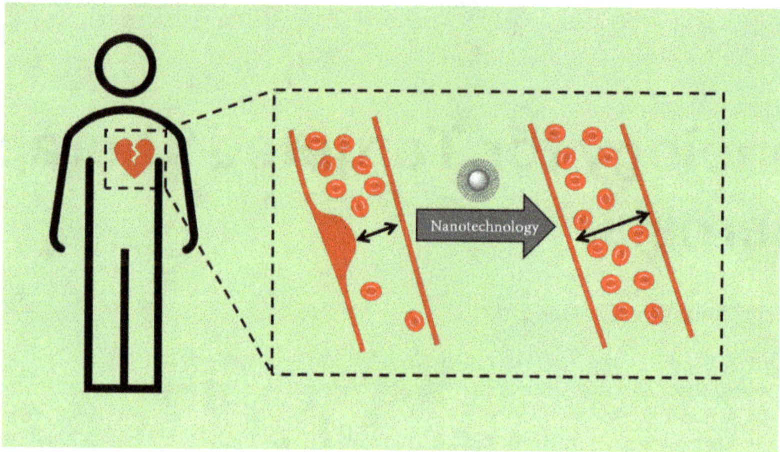

GRAPHICAL ABSTRACT |

Type 1 helper T (Th1) cells, type 2 helper T (Th2) cells, regulatory T (Treg) cells, $CD4^{+}$ T cells and $CD8^{+}$ T cells are the main contributors of the adaptive immune system involved in plaque formation and resolution (Roy et al., 2021). The understanding of the mechanisms of immune responses involved in pathophysiology of inflammatory atherosclerosis not only bring in a realistic perception of the complexity of the disease but also inspire the development of novel therapeutics (Ridker, 2021).

CURRENT ATHEROSCLEROTIC TREATMENT METHODS

Management of atherosclerosis typically involves drugs and/or surgery. Surgical intervention includes procedures such as angioplasty and bypass grafting. In angioplasty, a blocked or narrowed artery can be reopened and sometimes a physical device called stent is placed there to keep it open (Derdeyn and Chimowitz, 2007), while in bypass grafting, a healthy blood vessel is used to circumvent the area of atherosclerosis plaques (Martínez-González et al., 2017).

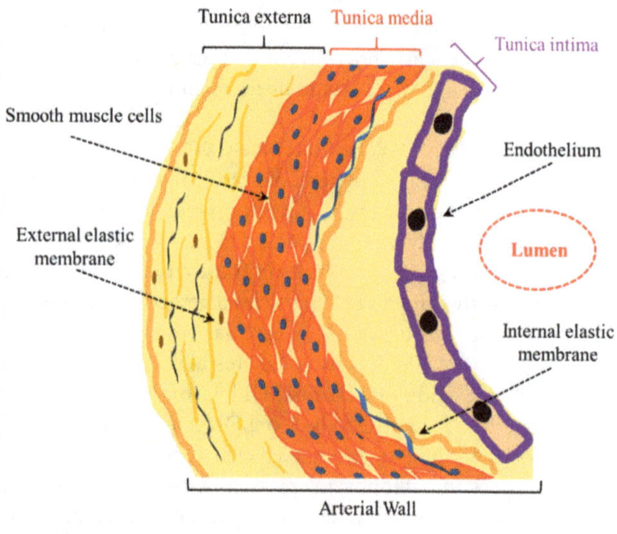

FIGURE 1 | Schematic demonstration of the arterial wall structure.

For pharmacological interventions, statins are one of the most important classes. Statins inhibit 3-hydroxy-3-methylglutaryl coenzyme A (HMG-CoA) reductase, which is a key enzyme for cholesterol biosynthesis (Cerqueira et al., 2016). Since a high cholesterol level in blood is an important risk factor for cardiovascular diseases (CVD), statins are believed to reduce possible CVD events through reduction of cholesterol (Taylor et al., 2013). In addition to their cholesterol modulating activities, statins can exert cardiovascular protecting effects through other pathways (Oesterle et al., 2017). These pleiotropic effects are mostly the result of isoprenylation inhibition that reduces the function of isoprenoids on targets such as Rho and Rac proteins. These proteins are involved in the expression of proinflammatory cytokines and transduction of signaling molecules. For instance, they can modulate reactive oxygen species (ROS) generation and their reduction can result in anti-inflammatory outcomes (Wolfrum et al., 2003). An important study that addressed anti-inflammatory effect of statins independent of their effect on LDL cholesterol level was conducted by Ridker and coworkers. In this study, Pravastatin was shown to reduce C-reactive protein (CRP) levels in people when assessed 12 and 24 weeks after taking the drug (Albert et al., 2001). CRP is known as a sensitive systemic marker for inflammation (Pepys and Baltz, 1983) and any acute inflammatory stimulus may cause a rapid rise of CRP level up to 1,000 folds (Black et al., 2004). Besides CRP, statins can reduce expression of cyclooxygenase-2 (Cox-2) in human endothelial cells (Massaro et al., 2010), murine macrophages (RAW264.7) (Shao et al., 2012) and atherosclerosis lesions in rabbits (Hernandez-Presa et al., 2002). Cox-2 is an inducible pro-inflammatory enzyme, which

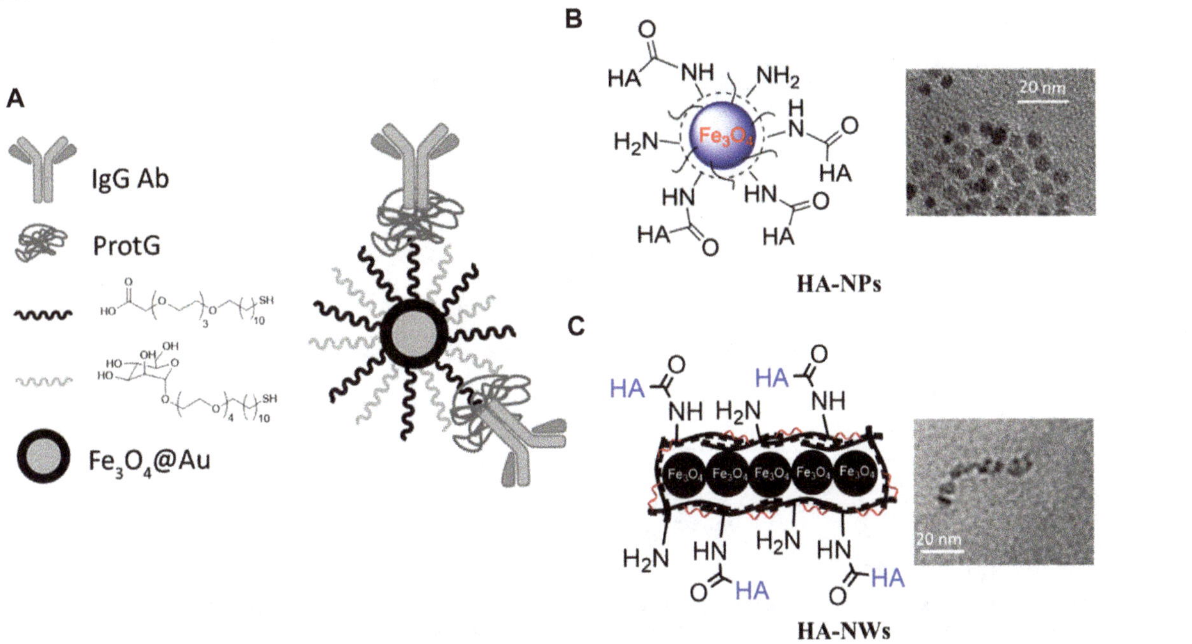

FIGURE 2 | Iron oxide nanoparticles for active targeting of atherosclerotic plaques. **(A)** Antibody directed nanoparticle for atherosclerotic plaque imaging. Gold coated iron oxide nanoparticles were first functionalized with mannose and carboxylic acid ending ligand, then protG was immobilized on nanoparticles. Finally, the nanoparticles were decorated with an anti-CD163 antibody. These nanoparticles were used for MRI and CT imaging of plaques (Tarin et al., 2015) **(B)** HA conjugated iron oxide NPs. These MRI probes were targeted towards the CD44 receptor for imaging of atherosclerotic plaques (El-Dakdouki et al., 2014). **(C)** HA conjugated worm shaped iron oxide nanoprobes. These HA-NWs induced lower inflammatory responses compared to the corresponding HA-NPs with a spherical morphology (Hossaini Nasr et al., 2018).

is mainly present (Gately and Li, 2004) in inflammatory macrophages in atherosclerotic plaques (Burleigh et al., 2005). Pro-inflammatory macrophages or M1 are known to propagate proinflammatory cytokines such as tumor necrosis factor-α (TNFα), interleukin (IL)-1 and IL-6 (Autieri, 2012). Statins can also alleviate proinflammatory cytokines effects. For instance, reduction of TNFα, IL-1 and IL-6 have been observed in hypercholesterolemic patients who received atorvastatin for 2 months (Ascer et al., 2004). High dose statin therapy can lead to the rapid reduction of atherosclerosis inflammation (Nissen et al., 2006; Tawakol et al., 2013) indicating the potential of this medicine for management of inflammatory atherosclerotic plaques. While statins have shown their beneficial effects, the therapeutic regimen should be carefully designed to prevent undesired outcomes. For example, discontinuation of statins results in rebound inflammation and increased short-term cardiovascular risks, even in the absence of changes in lipid levels (Heeschen et al., 2002; Spencer et al., 2004).

Besides statins, there are other therapeutic molecules for management of atherosclerosis. Proprotein convertase subtilisin/kexin type 9 (PCSK9) is an enzyme involved in LDL homeostasis. Agents that can block PCSK9 can enhance LDL degradation and lower cholesterol levels. Two PCSK9 inhibitors, alirocumab and evolocumab, were approved by the U.S. Food and Drug Administration to be used in patients not tolerant of statins. In addition, anti-inflammatory agents are entering the clinic for atherosclerosis complications. For instance, canakinumab, which targets human IL-1β, has shown promising results when evaluated in patients with CVD complications and high levels of CRP (Ridker et al., 2017). In addition, immunosuppressants such as methotrexate and rapamycin have shown promising effects to reduce atherosclerotic plaque sizes when studied in ApoE knockout mice (Zhang X. et al., 2017; Stigliano et al., 2017).

The incorporation of nanotechnology into atherosclerosis management is an exciting direction to pursue complementing the current treatment methods (Peters et al., 2021). While anti-inflammatory approach is a popular drug therapy regimen, the choice of suitable anti-inflammatory molecules requires consideration. Prednisolone, a corticosteroid drug, showed high accumulation in plaque macrophages when formulated in liposomal nanoparticle (LN-PLP) (Lobatto et al., 2010). However, further studies ruled out this medicine for atherosclerosis management. *In vitro* experiments showed lipotoxic effects of LN-PLP when incubated with macrophages (Van Der Valk et al., 2016). *In vivo* analysis indicated the drug accelerated atherosclerosis increasing the size of the necrotic areas. Another example is a study that compared the effect of anti-proliferative drugs used in vascular restenosis treatment (Chen et al., 2021). Although sirolimus and paclitaxel nanoparticles both exert anti-proliferation effects under normoxia conditions, sirolimus nanoparticle showed a significantly higher effect under the hypoxia condition. Therefore, sirolimus nanoparticle would be a better candidate for atherosclerosis treatment due to

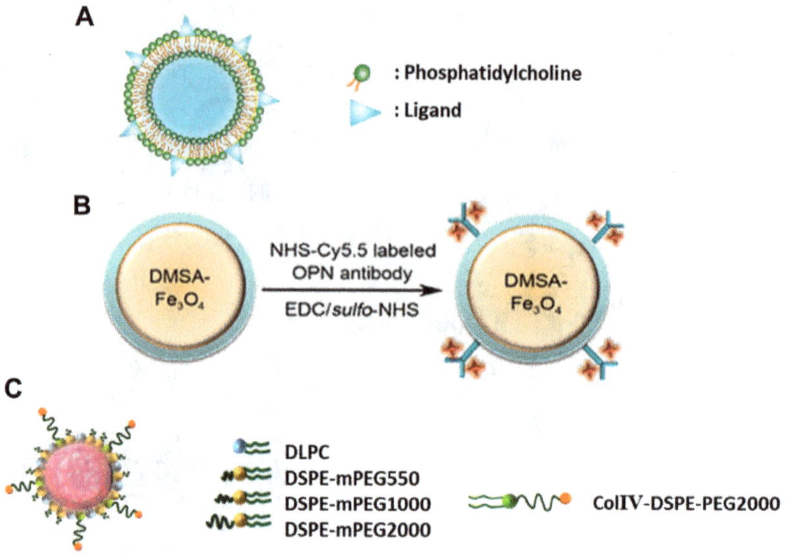

FIGURE 3 | (A) Liposome-like nanovesicle was prepared to target CD36 receptor through KOdiA-PC ligand. **(B)** Iron oxide nanoparticles were conjugated with an anti-osteopontin antibody labeled with Cy5.5 fluorescent dye for dual modality imaging of plaques. **(C)** Lipid-polymer hybrid nanoparticles contained three components: a biodegradable hydrophobic polymeric core, a lipid layer and a peptide decoration for collagen IV (ColIV) targeting.

the presence of hypoxic microenvironment in the plaques. These results highlight the importance of drug choice in treatment of atherosclerosis.

STRATEGIES FOR ACTIVE TARGETING OF ATHEROSCLEROSIS

Active Targeting of Macrophages

As mentioned earlier, macrophages and monocytes play important roles in the formation and progression of atherosclerosis. Not surprisingly, these cells have been considered extensively for imaging and/or therapeutic purposes of atherosclerosis. The phagocytic activities of macrophages together with their abilities to traffic into the inflammatory sites make them a good candidate for targeting atherosclerosis plaques (Kircher et al., 2008). Methods enabling active targeting of inflammatory macrophages can provide additional advantages. For example, while 500–1,000 μmol Fe/kg body weight was needed for magnetic resonance imaging (MRI) of atherosclerosis plaques in ApoE knockout mouse through non-targeted iron oxide nanoparticles (Klug et al., 2009), the amounts of agents needed could be reduced to 36 μmol Fe/kg when iron oxide nanoprobes were decorated with anti-CD163 mAb for active targeting of macrophages residing in inflammatory atherosclerotic plaques (**Figure 2A**) (Tarin et al., 2015). Moreover, polysaccharide hyaluronic acid (HA) conjugated iron oxide nanoparticles (HA-NP) (El-Dakdouki et al., 2014) have been developed for active targeting of macrophage CD44 receptor enabling *in vivo* imaging of atherosclerotic plaques in a rabbit model of atherosclerosis following injection of 3.75 μmol Fe/kg (**Figure 2B**). Other studies used at least 10 times higher amount of Fe/kg for imaging atherosclerosis plaques in this animal model without installing a recognition element on the nanoparticles capable of binding with a receptor on the surface of macrophages (Yu et al., 2011; Tsuchiya et al., 2013). Moreover, active targeting of atherosclerotic plaques by HA bearing iron oxide nanoparticles can be improved using worm shape morphology. For instance, HA conjugated iron oxide nanoworms (HA-NW) (Hossaini Nasr et al., 2018) showed a higher binding with CD44 expressing cells *in vitro* and induced lower inflammatory responses *in vivo*, when administered to ApoE knockout mice (**Figure 2C**).

Besides antibodies and carbohydrates, active targeting of atherosclerotic plaques has been studied through various other strategies. For instance, activated macrophages and foam cells residing in inflammatory atherosclerosis plaques overexpress myeloperoxidase (MPO) (Daugherty et al., 1994). Gd based MPO sensor was designed to detect inflammation in a rabbit model of atherosclerosis (Ronald et al., 2009). Another approach for active targeting of macrophages was the coating of nanocarrier with oxidized phosphatidylcholine (Nie et al., 2015). Interaction of macrophages with oxidized phosphatidylcholine [e.g., 1-(palmitoyl)-2-(5-keto-6-octene-dioyl)] through CD36 receptor has been explored (Collot-Teixeira et al., 2007; Seimon et al., 2010), due to the ability of the oxidized lipid to bind with CD36 (IC50: 3.9 μM) (**Figure 3A**) (Podrez et al., 2002). Another example is a cytokine known as osteopontin (OPN) expressed by foamy macrophages to recruit leukocytes and induce matrix metalloproteinase expression (Matsui et al., 2003; Scatena et al., 2007). An anti-OPN mAb has been used for imaging vulnerable atherosclerotic plaques with various engineered nanoprobes (**Figure 3B**) (Qiao H. et al., 2017; Qiao R. et al., 2017).

An additional molecule for targeting apoptotic macrophages in atherosclerotic plaques is annexin v (Sarai et al., 2007). Decoration of nanoprobes with annexin v protein can target phosphatidylserine present on membrane of apoptotic macrophages in atherosclerotic plaques (Li et al., 2016). Interestingly, virus like particles have also been used for targeting macrophages. For instance, Simian virus 40 (SV40) has been loaded with imaging and therapeutic molecules and targeted to p32 protein on macrophage surface through insertion of CGNKRTRGC peptide known as LyP-1 (Hamzah et al., 2011). In addition, a therapeutic peptide, Hirulog, has been incorporated, which is a thrombin inhibitor with anti-coagulant activities (Sun et al., 2016). Elaborate protein engineering was applied to insert the peptide to guide targeting with the Hirulog peptide pointing in after self-assembly of SV40 virus nanoparticles.

Physicochemical properties of a nanomedicine can be elaborately adjusted to exert atheroprotective effects. For instance, Lewis and coworkers synthesized nanoparticles that exhibited significant targeting and therapeutic effects when tested in ApoE knockout mice (Lewis et al., 2015). A library of composite nanoparticles with different shells consisted of sugar-based amphiphilic macromolecules (AMs) were prepared. Interestingly, the fully synthetic AM constructs could bind with the scavenger receptors on atherogenic macrophages through mimicking physicochemical properties (charge and hydrophobicity) of oxidized lipoproteins (Chnari et al., 2006) resulting in their accumulation in the plaques. They also competed with oxLDL uptake and downregulated the expression of primary scavenger receptors such as CD36 and macrophage scavenger receptor 1 (MSR1) to exert their atheroprotective effects for a site-directed treatment for atherosclerosis plaques.

Active Targeting Through Adhesion Molecules

Angiogenesis targeting is another strategy for imaging atherosclerotic lesions. Since integrin molecules such as αvβ3 play critical roles in angiogenesis, they could be targeted by an integrin receptor antagonist (Winter et al., 2003). In addition, endothelial cells over-express adhesion molecules such as vascular cell adhesion molecule-1 (VCAM-1), intracellular adhesion molecule-1 (ICAM-1) and selectins in atherosclerotic plaques (Khodabandehlou et al., 2017). Thus, various studies have targeted adhesion molecules to direct nanoprobes. For instance, VCAM-1 has been targeted by a short peptide (VHPKQHRAEEAK) (Bruckman et al., 2014) to image atherosclerotic plaques in ApoE knockout mice. Anti-ICAM-1 mAb is another approach for targeting endothelial cell adhesion molecules and delivering their payload through cell adhesion molecule-mediated endocytosis into the plaque site (Serrano et al., 2012). In other studies, microparticles containing atheroprotective microRNA (miR-146a/-181b) have been targeted to E-selectin through a thioaptamer molecule (Ma et al., 2016).

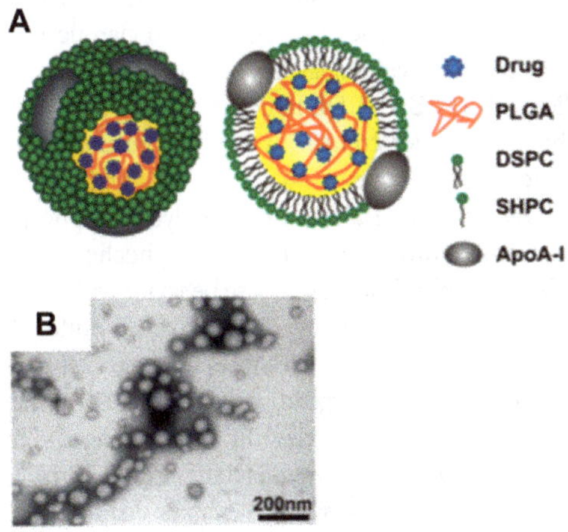

FIGURE 4 | HDL like nanoparticles. **(A)** Schematic demonstration of the PLGA-HDL nanoparticles with PLGA forming the polymeric core of this nanoparticle; **(B)** TEM images showed the spherical morphology of the nanoparticles.

Active Targeting of Extracellular Matrix

Collagen is an important target for atherosclerotic lesions especially since collagen IV forms the bases of blood vessels and it gets exposed during atherosclerosis progression (Murata et al., 1986). Phage display has been used to discover short peptides enabling the targeting of collagen IV (Chan et al., 2010). Theranostic nanoparticles have been engineered to deliver their payload into the atherosclerosis plaques through collagen IV binding peptide (**Figure 3C**) (Fredman et al., 2015; Kamaly et al., 2016; Yu et al., 2017). Another protein molecule for atherosclerosis targeting is profilin-1, which is an actin binding protein (Romeo et al., 2007). The over-expression of profilin-1 is associated with atherosclerosis and other cardiovascular complications. Subsequently, nanoparticles have been conjugated with anti-profilin-1 molecule to deliver therapeutics such as profilin-1 siRNA into the plaque sites. Profilin-1 silencing exerts its therapeutic properties by reducing mouse aorta smooth muscle cell proliferation and migration (Wang et al., 2016).

HDL LIKE NANOPARTICLES FOR DRUG DELIVERY TO ATHEROSCLEROTIC PLAQUES

In human bodies, two endogenous nanoparticles known as high-density lipoprotein (HDL) and LDL, play important roles in managing cholesterol homeostasis. LDL are small carriers of fat molecules to the cells, which can penetrate into arterial walls, get oxidized and cause inflammation. In contrast, HDL can interact with lipid-laden plaque macrophages, and mediate cholesterol removal from plaques by transporting them into the liver (Wang et al., 2004; Duong et al., 2006). The diameter of HDL is about 8–12 nm and hydrophobic lipids are located in the core while phospholipids and apolipoproteins such as apolipoprotein A (ApoA)-1 or ApoA-II form the outer layer (Gordon et al., 2010). Based on the knowledge of HDL structures and functions, scientists have investigated HDL and/or HDL mimetic nanoparticles to target atherosclerotic plaques. For instance, microfluidic technology has been used to build poly (lactic-co-glycolic acid) (PLGA)-HDL nanocarrier (Sanchez-Gaytan et al., 2015). This nanocarrier contains a PLGA core capable of loading hydrophobic drugs while it is decorated with ApoA-1 and phospholipids such as 1,2-distearoyl-sn-glycero-3-phosphocholine and 1-stearoyl-2-hydroxy-sn-glycero-3-phosphocholine (**Figure 4**). PLGA-HDL showed a slow drug release behavior with 60% release in 24 h and up to 90% release after 5 days in PBS buffer. Moreover, animal study on ApoE knockout mice showed 12.8-h half-life in blood circulation and their targeting property was confirmed by high accumulation of these particles in macrophages residing in atherosclerotic plaques (Sanchez-Gaytan et al., 2015). Although using PLGA core in this system enables loading of different therapeutic and/or imaging molecules, it can impose limitations on ApoA-I conformational flexibility resulting in impaired cholesterol efflux (Tall et al., 2008; Tang et al., 2016). Moreover, this artificial polymeric core induced changes in the shape of these nanoparticles to be more spherical rather than discoidal shape of native HDL, and their sizes increased significantly in comparison to the HDL.

In addition to the nanoparticle size and shape, the phospholipid core was studied and 1-palmitoyl-2-oleoyl-sn-glycero-3-phosphocholine based HDL nanoparticle showed the highest similarity to natural HDL (Tang et al., 2016). Such HDL like nanoparticles have been used to deliver statins into inflammatory atherosclerotic plaques. For instance, reconstituted HDL (rHDL) nanoparticles loaded with simvastatin [S]-rHDL have been designed and successfully employed to deliver the payload into inflammatory plaques in ApoE knockout mice (Duivenvoorden et al., 2014). A comparison was made for low doses of [S]-rHDL (15 mg/kg simvastatin, 10 mg/kg ApoA-I) that was administered intravenously biweekly for 12 weeks vs. orally administered simvastatin (15 mg/kg per day) and the results showed lower plaque macrophage content for the [S]-rHDL group. Interestingly, delivery of a high dose (60 mg/kg simvastatin, 40 mg/kg ApoA-I) by this nanosystem into ApoE knockout mice in four intravenous injections showed significant mitigation effects on plaque inflammation while rHDL alone could not decrease the sizes of plaque area based on histological analysis. The stronger effect for short term high [S]-rHDL group indicated the importance of delivering higher amounts of simvastatin for inhibiting atherosclerotic plaque inflammation.

Although rHDL is an attractive drug delivery system for cardiovascular diseases, undesired drug leakage is a drawback of this system. One reason for this leakage is believed to be the interaction of drug loaded rHDL with the lecithin cholesterol acyltransferase that can remodel this particle (Zhang et al., 2013). An approach to decrease r-HDL reactivity with the lecithin cholesterol acyltransferase is through the insertion of arachidonic acid into the phospholipid bilayers of rHDL (He et al., 2014). Such adjustment of physicochemical properties of rHDL could enhance nanocarrier design for drug delivery to atherosclerotic plaques (He et al., 2015).

In order to improve drug delivery property of HDL like particles, dextran sulfate (DXS) has been used to coat rHDL as DXS can bind with scavenge receptor AI highly expressed on activated macrophages and foam cells in inflammatory plaques through electrostatic interactions (De Winther et al., 2000; Chao et al., 2012). In this design, atorvastatin was loaded in a spherical PLGA core encapsulated in liposomes. Then, it was decorated by ApoA-I and finally coated with DXS (AT-DXS-LP-rHDL) (Zhao et al., 2017). Cellular study showed the ability of these particles to facilitate cholesterol efflux from macrophages (RAW264.7 and THP-1 cells). Moreover, these particles were able to reduce TNFα and IL-6 production in macrophages due to atorvastatin release. It is noteworthy that ApoA-I and DXS coating both helped retard atorvastatin release. In addition, ox-LDL uptake by macrophages was significantly reduced because high affinity DXS competes with ox-LDL for SR-AI binding.

Since the incorporation of ApoA-1 into a small molecule therapeutic agent can be challenging due to the hydrophobicity and large size (21–31 kDa) of ApoA-1, a mimetic peptide containing 18-amino acids, known as "4F" was employed by Mansukhani and coworkers to prepare peptide amphiphile nanofibers loaded with liver X receptor agonist GW3965 (LXR) (Mansukhani et al., 2019). Intravenous administration of this formulation (8-weeks, two injections per week) to ApoE knockout mice showed therapeutic effects comparable to the free drug (LXR) while the liver toxicity was reduced. Future work on this formulation would focus on physicochemical analysis on peptide amphiphile and covalently loading LXR to improve the overall therapeutic efficacy.

BLOOD CELLS AS TROJAN HORSES FOR ANTI-ATHEROSCLEROSIS DRUG DELIVERY

Harnessing blood cells for drug delivery has important features rendering it attractive for atherosclerosis therapy. For instance, the blood circulation time of nanomedicine will be increased due to the inherent abilities of cellular membrane enabling the cells to evade the phagocytic system. Accordingly, Wang and coworkers packed rapamycin (RAP) loaded PLGA nanoparticles in the membrane of red blood cells (RBC) termed RBC/RAP@PLGA (Wang et al., 2019). RAP is an immunosuppressant molecule with anti-atherogenic effects (Waksman et al., 2003; Castro et al., 2004). This formulation showed a significantly higher therapeutic effect in ApoE knockout mice following a 1-month treatment compared to the RAP@PLG nanoparticles lacking the RBC membrane. Similarly, Song and coworkers introduced RAP loaded PLGA nanoparticle coated with platelet membrane named RAP-PNP (Song et al., 2019). Platelets play important roles in the pathogenesis of atherosclerosis and they have inherent affinities to home to the plaques (Lindemann et al., 2007). Four-week treatment of ApoE knockout mice with RAP-PNP led to superior therapeutic effects compared to free RAP or RAP-NP with a favorite safety profile for long-term use. In a similar study, RAP loaded nanoparticles coated by macrophage membrane (MM), i.e., the MM/RAP NPs, showed an efficient accumulation in atherosclerotic plaques in ApoE knockout mice and inhibited the progression of disease (Wang et al., 2021). Moreover, MM/RAP NPs had an enhanced blood retention time compared to uncoated RAP NPs indicating the importance of MM coating to improve pharmacokinetics of the formulation.

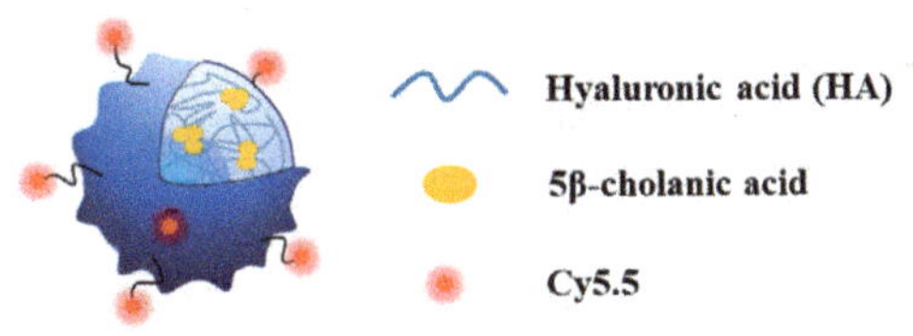

FIGURE 5 | Conjugation of hydrophobic 5-cholanic acid with hyaluronan resulted in self-assembled nanoparticle formation. This formulation could be a drug carrier for atherosclerotic plaques imaging and/or therapy.

Neutrophils can be recruited to atherosclerotic plaques through their interactions with ICAM-1, E-selectin, P-selectin, CXCL1/KC, CXCL2 and CXCL4 (Baetta and Corsini, 2010; Williams et al., 2011; Soehnlein, 2012; Kolaczkowska and Kubes, 2013). Xue and coworkers introduced cellular vehicles based on neutrophils as a novel strategy for targeting atherosclerotic plaques (Xue et al., 2019), which can be a potential strategy for delivering cargoes. Although this work showed excellent targeting properties of engineered neutrophils into the plaques in the ApoE knockout mouse model, the encapsulation of an anti-atherosclerotic compound for therapy has yet to be evaluated.

HA BASED NANOPARTICLES TARGETING CD44 FOR ATHEROSCLEROSIS TREATMENT

Overexpressed CD44 in atherosclerotic plaques is an important target for drug delivery. HA is a naturally occurring polysaccharide with high affinity for CD44, which has been used to decorate rHDL for targeting inflammatory atherosclerotic plaques (Slevin et al., 2007). Simvastatin loaded PLGA nanoparticles have been encapsulated into liposomes and decorated with ApoA-I and HA (ST-HA-PLGA-rHDL). HA immobilization was carried out by two different strategies. The first strategy includes covalent conjugation of HA onto available amine groups of ApoA-I through 1-ethyl-3-(3-dimethylaminopropyl) carbodiimide (EDC) and *N*-hydroxy-succinimide (NHS) coupling agents (ST-HA-(C)-PLGA-rHDL). The second strategy was electrostatic absorption of HA by cationic ST-PLGA-rHDL (ST-HA-(E)-PLGA-rHDL). Testing these nanostructures *in vivo* on a rabbit model of atherosclerosis indicated better atheroprotective activity for ST-HA-(C)-PLGA-rHDL. This observation has been explained through a better shielding effect of covalent HA coating that decreases their liver uptake (Zhang M. et al., 2017). In addition, HA coating enhanced nanoparticle accumulation in atherosclerotic plaques due to its interaction with CD44. This effect has been shown in the rabbit model of atherosclerosis through quantification of DiR labeled HA-(C)-PLGA-rHDL in the aortic tree.

Huang and coworkers recently introduced HA conjugated atorvastatin nanoparticle (HA-ATV-NPs) capable of delivering atorvastatin into the inflammatory atherosclerotic plaques in ApoE knockout mice (Hossaini Nasr et al., 2020). HA-ATV-NPs were constructed through chemical conjugation of ATV to HA backbone, which enabled the loading of a significant amount of ATV (35% by weight) into the NPs rendering it attractive for statin therapy. The therapeutic effects by HA-ATV-NPs were observed following a 1-week treatment (8.5 mg ATV.kg^{-1}, one injection every other day). Moreover, the therapeutic effect could be monitored non-invasively by magnetic resonance imaging aided by a superparamagnetic iron oxide based nanoworms bearing HA (Hossaini Nasr et al., 2018), highlighting the utility of HA for plaque targeting.

HA has been utilized to reduce rHDL uptake by liver's scavenger receptor class B type I (SR-BI). Lovastatin loaded r-HDL (LT-rHDL) has been decorated with HA, which facilitated their interactions with up-regulated CD44 receptors in inflammatory plaques while reducing their liver uptake (Liu et al., 2014). Functionalizing the Apo proteins with HA helped LT-rHDL escape from the reticuloendothelial system (RES) and improved lovastatin circulation time *in vivo*.

In addition to HA-rHDL, another type of HA nanoparticle has been prepared by conjugation of hydrophobic 5β-cholanic acid to HA through NHS, EDC chemistry *via* a diamine linker. The resulting conjugate can self-assemble to nanoparticles in water due to the hydrophilic nature of HA backbone and hydrophobic property of 5β-cholanic acid (**Figure 5**). Labeling this NP system with fluorescent molecules such as Cy5.5 and fluorescein isothiocyanate demonstrated that this HA-NP could be selectively taken up by CD44 expressing cells *in vitro* through receptor mediated endocytosis. Moreover, injection of this nanoparticle to ApoE knockout mice showed its accumulation in atherosclerotic plaques and further immunohistochemistry studies confirmed co-localization of HA-NPs with CD44 and another HA receptor, i.e., hyaluronic acid receptor for endocytosis (HARE) in atherosclerotic lesions (Lee et al., 2015).

In nature, HA can vary significantly in length, and its molecular weight can significantly impact its biological activities. For example, high molecular weight HA (megadaltons, MDa) can suppress inflammation and angiogenesis, while low molecular HA oligomers are inflammatory and angiogenic (Rooney et al., 1995; Masuko et al., 2009). Subsequently, in addition to their CD44 targeting property, HA atheroprotective effect has been investigated through PET/MRI. HA (MW 66–99 kDa) has been used to prepare radiolabeled HA-NP (^{89}Zr-HA-NP) and administered to ApoE knockout mouse and rabbit models of atherosclerosis (Beldman et al., 2017). HA-NP inhibited the production of TNFα, IL-2, IL-6 and nitric oxide by macrophages *in vitro*. Furthermore, HA-NP treatment stabilized plaques *in vivo*, which increased collagen content of plaques up to 30–40% while reducing macrophage content by 30% in comparison with control groups. One hypothesis to explain these observations is that aggregation of HA polymer to form HA-NPs might imitate the anti-inflammatory effect of high molecular weight (MDa) HA.

SOLID LIPID NANOPARTICLES AND NANOFIBERS FOR ATHEROSCLEROSIS TREATMENT

Methotrexate (MTX) is an immunomodulatory drug that is often used for chronic inflammatory disease (Chan and Cronstein, 2002) and its atheroprotective effect in the presence of systemic inflammation has been the subject of several studies (Bulgarelli et al., 2012; Ronda et al., 2015). MTX can decrease inflammatory cytokine production and downregulate the expression of adhesion molecules although the specific mechanism is not fully understood (Chan and Cronstein, 2002; Gerards et al., 2003). MTX has been formulated in solid lipid nanoparticle (MTX SPN) for targeted delivery to atherosclerotic plaques. In this formulation, MTX has been loaded into the hydrophobic PLGA core and decorated with phospholipids, which were found to decrease inflammatory cytokines production (IL-6 and TNFα) upon *in vitro* incubation with J774.A1 macrophages. Moreover, MTX SPN has been labeled with DiD and rhodamine for fluorescent imaging and radiolabeled with ^{64}Cu for further *in vivo* studies. These particles were taken up by macrophages releasing their cargo inside the cells. In addition, circulating monocytes can take up them and infiltrate into atherosclerotic plaques. *In vivo* evaluation of MTX SPN on ApoE knockout mice showed 50% reduction of plaque burden following biweekly administration of 1 mg/kg MTX in 1 month (Stigliano et al., 2017).

As discussed earlier, macrophage targeting is a known strategy for atherosclerosis therapy and/or imaging. Lipid-latex (LiLa) hybrid nanoparticles have been designed for targeting inflammatory macrophages. In this design, a hydrophobic polymer latex serves as a drug reservoir, while lipids bring colloidal stability to the system as well as targeting properties. Phosphatidylserine and cholesterol-9-carboxynonanoate have been used as lipid coating. These molecules served as "eat me" signal for macrophages enhancing macrophage uptake (Poon et al., 2014). In addition, over-expression of phospholipase A2 (Goncalves et al., 2012) in inflammatory macrophages could disrupt lipid coating and trigger drug release inside the macrophages (Bagalkot et al., 2015). Testing LiLa NP for imaging atherosclerotic plaques in ApoE knockout mice showed their accumulation in plaques while control bare latex nanoparticle mostly accumulated in the liver. However, LiLa NP may not be a good candidate for clinical translation to humans due to the poor biodegradability properties of polystyrene latex.

The immune system can be regulated to reduce the plaque burden. Accordingly, Flores and coworkers developed single-walled carbon nanotubes (SWNTs) loaded with SHP-1 inhibitor termed as SWNT-SHP1i (Flores et al., 2020). SHP-1i is a small molecule inhibitor of CD47's downstream effector molecule, resulting in phagocytic function recovery that was suppressed in the plaques. It is important to note that the impairment of phagocytic activity in inflammatory sites contribute to the pathology of atherosclerosis. SWNT-SHP1i was able to restore the phagocytic activity of macrophages in the plaques, resulting in plaque expansion inhibition and reduction of inflammation.

ADMINISTRATION ROUTES OF ATHEROPROTECTIVE NANOMEDICINE

Route of nanoparticle administration is an important consideration. While intravenous (iv) administration of nanoparticles is commonly utilized, formulations for oral delivery of nanoparticles have been investigated. For example, rosuvastatin was incorporated into solid lipid nanoparticles for oral administration and it led to not only better bioavailability of drug, but also higher decrease of plasma cholesterol and LDL levels compared with the free drug (Beg et al., 2017). However, these rosuvastatin loaded solid lipid nanoparticles have only been investigated under hyperlipidemia-like condition, not in atherosclerotic models.

In another study for oral delivery, RAP loaded nanoparticles have been prepared through self-assembly of cationic polymer polyethyleneimine. These positively charged nanoparticles have been packed into microcapsule obtained from yeast *Saccharomyces cerevisiae* to form complex yeast-derived microcapsule (YC) (Zhang X. et al., 2017). Through the transcytosis mechanism, the YC could be absorbed by M cells in Peyer's patches, which are aggregated lymphoid follicles in the gut (Jung et al., 2010). Following the absorption, monocytes and/or macrophages are able to uptake them by endocytosis and relocate them in inflammatory atherosclerotic plaques. In addition to RAP, this nanoparticle system has been tuned to deliver other drugs such as ursodeoxycholic acid and sulindac to atherosclerotic plaques. Using an oral formulation that can target inflammatory atherosclerotic plaques efficiently is much more convenient than iv injections, which is advantageous for future clinical translation.

Intraperitoneal (ip) injection of nanoparticle is another common route of administration for atheroprotective nanoparticles (Guo et al., 2018). Interestingly, superiority of ip over iv injection of an HDL like nanoparticle was reported by Jung and coworkers (Jung et al., 2014). However, other HDL like nanoparticles reported in the same work were administered iv, indicating that individual characteristic of HDL like nanoparticles, such as size and surface charge, likely dictated the best route of their administration. Finally, subcutaneous (sc) injection of hydrogel has been studied for sustained delivery of anti-inflammatory nanoparticles (Yi et al., 2020). In another study, insulin-like growth factor (IGF)-1 was formulated in nanofibers/hydrogel showed atherosclerosis inhibition *in vivo* following sc administration in ApoE knockout mice (Shang et al., 2020). In general, most nanoparticles designed for active targeting of atherosclerosis have been administered iv and other routes of administration take advantage of the abilities of macrophages to take up the particles and traffic to the inflammatory sites including atherosclerotic plaques.

CONCLUSION AND FUTURE DIRECTIONS

Increasing and improving the stability of a rupture prone plaque should be the first high priority target for an atheroprotective nanoparticle. Obviously, this is the main reason why the majority of the research in this area focuses on inflammatory aspect of atherosclerosis, the major contributor of plaque instability. Another key step towards management of inflammatory atherosclerotic plaques is the diagnosis of unstable plaques by imaging. Therefore, designing of imaging probes for detection of unstable plaques is important (Vazquez-Prada et al., 2021). One of the future directions for this field would be to develop theranostic nanoparticle that not only impose therapeutic effects on plaques but also help clinicians to monitor the treatment progress. It is noteworthy to mention that a lack of proper animal models resembling the unstable plaque features with human is an important limitation factor for the field. Finally, another challenge that has not been fully addressed yet, is adjusting pharmacokinetic of nanoparticles targeting atherosclerosis. Therefore, optimizing the blood circulation time, minimizing the liver uptake through elaborated physicochemical design, and introducing specified ligands targeting unstable plaques will introduce more nanomedicine candidates to the clinical trials in the future.

Targeting of inflammatory atherosclerosis plaques is highly desired for delivering therapeutic molecules to the sites of action. To achieve this goal, a multitask nanocarrier should be designed with the capability of reaching atherosclerosis plaques selectively and releasing its payload. Although, HDL, the naturally occurring nanoparticle, has inspired scientists to fabricate HDL mimetic nanoparticles, the challenges have not been fully addressed due to the high affinity of liver for these particles as well as the high cost of ApoA (1 mg costs $333 from Sigma-Aldrich). In addition, physicochemical properties of these nanoparticles should be carefully tuned to get the highest HDL like activity. Therefore, researchers have investigated other nanocarriers to deliver anti-inflammatory or anti-proliferative molecules. Among anti-inflammatory therapeutics, statins have been investigated the most due to their applications in the clinic for management of atherosclerosis. With suitably designed nanoparticle systems, significant therapeutic effects towards atherosclerotic plaques can be achieved to reduce the adverse impacts of atherosclerosis.

AUTHOR CONTRIBUTIONS

SH searched the literature and wrote the manuscript while XH gave ideas and edited the manuscript.

REFERENCES

Albert, M. A., Danielson, E., Rifai, N., and Ridker, P. M. (2001). Effect of Statin Therapy on C-Reactive Protein Levels: the Pravastatin Inflammation/CRP Evaluation (PRINCE): a Randomized Trial and Cohort Study. *JAMA* 286, 64–70. doi:10.1001/jama.286.1.64

Ascer, E., Bertolami, M. C., Venturinelli, M. L., Buccheri, V., Souza, J., Nicolau, J. C., et al. (2004). Atorvastatin Reduces Proinflammatory Markers in Hypercholesterolemic Patients. *Atherosclerosis* 177, 161–166. doi:10.1016/j.atherosclerosis.2004.07.003

Autieri, M. V. (2012). Pro- and Anti-inflammatory Cytokine Networks in Atherosclerosis. *ISRN Vasc. Med.* 2012, 1–17. doi:10.5402/2012/987629

Baetta, R., and Corsini, A. (2010). Role of Polymorphonuclear Neutrophils in Atherosclerosis: Current State and Future Perspectives. *Atherosclerosis* 210, 1–13. doi:10.1016/j.atherosclerosis.2009.10.028

Bagalkot, V., Badgeley, M. A., Kampfrath, T., Deiuliis, J. A., Rajagopalan, S., and Maiseyeu, A. (2015). Hybrid Nanoparticles Improve Targeting to Inflammatory Macrophages through Phagocytic Signals. *J. Control Release* 217, 243–255. doi:10.1016/j.jconrel.2015.09.027

Beg, S., Jain, S., Kushwah, V., Bhatti, G. K., Sandhu, P. S., Katare, O. P., et al. (2017). Novel Surface-Engineered Solid Lipid Nanoparticles of Rosuvastatin Calcium for Low-Density Lipoprotein-Receptor Targeting: a Quality by Design-Driven Perspective. *Nanomedicine (Lond)* 12, 333–356. doi:10.2217/nnm-2016-0336

Beldman, T. J., Senders, M. L., Alaarg, A., Pérez-Medina, C., Tang, J., Zhao, Y., et al. (2017). Hyaluronan Nanoparticles Selectively Target Plaque-Associated Macrophages and Improve Plaque Stability in Atherosclerosis. *ACS Nano* 11, 5785–5799. doi:10.1021/acsnano.7b01385

Benjamin, E. J., Blaha, M. J., Chiuve, S. E., Cushman, M., Das, S. R., Deo, R., et al. (2017). Heart Disease and Stroke Statistics-2017 Update: A Report from the American Heart Association. *Circulation* 135, e146–e603. doi:10.1161/cir.0000000000000485

Berliner, J. A., Navab, M., Fogelman, A. M., Frank, J. S., Demer, L. L., Edwards, P. A., et al. (1995). Atherosclerosis: Basic Mechanisms. Oxidation, Inflammation, and Genetics. *Circulation* 91, 2488–2496. doi:10.1161/01.cir.91.9.2488

Black, S., Kushner, I., and Samols, D. (2004). C-reactive Protein. *J. Biol. Chem.* 279, 48487–48490. doi:10.1074/jbc.R400025200

Bruckman, M. A., Jiang, K., Simpson, E. J., Randolph, L. N., Luyt, L. G., Yu, X., et al. (2014). Dual-Modal Magnetic Resonance and Fluorescence Imaging of Atherosclerotic Plaques *In Vivo* Using VCAM-1 Targeted Tobacco Mosaic Virus. *Nano Lett.* 14, 1551–1558. doi:10.1021/nl404816m

Bulgarelli, A., Martins Dias, A. A., Caramelli, B., and Maranhão, R. C. (2012). Treatment with Methotrexate Inhibits Atherogenesis in Cholesterol-Fed Rabbits. *J. Cardiovasc. Pharmacol.* 59, 308–314. doi:10.1097/FJC.0b013e318241c385

Burleigh, M. E., Babaev, V. R., Yancey, P. G., Major, A. S., Mccaleb, J. L., Oates, J. A., et al. (2005). Cyclooxygenase-2 Promotes Early Atherosclerotic Lesion Formation in ApoE-Deficient and C57BL/6 Mice. *J. Mol. Cel. Cardiol.* 39, 443–452. doi:10.1016/j.yjmcc.2005.06.011

Castro, C., Campistol, J. M., Sancho, D., Sánchez-Madrid, F., Casals, E., and Andrés, V. (2004). Rapamycin Attenuates Atherosclerosis Induced by Dietary Cholesterol in Apolipoprotein-Deficient Mice through a P27 Kip1 -independent Pathway. *Atherosclerosis* 172, 31–38. doi:10.1016/j.atherosclerosis.2003.09.003

Cerqueira, N. M., Oliveira, E. F., Gesto, D. S., Santos-Martins, D., Moreira, C., Moorthy, H. N., et al. (2016). Cholesterol Biosynthesis: A Mechanistic Overview. *Biochemistry* 55, 5483–5506. doi:10.1021/acs.biochem.6b00342

Chan, E. S., and Cronstein, B. N. (2002). Molecular Action of Methotrexate in Inflammatory Diseases. *Arthritis Res.* 4, 266–273. doi:10.1186/ar419

Chan, J. M., Zhang, L., Tong, R., Ghosh, D., Gao, W., Liao, G., et al. (2010). Spatiotemporal Controlled Delivery of Nanoparticles to Injured Vasculature. *Proc. Natl. Acad. Sci. U S A.* 107, 2213–2218. doi:10.1073/pnas.0914585107

Chao, Y., Makale, M., Karmali, P. P., Sharikov, Y., Tsigelny, I., Merkulov, S., et al. (2012). Recognition of Dextran-Superparamagnetic Iron Oxide Nanoparticle Conjugates (Feridex) via Macrophage Scavenger Receptor Charged Domains. *Bioconjug. Chem.* 23, 1003–1009. doi:10.1021/bc200685a

Chelly, J., Mongardon, N., Dumas, F., Varenne, O., Spaulding, C., Vignaux, O., et al. (2012). Benefit of an Early and Systematic Imaging Procedure after Cardiac Arrest: Insights from the PROCAT (Parisian Region Out of Hospital Cardiac Arrest) Registry. *Resuscitation* 83, 1444–1450. doi:10.1016/j.resuscitation.2012.08.321

Chen, Y., Zeng, Y., Zhu, X., Miao, L., Liang, X., Duan, J., et al. (2021). Significant Difference between Sirolimus and Paclitaxel Nanoparticles in Anti-proliferation Effect in Normoxia and Hypoxia: The Basis of Better Selection of Atherosclerosis Treatment. *Bioact. Mater.* 6, 880–889. doi:10.1016/j.bioactmat.2020.09.005

Chnari, E., Nikitczuk, J. S., Wang, J., Uhrich, K. E., and Moghe, P. V. (2006). Engineered Polymeric Nanoparticles for Receptor-Targeted Blockage of Oxidized Low Density Lipoprotein Uptake and Atherogenesis in Macrophages. *Biomacromolecules* 7, 1796–1805. doi:10.1021/bm0600872

Collot-Teixeira, S., Martin, J., Mcdermott-Roe, C., Poston, R., and Mcgregor, J. L. (2007). CD36 and Macrophages in Atherosclerosis. *Cardiovasc. Res.* 75, 468–477. doi:10.1016/j.cardiores.2007.03.010

Daugherty, A., Dunn, J. L., Rateri, D. L., and Heinecke, J. W. (1994). Myeloperoxidase, a Catalyst for Lipoprotein Oxidation, Is Expressed in Human Atherosclerotic Lesions. *J. Clin. Invest.* 94, 437–444. doi:10.1172/jci117342

De Winther, M. P., Van Dijk, K. W., Havekes, L. M., and Hofker, M. H. (2000). Macrophage Scavenger Receptor Class A: A Multifunctional Receptor in Atherosclerosis. *Arterioscler. Thromb. Vasc. Biol.* 20, 290–297. doi:10.1161/01.atv.20.2.290

Derdeyn, C. P., and Chimowitz, M. I. (2007). Angioplasty and Stenting for Atherosclerotic Intracranial Stenosis: Rationale for a Randomized Clinical Trial. *Neuroimaging Clin. N. Am.* 17, 355–ix. doi:10.1016/j.nic.2007.05.001

Duivenvoorden, R., Tang, J., Cormode, D. P., Mieszawska, A. J., Izquierdo-Garcia, D., Ozcan, C., et al. (2014). A Statin-Loaded Reconstituted High-Density Lipoprotein Nanoparticle Inhibits Atherosclerotic Plaque Inflammation. *Nat. Commun.* 5, 3065. doi:10.1038/ncomms4065

Duong, M., Collins, H. L., Jin, W., Zanotti, I., Favari, E., and Rothblat, G. H. (2006). Relative Contributions of ABCA1 and SR-BI to Cholesterol Efflux to Serum from Fibroblasts and Macrophages. *Arterioscler. Thromb. Vasc. Biol.* 26, 541–547. doi:10.1161/01.Atv.0000203515.25574.19

El-Dakdouki, M. H., El-Boubbou, K., Kamat, M., Huang, R., Abela, G. S., Kiupel, M., et al. (2014). CD44 Targeting Magnetic Glyconanoparticles for Atherosclerotic Plaque Imaging. *Pharm. Res.* 31, 1426–1437. doi:10.1007/s11095-013-1021-8

Flores, A. M., Hosseini-Nassab, N., Jarr, K. U., Ye, J., Zhu, X., Wirka, R., et al. (2020). Pro-efferocytic Nanoparticles Are Specifically Taken up by Lesional Macrophages and Prevent Atherosclerosis. *Nat. Nanotechnol.* 15, 154–161. doi:10.1038/s41565-019-0619-3

Fredman, G., Kamaly, N., Spolitu, S., Milton, J., Ghorpade, D., Chiasson, R., et al. (2015). Erratum for the Research Article: "Targeted Nanoparticles Containing the Proresolving Peptide Ac2-26 Protect against Advanced Atherosclerosis in Hypercholesterolemic Mice" by G. Fredman, N. Kamaly, S. Spolitu, J. Milton, D. Ghorpade, R. Chiasson, G. Kuriakose, M. Perretti, O. Farokzhad, I. Tabas. *Sci. Transl. Med.* 7, 277er2. doi:10.1126/scitranslmed.aaa106510.1126/scitranslmed.aaa9877

Gately, S., and Li, W. W. (2004). Multiple Roles of COX-2 in Tumor Angiogenesis: a Target for Antiangiogenic Therapy. *Semin. Oncol.* 31, 2–11. doi:10.1053/j.seminoncol.2004.03.040

Gerards, A. H., De Lathouder, S., De Groot, E. R., Dijkmans, B. A., and Aarden, L. A. (2003). Inhibition of Cytokine Production by Methotrexate. Studies in Healthy Volunteers and Patients with Rheumatoid arthritisStudies in Healthy Volunteers and Patients with Rheumatoid Arthritis. *Rheumatology (Oxford)* 42, 1189–1196. doi:10.1093/rheumatology/keg323

Gonçalves, I., Edsfeldt, A., Ko, N. Y., Grufman, H., Berg, K., Björkbacka, H., et al. (2012). Evidence Supporting a Key Role of Lp-PLA2-Generated Lysophosphatidylcholine in Human Atherosclerotic Plaque Inflammation. *Arterioscler. Thromb. Vasc. Biol.* 32, 1505–1512. doi:10.1161/atvbaha.112.249854

Gordon, S. M., Deng, J., Lu, L. J., and Davidson, W. S. (2010). Proteomic Characterization of Human Plasma High Density Lipoprotein Fractionated by Gel Filtration Chromatography. *J. Proteome. Res.* 9, 5239–5249. doi:10.1021/pr100520x

Guo, Y., Yuan, W., Yu, B., Kuai, R., Hu, W., Morin, E. E., et al. (2018). Synthetic High-Density Lipoprotein-Mediated Targeted Delivery of Liver X Receptors Agonist Promotes Atherosclerosis Regression. *EBioMedicine* 28, 225–233. doi:10.1016/j.ebiom.2017.12.021

Hamzah, J., Kotamraju, V. R., Seo, J. W., Agemy, L., Fogal, V., Mahakian, L. M., et al. (2011). Specific Penetration and Accumulation of a Homing Peptide within Atherosclerotic Plaques of Apolipoprotein E-Deficient Mice. *Proc. Natl. Acad. Sci. U S A.* 108, 7154–7159. doi:10.1073/pnas.1104540108

He, H., Liu, L., Bai, H., Wang, J., Zhang, Y., Zhang, W., et al. (2014). Arachidonic Acid-Modified Lovastatin Discoidal Reconstituted High Density Lipoprotein Markedly Decreases the Drug Leakage during the Remodeling Behaviors Induced by Lecithin Cholesterol Acyltransferase. *Pharm. Res.* 31, 1689–1709. doi:10.1007/s11095-013-1273-3

He, H., Zhang, M., Liu, L., Zhang, S., Liu, J., and Zhang, W. (2015). Suppression of Remodeling Behaviors with Arachidonic Acid Modification for Enhanced *In Vivo* Antiatherogenic Efficacies of Lovastatin-Loaded Discoidal Recombinant High Density Lipoprotein. *Pharm. Res.* 32, 3415–3431. doi:10.1007/s11095-015-1719-x

Heeschen, C., Hamm, C. W., Laufs, U., Snapinn, S., Böhm, M., and White, H. D. (2002). Withdrawal of Statins Increases Event Rates in Patients with Acute Coronary Syndromes. *Circulation* 105, 1446–1452. doi:10.1161/01.cir.0000012530.68333.c8

Hernández-Presa, M. A., Martín-Ventura, J. L., Ortego, M., Gómez-Hernández, A., Tuñón, J., Hernández-Vargas, P., et al. (2002). Atorvastatin Reduces the Expression of Cyclooxygenase-2 in a Rabbit Model of Atherosclerosis and in Cultured Vascular Smooth Muscle Cells. *Atherosclerosis* 160, 49–58. doi:10.1016/s0021-9150(01)00547-0

Herrero-Fernandez, B., Gomez-Bris, R., Somovilla-Crespo, B., and Gonzalez-Granado, J. M. (2019). Immunobiology of Atherosclerosis: A Complex Net of Interactions. *Int. J. Mol. Sci.* 20, 5293. doi:10.3390/ijms20215293

Hossaini Nasr, S., Rashidijahanabad, Z., Ramadan, S., Kauffman, N., Parameswaran, N., Zinn, K. R., et al. (2020). Effective Atherosclerotic Plaque Inflammation Inhibition with Targeted Drug Delivery by Hyaluronan Conjugated Atorvastatin Nanoparticles. *Nanoscale* 12, 9541–9556. doi:10.1039/D0NR00308E

Hossaini Nasr, S., Tonson, A., El-Dakdouki, M. H., Zhu, D. C., Agnew, D., Wiseman, R., et al. (2018). Effects of Nanoprobe Morphology on Cellular Binding and Inflammatory Responses: Hyaluronan-Conjugated Magnetic Nanoworms for Magnetic Resonance Imaging of Atherosclerotic Plaques. *ACS Appl. Mater. Inter.* 10, 11495–11507. doi:10.1021/acsami.7b19708

Jung, C., Hugot, J. P., and Barreau, F. (2010). Peyer's Patches: The Immune Sensors of the Intestine. *Int. J. Inflam* 2010, 823710. doi:10.4061/2010/823710

Jung, C., Kaul, M. G., Bruns, O. T., Dučić, T., Freund, B., Heine, M., et al. (2014). Intraperitoneal Injection Improves the Uptake of Nanoparticle-Labeled High-Density Lipoprotein to Atherosclerotic Plaques Compared with Intravenous Injection: a Multimodal Imaging Study in ApoE Knockout Mice. *Circ. Cardiovasc. Imaging* 7, 303–311. doi:10.1161/CIRCIMAGING.113.000607

Kamaly, N., Fredman, G., Fojas, J. J., Subramanian, M., Choi, W. I., Zepeda, K., et al. (2016). Targeted Interleukin-10 Nanotherapeutics Developed with a Microfluidic Chip Enhance Resolution of Inflammation in Advanced Atherosclerosis. *ACS Nano* 10, 5280–5292. doi:10.1021/acsnano.6b01114

Khodabandehlou, K., Masehi-Lano, J. J., Poon, C., Wang, J., and Chung, E. J. (2017). Targeting Cell Adhesion Molecules with Nanoparticles Using *In Vivo* and Flow-Based *In Vitro* Models of Atherosclerosis. *Exp. Biol. Med. (Maywood)* 242, 799–812. doi:10.1177/1535370217693116

Kircher, M. F., Grimm, J., Swirski, F. K., Libby, P., Gerszten, R. E., Allport, J. R., et al. (2008). Noninvasive *In Vivo* Imaging of Monocyte Trafficking to Atherosclerotic Lesions. *Circulation* 117, 388–395. doi:10.1161/circulationaha.107.719765

Klug, G., Kampf, T., Ziener, C., Parczyk, M., Bauer, E., Herold, V., et al. (2009). Murine Atherosclerotic Plaque Imaging with the USPIO Ferumoxtran-10. *Front. Biosci. (Landmark Ed.* 14, 2546–2552. doi:10.2741/3396

Kolaczkowska, E., and Kubes, P. (2013). Neutrophil Recruitment and Function in Health and Inflammation. *Nat. Rev. Immunol.* 13, 159–175. doi:10.1038/nri3399

Lee, G. Y., Kim, J. H., Choi, K. Y., Yoon, H. Y., Kim, K., Kwon, I. C., et al. (2015). Hyaluronic Acid Nanoparticles for Active Targeting Atherosclerosis. *Biomaterials* 53, 341–348. doi:10.1016/j.biomaterials.2015.02.089

Lewis, D. R., Petersen, L. K., York, A. W., Zablocki, K. R., Joseph, L. B., Kholodovych, V., et al. (2015). Sugar-based Amphiphilic Nanoparticles Arrest Atherosclerosis *In Vivo*. *Proc. Natl. Acad. Sci. U S A.* 112, 2693–2698. doi:10.1073/pnas.1424594112

Li, X., Wang, C., Tan, H., Cheng, L., Liu, G., Yang, Y., et al. (2016). Gold Nanoparticles-Based SPECT/CT Imaging Probe Targeting for Vulnerable Atherosclerosis Plaques. *Biomaterials* 108, 71–80. doi:10.1016/j.biomaterials.2016.08.048

Lindemann, S., Krämer, B., Seizer, P., and Gawaz, M. (2007). Platelets, Inflammation and Atherosclerosis. *J. Thromb. Haemost.* 5 (Suppl. 1), 203–211. doi:10.1111/j.1538-7836.2007.02517.x

Liu, L., He, H., Zhang, M., Zhang, S., Zhang, W., and Liu, J. (2014). Hyaluronic Acid-Decorated Reconstituted High Density Lipoprotein Targeting Atherosclerotic Lesions. *Biomaterials* 35, 8002–8014. doi:10.1016/j.biomaterials.2014.05.081

Lobatto, M. E., Fayad, Z. A., Silvera, S., Vucic, E., Calcagno, C., Mani, V., et al. (2010). Multimodal Clinical Imaging to Longitudinally Assess a Nanomedical Anti-inflammatory Treatment in Experimental Atherosclerosis. *Mol. Pharm.* 7, 2020–2029. doi:10.1021/mp100309y

Ma, S., Tian, X. Y., Zhang, Y., Mu, C., Shen, H., Bismuth, J., et al. (2016). E-selectin-targeting Delivery of microRNAs by Microparticles Ameliorates Endothelial Inflammation and Atherosclerosis. *Sci. Rep.* 6, 22910. doi:10.1038/srep22910

Maiolino, G., Rossitto, G., Caielli, P., Bisogni, V., Rossi, G. P., and Calò, L. A. (20132013). The Role of Oxidized Low-Density Lipoproteins in Atherosclerosis: The Myths and the Facts. *Mediators Inflamm.* 2013, 714653. doi:10.1155/2013/714653

Mansukhani, N. A., Peters, E. B., So, M. M., Albaghdadi, M. S., Wang, Z., Karver, M. R., et al. (2019). Peptide Amphiphile Supramolecular Nanostructures as a Targeted Therapy for Atherosclerosis. *Macromol. Biosci.* 19, e1900066. doi:10.1002/mabi.201900066

Martínez-González, B., Reyes-Hernández, C. G., Quiroga-Garza, A., Rodríguez-Rodríguez, V. E., Esparza-Hernández, C. N., Elizondo-Omaña, R. E., et al. (2017). Conduits Used in Coronary Artery Bypass Grafting: A Review of Morphological Studies. *Ann. Thorac. Cardiovasc. Surg.* 23, 55–65. doi:10.5761/atcs.ra.16-00178

Massaro, M., Zampolli, A., Scoditti, E., Carluccio, M. A., Storelli, C., Distante, A., et al. (2010). Statins Inhibit Cyclooxygenase-2 and Matrix Metalloproteinase-9 in Human Endothelial Cells: Anti-angiogenic Actions Possibly Contributing to Plaque Stability. *Cardiovasc. Res.* 86, 311–320. doi:10.1093/cvr/cvp375

Masuko, K., Murata, M., Yudoh, K., Kato, T., and Nakamura, H. (2009). Anti-inflammatory Effects of Hyaluronan in Arthritis Therapy: Not Just for Viscosity. *Int. J. Gen. Med.* 2, 77–81. doi:10.2147/ijgm.s5495

Matsui, Y., Rittling, S. R., Okamoto, H., Inobe, M., Jia, N., Shimizu, T., et al. (2003). Osteopontin Deficiency Attenuates Atherosclerosis in Female Apolipoprotein E-Deficient Mice. *Arterioscler Thromb. Vasc. Biol.* 23, 1029–1034. doi:10.1161/01.Atv.0000074878.29805.D0

Mescher, A. L. (2016). "The Circulatory System," in *Junqueira's Basic Histology*. 14e. (New York, NY: McGraw-Hill Education).

Miteva, K., Madonna, R., De Caterina, R., and Van Linthout, S. (2018). Innate and Adaptive Immunity in Atherosclerosis. *Vascul Pharmacol.* 107, 67–77. doi:10.1016/j.vph.2018.04.006

Murata, K., Motayama, T., and Kotake, C. (1986). Collagen Types in Various Layers of the Human Aorta and Their Changes with the Atherosclerotic Process. *Atherosclerosis* 60, 251–262. doi:10.1016/0021-9150(86)90172-3

Nie, S., Zhang, J., Martinez-Zaguilan, R., Sennoune, S., Hossen, M. N., Lichtenstein, A. H., et al. (2015). Detection of Atherosclerotic Lesions and Intimal Macrophages Using CD36-Targeted Nanovesicles. *J. Control Release* 220, 61–70. doi:10.1016/j.jconrel.2015.10.004

Nissen, S. E., Nicholls, S. J., Sipahi, I., Libby, P., Raichlen, J. S., Ballantyne, C. M., et al. (2006). Effect of Very High-Intensity Statin Therapy on Regression of Coronary Atherosclerosis: The Asteroid Trial. *JAMA* 295, 1556–1565. doi:10.1001/jama.295.13.jpc60002

Oesterle, A., Laufs, U., and Liao, J. K. (2017). Pleiotropic Effects of Statins on the Cardiovascular System. *Circ. Res.* 120, 229–243. doi:10.1161/circresaha.116.308537

Pepys, M. B., and Baltz, M. L. (1983). Acute Phase Proteins with Special Reference to C-Reactive Protein and Related Proteins (Pentaxins) and Serum Amyloid A Protein. *Adv. Immunol.* 34, 141–212. doi:10.1016/s0065-2776(08)60379-x

Peters, L. J. F., Jans, A., Bartneck, M., and Van Der Vorst, E. P. C. (2021). Immunomodulatory Nanomedicine for the Treatment of Atherosclerosis. *J. Clin. Med.* 10, 3185. doi:10.3390/jcm10143185

Podrez, E. A., Poliakov, E., Shen, Z., Zhang, R., Deng, Y., Sun, M., et al. (2002). Identification of a Novel Family of Oxidized Phospholipids that Serve as Ligands for the Macrophage Scavenger Receptor CD36. *J. Biol. Chem.* 277, 38503–38516. doi:10.1074/jbc.M203318200

Poon, I. K., Lucas, C. D., Rossi, A. G., and Ravichandran, K. S. (2014). Apoptotic Cell Clearance: Basic Biology and Therapeutic Potential. *Nat. Rev. Immunol.* 14, 166–180. doi:10.1038/nri3607

Qiao, H., Wang, Y., Zhang, R., Gao, Q., Liang, X., Gao, L., et al. (2017a). MRI/optical Dual-Modality Imaging of Vulnerable Atherosclerotic Plaque with an Osteopontin-Targeted Probe Based on Fe3O4 Nanoparticles. *Biomaterials* 112, 336–345. doi:10.1016/j.biomaterials.2016.10.011

Qiao, R., Qiao, H., Zhang, Y., Wang, Y., Chi, C., Tian, J., et al. (2017b). Molecular Imaging of Vulnerable Atherosclerotic Plaques *In Vivo* with Osteopontin-specific Upconversion Nanoprobes. *ACS Nano* 11, 1816–1825. doi:10.1021/acsnano.6b07842

Ridker, P. M., Everett, B. M., Thuren, T., Macfadyen, J. G., Chang, W. H., Ballantyne, C., et al. (2017). Antiinflammatory Therapy with Canakinumab for Atherosclerotic Disease. *N. Engl. J. Med.* 377, 1119–1131. doi:10.1056/NEJMoa1707914

Ridker, P. M. (2021). From RESCUE to ZEUS: Will Interleukin-6 Inhibition with Ziltivekimab Prove Effective for Cardiovascular Event Reduction. *Cardiovasc. Res.* 117, e138–e140. doi:10.1093/cvr/cvab231

Romeo, G. R., Moulton, K. S., and Kazlauskas, A. (2007). Attenuated Expression of Profilin-1 Confers protection from Atherosclerosis in the LDL Receptor Null Mouse. *Circ. Res.* 101, 357–367. doi:10.1161/circresaha.107.151399

Ronald, J. A., Chen, J. W., Chen, Y., Hamilton, A. M., Rodriguez, E., Reynolds, F., et al. (2009). Enzyme-sensitive Magnetic Resonance Imaging Targeting Myeloperoxidase Identifies Active Inflammation in Experimental Rabbit Atherosclerotic Plaques. *Circulation* 120, 592–599. doi:10.1161/circulationaha.108.813998

Ronda, N., Greco, D., Adorni, M. P., Zimetti, F., Favari, E., Hjeltnes, G., et al. (2015). Newly Identified Antiatherosclerotic Activity of Methotrexate and Adalimumab: Complementary Effects on Lipoprotein Function and Macrophage Cholesterol Metabolism. *Arthritis Rheumatol.* 67, 1155–1164. doi:10.1002/art.39039

Rooney, P., Kumar, S., Ponting, J., and Wang, M. (1995). The Role of Hyaluronan in Tumour Neovascularization (Review). *Int. J. Cancer* 60, 632–636. doi:10.1002/ijc.2910600511

Roy, P., Orecchioni, M., and Ley, K. (Forthcoming 2021). How the Immune System Shapes Atherosclerosis: Roles of Innate and Adaptive Immunity. *Nat. Rev. Immunol.* 21. doi:10.1038/s41577-021-00584-1

Sakakura, K., Nakano, M., Otsuka, F., Ladich, E., Kolodgie, F. D., and Virmani, R. (2013). Pathophysiology of Atherosclerosis Plaque Progression. *Heart Lung Circ.* 22, 399–411. doi:10.1016/j.hlc.2013.03.001

Sanchez-Gaytan, B. L., Fay, F., Lobatto, M. E., Tang, J., Ouimet, M., Kim, Y., et al. (2015). HDL-mimetic PLGA Nanoparticle to Target Atherosclerosis Plaque Macrophages. *Bioconjug. Chem.* 26, 443–451. doi:10.1021/bc500517k

Sarai, M., Hartung, D., Petrov, A., Zhou, J., Narula, N., Hofstra, L., et al. (2007). Broad and Specific Caspase Inhibitor-Induced Acute Repression of Apoptosis in Atherosclerotic Lesions Evaluated by Radiolabeled Annexin A5 Imaging. *J. Am. Coll. Cardiol.* 50, 2305–2312. doi:10.1016/j.jacc.2007.08.044

Scatena, M., Liaw, L., and Giachelli, C. M. (2007). Osteopontin: a Multifunctional Molecule Regulating Chronic Inflammation and Vascular Disease. *Arterioscler. Thromb. Vasc. Biol.* 27, 2302–2309. doi:10.1161/atvbaha.107.144824

Seimon, T. A., Nadolski, M. J., Liao, X., Magallon, J., Nguyen, M., Feric, N. T., et al. (2010). Atherogenic Lipids and Lipoproteins Trigger CD36-TLR2-dependent Apoptosis in Macrophages Undergoing Endoplasmic Reticulum Stress. *Cell Metab* 12, 467–482. doi:10.1016/j.cmet.2010.09.010

Serrano, D., Bhowmick, T., Chadha, R., Garnacho, C., and Muro, S. (2012). Intercellular Adhesion Molecule 1 Engagement Modulates Sphingomyelinase and Ceramide, Supporting Uptake of Drug Carriers by the Vascular Endothelium. *Arterioscler. Thromb. Vasc. Biol.* 32, 1178–1185. doi:10.1161/atvbaha.111.244186

Shang, Y., Ma, C., Zhang, J., Wang, Z., Ren, C., Luo, X., et al. (2020). Bifunctional Supramolecular Nanofiber Inhibits Atherosclerosis by Enhancing Plaque Stability and Anti-inflammation in apoE-/- Mice. *Theranostics* 10, 10231–10244. doi:10.7150/thno.48410

Shao, Q., Shen, L. H., Hu, L. H., Pu, J., Jing, Q., and He, B. (2012). Atorvastatin Suppresses Inflammatory Response Induced by oxLDL through Inhibition of ERK Phosphorylation, IκBα Degradation, and COX-2 Expression in Murine Macrophages. *J. Cel. Biochem.* 113, 611–618. doi:10.1002/jcb.23388

Slevin, M., Krupinski, J., Gaffney, J., Matou, S., West, D., Delisser, H., et al. (2007). Hyaluronan-mediated Angiogenesis in Vascular Disease: Uncovering RHAMM and CD44 Receptor Signaling Pathways. *Matrix Biol.* 26, 58–68. doi:10.1016/j.matbio.2006.08.261

Soehnlein, O. (2012). Multiple Roles for Neutrophils in Atherosclerosis. *Circ. Res.* 110, 875–888. doi:10.1161/circresaha.111.257535

Song, Y., Huang, Z., Liu, X., Pang, Z., Chen, J., Yang, H., et al. (2019). Platelet Membrane-Coated Nanoparticle-Mediated Targeting Delivery of Rapamycin Blocks Atherosclerotic Plaque Development and Stabilizes Plaque in Apolipoprotein E-Deficient (ApoE-/-) Mice. *Nanomedicine* 15, 13–24. doi:10.1016/j.nano.2018.08.002

Spencer, F. A., Fonarow, G. C., Frederick, P. D., Wright, R. S., Every, N., Goldberg, R. J., et al. (2004). Early Withdrawal of Statin Therapy in Patients with Non-ST-segment Elevation Myocardial Infarction: National Registry of Myocardial Infarction. *Arch. Intern. Med.* 164, 2162–2168. doi:10.1001/archinte.164.19.2162

Stigliano, C., Ramirez, M. R., Singh, J. V., Aryal, S., Key, J., Blanco, E., et al. (2017). Methotraxate-Loaded Hybrid Nanoconstructs Target Vascular Lesions and Inhibit Atherosclerosis Progression in ApoE-/- Mice. *Adv. Healthc. Mater.* 6, 1601286. doi:10.1002/adhm.201601286

Sun, X., Li, W., Zhang, X., Qi, M., Zhang, Z., Zhang, X. E., et al. (2016). *In Vivo* Targeting and Imaging of Atherosclerosis Using Multifunctional Virus-like Particles of Simian Virus 40. *Nano Lett.* 16, 6164–6171. doi:10.1021/acs.nanolett.6b02386

Tall, A. R., Yvan-Charvet, L., Terasaka, N., Pagler, T., and Wang, N. (2008). HDL, ABC Transporters, and Cholesterol Efflux: Implications for the Treatment of Atherosclerosis. *Cel Metab* 7, 365–375. doi:10.1016/j.cmet.2008.03.001

Tang, J., Baxter, S., Menon, A., Alaarg, A., Sanchez-Gaytan, B. L., Fay, F., et al. (2016). Immune Cell Screening of a Nanoparticle Library Improves Atherosclerosis Therapy. *Proc. Natl. Acad. Sci. U S A.* 113, E6731–E6740. doi:10.1073/pnas.1609629113

Tarin, C., Carril, M., Martin-Ventura, J. L., Markuerkiaga, I., Padro, D., Llamas-Granda, P., et al. (2015). Targeted Gold-Coated Iron Oxide Nanoparticles for CD163 Detection in Atherosclerosis by MRI. *Sci. Rep.* 5, 17135. doi:10.1038/srep17135

Tawakol, A., Fayad, Z. A., Mogg, R., Alon, A., Klimas, M. T., Dansky, H., et al. (2013). Intensification of Statin Therapy Results in a Rapid Reduction in Atherosclerotic Inflammation: Results of a Multicenter Fluorodeoxyglucose-Positron Emission Tomography/computed Tomography Feasibility Study. *J. Am. Coll. Cardiol.* 62, 909–917. doi:10.1016/j.jacc.2013.04.066

Taylor, F., Huffman, M. D., Macedo, A. F., Moore, T. H., Burke, M., Davey Smith, G., et al. (2013). Statins for the Primary Prevention of Cardiovascular Disease. *Cochrane Database Syst. Rev.* 1, CD004816. doi:10.1002/14651858.CD004816.pub5

Tsuchiya, K., Nitta, N., Sonoda, A., Otani, H., Takahashi, M., Murata, K., et al. (2013). Atherosclerotic Imaging Using 4 Types of Superparamagnetic Iron Oxides: New Possibilities for Mannan-Coated Particles. *Eur. J. Radiol.* 82, 1919–1925. doi:10.1016/j.ejrad.2013.07.017

Van Der Valk, F. M., Schulte, D. M., Meiler, S., Tang, J., Zheng, K. H., Van Den Bossche, J., et al. (2016). Liposomal Prednisolone Promotes Macrophage Lipotoxicity in Experimental Atherosclerosis. *Nanomedicine* 12, 1463–1470. doi:10.1016/j.nano.2016.02.022

Vazquez-Prada, K. X., Lam, J., Kamato, D., Xu, Z. P., Little, P. J., and Ta, H. T. (2021). Targeted Molecular Imaging of Cardiovascular Diseases by Iron Oxide Nanoparticles. *Arterioscler. Thromb. Vasc. Biol.* 41, 601–613. doi:10.1161/ATVBAHA.120.315404

Waksman, R., Pakala, R., Burnett, M. S., Gulick, C. P., Leborgne, L., Fournadjiev, J., et al. (2003). Oral Rapamycin Inhibits Growth of Atherosclerotic Plaque in apoE Knock-Out Mice. *Cardiovasc. Radiat. Med.* 4, 34–38. doi:10.1016/S1522-1865(03)00121-5

Wang, N., Lan, D., Chen, W., Matsuura, F., and Tall, A. R. (2004). ATP-binding Cassette Transporters G1 and G4 Mediate Cellular Cholesterol Efflux to High-Density Lipoproteins. *Proc. Natl. Acad. Sci. U S A.* 101, 9774–9779. doi:10.1073/pnas.0403506101

Wang, Y., Chen, J., Yang, B., Qiao, H., Gao, L., Su, T., et al. (2016). *In Vivo* MR and Fluorescence Dual-Modality Imaging of Atherosclerosis Characteristics in Mice Using Profilin-1 Targeted Magnetic Nanoparticles. *Theranostics* 6, 272–286. doi:10.7150/thno.13350

Wang, Y., Zhang, K., Li, T., Maruf, A., Qin, X., Luo, L., et al. (2021). Macrophage Membrane Functionalized Biomimetic Nanoparticles for Targeted Anti-atherosclerosis Applications. *Theranostics* 11, 164–180. doi:10.7150/thno.47841

Wang, Y., Zhang, K., Qin, X., Li, T., Qiu, J., Yin, T., et al. (2019). Biomimetic Nanotherapies: Red Blood Cell Based Core-Shell Structured Nanocomplexes for Atherosclerosis Management. *Adv. Sci. (Weinh)* 6, 1900172. doi:10.1002/advs.201900172

Weber, C., and Noels, H. (2011). Atherosclerosis: Current Pathogenesis and Therapeutic Options. *Nat. Med.* 17, 1410–1422. doi:10.1038/nm.2538

Williams, M. R., Azcutia, V., Newton, G., Alcaide, P., and Luscinskas, F. W. (2011). Emerging Mechanisms of Neutrophil Recruitment across Endothelium. *Trends Immunol.* 32, 461–469. doi:10.1016/j.it.2011.06.009

Winter, P. M., Morawski, A. M., Caruthers, S. D., Fuhrhop, R. W., Zhang, H., Williams, T. A., et al. (2003). Molecular Imaging of Angiogenesis in Early-Stage Atherosclerosis with Alpha(v)beta3-Integrin-Targeted Nanoparticles. *Circulation* 108, 2270–2274. doi:10.1161/01.Cir.0000093185.16083.95

Wolfrum, S., Jensen, K. S., and Liao, J. K. (2003). Endothelium-Dependent Effects of Statins. *Arterioscler Thromb. Vasc. Biol.* 23, 729–736. doi:10.1161/01.Atv.0000063385.12476.A7

Xue, Y., Wu, Y., Wang, Q., Xue, L., Su, Z., and Zhang, C. (2019). Cellular Vehicles Based on Neutrophils Enable Targeting of Atherosclerosis. *Mol. Pharm.* 16, 3109–3120. doi:10.1021/acs.molpharmaceut.9b00342

Yi, S., Karabin, N. B., Zhu, J., Bobbala, S., Lyu, H., Li, S., et al. (2020). An Injectable Hydrogel Platform for Sustained Delivery of Anti-inflammatory Nanocarriers and Induction of Regulatory T Cells in Atherosclerosis. *Front. Bioeng. Biotechnol.* 8, 542. doi:10.3389/fbioe.2020.00542

Yu, M., Amengual, J., Menon, A., Kamaly, N., Zhou, F., Xu, X., et al. (2017). Targeted Nanotherapeutics Encapsulating Liver X Receptor Agonist GW3965 Enhance Antiatherogenic Effects without Adverse Effects on Hepatic Lipid Metabolism in Ldlr-/- Mice. *Adv. Healthc. Mater.* 6, 1700313. doi:10.1002/adhm.201700313

Yu, Z., Geng, J., Tan, Y., Wang, Q., Zhu, J., and Zhang, M. (2011). Non-invasive Assessment of Acute Vascular Inflammation after PCI Using USPIO Enhanced MRI *In Vivo*. *Int. J. Cardiol.* 151, 110–112. doi:10.1016/j.ijcard.2011.06.021

Zhang, M., He, J., Jiang, C., Zhang, W., Yang, Y., Wang, Z., et al. (2017a). Plaque-hyaluronidase-responsive High-Density-Lipoprotein-Mimetic Nanoparticles for Multistage Intimal-Macrophage-Targeted Drug Delivery and Enhanced Anti-atherosclerotic Therapy. *Int. J. Nanomedicine* 12, 533–558. doi:10.2147/IJN.S124252

Zhang, M., Jia, J., Liu, J., He, H., and Liu, L. (2013). A Novel Modified Paclitaxel-Loaded Discoidal Recombinant High-Density Lipoproteins: Preparation, Characterizations and *In Vivo* Evaluation. *Asian J. Pharm. Sci.* 8, 11–18. doi:10.1016/j.ajps.2013.07.002

Zhang, X., Xu, X., Chen, Y., Dou, Y., Zhou, X., Li, L., et al. (2017b). Bioinspired Yeast Microcapsules Loaded with Self-Assembled Nanotherapies for Targeted Treatment of Cardiovascular Disease. *Mater. Today* 20, 301–313. doi:10.1016/j.mattod.2017.05.006

Zhao, Y., Jiang, C., He, J., Guo, Q., Lu, J., Yang, Y., et al. (2017). Multifunctional Dextran Sulfate-Coated Reconstituted High Density Lipoproteins Target Macrophages and Promote Beneficial Antiatherosclerotic Mechanisms. *Bioconjug. Chem.* 28, 438–448. doi:10.1021/acs.bioconjchem.6b00600

Permissions

All chapters in this book were first published by Frontiers; hereby published with permission under the Creative Commons Attribution License or equivalent. Every chapter published in this book has been scrutinized by our experts. Their significance has been extensively debated. The topics covered herein carry significant findings which will fuel the growth of the discipline. They may even be implemented as practical applications or may be referred to as a beginning point for another development.

The contributors of this book come from diverse backgrounds, making this book a truly international effort. This book will bring forth new frontiers with its revolutionizing research information and detailed analysis of the nascent developments around the world.

We would like to thank all the contributing authors for lending their expertise to make the book truly unique. They have played a crucial role in the development of this book. Without their invaluable contributions this book wouldn't have been possible. They have made vital efforts to compile up to date information on the varied aspects of this subject to make this book a valuable addition to the collection of many professionals and students.

This book was conceptualized with the vision of imparting up-to-date information and advanced data in this field. To ensure the same, a matchless editorial board was set up. Every individual on the board went through rigorous rounds of assessment to prove their worth. After which they invested a large part of their time researching and compiling the most relevant data for our readers.

The editorial board has been involved in producing this book since its inception. They have spent rigorous hours researching and exploring the diverse topics which have resulted in the successful publishing of this book. They have passed on their knowledge of decades through this book. To expedite this challenging task, the publisher supported the team at every step. A small team of assistant editors was also appointed to further simplify the editing procedure and attain best results for the readers.

Apart from the editorial board, the designing team has also invested a significant amount of their time in understanding the subject and creating the most relevant covers. They scrutinized every image to scout for the most suitable representation of the subject and create an appropriate cover for the book.

The publishing team has been an ardent support to the editorial, designing and production team. Their endless efforts to recruit the best for this project, has resulted in the accomplishment of this book. They are a veteran in the field of academics and their pool of knowledge is as vast as their experience in printing. Their expertise and guidance has proved useful at every step. Their uncompromising quality standards have made this book an exceptional effort. Their encouragement from time to time has been an inspiration for everyone.

The publisher and the editorial board hope that this book will prove to be a valuable piece of knowledge for researchers, students, practitioners and scholars across the globe.

List of Contributors

Xushan Yang, Hong Deng, Yuting Hao, Lianzhi Mao, Rongjun Zhang and Wenzhen Liao
Department of Nutrition and Food Hygiene, Guangdong Provincial Key Laboratory of Tropical Disease Research, School of Public Health, Southern Medical University, Guangzhou, China

Miaomiao Yuan
The Eighth Affiliated Hospital, Sun Yat-sen University, Shenzhen, China

Xiaoshan Liao
Department of Nutrition and Food Hygiene, Guangdong Provincial Key Laboratory of Tropical Disease Research, School of Public Health, Southern Medical University, Guangzhou, China
The Eighth Affiliated Hospital, Sun Yat-sen University, Shenzhen, China

Jinfu Yang and Chengming Fan
Department of Cardiovascular Surgery, The Second Xiangya Hospital, Central South University, Changsha, China

Jyotsna Joshi, Fan Li and Bing Xu
Department of Cardiovascular Diseases, Mayo Clinic, Scottsdale, AZ, United States

Mahmood Khan
Department of Emergency Medicine, The Ohio State University Wexner Medical Center, Columbus, OH, United States

Wuqiang Zhu
Department of Cardiovascular Diseases, Mayo Clinic, Scottsdale, AZ, United States
Department of Physiology and Biomedical Engineering, Mayo Clinic, Rochester, MN, United States

Caroline Hu and Cynthia Alcazar
Veterans Affairs Palo Alto Health Care System, Palo Alto, CA, United States

Tatiana S. Zaitseva, Peter Tabada, Steve Sawamura and Michael V. Paukshto
Fibralign Corporation, Inc., Union City, CA, United States

Guang Yang
The Stanford Cardiovascular Institute, Stanford University, Palo Alto, CA, United States
Department of Cardiothoracic Surgery, Stanford University, Palo Alto, CA, United States

Ngan F. Huang
Veterans Affairs Palo Alto Health Care System, Palo Alto, CA, United States
The Stanford Cardiovascular Institute, Stanford University, Palo Alto, CA, United States
Department of Cardiothoracic Surgery, Stanford University, Palo Alto, CA, United States

Mimi R. Borrelli, Derrick C. Wan and Dung H. Nguyen
Division of Plastic and Reconstructive Surgery, Stanford University, Palo Alto, CA, United States

Xudong Zhang, Haibin Shen, Qiangnan He and Zijian Wu
Guangdong Provincial Key Laboratory of Tropical Disease Research, Department of Nutrition and Food Hygiene, School of Public Health, Southern Medical University, Guangzhou, China

Yudi Deng
The Eighth Affiliated Hospital, Sun Yat-sen University, Shenzhen, China
Guangdong Provincial Key Laboratory of Tropical Disease Research, Department of Nutrition and Food Hygiene, School of Public Health, Southern Medical University, Guangzhou, China

Sijia Yi, Nicholas B. Karabin, Jennifer Zhu, Sharan Bobbala, Huijue Lyu, Sophia Li, Yugang Liu, Molly Frey, Michael Vincent and Evan A. Scott
Department of Biomedical Engineering, Northwestern University, Evanston, IL, United States

Ho Pan Bei, Yuhe Yang, Yu Liu and Xin Zhao
Department of Biomedical Engineering, The Hong Kong Polytechnic University, Hong Kong, China

Jingdong Rao
Department of Biomedical Engineering, The Hong Kong Polytechnic University, Hong Kong, China
State Key Laboratory of Molecular Engineering of Polymers, Department of Orthopedic Surgery, Fudan University, Shanghai, China

Haodong Lin
General Hospital, Shanghai Jiaotong University School of Medicine, Shanghai, China

Tong Sun, Xi Guo and Hao Liu
Neurosurgery Research Laboratory, National Clinical Research Center for Geriatrics, West China Hospital, Sichuan University, Chengdu, China
Department of Neurosurgery, West China Hospital, Sichuan University, Chengdu, China

Hao Li, Lu Ma and Junwen Guan
Department of Neurosurgery, West China Hospital, Sichuan University, Chengdu, China

Chao You and Meng Tian
Neurosurgery Research Laboratory, National Clinical Research Center for Geriatrics, West China Hospital, Sichuan University, Chengdu, China
Department of Neurosurgery, West China Hospital, Sichuan University, Chengdu, China
West China Brain Research Centre, West China Hospital, Sichuan University, Chengdu, China

Rui Zhong
Institute of Blood Transfusion, Chinese Academy of Medical Sciences and Peking Union Medical College, Chengdu, China

Chengwei Wang
Neurosurgery Research Laboratory, National Clinical Research Center for Geriatrics, West China Hospital, Sichuan University, Chengdu, China
Department of Integrated Traditional Chinese and Western Medicine, West China Hospital, Sichuan University, Chengdu, China

Chuanchao He
Department of Surgery, School of Medicine, University of California, Davis, Sacramento, CA, United States

Hila Shimshi Swindell, Lalithasri Ramasubramanian, Dake Hao, Kewa Gao, Siqi He and Diana L. Farmer
Department of Surgery, School of Medicine, University of California, Davis, Sacramento, CA, United States
Institute for Pediatric Regenerative Medicine, Shriners Hospitals for Children, Sacramento, CA, United States

Alyssa Panitch
Department of Surgery, School of Medicine, University of California, Davis, Sacramento, CA, United States
Department of Biomedical Engineering, University of California, Davis, Davis, CA, United States

Aijun Wang
Department of Surgery, School of Medicine, University of California, Davis, Sacramento, CA, United States
Institute for Pediatric Regenerative Medicine, Shriners Hospitals for Children, Sacramento, CA, United States
Department of Biomedical Engineering, University of California, Davis, Davis, CA, United States

Kit S. Lam and Ruiwu Liu
Department of Biochemistry and Molecular Medicine, School of Medicine, University of California, Davis, Sacramento, CA, United States

Cunyi Zhao and Gang Sun
Department of Biological and Agricultural Engineering, University of California, Davis, Davis, CA, United States

Jiaqi Liang, Shuangying Gu, Xiuli Mao, Yiling Tan, Huanli Wang and Yue Zhou
Shanghai Jiao Tong University Affiliated Sixth People's Hospital, School of Biomedical Engineering, Med-X Research Institution, Shanghai Jiao Tong University, Shanghai, China

Song Li
Department of Bioengineering, Department of Medicine, University of California, Los Angeles, Los Angeles, CA, United States

Jing Bai
School of Chemistry and Chemical Engineering, State Key Laboratory of Metal Matrix Composite Materials and Shanghai Key Lab of Electrical Insulation and Thermal Ageing, Shanghai Jiao Tong University, Shanghai, China

Juanjuan Tan
School of Chemistry and Chemical Engineering, State Key Laboratory of Metal Matrix Composite Materials and Shanghai Key Lab of Electrical Insulation and Thermal Ageing, Shanghai Jiao Tong University, Shanghai, China
Joint Research Center for Precision Medicine, Shanghai Jiao Tong University Affiliated Sixth People's Hospital South Campus, Shanghai, China

Zhiqiang Yan
Central Laboratory, Southern Medical University affiliated Fengxian Hospital, Shanghai, China

Chaohong Shi
Department of Rehabilitation Medicine, The First People's Hospital of Wenling, Wenzhou Medical University, Wenling, China,

Haotian Xie
Department of Mathematics, The Ohio State University, Columbus, OH, United States,

Yifan Ma and Jingjing Zhang
Department of Chemical and Biomolecular Engineering, The Ohio State University, Columbus, OH, United States

Zhaogang Yang
Department of Radiation Oncology, University of Texas Southwestern Medical Center, Dallas, TX, United States

Wencheng Zhou
Neurosurgery Research Laboratory, National Clinical Research Center for Geriatrics, West China Hospital, Sichuan University, Chengdu, China
Department of Burns and Plastic Surgery, West China Hospital, Sichuan University, Chengdu, China

Ying Cen
Department of Burns and Plastic Surgery, West China Hospital, Sichuan University, Chengdu, China

Liu Zi
Neurosurgery Research Laboratory, National Clinical Research Center for Geriatrics, West China Hospital, Sichuan University, Chengdu, China
Department of Integrated Traditional and Western Medicine, West China Hospital, Sichuan University, Chengdu, China

Chao You
Neurosurgery Research Laboratory, National Clinical Research Center for Geriatrics, West China Hospital, Sichuan University, Chengdu, China
Department of Neurosurgery, West China Hospital, Sichuan University, Chengdu, China
West China Brain Research Centre, West China Hospital, Sichuan University, Chengdu, China

Meng Tian
Neurosurgery Research Laboratory, National Clinical Research Center for Geriatrics, West China Hospital, Sichuan University, Chengdu, China
Department of Burns and Plastic Surgery, West China Hospital, Sichuan University, Chengdu, China
Department of Neurosurgery, West China Hospital, Sichuan University, Chengdu, China
West China Brain Research Centre, West China Hospital, Sichuan University, Chengdu, China

Naresh Kumar, Divya Sridharan, Arunkumar Julie A. Dougherty, Muhamad Mergaye and Mark G. Angelos
Department of Emergency Medicine, The Ohio State University Wexner Medical Center, Columbus, OH, United States
Dorothy M. Davis Heart & Lung Research Institute, The Ohio State University Wexner Medical Center, Columbus, OH, United States

Palaniappan
Department of Emergency Medicine, The Ohio State University Wexner Medical Center, Columbus, OH, United States
Dorothy M. Davis Heart & Lung Research Institute, The Ohio State University Wexner Medical Center, Columbus, OH, United States
Centre for Biomaterials, Cellular and Molecular Theranostics, Vellore Institute of Technology, Vellore, India

Andras Czirok
Department of Anatomy and Cell Biology, University of Kansas Medical Center, Kansas City, KS, United States

Dona Greta Isai
Department of Biomedical Engineering, The Ohio State University, Columbus, OH, United States

Heather M. Powell
Department of Biomedical Engineering, The Ohio State University, Columbus, OH, United States
Department of Materials Science and Engineering, The Ohio State University, Columbus, OH, United States
Research Department, Shriners Hospitals for Children, Cincinnati, OH, United States

Mahmood Khan
Department of Emergency Medicine, The Ohio State University Wexner Medical Center, Columbus, OH, United States
Dorothy M. Davis Heart & Lung Research Institute, The Ohio State University Wexner Medical Center, Columbus, OH, United States
Department of Physiology and Cell Biology, The Ohio State University Wexner Medical Center, Columbus, OH, United States

Lucas Antônio Miranda Ferreira
Departamento de Produtos Farmacêuticos, Faculdade de Farmácia, Universidade Federal de Minas Gerais, Belo Horizonte, Brazil

Gabriel Silva Marques Borges and Eduardo Burgarelli Lages
Departamento de Produtos Farmacêuticos, Faculdade de Farmácia, Universidade Federal de Minas Gerais, Belo Horizonte, Brazil
PhyMedExp, Université de Montpellier, INSERM, CNRS, Montpellier, France

Pierre Sicard and Sylvain Richard
PhyMedExp, Université de Montpellier, INSERM, CNRS, Montpellier, France
IPAM, Bio Campus, CNRS, INSERM, Université de Montpellier, Montpellier, France

Xuejun Du and Wei Han
Emergency Department, Shenzhen University General Hospital, Shenzhen University, Shenzhen, China

Huihua Huang
Emergency Department, Shenzhen University General Hospital, Shenzhen University, Shenzhen, China
Guangdong Key Laboratory for Biomedical Measurements and Ultrasound Imaging, School of Biomedical Engineering, Shenzhen University, Health Science Center, Shenzhen, China

Zhiguo He and Zifeng Yan
Advanced Materials Institute, Graduate School at Shenzhen, Tsinghua University, Shenzhen, China

Weimin Huang
Baotou Clinical Medical College, Inner Mongolia Medical University, Hohhot, China
Department of Cardiac Surgery, Chinese PLA General Hospital, Beijing, China

Nan Cheng and Rong Wang
Department of Cardiac Surgery, Chinese PLA General Hospital, Beijing, China

Mengen Huo
Institute of Poisons and Drugs, Beijing Academy of Military Medical Sciences, Beijing, China

Tetsuya Matoba
Department of Cardiovascular Medicine, Kyushu University Graduate School of Medical Sciences, Fukuoka, Japan

Shunsuke Katsuki
Department of Cardiovascular Medicine, Kyushu University Graduate School of Medical Sciences, Fukuoka, Japan
Center for Excellence in Vascular Biology, Division of Cardiovascular Medicine, Department of Medicine, Brigham and Women's Hospital, Harvard Medical School, Boston, MA, United States

Kaku Nakano
Department of Cardiovascular Research, Development, and Translational Medicine, Center for Cardiovascular Disruptive Innovation, Kyushu University, Fukuoka, Japan

Jun-ichiro Koga and Kensuke Egashira
Department of Cardiovascular Medicine, Kyushu University Graduate School of Medical Sciences, Fukuoka, Japan
Department of Cardiovascular Research, Development, and Translational Medicine, Center for Cardiovascular Disruptive Innovation, Kyushu University, Fukuoka, Japan

Shenjie Liao and Xiaoshen Zhang
Department of Cardiovascular Surgery, The First Affiliated Hospital, Jinan University, Guangzhou, China

Yun Liang
Department of Cardiovascular Surgery, The First Affiliated Hospital, Jinan University, Guangzhou, China
Academician Workstation, Affiliated Hospital of North Sichuan Medical College, Nanchong, China

Seyedmehdi Hossaini Nasr
Department of Chemistry, Michigan State University, East Lansing, MI, United States
Institute for Quantitative Health Science and Engineering, Michigan State University, East Lansing, MI, United States

Xuefei Huang
Department of Chemistry, Michigan State University, East Lansing, MI, United States
Institute for Quantitative Health Science and Engineering, Michigan State University, East Lansing, MI, United States
Department of Biomedical Engineering, Michigan State University, East Lansing, MI, United States

Index

Printed in the USA
CPSIA information can be obtained
at www.ICGtesting.com
LVHW080035211023
761596LV00010BA/1777

9 781646 465842